Churchill Livingstone's

DICTIONARY of NURSING

Personal Information

Name ....

Address ....

....

....

Job/Course Title ....

Work/College Address ....

....

....

National Insurance No. ....

RCN Membership No. ....

UKCC PIN No. ....

Date of Registration ....

Date for Re-registration ....

Churchill Livingstone's

DICTIONARY of NURSING

SEVENTEENTH EDITION

Prepared in collaboration with the Royal College of Nursing

Head of Royal College of Nursing Advisory Team

Sue Hinchliff BA RGN RNT

Head of Continuing Professional Development
Royal College of Nursing Institute, London

Foreword by

Christine Hancock

General Secretary
Royal College of Nursing

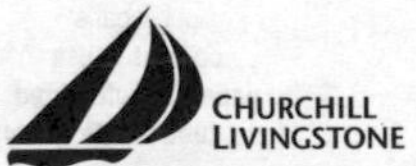

New York Edinburgh London Madrid Melbourne San Francisco and Tokyo 1996

CHURCHILL LIVINGSTONE
Medical Division of Pearson Professional Limited

Distributed in the United States of America by Churchill Livingstone Inc., 650 Avenue of the Americas, New York, NY 10011, and by associated companies, branches and representatives throughout the world.

First edition 1932
Second edition 1933
Third edition 1934
Fourth edition 1936
Fifth edition 1938
Sixth edition 1940
Seventh edition 1941
Eighth edition 1943
Ninth edition 1946
Tenth edition 1949
Eleventh edition 1961
Twelfth edition 1966
Thirteenth edition 1969
Fourteenth edition 1973
Fifteenth edition 1978
Sixteenth edition 1989
Seventeenth edition 1996

Standard edition ISBN 0443 05534 3

International edition ISBN 0443 05578 5

British Library Cataloguing in Publication Data
A catalogue record for this book is available from the British Library.

Library of Congress Cataloging in Publication Data
A catalog record for this book is available from the Library of Congress.

Printed in Hong Kong
EPC/01

For Churchill Livingstone:

Commissioning editor: Ellen Green
Project manager: Valerie Burgess
Project development editor: Valerie Bain
Illustrator: Ethan Danielson
Designer: Judith Wright
Pre-press manager: Alex Watson
Promotions executive: Hilary Brown

The publisher's policy is to use **paper manufactured from sustainable forests**

Contents

Foreword

Nursing is changing every day. Today, nurses are taking on new roles and responsibilities, challenging old assumptions about health care. Nurses are increasingly confident, educated, flexible and independent professionals, more than capable of finding new solutions to long-standing problems in our health services.

Nurses are not just responding to changes in the way health care is structured. So much of the momentum for change has come from nursing's growing understanding of its own contribution to patient care. An expanding body of evidence proves that people who are cared for by registered nurses get better quicker. More and more nurses have realised that equipped with this knowledge, and a thorough understanding of the health environment in which they work, they can make a real and lasting impact on the way in which health care is delivered.

The *Dictionary of Nursing* meets the information needs of today's nurses. It focuses on professional and personal development, containing information about education and career issues as well as clinical information and networking opportunities. It is an invaluable tool for all nurses who want to make a difference in today's health services.

Christine Hancock
General Secretary
Royal College of Nursing

Preface

Nursing and the environment in which it takes place have changed enormously over the past decade. The time therefore seemed ripe for a major revision of this well-established dictionary. A team of advisers from the Royal College of Nursing Institute and various other universities and institutions have worked to bring the dictionary up to date by revising definitions, deleting those which have become redundant and introducing new terminology relevant to modern nursing practice.

A feature of this new edition is the introduction of a few carefully chosen longer entries, set off in boxes, where it seemed important to go into more detail than an average-sized definition permits. The appendices have also been considerably revised, and many totally new ones have been added. A practical change to a more hardwearing cover and a slightly larger and slimmer format should increase the dictionary's lifespan and make it easier to carry around in bag or pocket. The new title, *Dictionary of Nursing*, is intended to signal a greater emphasis on nursing information and terminology, in keeping with the emergence of a more confident and better educated nursing professional.

We hope the dictionary will continue to provide a valuable reference source for all student nurses, and that it will find a new market among registered nurses in helping them to fulfil their continuing professional development responsibilities.

Sue Hinchliff London, 1996
Head of Continuing Professional Development
Royal College of Nursing Institute

Acknowledgement

The Publishers wish to pay tribute to Miss Nancy Roper, whose association with the *Nurses' Dictionary* spanned more than 30 years. Miss Roper's work is recognised and admired by an international nursing audience. Her publications include *Man's Anatomy, Physiology, Health and Environment, Principles of Nursing in Process Context* and, with Winifred W. Logan and Alison J. Tierney, *The Elements of Nursing*. She is also a well-known lecturer whose insights into nursing are valued throughout the world.

Panel of Advisers

Chief advisory editor:

Rosemary Rogers BA (Hons) RGN
Continuing Professional Development Editor, *Nursing Standard*

Nursing advisers:

Philip Burnard MSc PhD CertEd RMN SRN RNT
Reader, University of Wales College of Medicine, Cardiff

Christopher Goodall RGN DipN RNT
Visiting Lecturer, North Yorkshire College of Health Studies, York

Specialist advisers:

Ivy A. Andrews RN ENB
264 (Burns & Plastic Surgery)

Elizabeth Armstrong RGN RHV
Mental Health Training Officer, National Primary Care Facilitation Programme

Margaret McAllister Banning BSc(Hons) MSc PGDE SRN SCM
Lecturer, Royal College of Nursing Institute, London

Gillian D. Barber MA(Educ) PGCEA MTD ADM RGN RM
Lecturer, Midwifery, Royal College of Nursing Institute, London

Helen M Barker BSc SRD,
Community Dietician, Solihull Hospital, West Midlands

Philip Beed RGN DPSN OND
Lecturer Practitioner, Oxford Brookes University, Oxford

Gosia Brykczynska BSc BA RGN RSCN DipPH Cert Ed ONC
Lecturer in Ethics, Royal College of Nursing Institute, London

Lesley J Cavalli BSc(Hons) MSc MCSLT
Tutor/Lecturer, Dept of Human Communication Science, University College London, London

Elisabeth Clark BA(Hons) PhD
Distance Learning Programme Coordinator, Royal College of Nursing Institute, London

Sue Coombes BA DipEd SRN HVCert RNT
Formerly Nurse Teacher, North Yorkshire College of Health Studies, York

Ann Cuthill RGN CertEd
Senior Nurse, Day Care Unit, Joyce Green Hospital, Dartford, Kent

Peter S. Davis MA BEd(Hons) CertEd RN DN ONC
Principal Lecturer, Nurse Education Dept., Royal National Orthopaedic Hospital NHS Trust, Stanmore, Middlesex

Elizabeth Gangar RGN RM
Research Sister, Ashford Hospital, Middlesex

Stephen Firn MSc BSc RMN
Director of Nursing, Bexley Hospital, Kent

Agnes Hibbert BSc(Hons) MSc CertEd RGN
Lecturer, Applied Physiology, Royal College of Nursing Institute, London

Hilary Hiscox RGN
Clinical ENT Manager, St Michael's Hospital, Bristol

Clephane Hume BA DipCOT CertFE
Lecturer, Queen Margaret College, Edinburgh

Alan Jacques MB BCh DPM MRCPsych
Medical Commissioner, Mental Welfare Commission for Scotland, Edinburgh

A. M. McConnachie BSc(Hons) MSc MRPS MCPP
Principal Pharmacist, Tayside Drug Information Service, Dundee Teaching Hospitals NHS Trust, Dundee

Anne MacDonald RGN RSCN DipN(Lond) OBE
Paediatric Nursing Consultant, Lymm, Cheshire

Judy J. Mewburn RGN
Theatre Sister

Siva Murugiah BSc(Hons) MSc RMN RGN DipN RCNT RNT
Lecturer, Royal College of Nursing Institute, London

Joy Norton RGN
Sister, Imaging Department, Luton & Dunstable Hospitals Trust, Luton

Gill Oliver BA RGN DipN ONCNurCert
Director of Patient Services, Clatterbridge Centre for Oncology, Clatterbridge

Hilary Oliver RGN FETC
Continence Service Manager, Bradford Community NHS Trust, Bradford

Roz Osborne MA BA(Hons) RGN
Adviser, Association of Nursing Students, Royal College of Nursing, London

Cliff Roberts BSc(Hons) PGDE RGN
Lecturer, Life Sciences, Royal College of Nursing Institute, London

Ros Rundle MA BA(Hons) PGCEA RGN RHV RM
Lecturer, Behavioural Sciences, Royal College of Nursing Institute, London

Julie Smith BSc PGCE RGN RHV
Lecturer and Clinical Nurse Specialist in Diabetes

Ellis Snitcher MB ChB
Senior Lecturer in Clinical Sciences, Middlesex University, Middlesex

Caroline Stevenson BA(Hons) RGN
Macmillan Specialist in Complementary Therapies, National Homoeopathic Hospital, London; Vice-Chair of Royal College of Nursing Complementary Therapies Forum

Stephen Thomas
Editor, *Cardiology Update*

Greta Thornbory MSc PGCEA RCN OHNC DipNOH
Lecturer, Continuing Professional Development, Royal College of Nursing Institute, London

Philippa H. Trnobranski BSc(Hons) MSc CertEd RN RHV
Lecturer in Nursing Studies, Department of Nursing & Midwifery Studies, Queen's Medical Centre, Nottingham

John Wilkinson BSc(Hons) DipNEd RGN RMN RNT
Lecturer, Royal College of Nursing Institute, London

Rosemary Wilkinson RGN OND RNT CertEd CMS DipEthics
Adviser in Nursing Practice, Department of Nursing Policy and Practice, Royal College of Nursing, London

Colin Selby DM MRCP
Consultant Physician, Respiratory and Intensive Care Medicine, Queen Margaret Hospital, Dunfermline

Lynn Young
Adviser, Department of Nursing Policy and Practice, Royal College of Nursing, London

Code of Professional Conduct for the Nurse, Midwife and Health Visitor

Third edition 1992

Each registered nurse, midwife and health visitor shall act, at all times, in such a manner as to:

- safeguard and promote the interests of individual patients and clients;
- serve the interests of society;
- justify public trust and confidence and
- uphold and enhance the good standing and reputation of the professions.

As a registered nurse, midwife or health visitor, you are personally accountable for your practice and, in the exercise of your professional accountability, must:

1 act always in such a manner as to promote and safeguard the interests and well-being of patients and clients;

2 ensure that no action or omission on your part, or within your sphere of responsibility, is detrimental to the interests, condition or safety of patients and clients;

3 maintain and improve your professional knowledge and competence;

4 acknowledge any limitations in your knowledge and competence and decline any duties or responsibilities unless able to perform them in a safe and skilled manner;

5 work in an open and co-operative manner with patients, clients and their families, foster their independence and recognise and respect their involvement in the planning and delivery of care;

6 work in a collaborative and co-operative manner with health care professionals and others involved in providing care, and recognise and respect their particular contributions within the care team;

7 recognise and respect the uniqueness and dignity of each patient and client, and respond to their need for care, irrespective of their ethnic origin, religious beliefs, personal attributes, the nature of their health problems or any other factor;

8 report to an appropriate person or authority, at the earliest possible time, any conscientious objection which may be relevant to your professional practice;

9 avoid any abuse of your privileged relationship with patients and clients and of the privileged access allowed to their person, property, residence or workplace;

10 protect all confidential information concerning patients and clients obtained in the course of professional practice and make disclosures only with consent, where required by the order of a court or where you can justify disclosure in the wider public interest;

11 report to an appropriate person or authority, having regard to the physical, psychological and social effects on patients and clients, any circumstances in the environment of care which could jeopardise standards of practice;

12 report to an appropriate person or authority any circumstances in which safe and appropriate care for patients and clients cannot be provided;

13 report to an appropriate person or authority where it appears that the health or safety of colleagues is at risk, as such circumstances may compromise standards of practice and care;

14 assist professional colleagues, in the context of your own knowledge, experience and sphere of responsibility, to develop their professional competence, and assist others in the care team, including informal carers, to contribute safely and to a degree appropriate to their roles;

15 refuse any gift, favour or hospitality from patients or clients currently in your care which might be interpreted as seeking to exert influence to obtain preferential consideration and

16 ensure that your registration status is not used in the promotion of commercial products or services, declare any financial or other interests in relevant organisations providing such goods or services and ensure that your professional judgement is not influenced by any commercial considerations.

Notice to all Registered Nurses, Midwives and Health Visitors

This Code of Professional Conduct for the Nurse, Midwife and Health Visitor is issued to all registered nurses, midwives and health visitors by the United Kingdom Central Council for Nursing, Midwifery and Health Visiting. The Council is the regulatory body responsible for the standards of these professions and it requires members of the professions to practice and conduct themselves within the standards and framework provided by the Code.

The Council's Code is kept under review and any recommendations for change and improvement would be welcomed and should be addressed to the:

Registrar and Chief Executive
United Kingdom Central Council
for Nursing, Midwifery and Health Visiting
23 Portland Place
London
W1N 3AF

How to use this dictionary

Main entries

These are listed in alphabetical order and appear in bold type. Derivative forms of the main entry also appear in bold type and along with their parts of speech are to be found at the end of the definition.

Separate meanings of main entry

Different meanings of the same word are separated by means of a bold Arabic numeral before each meaning. For example:

acme *n* **1** highest point. **2** crisis or critical state of a disease.

Subentries

Subentries relating to the defined headword are listed in alphabetical order and appear in italic type following the main definition. For example:

intelligence *n* inborn mental ability. *intelligence tests* designed to determine the level of intelligence. *intelligence quotient (IQ)* the ratio of mental age to chronological (actual) age.

Parts of speech

The part of speech follows single word main entries and derivative forms of the main entry and appears in italic type. The parts of speech used in the dictionary are:

abbr	abbreviation
adj	adjective
adv	adverb
Am	American
e.g.	for example
i.e.	that is
i.m.	intramuscular
i.v.	intravenous
n	noun
npl	plural noun
opp	opposite
pl	plural
sing	singular
syn	synonym
v	verb

vi	intransitive verb
vt	transitive verb

Cross-references

Cross-references alert you to related words and additional information elsewhere in the dictionary. Two symbols have been used for this purpose–an arrow ⇒ and an asterisk*. At the end of a definition, the arrow indicates the word you can then look up for related subject matter. Within a definition, an asterisk placed at the end of a word means that there is a separate entry in the dictionary may convey useful further information. For example:

hyperthyroidism *n* overaction of the parathyroid* glands with increase in serum calcium levels: may result in osteitis fibrosa cysteica with decalcification and spontaneous fracture of bones. ⇒ hypercalcaemia, hypercalciuria.

Boxed entries

These are longer entries set off from the text in a box; they are cross-referenced in the main entries.

List of illustrations

Prefixes which can be used as combining forms in compounded words

Prefix	Meaning
a-	without, not
ab-	away from
abdo-	
abdomino-	abdominal
acro-	extremity
ad-	towards
adeno-	glandular
aer-	air
amb-	both, on both
ambi-	sides
amido-	NH_2 group united to an acid radical
amino-	NH_2 group united to a radical other than an acid radical
amphi-	on both sides, around
amyl-	starch
an-	not, without
ana-	up
andro-	male
angi-	vessel (blood)
aniso-	unequal
ant-	against,
anti-	counteracting
ante-	
antero-	before
antro-	antrum
aorto-	aorta
app-	away, from
arachn-	spider
arthro-	joint

Prefix	Meaning
auto-	self
bi-	twice, two
bili-	bile
bio-	life
blenno-	mucus
bleph-	eyelid
brachio-	arm
brachy-	short
brady-	slow
broncho-	bronchi
calc-	chalk
carcin-	cancer
cardio-	heart
carpo-	wrist
cata-	down
cav-	hollow
centi-	a hundredth
cephal-	head
cerebro-	brain
cervic-	neck, womb
cheil-	lip
cheir-	hand
chemo-	chemical
chlor-	green
chol-	bile
cholecysto-	gall bladder
choledocho-	common bile duct
chondro-	cartilage
chrom-	colour
cine-	film, motion
circum-	around
co-	
col-	together
com-	
con-	

Prefix	Meaning
coli-	bowel
colpo-	vagina
contra-	against
costo-	rib
cox-	hip
crani- cranio-	skull
cryo-	cold
crypt-	hidden, concealed
cyan-	blue
cysto-	bladder
cyto-	cell
dacryo-	tear
dactyl-	finger
de-	away, from, reversing
deca-	ten
deci-	tenth
demi-	half
dent-	tooth
derma- dermat-	skin
dextro-	to the right
dia-	through
dip-	double
dis-	separation, against
dorso-	dorsal
dys-	difficult, painful, abnormal
ecto-	outside, without, external
electro-	electricity
em-	in
en- end- endo-	in, into, within
ent-	within
entero-	intestine
epi-	on, above, upon

Prefix	Meaning
ery-	red
eu-	well, normal
ex- exo-	away from, out, out of
extra-	outside
faci-	face
ferri- ferro-	iron
fibro-	fibre, fibrous tissue
flav-	yellow
feto-	fetus
fore-	before, in front of
gala-	milk
gastro-	stomach
genito-	genitals, reproductive
ger-	old age
glosso-	tongue
glyco-	sugar
gnatho-	jaw
gynae-	female
haema- haemo-	blood
hemi-	half
hepa- hepatico- hepato-	liver
hetero-	unlikeness, dissimilarity
hexa-	six
histo-	tissue
homeo-	like
homo-	same
hydro-	water
hygro-	moisture
hyper-	above
hypo-	below
hypno-	sleep
hystero-	uterus

Prefixes

Prefix	Meaning
iatro-	physician
idio-	peculiar to the individual
ileo-	ileum
ilio-	ilium
immuno-	immunity
in-	not, in, into, within
infra-	below
inter-	between
intra-	within
intro-	inward
ishio-	ischium
iso-	equal
karyo-	nucleus
kerato-	horn, skin, cornea
kypho-	rounded, humped
lact-	milk
laparo-	flank
laryngo-	larynx
lepto-	thin, soft
leuco- leuko-	white
lympho-	lymphatic
macro-	large
mal-	abnormal, poor
mamm- mast-	breast
medi-	middle
mega-	large
melano-	pigment, dark
meso-	middle
meta-	between
metro-	uterus
micro-	small
milli-	a thousandth
mio-	smaller
mono-	one, single
muco-	mucus
multi-	many

Prefix	Meaning
myc-	fungus
myelo-	spinal cord, bone marrow
myo-	muscle
narco-	stupor
naso-	nose
necro-	corpse
neo-	new
nephro-	kidney
neuro-	nerve
noct-	night
normo-	normal
nucleo-	nucleus
nyc-	night
oculo-	eye
odonto-	tooth
oligi-	deficiency, diminution
onc-	mass
onycho-	nail
oo-	egg, ovum
oophor-	ovary
ophthalmo-	eye
opisth-	backward
orchido-	testis
oro-	mouth
ortho-	straight
os-	bone, mouth
osteo-	bone
oto-	ear
ova-	egg
ovari-	ovary
pachy-	thick
paed-	child
pan-	all
para-	beside
patho-	disease
ped-	child, foot
penta- pento-	five
per-	by, through
peri-	around

Prefix	Meaning
perineo-	perineum
pharma-	drug
pharyngo-	pharynx
phlebo-	vein
phono-	voice
photo-	light
phren-	diaphragm, mind
physio-	form, nature
pleuro-	pleura
pluri-	many
pneumo-	lung
podo-	foot
polio-	grey
poly-	many, much
post-	after
pre- pro-	before
proct-	anus
proto-	first
pseudo-	false
psycho-	mind
pyelo-	pelvis of the kidney
pyo-	pus
pyr-	fever
quadri-	four
radi-	ray
radio-	radiation
re-	again, back
ren-	kidney
retro-	backward
rhin-	nose
rub-	red
sacchar-	sugar
sacro-	sacrum
salpingo-	Fallopian tube
sapro-	dead, decaying
sarco-	flesh
sclero-	hard
scota-	darkness
semi-	half

Prefix	Meaning
sept-	seven
sero-	serum
socio-	sociology
sphygm-	pulse
spleno-	spleen
spondy-	vertebra
steato-	fat
sterno-	sternum
sub-	below
supra-	above
syn-	together, union, with
tabo-	tabes
tachy-	fast
tarso-	foot, edge of eyelid
teno-	tendon
tetra-	four
thermo-	heat
thoraco-	thorax
thrombo-	blood clot
thyro-	thyroid gland
tibio-	tibia
tox-	poison
tracheo-	trachea
trans-	across, through
tri-	three
trich-	hair
tropho-	nourishnment
ultra-	beyond
uni-	one
uretero-	ureter
urethro-	urethra
uri-	urine
uro-	urine, urinary organs
utero-	uterus
vaso-	vessel
veno-	vein
vesico-	bladder
xanth-	yellow

Prefix	Meaning
xero-	dry
xiphi- xipho-	ensiform cartilage of sternum
zoo-	animal

Suffixes which can be used as combining forms in compounded words

Sufix	Meaning
-able	able to, capable of
-aemia	blood
-aesthesia	sensibility, sense-perception
-agra	attack, severe pain
-al	characterized by, pertaining to
-algia	pain
-an	belonging to, pertaining to
-ase	catalyst, enzyme, ferment
-asis	state of
-blast	cell
-caval	pertaining to venae cavae
-cele	tumour, swelling
-centesis	to puncture
-cide	destructive, killing
-clysis	infusion, injection
-coccus	spherical cell
-cule	little
-cyte	cell
-derm	skin
-desis	to bind together
-dynia	pain

Sufix	Meaning
-ectasis	dilation, extension
-ectomy	removal of
-facient	making
-form	having the form of
-fuge	expelling
-genesis -genetic	formation, origin
-genic	capable of causing
-gogue	increasing flow
-gram	a tracing
-graph	description, treatise, writing
-iasis	condition of, state
-iatric	practice of healing
-itis	inflammation of
-kinesis -kinetic	motion
-lith	calculus, stone
-lithiasis	presence of stones
-logy	science of, study of
-lysis -lytic	breaking down, disintegration

Suffixes

Sufix	Meaning
-malacia	softening
-megaly	enlargement
-meter	measure
-morph	form
-odynia	pain
-ogen	precursor
-oid	likeness, resemblance
-ol	alcohol
-ology	the study of
-oma	tumour
-opia	eye
-opsy	looking
-ose	sugar
-osis	condition, disease, excess
-ostomy	to form an opening or outlet
-otomy	incision of
-ous	like, having the nature of
-pathy	disease
-penia	lack of
-pexy	fixation
-phage	ingesting
-phagia	swallowing
-phasia	speech
-philia	affinity for, loving
-phobia	fear
-phylaxis	protection
-plasty	reconstructive surgery
-plegia	paralysis
-pnoea	breathing
-poiesis	making
-ptosis	falling
-rhage	to burst forth
-rhaphy	suturing
-rhoea	excessive discharge

Sufix	Meaning
-rhythmia	rhythm
-saccharide	basic carbohydrate molecule
-scope	instrument for visual examination
-scopy	to examine visually
-somatic	pertaining to the body
-somy	pertaining to chromosomes
-sonic	sound
-stasis	stagnation, cessation of movement
-sthenia	strength
-stomy	to form an opening or outlet
-taxia -taxis -taxy	arrangement, coordination, order
-tome	cutting instrument
-tomy	incision of
-trophy	nourishment
-trophy	turning
-uria	urine

A

AA *abbr* Alcoholics* Anonymous.

abdomen *n* the largest body cavity, immediately below the thorax, from which it is separated by the diaphragm*. It is enclosed largely by muscle and fascia, and is therefore capable of change in size and shape. It is lined with a serous membrane, the peritoneum*, which is reflected as a covering over most of the organs. *acute abdomen* pathological condition within the abdomen requiring immediate surgical intervention. *pendulous abdomen* a relaxed condition of the anterior wall, allowing it to hang down over the pubis. *scaphoid abdomen* (navicular) concavity of the anterior wall.

abdominal *adj* pertaining to the abdomen*. *abdominal breathing* more than usual use of the diaphragm and abdominal muscles to increase the input of air to and output from the lungs. It can be done voluntarily in the form of exercises. When it occurs in disease it is a compensatory mechanism for inadequate oxygenation. *abdominal excision of the rectum, normally for a tumour* usually performed by two surgeons working at the same time. The rectum is mobilized through an abdominal incision. The bowel is divided well proximal to the tumour. The proximal end is brought out as a permanent colostomy. Excision of the distal bowel containing the tumour together with the anal canal is completed through a perineal incision. *abdominal migraine* recurrent bouts of tummy ache and nausea in children; often associated with headaches. *abdominal pregnancy* condition where the embryo/fetus develops in the abdominal cavity, the placenta adhering to the gut, peritoneum and other organs. Rare, occasionally results in the operative birth of a live baby but normally the fetus will die. ⇒ lithopaedion.

abdominocentesis *n* aspiration* of the peritoneal cavity. ⇒ amniocentesis, colpocentesis, thoracentesis.

abdominopelvic *adj* pertaining to the abdomen* and pelvis* or pelvic cavity.

abdominoperineal *adj* pertaining to the abdomen* and perineum*.

abduct *vt* to draw away from the median line of the body. ⇒ adduct *opp.*

abduction *n* the act of abducting away from the midline. ⇒ adduction *opp.*

abductor *n* a muscle which, on contraction, draws a part away from the median line of the body. ⇒ adductor *opp.*

aberrant *adj* abnormal; usually applied to a blood vessel or nerve which does not follow the normal course.

aberration *n* a deviation from normal—**aberrant** *adj. chromosomal aberration* loss, gain or exchange of genetic material in the chromosomes of a cell resulting in deletion, duplication, inversion or translocation of genes. *mental aberration* ⇒ mental. *optical aberration* imperfect focus of light rays by a lens.

ablation *n* removal. In surgery, the word means excision, amputation or destruction by chemical means, e.g. phenol to destroy the nail bed after removal of the great toe nail—**ablative** *adj.*

abort *vt, vi* to terminate before full development.

abortifacient *adj* causing abortion. A drug or agent inducing expulsion of a nonviable fetus.

abortion *n* **1** abrupt termination of a process. **2** expulsion from a uterus of the product of conception before it is viable. In English law, a fetus is viable at 24 weeks but some infants born before this survive because of advances in neonatal intensive care. Health professionals are encouraged to use the word miscarriage rather than abortion to describe spontaneous pregnancy loss. ⇒ abortus—**abortive** *adj. complete abortion* the entire contents of the uterus are expelled. *criminal abortion* intentional evacuation of uterus by other than trained, licensed medical personnel, and/or when abortion is prohibited by law. *habitual abortion* (preferable syn.) *recurrent abortion* term used when abortion recurs in successive pregnancies. *incomplete abortion* part of the fetus or placenta is retained within the uterus. *induced abortion* (also called 'artificial') intentional evacuation of uterus. *inevitable abortion* one which has advanced to a stage where termination of pregnancy cannot be prevented. *missed abortion* early signs and symptoms of pregnancy disappear and the fetus dies, but is not expelled for some time. ⇒ carneous mole. *septic abortion* one associated with uterine infection and rise in body temperature. *spontaneous abortion* one which occurs naturally without intervention. *therapeutic abortion* intentional termination of a pregnancy which is a hazard to the mother's life and health. *threatened abortion* slight blood loss per vaginam whilst cervix remains closed. May be accompanied by abdominal pain. *tubal abortion* an ectopic* pregnancy that dies and is expelled from the fimbriated end of the uterine tube. ⇒ Ethics box, p. 134.

abortus *n* an aborted fetus weighing less than 500 g. It is either dead or incapable of surviving.

abrasion *n* **1** superficial injury to skin or mucous membrane from scraping or rubbing; excoriation. **2** can be used therapeutically for removal of scar tissue (dermabrasion).

abreaction *n* an emotional reaction resulting from recall of past painful experiences relived in speech and action during psychoanalysis or under the influence of light anaesthesia, or drugs. ⇒ narcoanalysis, catharsis.

abscess *n* localized collection of pus produced by pyogenic organisms. May be acute or chronic. ⇒ quinsy. *alveolar abscess* at the root of a tooth. *amoebic abscess* one caused by *Entamoeba hystolitica;* usual site is the liver, other sites are lung, brain and spleen. ⇒ amoebiasis. *Brodie's abscess* chronic osteomyelitis* occurring without previous acute phase. *cold abscess* one occurring with few signs of inflammation and may be due to *Mycobacterium tuberculosis. psoas abscess* ⇒ psoas.

absorption *n* the passage of substances into and out of body cells, e.g. digested food in the small intestine into blood and lymph.

abuse *n* deliberate injury to another person—either physical, sexual, psychological or through neglect. The groups of people most vulnerable are children, women and older people. ⇒ child abuse, nonaccidental injury.

abused child ⇒ abuse, nonaccidental injury.

acalulia *n* inability to do simple arithmetic.

acatalasia *n* genetically determined absence of the enzyme catalase; predisposes to oral sepsis.

accident form a form designed by a health authority or NHS Trust to be used as soon as possible after an accident to any person on its premises. The signed forms (data) are collected centrally and analysed to provide information such as the most common type of accident, to whom it occurred, where and when and so on. Such factual information is essential to the trade union Health and Safety Representatives as well as to managers. ⇒ accidental inoculation, accidents, prevention of.

accidents, prevention of part of the nursing role. Nurses must ensure that their fear of accidents does not prevent patients, especially those who are elderly, from taking reasonable risk, thereby lowering their level of independence. Nurses are encouraged, for example, to have an uncluttered space before attempting to lift or transfer patients, to use lifting aids wherever possible, and to use the large muscle groups if manual lifting is unavoidable. ⇒ accident form.

accommodation *n* adjustment, e.g. the power of the eye to alter the convexity of the lens according to the nearness or distance of objects, so that a distinct image is always achieved—**accommodative** *adj.*

accountability *n* a nurse has a duty to care according to law. In some countries the statutory body, and/or the professional organisation, elaborate a code of conduct via which each qualified nurse can accept responsibility and accountability for the nursing service delivered to each patient/client. ⇒ UKCC, RCN.

accretion *n* an increase of substance or deposit round a central object; in dentistry, an accumulation of tartar or calculus around the teeth.—**accrete** *vt, vi,* **accretive** *adj.*

acetabuloplasty *n* an operation to improve the depth and shape of the hip socket (acetabulum); necessary in such conditions as congenital dislocation of the hip and osteoarthritis of the hip.

acetabulum *n* a cup-like socket on the external lateral surface of the pelvis into which the head of the femur fits to form the hip joint—**acetabula** *pl.*

acetate *n* a salt of acetic acid (the acid present in vinegar).

acetoacetic acid *n* (*syn* diacetic acid) a monobasic keto acid. Produced at an interim stage in the oxidation of fats in the human body. In some metabolic upsets, e.g. acidosis and diabetes mellitus, it is present in excess in the blood and escapes in the urine. (It changes to acetone if urine is left standing.) The excess acid in the blood can produce coma.

acetonaemia *n* acetone bodies in the blood—**acetonaemic** *adj.*

acetone *n* inflammable liquid with characteristic odour; valuable as a solvent. *ketone bodies* ⇒ ketone.

acetonuria *n* excess acetone bodies in the urine, causing a characteristic sweet smell—**acetonuric** *adj.*

acetylcholine *n* a chemical substance released from nerve endings to activate muscle, secretory glands and other nerve cells. The nerve fibres releasing this chemical are termed 'cholinergic'. Hydrolysed into choline and acetate by the enzyme acetylcholinesterase, which is present around the synaptic cleft.

achalasia *n* failure to relax. *cardiac achalasia* ⇒ cardiac.

Achilles tendon *n* tendon of the muscles of the calf of the leg (gastrocnemius and soleus) situated at the back of the ankle and attached to the heel. Named after the figure in Greek mythology who could only be wounded in the heel.

achlorhydria *n* the absence of free hydrochloric acid in the stomach. Found in pernicious anaemia and gastric cancer—**achlorhydric** *adj.*

acholia *n* the absence of bile*—**acholic** *adj.*

acholuria *n* the absence of bile* pigment from the urine. ⇒ jaundice—**acholuric** *adj.*

achondroplasia *n* a genetically inherited disorder characterized by arrested growth of the long bones resulting in short-limbed dwarfism with a big head. The intellect is not impaired. Inheritance is dominant—**achondroplastic** *adj.*

achylia *n* absence of chyle*—**achylic** *adj.*

acid *n* any substance which in solution gives rise to an excess of hydrogen ions. Identified (a) by turning blue litmus paper red (b) by being neutralized by an alkali with the formation of a salt.

acidaemia *n* abnormal acidity of the blood, giving increased hydrogen ions, and a below normal pH*.—**acidaemic** *adj.*

acid-alcohol fast *adj* in bacteriology, describes an organism which, when stained, is resistant to decolourization by alcohol as well as acid, e.g. *Mycobacterium tuberculosis.*

acid-base balance equilibrium between the acid and base elements of the blood and body fluids.

acid-fast *adj* in bacteriology, describes an organism which, when stained, is able to retain dyes despite washing with acid.

acidity *n* the state of being acid or sour. The degree of acidity can be determined and interpreted on the pH* scale, pH 6.69 denoting a very weak acid and pH 1 a strong acid.

acidosis *n* depletion of the body's alkali reserve, with resulting disturbance of the acid-base balance. ⇒ acidaemia, ketosis. *metabolic acidosis* caused by increased lactic acid production in muscles. *respiratory acidosis* may result from hypoventilation or excess carbon dioxide production—**acidotic** *adj.*

acid phosphatase *n* an enzyme which synthesizes phosphate esters of carbohydrates in an acid medium. *acid phosphatase test* an increase of this enzyme in the blood is indicative of carcinoma of the prostate gland.

acini *n* minute saccules* or alveoli*, lined or filled with secreting cells. Several acini combine to form a lobule—**acinus** *sing,* **acinous, acinar** *adj.*

acme *n* **1** highest point. **2** crisis or critical state of a disease.

acne, acne vulgaris *n* a condition in which the pilosebaceous glands are overstimulated by circulating androgens and the excessive sebum is trapped by a plug of keratin, one of the protein constituents of human hair. Skin bacteria then colonize the glands and convert the trapped sebum into irritant fatty acids responsible for the swelling and inflammation (pustules) which follow.

acneiform *adj* resembling acne.

acoustic neuroma benign tumour of the auditory nerve.

acquired immune deficiency syndrome (AIDS) caused by Human Immunodeficiency Virus (HIV), which belongs to the retrovirus group. Classified into four stages: (a) acute primary HIV infection, the fever-like illness seen in some individuals 2–6 weeks after initial infection, at the end of which the person will start to produce antibodies to HIV; (b) antibody positive stage, phase following seroconversion–may last several years and may be entirely asymptomatic or accompanied by persistent* generalized lymphadenopathy (PGL); (c) early symptomatic disease, also known as AIDS-related complex (ARC), when the individual may display a range of minor opportunistic infections; (d) late symptomatic disease, when the patient is infected with a range of opportunistic infections causing clinical illness. *Pneumocystis carinii* pneumonia (PCP) is the main presenting disease seen in AIDS and the most frequent cause of death.

acrocyanosis *n* coldness and blueness of the extremities due to circulatory disorder–**acrocyanotic** *adj.*

acrodynia *n* painful reddening of the extremities such as occurs in erythroedema polyneuritis ('pink disease').

acromegaly *n* enlargement of the hands, face and feet, occurring in an adult due to excess growth hormone. In a child this causes gigantism*. ⇒ growth hormone test–**acromegalic** *adj.*

acromicria *n* smallness of the hands, face and feet, probably due to deficiency of growth hormone from the pituitary gland.

acromioclavicular *adj* pertaining to the acromion process (of scapula) and the clavicle.

acromion *n* the point or summit of the shoulder: the triangular process at the extreme outer end of the spine of the scapula–**acromial** *adj.*

acroparaesthesia *n* tingling and numbness of the hands.

acrophobia *n* irrational fear of being at a height.

ACTH *abbr* adrenocorticotrophic hormone ⇒ corticotrophin.

acting out *n* reduction of emotional distress by the release of disturbed or violent behaviour, which is unconsciously determined and reflects previous unresolved conflicts and attitudes.

actinic dermatoses skin conditions in which the integument is abnormally sensitive to ultraviolet light.

Actinomyces *n* a genus of parasitic fungus-like bacteria exhibiting a radiating mycelium. Also called 'ray fungus'. Many of the antibiotic drugs are produced from this genus.

actinomycosis *n* a disease caused by the bacterium *Actinomyces israeli,* sites most affected being the lung, jaw and intestine. Granulomatous tumours form which usually suppurate, discharging a thick, oily pus containing yellowish granules ('sulphur granules')–**actinomycotic** *adj.*

action *n* the activity or function of any part of the body. *antagonistic action* performed by those muscles which limit the movement of an opposing group. *compulsive action* an overwhelming need to perform an act which is not necessarily rational *impulsive action* resulting from a sudden urge rather than the will. *reflex action* ⇒ reflex. *sexual action* coitus, sexual intercourse. *specific action* that brought about by certain remedial agents in a particular disease, e.g. salicylates in acute rheumatism. *specific dynamic action* the stimulating effect upon the metabolism produced by the ingestion of food, especially proteins, causing the metabolic rate to rise above basal levels. *synergistic action* that brought about by the cooperation of two or more muscles, neither of which could bring about the action alone.

actin *n* one of the proteins in muscle cells; it reacts with myosin to cause contraction.

Actisorb *n* activated charcoal pads for preventing odour from discharging wounds.

activator *n* a substance which renders something else active, e.g. the hormone secretin*, the enzyme enterokinase*–**activate** *v.*

active *adj* energetic. ⇒ passive *opp. active hyperaemia* ⇒ hyperaemia. *active immunity* ⇒ immunity. *active movements* those produced by the patient using his neuromuscular mechanism. *active principle* an ingredient which gives a complex drug its chief therapeutic value, e.g. atropine is the active principle in belladonna.

Activities of Daily Living (ADLs) most nurses include the usual hygiene activities associated with washing and dressing; and maintenance activities such as eating and drinking. Occupational therapists recognize the following ADLs: Self-care skills–eating and drinking, washing and bathing, dressing/undressing, grooming, toilet management; Home-care skills–cooking and kitchen skills, cleaning, laundry, budgeting and shopping, gardening; Work skills; Leisure and recreation; Mobility; Community and personal relationships.

Activities of Living (ALs) on the grounds that not all activities are carried out daily, some nurses prefer the term activities of living to that of activities of daily living. Roper, Logan and Tierney selected 12 ALs as the focus for their model for nursing based on a model of living; they are: maintaining a safe environment, communicating, breathing, eating and drinking, eliminating, personal cleansing and dressing, controlling body temperature, mobilising, working and playing, expressing sexuality, sleeping and dying.

activity tolerance graded exercise including walking, cycling and going up stairs so that confidence is gained in the convalescent phase after an illness–an important aspect of any rehabilitation programme.

acuity *n* sharpness, clearness, keenness, distinctness. *auditory acuity* ability to hear clearly and distinctly. Tests include the use of tuning fork, whispered voice and audiometer. In infants, simple sounds, e.g. bells, rattles, cup and spoon are utilized. *visual acuity* the extent of visual perception is dependent on the clarity of retinal focus, integrity of nervous elements and cerebral interpretation of the stimulus. Usually tested by Snellen's* test types at 6 metres.

acupuncture *n* a technique of insertion of special needles into particular parts of the body for the treatment of disease, relief of pain or production of anaesthesia.

acute *adj* short and severe; not long drawn out or chronic. *acute abdomen* a pathological condition within the belly requiring immediate surgical intervention. *acute defibrination syndrome (ADS)* (*syn* hypofibrinogenaemia), excessive bleeding due to maternal absorption of thromboplastins from retained blood clot or damaged placenta within the uterus. A missed abortion, placental abruption, amniotic fluid embolus, prolonged retention in utero of a dead fetus and the intravenous administration of dextran can lead to ADS. *acute dilatation of the stomach* sudden enlargement of this organ due to paralysis of the muscular wall ⇒ paralytic ileus. *acute haemorrhagic fevers* include Embola fever, Lassa fever and Marburg fever. Also called the viral haemorrhagic fevers. *acute heart failure* cessation or impairment of heart action, in previously undiagnosed heart disease, or in the course of another disease. *acute lymphoblastic leukaemia* proliferation of circulating lymphoblasts (abnormal cells). The outlook is increasingly favourable in children and many can expect to be cured after a 2 year course of treatment. *acute myeloblastic leukaemia* proliferation of circulating myeloblasts. The condition is rapidly fatal if not treated: it requires intensive inpatient chemotherapy in a protected environment. The average duration of the first remission is 14 months. *acute yellow atrophy* acute diffuse necrosis of the liver; icterus gravis; malignant jaundice.

acyanosis *n* without cyanosis*–**acyanotic** *adj* used to differentiate congenital cardiovascular defects.

acyclovir *n* an antiviral drug used to treat herpes simplex infections.

acyesis *n* absence of pregnancy–**acyetic** *adj.*

acystia *n* congenital absence of the bladder–**acystic** *adj.*

Adam's apple *n* the laryngeal prominence in front of the neck, especially in the adult male, formed by the junction of the two wings of the thyroid cartilage.

adaptability *n* the capacity to adjust mentally and physically to circumstances in a flexible way.

addiction *n* craving for chemical substances such as drugs, alcohol and tobacco which the addicted person finds difficult to control. ⇒ dependence.

Addison's disease a condition due to deficient secretion of cortisol and aldosterone by the adrenal cortex, causing electrolytic upset, diminution of blood volume, lowered blood pressure, weight loss, hypoglycaemia, great muscular weakness, gastrointestinal upsets and pigmentation of skin.

adduct *vt* to draw towards the midline of the body. ⇒ abduct *opp.*

adduction *n* the act of adducting, drawing towards the midline. ⇒ abduction *opp.*

adductor *n* any muscle which moves a part toward the median axis of the body. ⇒ abductor *opp.*

adenectomy *n* surgical removal of a gland.

adenitis *n* inflammation of a gland or lymph node. *hilar adenitis* inflammation of bronchial lymph nodes.

adenocarcinoma *n* a malignant growth of glandular tissue–**adenocarcinomata** *pl,* **adenocarcinomatous** *adj.*

adenoid *adj* resembling a gland.⇒ adenoids.

adenoidectomy *n* surgical removal of adenoid tissue from nasopharynx.

adenoids *npl* (pharyngeal tonsils) a mass of lymphoid tissue in the nasopharynx which can obstruct breathing and interfere with hearing.

adenoma *n* a benign tumour of glandular epithelium*–**adenomata** *pl,* **adenomatous** *adj.*

adenomyoma *n* a benign tumour composed of muscle and glandular epithelium, usually applied to benign growths of the uterus–**adenomyomata** *pl,* **adenomyomatous** *adj.*

adenopathy *n* any disease of a

gland, especially a lymphatic gland—**adenopathic** *adj.*

adenosclerosis *n* hardening of a gland with or without swelling, usually due to replacement by fibrous tissue or calcification*—**adenosclerotic** *adj.*

adenosine diphosphate (ADP) an important cellular metabolite involved in energy exchange within the cell. Chemical energy is conserved in the cell, by the phosphorylation of ADP to ATP primarily in the mitochondrion, as a high energy phosphate bond.

adenosine triphosphate (ATP) an intermediate high energy compound which on hydrolysis to ADP releases chemically useful energy. ATP is generated during catabolism and utilized during anabolism.

adenotonsillectomy *n* surgical removal of the adenoids and tonsils.

adenovirus *n* a group of DNA-containing viruses composed of 47 serologically distinct types: 31 serotypes have been found in man, and many in various animal species. Some cause upper respiratory infection, others pneumonia, others epidemic keratoconjunctivitis.

ADH *abbr* antidiuretic hormone.⇒ vasopressin.

adhesion *n* abnormal union of two parts, occurring after inflammation; a band of fibrous tissue which joins such parts. In the abdomen such a band may cause intestinal obstruction; in joints it restricts movement; between two surfaces of pleura it prevents complete pneumothorax—**adherent** *adj,* **adherence** *n,* **adhere** *vi.*

adipose *n, adj* fat; of a fatty nature. The cells constituting adipose tissue contain either white or brown fat.

adiposity *n* excessive accumulation of fat in the body.

adjustment *n* stability within an individual and a satisfactory relationship between the individual and his environment.

adjuvant *n* a substance included in a prescription to aid the action of other drugs. *adjuvant therapy* a treatment (usually refers to a cancer treatment) given in conjunction with another, usually after any obvious tumour has been removed either by surgery or radiotherapy. The aim is to improve cure rate and prevent recurrence. ⇒ neoadjuvant therapy.

ADLs *abbr* Activities* of Daily Living.

admissions *npl* the word is usually reserved for admission to a hospital. The admission may be planned, from a waiting list, or as an emergency, either from an outpatient clinic or via the Accident and Emergency Department.

adolescence *n* the period between the onset of puberty and full maturity; youth. The special needs of this age group as patients are being increasingly recognized, with the provision, in some hospitals, of special facilities and/or separate units—**adolescent** *adj, n.*

adoption *n* the acquisition of legal responsibility for a child who is not a natural offspring of the adopter.

ADP *abbr* adenosine diphosphate*.

adrenal *adj* near the kidney, by custom referring to the adrenal glands, one lying above each kidney. The *adrenal cortex* secretes mineral and glucocorticoids which control the chemical constitution of body fluids, metabolism and secondary sexual characteristics. Under the control of the pituitary gland via the secretion of corticotrophin*. The *adrenal medulla* secretes noradrenaline and adrenaline. ⇒ adrenalectomy.

adrenalectomy *n* removal of an adrenal gland, usually due to a tumour. If both adrenal glands are removed, replacement administration of cortical hormones is required.

adrenal function tests abnormal adrenal–cortical function can be detected by measuring plasma cortisol. If hypoadrenalism is suspected the estimations can be repeated following the administration of synthetic ACTH (Synacthen*). Increased adrenal medullary function may be detected by measuring urinary vanyl* mandelic acid (VMA) excretion, Synacthen test.

adrenaline *n* a hormone produced by the adrenal medulla in mammals to prepare the body for fight or flight. It can be prepared synthetically. *liquor adrenaline* applied locally in epistaxis; given by subcutaneous injection, it is invaluable in relieving serum sickness, asthmatic attacks, urticaria and other allergic states. It is added to local anaesthetic solutions to reduce diffusion and so prolong the anaesthetic effect. Also used in circulatory collapse, but only in very dilute solution (1:100000) by slow intravenous infusion.

adrenergic *adj* describes nerves which liberate either noradrenaline* or adrenaline* from their endings. Most sympathetic nerves release noradrenaline. ⇒ cholinergic *opp.*

adrenocorticotrophic hormone (ACTH) ⇒ corticotrophin.

adrenogenital syndrome an endocrine disorder, usually congenital, resulting from abnormal activity of the adrenal cortex. A female child will show enlarged clitoris and possibly labial fusion, perhaps being confused with a male. The male child may show pubic hair and enlarged penis. In both male and female there is rapid growth, muscularity and advanced bone age.

adsorbents *npl* solids which bind gases or dissolved substances on their surfaces. Charcoal adsorbs gases and acts as a deodorant. Kaolin adsorbs bacterial and other toxins, hence used in cases of food poisoning.

adsorption *n* the property of a substance to attract and to hold to its surface a gas, liquid or solid in solution or suspension—**adsorptive** *adj,* **adsorb** *vt.*

advanced nursing practice a higher level of nursing practice agreed by the UKCC as part of its framework for postregistration education and practice. Advanced practice is defined as that which is concerned with 'adjusting the boundaries for the development of future practice, pioneering and developing new roles responsive to changing needs and with advancing clinical practice, research and education to enrich professional practice as a whole'. ⇒ specialist* nursing practice.

adventitia *n* the external coat, especially of an artery or vein—**adventitious** *adj.*

Aedes *n* a genus of mosquito which includes *Aedes aegypti,* the principal vector* of yellow* fever and dengue*.

aerobe *n* a microorganism which requires O_2 to grow and to maintain life—**aerobic** *adj.*

aerogenous *adj* gas producing.

aerophagia, aerophagy *n* excessive air swallowing*.

aerosol *n* small particles finely dispersed in a gas phase. Commercial aerosol sprays may be used: (a) as inhalation therapy (b) to sterilize the air (c) in insect control (d) for skin application. Some aerosol sources (e.g. sneezing) are responsible for the spread of infection.

aetiology *n* (etiology) a science dealing with the causation of disease—**aetiological** *adj*, **aetiologically** *adv*.

afebrile *adj* without fever.

affect *n* emotion or mood.

affection *n* the feeling or emotional aspect of mind; one of the three aspects. ⇒ cognition, conation.

affective *adj* pertaining to emotions or moods. *affective psychosis* major mental illness in which there is grave disturbance of the emotions or mood with psychotic features such as hallucinations or delusions.⇒ psychosis.

afferent *adj* conducting inward to a part or organ; used to describe nerves, blood and lymphatic vessels. ⇒ efferent *opp.* afferent degeneration that which spreads up sensory nerves.

affiliation *n* settling of the paternity of an illegitimate child on the putative father.

affinity *n* a chemical attraction between two substances, e.g. oxygen and haemoglobin.

afibrinogenaemia *n* rare genetic disorder in which fibrinogen is not produced—**afibrinogenaemic** *adj*.

aflatoxin *n* carcinogenic metabolites of certain strains of *Aspergillus flavus* which can infect peanuts and carbohydrate foods stored in warm humid climates. Four major aflatoxins: B_1, B_2, G_1 and G_2. Human liver cells contain the enzymes necessary to produce the metabolites of aflatoxins which predispose to liver cancer.

AFP *abbr* alphafetoprotein*.

afterbirth *n* the placenta, cord and membranes which are expelled from the uterus after childbirth.

aftereffect *n* a response which occurs after the initial effect of a stimulus.

afterimage *n* a visual impression of an object which persists after the object has been removed. This is called 'positive' when the image is seen in its natural bright colours; 'negative' when the bright parts become dark, while the dark parts become light.

afterpains *npl* the pains felt after childbirth, due to contraction and retraction of the uterine muscle fibres.

agammaglobulinaemia *n* absence of gammaglobulin in the blood, with consequent inability to produce immunity to infection ⇒ dysgammaglobulinaemia—**agammaglobulinaemic** *adj*.

aganglionosis *n* absence of ganglia, as those of the distant bowel. ⇒ Hirschsprung's disease, megacolon.

agar *n* a gelatinous substance obtained from certain seaweeds. It is used as a bulk-increasing laxative and as a solidifying agent in bacterial culture media.

age *n* ⇒ mental age, physiological age.

ageism *n* stereotyping people according to chronological age: overemphasizing negative aspects to the detriment of positive aspects.

agenesis *n* incomplete and imperfect development—**agenetic** *adj*.

agglutination *n* the clumping of bacteria, red blood cells or antigen-coated particles by antibodies called 'agglutinins', developed in the blood serum of a previously infected or sensitized person or animal. Agglutination forms the basis of many laboratory tests—**agglutinable, agglutinative,** *adj*, **agglutinate** *vt, vi*.

agglutinins *npl* antibodies which agglutinate or clump organisms or particles.

agglutinogen *n* an antigen which stimulates production of agglutinins*, used in the production of immunity, e.g. dead bacteria as in vaccine, particulate protein as in toxoid.

aggressin *n* a metabolic substance, produced by certain bacteria to enhance their aggressive action against their host.

aggression *n* a feeling of anger or hostility—**aggressive** *adj.*

agitated depression persistent restlessness, with deep depression and apprehension. Occurs in affective psychoses.

aglossia *n* absence of the tongue—**aglossic** *adj.*

aglutition *n* dysphagia*.

agnosia *n* inability to organise sensory information so as to recognize objects (visual agnosia) or parts of the body (somatoagnosia)—**agnosic** *adj.*

agonist *n* a muscle which shortens to perform a movement. ⇒ antagonist *opp.*

agoraphobia *n* irrational fear of being alone in large open places or in places from which escape might be difficult or embarrassing, e.g. on public transport or in a supermarket queue—**agoraphobic** *adj.*

agranulocyte *n* a nongranular leucocyte (white blood cell).

agranulocytosis *n* marked reduction in or complete absence of granulocytes*. Usually results from bone marrow depression caused by (a) hypersensitivity to drugs (b) cytotoxic drugs or (c) irradiation. It is characterized by fever, ulceration of the mouth and throat and may be fatal—**agranulocytic** *adj.*

agraphia *n* loss of language facility. *motor agraphia* inability to express thoughts in writing, usually due to left precentral cerebral lesions. *sensory agraphia* inability to interpret the written word, due to lesions in the posterior part of the left parietooccipital region—**agraphic** *adj.*

ague *n* malaria*.

AHF *abbr* antihaemophilic* factor.

AID *abbr* artificial* insemination of a female with donor semen. More often now known as donor* insemination (DI).

AIDS *abbr* acquired* immune deficiency syndrome.

AIDS-related complex also known as early symptomatic disease. Third phase (phase C) in the clinical manifestation of AIDS. Individuals appear chronically ill and display minor opportunistic infections. ⇒ AIDS.

aids to independence any articles which enable a person to retain or regain independence. They include those used for preparation, cooking, serving and eating food, as well as swallowing liquids; those used for personal hygiene, dressing and undressing; those used to accomplish walking, ascending stairs and so on; and those used for transit. Their use is explicit in the concept 'aided independence'. ⇒ Zimmer aids.

AIH *abbr* artificial* insemination of a female with her husband's semen.

air *n* the gaseous mixture which makes up the atmosphere surrounding the Earth. It consists of approximately 78% nitrogen, 20% oxygen, 0.04% carbon dioxide, 1% argon, and traces of ozone, neon, helium, etc. and a variable amount of water vapour. *air-bed* a rubber mattress inflated with air. *air hunger* a deep indrawing of breath which characterizes the late stages of uncontrolled haemorrhage. *air swallowing* swallowing of excessive air particularly when eating: it may result in belching or expulsion of gas via the anus.

airway *n* a word used to describe the entry to the larynx from the pharynx. *artificial airway* a flexible oval tube which can be placed along the upper surface of the tongue; it is held in position by a metal ending which rests between the front teeth and the lips. It prevents a flaccid tongue from resting against the posterior pharyngeal wall, thereby obstructing the airway, and is commonly used during general anaesthesia. *Brook airway* a popular oropharyngeal airway used in expired air resuscitation. It has a one-way valve providing a barrier to infection passing in either direction. *Dual Aid airway* designed for both nasal and oral application in expired air resuscitation. It, too, has a one-way protective valve; it has a longer mouthpiece than the Brook airway, allowing good support for the tongue when used orally. It is unique in that a self-inflating bag such as an Ambubag can be attached to it for inflation of the lungs.

akathisia *n* a state of persistent motor restlessness: it can occur as a side-effect of neuroleptic drugs.

akinetic *adj* literally 'without movement'. A word applied to states or conditions where there is lack of movement—**akinesia** *n*.

Albers-Schönberg disease ⇒ osteopetrosis.

albinism *n* congenital absence, either partial or complete, of normal pigmentation, so that the skin is fair, the hair white and the eyes pink: due to a defect in melanin synthesis.

albino *n* a person affected with albinism*—**albinotic** *adj*.

albumin *n* a variety of protein found in animal and vegetable matter. It is soluble in water and coagulates on heating. *serum albumin* the chief protein of blood plasma and other serous fluids. ⇒ lactalbumin—**albuminous, albuminoid** *adj*.

albuminuria *n* the presence of albumin (protein) in the urine. The condition is frequently benign and temporary, as in many febrile states, but it may be an indication of renal disease. ⇒ orthostatic albuminuria—**albuminuric** *adj*. *chronic albuminuria* leads to hypoproteinaemia*.

albumose *n* an early product of proteolysis. It resembles albumin, but is not coagulated by heat.

albumosuria *n* the presence of albumose in the urine—**albumosuric** *adj*.

alcohol *n* (*syn* ethanol) a constituent of wines and spirits. Methylated spirit contains 95% alcohol with wood naphtha and is for external application only. Enhances the action of hypnotics and tranquillizers. *alcohol psychosis* Korsakoff* psychosis, syndrome.

alcohol-fast *adj* in bacteriology, describes an organism which, when stained, is resistant to decolourization by alcohol.

Alcoholics Anonymous (AA) a voluntary , locally based organization which helps people with alcohol dependency deal with their urge to drink, particularly through a system of mutual support.

alcoholism *n* poisoning resulting from alcoholic addiction. In its chronic form it causes severe disturbances of the nervous and digestive systems.

alcoholuria *n* alcohol in the urine. It is the basis of one test for fitness to drive after drinking alcohol.

aldolase test an enzyme test: the serum enzyme aldolase is increased in diseases affecting muscle.

aldosterone *n* an adrenocortical steroid which, by its action on renal tubules, regulates electrolyte metabolism; hence described as a 'mineralocorticoid'. Secretion is regulated by the renin*–angiotensin system. It increases excretion of potassium and conserves sodium and chloride.

aldosteronism *n* a condition resulting from tumours of the adrenal cortex in which the electrolyte imbalance is marked and alkalosis and tetany may ensue.

Aleppo boil ⇒ leishmaniasis.

Alexander technique based on the theory that the imbalanced use of the body can contribute to ill health, injury and chronic pain. The technique aims to promote postural improvement through self-awareness.

algesia *n* excessive sensitivity to pain; hyperaesthesia. ⇒ analgesia *opp*—**algesic** *adj.*

alginates *npl* seaweed derivatives which, when applied locally, encourage the clotting of blood. They are available in solution and in specially impregnated gauze.

alienation *n* in psychology and sociology, estrangement from people.

alimentary *adj* pertaining to food. *alimentary tract* comprises the mouth, oesophagus, stomach, small and large intestine*.

alimentation *n* the act of nourishing with food; feeding.

alkali *n* soluble corrosive bases, including soda, potash and ammonia, which neutralize acids forming salts and combine with fats to form soaps. Alkaline solutions turn red litmus blue. *alkaline reserve* a biochemical term denoting the amount of buffered alkali (normally bicarbonate) available in the blood for the neutralization of acids (normally dissolved CO_2) formed in or introduced into the body.

alkaline *adj* **1** possessing the properties of or pertaining to an alkali. 2 containing an excess of hydroxyl over hydrogen ions. *alkaline phosphatase test* an increase in the enzyme alkaline phosphatase in the blood is indicative of such conditions as obstructive jaundice and is also indicative of osteoblastic activity.

alkalinuria *n* alkalinity of urine—**alkalinuric** *adj.*

alkaloid *n* resembling an alkali. A name often applied to a large group of organic bases found in plants and which possess important physiological actions. Morphine, quinine, caffeine, atropine and strychnine are well-known examples of alkaloids—**alkaloidal** *adj.*

alkalosis *n* (*syn* alkalaemia) excess of alkali or reductions of acid in the body. Develops from a variety of causes such as overdosage with alkali, excessive vomiting or diarrhoea and hyperventilation. Results in neuromuscular excitability expressed clinically as tetany*.

alkaptonuria *n* the presence of alkaptone (homogentisic acid) in the urine, resulting from only partial oxidation of phenylalanine and tyrosine. Condition usually noticed because urine goes black in the nappies, or when left to stand. Apart from this, and a tendency to arthritis in later life, there are no ill-effects from alkaptonuria.

alkylating agents disrupt the process of cell division by affecting DNA in the nucleus, probably by adding to it alkyl group—hence the name alkylating agents. Some are useful against malignant cell growth.

allantois *n* a ventral outgrowth of the hindgut of the early embryo which becomes a small vestigial structure in the developing fetus. Stretching from the uractus at the apex of the bladder to the umbilicus, its blood vessels develop into those of the umbilical cord and, later, the placenta—**allantoic, allantoid** *adj.*

alleles *npl* originally used to denote inherited characteristics that are alternative and contrasting, such as normal colour vision contrasting with colour blindness, or the ability to taste or not to taste certain substances, or different blood groups. The basis of Mendelian inheritance of dominants and recessives. In modern usage allelomorph(s) is equivalent to allele(s), namely alternative forms of a gene at the same chromosomal location (locus).

allelomorph ⇒ allele.

allergen *n* any antigen* capable of producing an altered state or manifestation of an immune response—**allergenic** *adj*, **allergenicity** *n*.

allergic rhinitis attacks of catarrh of the conjunctiva, nose and throat precipitated by exposure to pollen (hay fever) or allergy to house dust or animal dander.

allergy *n* an altered or exaggerated susceptibility to various foreign substances or physical agents. Colloquially, implies that an individual has become overreactive to an antigen* which would not normally produce an adverse response (often difficult to prove). Sometimes caused by the interaction of an antigen with IgE antibody on the surface of mast cells. Scientifically, describes diseases due to an altered immune response, a state of altered reactivity. Some drug reactions, hay fever, insect bite reactions, urticarial reactions and asthma are classed as allergic diseases—**allergic** *adj*. ⇒ anaphylaxis, sensitization.

alloantibody *n* ⇒ isoantibody.

allocation *n* **1** patient allocation is the term used when one or more patients are assigned to one nurse for a spell of duty. The nurse is able to address the total care needs of each patient. **2** task allocation is the term used when one nurse is allocated to carry out one nursing activity for all patients. This method of organizing care is no longer considered to be in the patient's best interests and individualized nursing is preferred. **3** ward allocation ⇒ placement.

allopurinol *n* a substance which prevents the formation of deposits of crystals of insoluble uric acid. Diminishes tophus* in gout and substantially reduces the frequency and severity of further attacks. Can cause skin rash.

alopecia *n* baldness, which can be congenital, premature or senile. *alopecia areata* a patchy baldness, usually of a temporary nature. Cause unknown, probably autoimmune, but shock and anxiety are common precipitating factors. Exclamation mark hairs are diagnostic. *cicatrical alopecia* progressive alopecia of the scalp in which tufts of normal hair occur between many bald patches. Folliculitis decalvans is an alopecia of the scalp characterized by pustulation and scars.

alphafetoprotein *n* present in maternal serum and amniotic fluid in some cases of fetal abnormality.

altered consciousness the level of consciousness* is normally changed during sleep; it can also be altered by some drugs, alcohol, general anaesthesia, head injuries, strokes and other neurological diseases. ⇒ coma, Glasgow coma scale, stupor.

alveolar abscess ⇒ abscess.

alveolar–capillary block syndrome a rare syndrome of unknown aetiology characterized by breathlessness, cyanosis* and right heart failure, due to thickening of the alveolar cells of the lungs, thus impairing diffusion of oxygen.

alveolitis *n* inflammation of alveoli, by custom usually referring to those in the lung; when caused by inhalation of an allergen such as pollen, it is termed *extrinsic allergic alveolitis*.

alveolus *n* **1** an air vesicle in the

lung. 2 bone of the tooth socket, providing support for the tooth, partially absorbed when the teeth are lost. 3 a gland follicle or acinus—**alveoli** *pl,* **alveolar** *adj.*

Alzheimer's disease *n* a dementing disease, also referred to as presenile dementia*; there are specific brain abnormalities. A protein called A-68 has appeared in the spinal fluid of living patients thought to have Alzheimer's disease.

amalgam *n* a mixture or combination. *dental amalgam* an alloy of mercury and another metal or metals used for filling teeth.

amastia *n* congenital absence of the breasts.

ambidextrous *adj* able to perform skilled movements, such as writing, with either hand, equally well.—**ambidexterity** *n.*

ambisexual *adj* denoting sexual characteristics common to both sexes before sexual differentiation occurs at about 6 weeks after fertilization.

ambivalence *n* coexistence of opposite feelings at the same time in one person, e.g. love and hate—**ambivalent** *adj.*

amblyopia *n* defective vision approaching blindness in a pathologically normal eye. ⇒ smoker's blindness—**amblyopic** *adj.*

ambulant *adj* able to walk. ⇒ ambulation.

ambulation a term which was introduced in the 50s and 60s after identification of complications associated with bedrest. The concept is of gentle unhurried exercise to improve circulation and prevent phlebothrombosis*, also called deep vein thrombosis (DVT). Professional judgement has to be exercised to prevent overactivity which exhausts the patient who then lies immobile in an attempt to recover, during which time the person is at risk of developing DVT.

ambulatory *adj* mobile, walking about. *ambulatory treatment* describes the monitoring of a patient at intermittent visits to the outpatients' department of a hospital.

amelia *n* congenital absence of a limb or limbs. *complete amelia* absence of both arms and legs ⇒ phocomelia.

amelioration *n* reduction of the severity of symptoms.

amenorrhoea *n* absence of the menses. When menstruation has not been established at the time when it should have been, it is *primary amenorrhoea;* absence of the menses after they have once commenced is referred to as *secondary amenorrhoea*—**amenorrhoeal** *adj.*

amentia *n* mental disability from birth; to be distinguished from dementia which is acquired mental impairment.

ametria *n* congenital absence of the uterus.

ametropia *n* defective sight due to imperfect refractive power of the eye—**ametropic** *adj,* **ametrope** *n.*

aminoacidopathy *n* disease caused by imbalance of amino acids.

amino acids *npl* organic acids in which one or more of the hydrogen atoms is replaced by the amino group, NH_2. They are the end product of protein hydrolysis and from them the body resynthesizes its own proteins. Ten cannot be elaborated in the body and are therefore essential in the diet—arginine, histidine, isoleucine, leucine, lysine, methionine, phenylalanine, threonine, tryptophan and valine. The remainder are designated nonessential amino acids—alanine, asparagine, aspartic acid, cystine, glutamic acid, glutamine, glycine, hydroxyproline, proline, serine and tyrosine.

aminoaciduria *n* the abnormal presence of amino acids in the urine; it usually indicates an inborn error of metabolism as in cystinosis* and Fanconi syndrome*—**aminoaciduric** *adj.*

ammonia *n* a naturally occurring compound of nitrogen and hydrogen. In the human, several inborn errors of ammonia metabolism can cause mental retardation, neurological signs and seizures. *ammonia solution* (Liq. ammon) colourless liquid with a characteristic pungent odour—**ammoniated, ammoniacal** *adj.*

amnesia *n* complete loss of memory; can occur after concussion, in dementia, hysterical neurosis and following ECT. The term *anterograde* amnesia* is used when there is impairment of memory for recent events after an accident etc., and *retrograde amnesia* when the impairment is for past events—**amnesic** *adj.*

amniocentesis *n* piercing the amniotic cavity through the abdominal wall for the purpose of withdrawing a sample of fluid for examination to establish prenatal diagnosis of chromosomal abnormalities, spina bifida, metabolic errors, fetal haemolytic disease and so on.

amniochorial *adj* pertaining to the amnion* and chorion*.

amniogenesis *n* development of the amnion*.

amniography *n* X-ray of the amniotic sac after injection of opaque medium into same: outlines the umbilical cord and placenta—**amniographical** *adj,* **amniographically** *adv.*

amnion *n* the innermost membrane enclosing the developing fetus and containing the amniotic* fluid. It ensheaths the umbilical cord and is connected with the fetus at the umbilicus—**amnionic, amniotic** *adj.*

amnionitis *n* inflammation of the amnion*.

amnion nodosum a nodular condition of the fetal surface of the amnion*, observed in oligohydramnios*, which may be associated with the absence of kidneys in the fetus.

amniorrhoea *n* escape of amniotic fluid.

amniorrhoexia *n* rupture of the amnion*.

amnioscopy *n* amnioscope (endoscope*) passed through the abdominal wall enables viewing of the fetus and amniotic fluid. Clear, colourless fluid is normal; yellow or green staining is due to meconium and occurs in cases of fetal hypoxia—**amnioscopic** *adj,* **amnioscopically** *adv. cervical amnioscopy* can be performed late in pregnancy. A different instrument is inserted via the vagina and cervix for the same reasons.

amniotic cavity the fluid-filled cavity between the embryo/fetus and the amnion.

amniotic fluid a liquid produced by the fetal membranes and the fetus which surrounds the fetus throughout pregnancy. As well as providing the fetus with physical protection, the amniotic fluid is a medium of active chemical exchange. It is secreted and reabsorbed by cells lining the amniotic cavity and is swallowed, metabolized and excreted as fetal urine. ⇒ amnioscopy. *amniotic fluid embolism* formation of an embolus in the amniotic sac and its transference in the blood circulation of mother to lung or brain. A rare complication of pregnancy. *amniotic fluid infusion* escape of amniotic fluid into the maternal circulation.

amniotome *n* an instrument for rupturing the fetal membranes.

amniotomy *n* artificial rupture of

the fetal membranes to induce or expedite labour.

amoeba *n* a protozoon. An elementary, unicellular form of life. The single cell is capable of ingestion and absorption, respiration, excretion, movement and reproduction by amitotic fission. One strain, *Entamoeba histolytica,* is the parasitic pathogen which produces amoebic dysentery* in man. ⇒ protozoon—**amoebae** *pl,* **amoebic** *adj.*

amoebiasis *n* infestation of large intestine by the protozoon *Entamoeba histolytica,* where it causes ulceration by invasion of the mucosa. This results in passage per rectum of necrotic mucous membrane and blood, hence the term 'amoebic dysentery'. If the amoebae enter the portal circulation they may cause liver necrocrosis (hepatic abscess). Diagnosis is by isolating the amoebae in the stools. Regarded as a sexually transmitted disease among homosexual men.

amoebicide *n* an agent which kills amoebae—**amoebicidal** *adj.*

amoeboid *adj* resembling an amoeba in shape or in mode of movement, e.g. white blood cells.

amoeboma *n* a tumour in the caecum or rectum caused by *Entamoeba hystolytica.* Fibrosis may occur and obstruct the bowel.

amorphous *adj* having no regular shape.

amphetamine *n* a sympathomimetic agent which is a potent CNS stimulant. The stimulant action of amphetamine has led to abuse and it is now rarely prescribed—the risks of misuse and dependence far outweigh any beneficial effects it might have.

ampoule *n* a hermetically sealed glass or plastic phial containing a single sterile dose of a drug.

ampulla *n* any flask-like dilatation—**ampullae** *pl,* **ampullar, ampullary, ampullate** *adj. ampulla of Vater* the enlargement formed by the union of the common bile duct with the pancreatic duct where they enter the duodenum.

amputation *n* removal of an appending part, e.g. breast, limb.

amputee *n* a person who has undergone amputation*.

amylase *n* any enzyme which converts starches into sugars. *pancreatic amylase* amylopsin*, *salivary amylase* ptyalin*. *amylase test* the urine is tested for starch to assess kidney function. Levels of serum amylase can be high in pancreatitis.

amyloid/beta-pleated sheets of protein *adj, n* resembling starch. An abnormal complex of protein which accumulates in tissues in certain disorders known as amyloidosis*.

amyloidosis *n* formation and deposit of amyloid* in any organ, notably the liver and kidney. *primary amyloidosis* has no apparent cause. *secondary amyloidosis* can occur in any prolonged toxic condition such as tuberculosis and leprosy. It is common in the genetic disease familial Mediterranean* fever.

amylolysis *n* the digestion of starch—**amylolytic** *adj.*

amylopsin *n* a pancreatic enzyme, which in an alkaline medium converts insoluble starch into soluble maltose.

anabolism *n* the series of chemical reactions in the living body requiring energy to change simple substances into complex ones. ⇒ adenosine diphosphate, adenosine triphosphate, metabolism.

anacidity *n* lack of normal acidity, especially in the gastric juice. ⇒ achlorhydria.

anacrotism *n* an oscillation in the ascending curve of a sphygmographic pulse tracing, occurring in aortic stenosis—**anacrotic** *adj.*

anaemia *n* a deficiency of haemoglobin in the blood due to lack of red blood cells and/or their haemoglobin content. May produce clinical manifestations arising from hypoxaemia*, such as lassitude and breathlessness on exertion. Treatment is according to the cause and severity–**anaemic** *adj. aplastic anaemia* is the result of complete bone marrow failure. *haemolytic anaemia* results from premature destruction of red blood cells, as in some inherited red cell disorders, or it can occur as a response to drugs or toxic agents. *iron deficiency anaemia* the commonest form of anaemia; due to lack of absorbable iron in the diet, poor absorption of dietary iron or chronic bleeding. Oral iron-containing medications usually correct the condition. *pernicious anaemia* results from the inability of the bone marrow to produce normal red cells because of the deprivation of a protein released by gastric glands, called the intrinsic factor, which is necessary for the absorption of vitamin B_{12} from food. An autoimmune mechanism may be responsible. *sickle-cell anaemia* familial, hereditary haemolytic anaemia. The red cells are crescent-shaped. Commonly occurring in people living in and originating from Africa, Middle East and the Mediterranean region. *splenic anaemia* (*syn* Banti's disease) leucopenia, thrombocytopenia, alimentary bleeding, and splenomegaly which in turn is caused by portal hypertension.⇒ haemolytic disease of the newborn, thalassaemia.

anaerobe *n* a microorganism which will not grow in the presence of molecular oxygen. When this is strictly so, it is termed an *obligatory anaerobe*. The majority of pathogens are indifferent to atmospheric conditions and will grow in the presence or absence of oxygen and are therefore termed *facultative anaerobes*–**anaerobic** *adj*.

anaerobic respiration occurs when oxygen available to the fetus is limited, with the consequent production of lactic and pyruvic acids and a fall in the pH value of fetal blood. This can be measured in labour once the cervix has dilated–by taking a microsample of blood from the fetal scalp.

anaesthesia *n* loss of sensation. *general anaesthesia* loss of sensation with loss of consciousness. In *local anaesthesia* the nerve conduction is blocked directly and painful impulses fail to reach the brain. *spinal anaesthesia* may be caused by (a) injection of a local anaesthetic into the spinal subarachnoid space (b) a lesion of the spinal cord.

anaesthesiology *n* the science dealing with anaesthetics, their administration and effect.

anaesthetic *n* insensible to stimuli–**anaesthetize** *vt. general anaesthetic* a drug which produces general anaesthesia by inhalation or injection. *local anaesthetic* a drug which injected into the tissues or applied topically causes local insensibility to pain. *spinal anaesthetic* ⇒ spinal.

anaesthetist *n* a person who is medically qualified to administer anaesthetics.

anal *adj* pertaining to the anus*. *anal canal* 3.8 cm long, forming the terminal part of the gastrointestinal tract. The internal anal sphincter muscle is covered by mucous membrane and controlled by the autonomic nervous system. The external anal sphincter muscle is covered by skin and is under voluntary nerve control. The tissues are puckered so that they can distend for the passing of faeces. ⇒ haemorrhoids. A clinical thermometer can be placed in the anal canal to measure the body's core temperature, by custom inaccurately called rectal temperature. *anal eroticism* sexual pleasure derived from stimulation and possible penetration of the anus. *anal fissure* ⇒ fissure. *anal fistula* ⇒ fistula.

analeptic *adj, n* restorative. Analeptics in current use include caffeine, amphetamines, monoamine oxidase inhibitors and tricyclic antidepressants.

analgesia *n* loss of painful impressions without loss of tactile sense. ⇒ algesia *opp*–**analgesic** *adj. patient controlled analgesia* at the push of a button the patient receives a preset dose and safety precautions prevent overdose.

analgesic *n* a drug which relieves pain. Can be administered locally, topically or systemically.

analogous *adj* similar in function but not in origin.

analysis *n* a term used in chemistry to denote the determination of the composition of a compound substance.–**analyses** *pl,* **analytic** *adj,* **analytically** *adv.*

anaphylactic reaction an adverse reaction due to the release of the constituents of acute inflammatory cells, generally as a result of antigens binding to IgE on mast cells and basophils. In hay fever* the reaction occurs mainly in the nose; in asthma* it occurs in the lower respiratory tract. In anaphylaxis* it occurs in many tissues throughout the body. ⇒ anaphylaxis.

anaphylactoid *adj* pertaining to or resembling anaphylaxis.

anaphylaxis *n* (*syn* anaphylactic shock, serum sickness) a hypersensitive state of the body to a foreign protein (e.g. horse serum) so that the injection of a second dose after 10 days brings about an acute reaction which may be fatal; in lesser degree it produces bronchospasm pallor and collapse. ⇒ allergy, sensitization–**anaphylactic** *adj.*

anaplasia *n* loss of the distinctive characteristics of a cell, associated with proliferative activity as in cancer–**anaplastic** *adj.*

anarthria *n* a severe form of dysarthria*. Loss of ability to produce the motor movements for speech. Muscle weakness involves the respiratory, phonatory, articulatory and resonatory systems of speech.

anasarca *n* serous infiltration of the cellular tissues and serous cavities; generalized oedema–**anasarcous** *adj.*

anastomosis *n* **1** the intercommunication of the branches of two or more arteries or veins. **2** in surgery, the establishment of an intercommunication between two hollow organs, vessels or nerves–**anastomoses** *pl,* **anastomotic** *adj,* **anastomose** *vt.*

anatomical position for the purpose of accurate description the anterior view is of the upright body facing forward, hands by the sides with palms facing forwards. The posterior view is of the back of the upright body in that position.

anatomy *n* the science which deals with the structure of the body by means of dissection–**anatomical** *adj,* **anatomically** *adv.*

Ancylostoma *n* (*syn* human hookworm). *Ancylostoma duodenale* is predominantly found in southern Europe and the Middle and Far East. *Necator americanus* is found in the New World and tropical Africa. Mixed infections are not uncommon. Only clinically significant when infestation is moderate or heavy. Worm inhabits duodenum and upper jejunum, eggs are passed in stools, hatch in moist soil and produce larvae which can penetrate bare feet and reinfect people. Prevention is by wearing shoes and using latrines.

ancylostomiasis *n* (*syn* hookworm disease) infestation of the human intestine with Ancylostoma* giving rise to malnutrition and severe anaemia.

androblastoma *n* (*syn* arrhenoblastoma) a tumour of the ovary; can produce male or female hormones and can cause masculinization in women or precocious puberty in girls.

androgens *npl* hormones secreted by the testes and adrenal cortex, or synthetic substances, which control the building up of protein and the male secondary sex characteristics, e.g. distribution of hair and deepening of voice. When given to females they have a masculinizing effect. ⇒ testosterone—**androgenic, androgenous** *adj.*

anencephaly *n* absence of the brain. Cerebral hemispheres completely or partially missing. The condition is incompatible with life: it may be detected during pregnancy by raised levels of alphafetoprotein in the amniotic fluid but more likely by a neural tube defect—**anencephalous, anencephalic** *adj.*

aneurysm *n* dilation of a blood vessel, usually an artery, due to local fault in the wall through defect, disease or injury, producing a pulsating swelling over which a murmur may be heard. True aneurysms may be saccular, fusiform, or dissecting, where the blood flows between the layers of the arterial wall—**aneurysmal** *adj.*

angiectasis *n* abnormal dilatation of blood vessels. ⇒ telangiectasis—**angiectatic** *adj.*

angiitis *n* inflammation of a blood or lymph vessel. ⇒ vasculitis—**angiitic** *adj.*

angina *n* sense of suffocation or constriction—**anginal** *adj. angina pectoris* severe but temporary attack of cardiac pain which may radiate to the arms. Results from myocardial ischaemia. Often the attack is induced by exercise (angina of effort).

angioblast *n* the earliest formative tissue from which blood vessels develop.

angiocardiography *n* demonstration of the chambers of the heart and great vessels after injection of a contrast medium—**angiocardiographic** *adj,* **angiocardiogram** *n,* **angiocardiograph** *n,* **angiocardiographically** *adv.*

angiofibroma *n* benign tumour arising from nasopharynx, most commonly seen in teenage boys.

angiogenesis *n* vascularization. Seen in oncology when new blood vessels may develop to supply a tumour.

angiography *n* demonstration of vessels (arteries, veins and lymph) after injection of a contrast medium—**angiographic** *adj,* **angiogram** *n,* **angiograph** *n,* **angiographically** *adv. digital subtraction angiography* (DSA) an imaging technique which produces clean, clear views of flowing blood, or its blockage by narrowed vessels.

angiology *n* the science dealing with blood and lymphatic vessels—**angiological** *adj,* **angiologically** *adv.*

angioma *n* ⇒ naevus.

angiooedema *n* (*syn* angioneurotic oedema) a severe form of urticaria* which may involve the skin of the face, hands or genitals and the mucous membrane of the mouth and throat: oedema of the glottis may be fatal. Immediately there is an abrupt local increase in vascular permeability, as a result of which fluid escapes from blood vessels into surrounding tissues.

Swelling may be due to an allergic hypersensitivity reaction to drugs, pollens or other known allergens, but in many cases no cause can be found.

angioplasty *n* surgical reconstruction of blood vessels—**angioplastic** *adj. percutaneous transluminal coronary angioplasty* a balloon is passed into a stenosed coronary artery and inflated with contrast medium; it presses the atheroma against the vessel wall, thereby increasing the lumen.

angiosarcoma *n* a malignant tumour arising from blood vessels—**angiosarcomata** *pl*, **angiosarcomatous** *adj*.

angiospasm *n* constricting spasm of blood vessels—**angiospastic** *adj*.

angiotensin an inactive substance formed by the action of renin* on a protein in the blood plasma. In the lungs angiotensin I is converted into angiotensin II, a highly active substance which constricts blood vessels and causes release of aldosterone* from the adrenal cortex.

angular stomatitis ⇒ stomatitis.

anhidrosis *n* deficient sweat secretion—**anhidrotic** *adj*.

anhidrotics *n* any agent which reduces perspiration.

anhydrous *adj* entirely without water, dry.

aniridia *n* lack or defect of the iris*; usually congenital.

anisocoria *n* inequality in diameter of the pupils.

anisocytosis *n* variation in size of red blood cells. Often seen on blood film in cases of anaemia.

anisomelia *n* unequal length of limbs—**anisomelous** *adj*.

anisometropia *n* a difference in the refraction* of the two eyes—**anisometropic** *adj*.

ankylosing spondylitis ⇒ spondylitis.

ankylosis *n* stiffness or fixation of a joint as a result of disease.⇒ spondylitis—**ankylosed** *adj*, **ankylose** *vt, vi*.

annular *adj* ring-shaped. *annular ligaments* hold two long bones in proximity, as in the wrist and ankle joints.

anogenital *adj* pertaining to the anus and the genital region.

anomaly *n* that which is unusual or differs from the normal—**anomalous** *adj*.

anomia *n* a difficulty in word finding occurring in many aphasic* patients. Most often demonstrated in naming tasks but also evident by the use of circumlocutions in spontaneous speech samples.

anomie *n* sociological term applied to a person who is lonely because he or she cannot relate to others and consequently no longer identifies with them.

anonychia *n* absence of nails.

anoperineal *adj* pertaining to the anus and perineum.

Anopheles *n* a genus of mosquito. The females of some species are the host of the malarial parasite, and their bite is the means of transmitting malaria* to man.

anophthalmos *n* congenital absence of a true eyeball.

anoplasty *n* plastic reconstructive surgery of the anus—**anoplastic** *adj*.

anorchism *n* congenital absence of one or both testes—**anorchic** *adj*.

anorectal *adj* pertaining to the anus and rectum, e.g. a fissure.

anorexia *n* loss of or impaired appetite for food. *anorexia nervosa* a complicated psychological illness, most common in female adolescents. There is minimal food intake leading to loss of weight and sometimes death from starvation ⇒ bulimia nervosa—**anorexic** *adj*.

anosmia *n* absence of sense of smell—**anosmic** *adj*.

anovular *n* absence of ovulation. *anovular menstruation* is the result of taking contraceptive pills. *anovular bleeding* occurs in metropathia* haemorrhagica. An endometrial biopsy following an *anovular cycle* shows no progestational changes.

anoxia *n* literally, no oxygen in the tissues. Usually used to signify hypoxia—**anoxic** *adj*.

antacid *n* a substance which neutralizes or counteracts acidity. Commonly used in alkaline stomach powders and mixtures.

antagonism *n* active opposition; a characteristic of some drugs; e.g. naloxone antagonizes and reverses all the effects of narcotic analgesics. Antagonism also characterizes some muscles and organisms—**antagonistic** *adj*, **antagonist** *n*.

antagonist *n* ⇒ antagonism.

antagonistic action ⇒ action.

anteflexion *n* the bending forward of an organ, commonly applied to the position of the uterus. ⇒ retroflexion *opp*.

antenatal *adj* prenatal*. ⇒ postnatal *opp*.—**antenatally** *adj*.

antepartum *adj* before birth. More generally confined to the 3 months preceding full-term delivery, i.e. the 6th to 9th month. ⇒ postpartum *opp*. antepartum haemorrhage* bleeding from the genital tract occurring after 24 weeks of pregnancy and before labour. May be due to placenta praevia*, placental abruption* or other causes.

anterior *adj* in front of; the front surface of; ventral. ⇒ posterior *opp*.—**anteriorly** *adv*. *anterior chamber of the eye* the space between the posterior surface of the cornea and the anterior surface of the iris. ⇒ aqueous. *anterior tibial syndrome* severe pain and inflammation over anterior tibial muscle group, with inability to dorsiflex the foot.

anterograde *adj* proceeding forward. ⇒ amnesia, retrograde *opp*.

anteversion *n* the normal forward tilting, or displacement forward, of an organ or part. ⇒ retroversion *opp*—**anteverted** *adj*, **antevert** *vt*.

anthelmintic *adj* (describes) any remedy for the destruction or elimination of intestinal worms.

anthracosis *n* accumulation of carbon in the lungs due to inhalation of coal dust; may cause fibrotic reaction. A form of pneumoconiosis*—**anthracotic** *adj*.

anthrax *n* a contagious disease of cattle, which may be transmitted to man by inoculation, inhalation and ingestion, causing malignant pustule, woolsorter's disease and gastrointestinal anthrax respectively. Causative organism is *Bacillus* anthracis*. Preventive measures include prophylactic immunization of cattle and man.

anthropoid *adj* resembling man. The word is also used to describe a pelvis that is narrow from side to side, a form of contracted pelvis*.

anthropology *n* the study of mankind. Subdivided into several specialities. ⇒ ethnology.

anthropometry *n* measurement of the human body and its parts for the purposes of comparison and establishing norms for sex, age, weight, race, etc.—**anthropometric** *adj*.

antiadrenergic *adj* neutralizing or lessening the effects of impulses produced by adrenergic postganglionic fibres of the sympathetic nervous system.

antialdosterone *n* any substance that acts as an aldosterone antagonist. Used in the treatment of oedema and ascites of hepatic cirrhosis, oedema of congestive heart failure and nephrotic syndrome.

antiallergic *adj* preventing or lessening allergy.

antiarrhythmic *adj* describes drugs

and treatments used in a variety of cardiac rhythm disorders.

antibacterial *adj* describes any agent which destroys bacteria or inhibits their growth.

antibilharzial *adj* against Bilharzia. ⇒ *Schistosoma*.

antibiosis *n* an association between organisms which is harmful to one of them. ⇒ symbiosis *opp*—**antibiotic** *adj*.

antibiotics *npl* antibacterial substances derived from fungi and bacteria, exemplified by penicillin*. Later antibiotics such as tetracycline* are active against a wider range of pathogenic organisms, and are also effective orally. Others, such as neomycin* and bacitracin*, are rarely used internally owing to high toxicity, but are effective when applied topically, and skin sensitization is uncommon.

antibodies *npl* ⇒ immunoglobulins.

anticholinergic *adj* inhibitory to the action of a cholinergic nerve* by interfering with the action of acetylcholine*, a chemical by which such a nerve transmits its impulses at neural or myoneural junctions.

anticholinesterase *n* enzyme that destroys/neutralizes cholinesterase enabling acetylcholine* to accumulate at nerve endings thus permitting resumption of normal muscle contraction.

anticoagulant *n* an agent which prevents or retards clotting of blood. Uses: (a) to obtain specimens suitable for pathological investigation and chemical analyses where whole blood or plasma is required instead of serum; the anticoagulant is usually oxalate (b) to obtain blood suitable for transfusion, the anticoagulant usually being sodium citrate (c) as a therapeutic agent in the treatment of various thromboses and as a preventive agent in cardiovascular surgery.

anticonvulsant *n* an agent which terminates a convulsion or prevents convulsions—**anticonvulsive** *adj*.

anti-D *n* anti-Rh_0, an immunoglobulin. A sterile solution of globulins derived from human plasma containing antibody to the erythrocyte factor Rh(D); used to suppress formation of active Rhesus antibodies in Rh-negative mothers after delivery or miscarriage of a Rh-positive baby or fetus.

antidepressants *npl* drugs which relieve depression. There are three main types: (a) tricyclic antidepressants (TCAs), e.g. amitryptilline; (b) selective serotonin re-uptake inhibitors (SSRIs), e.g. fluoxetine; (c) monoamine* oxidase inhibitors (MAOIs), e.g. nardil. All antidepressants are equally effective in relieving symptoms of major depression but side-effect profiles and toxicity vary widely. MAOIs are less widely used because of severe reaction to some foods (but new ones may be less toxic).

antidiabetic *adj* literally 'against diabetes'. Used to describe therapeutic measures in diabetes mellitus; the hormone insulin*, oral diabetic agents, e.g. tolbutamide*.

antidiphtheritic *adj* against diphtheria. Describes preventive measures such as immunization to produce active immunity; therapeutic measures, e.g. serum, used to give passive immunity.

antidiuretic *adj* reducing the volume of urine. *antidiuretic hormone (ADH)* vasopressin*.

antidote *n* a remedy which counteracts or neutralizes the action of a poison.

antiembolic *adj* against embolism*. Antiembolic stockings are worn to decrease the risk of deep vein thrombosis, especially after surgery.

antiemetic *adj* against emesis*. Any agent which prevents nausea and vomiting.
antienzyme *n* a substance which exerts a specific inhibiting action on an enzyme. Found in the digestive tract to prevent digestion of its lining, in blood where they act as immunoglobulins*.
antiepileptic *adj* describes drugs which reduce the frequency of epileptic attacks.
antifebrile *adj* describes any agent which reduces or allays fever.
antifibrinolytic *adj* describes any agent which prevents fibrinolysis*.
antifungal *adj* describes any agent which destroys fungi.
antigen *n* any substance which is capable, under appropriate conditions, of inducing a specific immune response and of reacting with the products of that response: that is with specific antibody or specifically sensitized T-lymphocytes, or both. *carcinoembryonic antigen* originally thought to be specific for adenocarcinoma of the colon, but now known to be found in many other cancers and some nonmalignant conditions. Its primary use is in monitoring the response of patients to cancer treatment. *conjugated antigen* antigen produced by coupling a heptan to a protein carrier molecule through covalent bonds; when it induces immunization, the resultant immune response is directed against both the heptan and the carrier—**antigenic** *adj*.
antihaemophilic factor (AHF) factor VIII involved in blood* clotting, deficiency of which produces haemophilia (classical or Type A).
antihaemorrhagic *adj* describes any agent which prevents haemorrhage; used to describe vitamin* K.
antihistamines *npl* drugs which suppress some of the effects of released histamine*. They are widely used in the palliative treatment of hay fever, urticaria, angioneurotic oedema and some forms of pruritus. They also have antiemetic* properties, and are effective in motion and radiation sickness. Side-effects include drowsiness, although preparations are now available without this side-effect.
antihypertensive *adj* describes any agent which reduces high blood pressure.
antiinfective *adj* describes any agent which prevents infection; used to describe vitamin* A.
antiinflammatory *adj* tending to reduce or prevent inflammation.
antilymphocyte globulin immunoglobulin* containing antibodies to lymphocyte membrane antigens, causing their inactivation or lysis and thus diminishing immune responses.
antilymphocyte serum (ALS) serum containing antibodies which bind to lymphocytes, inhibiting their function. Used to induce immunosuppression in a patient undergoing organ transplant.
antimalarial *adj* against malaria.
antimetabolite *n* a compound which is sufficiently similar to the chemicals needed by a cell to be incorporated into the nucleoproteins* of that cell, thereby preventing its development. Examples are methotrexate, a folic acid antagonist, and mercaptopurine, a purine antagonist. Antimetabolites are used in the treatment of cancer.
antimicrobial *adj* against microbes.
antimitotic *adj* preventing reproduction of a cell by mitosis. Describes many of the drugs used to treat cancer.
antimutagen *n* a substance which nullifies the action of a mutagen*—**antimutagenic** *adj*.

antimycotic *adj* describes any agent which destroys fungi.

antineoplastic *adj* describes any substance or procedure which works against neoplasms. ⇒ alkylating agents, cytotoxic, radiotherapy.

antineuritic *adj* describes any agent which prevents neuritis. Specially applied to vitamin* B complex.

antioxidants *npl* describes any substances which delay the process of oxidation.

antiparasitic *adj* describes any agent which prevents or destroys parasites.

antiparkinson(ism) drugs *npl* name given to the major tranquillizing drugs such as the phenothiazines. They counter the side-effects of the neuroleptic or antipsychotic drugs.

antiperiodic *n* an agent which prevents the periodic return of a disease, e.g. the use of proquanil in malaria.

antiperistalsis *n* reversal of the normal peristaltic* action—**antiperistaltic** *adj.*

antiprothrombin *n* arrests blood clotting by preventing conversion of prothrombin into thrombin. Anticoagulant.

antipruritic *adj* describes any agent which relieves or prevents itching.

antipsychotic *adj* literally against psychosis. Describes drugs, also known as neuroleptics or major tranquillizers, used in psychotic illness and electroconvulsive therapy*. ⇒ hyperprolactinaemia, parkinsonism.

antipyretic *adj* describes any agent which allays or reduces fever.

antirabic *adj* describes any agent which prevents or cures rabies.

antireflux *adj* against backward flow. Usually refers to reimplantation of ureters into bladder in cases of chronic pyelonephritis* with associated vesicoureteric reflux.

antirheumatic *adj* describes any agent which prevents or lessens rheumatism.

antischistosomal *adj* describes any agent which works against *Schistosoma.*

antisepsis *n* prevention of infection of tissues or body surfaces by the application of nonantibiotic chemicals (antiseptics). Introduced into surgery in 1880 by Lord Lister, who used carbolic acid—**antiseptic** *adj.*

antiseptics *npl* nonantibiotic substances which destroy or inhibit the growth of microorganisms. They can be applied to living tissues.

antiserotonin *n* a substance which neutralizes or lessens the effect of serotonin*.

antiserum *n* a substance prepared from the blood of an animal which has been immunized by the requisite antigen; it contains a high concentration of antibodies.

antisialagogue *n* a substance which inhibits salivation.

antisocial *adj* against society. A term used to denote a psychopathic state in which the individual cannot accept the obligations and restraints imposed on a community by its members—**antisocialism** *n.*

antispasmodic *adj* describes any measure used to relieve spasm in muscle.

antistatic *adj* preventing the accumulation of static electricity.

antistreptolysin *adj* against streptolysins*. A raised antistreptolysin titre in the blood is indicative of recent streptococcal infection.

antisyphilitic *adj* describes any measures taken to combat syphilis*.

antithrombin III *n* a protease inhibitor of coagulation, synthesized in the liver. It reacts with several clotting factors and is the cofactor for heparin ⇒ thrombin.

antithrombotic *adj* describes any measures that prevent or cure thrombosis*.

antithymocyte globulin (ATG) an immunoglobulin* which binds to antigens on thymic lymphocytes and inhibits lymphocyte-dependent immune responses.

antithyroid *n* any agent used to decrease the activity of the thyroid gland.

antitoxin *n* an antibody which neutralizes a given toxin. Made in response to the invasion by toxin-producing bacteria, or the injection of toxoids—**antitoxic** *adj.*

antitreponemal *adj* describes any measures used against infections caused by *Treponema.*

antitumour *adj* against tumour formation; describes an agent which inhibits growth of tumour.

antitussive *adj* describes any measures which suppress cough.

antiviral *adj* acting against viruses.

antrectomy *n* excision of pyloric antrum* of stomach thus removing the source of the hormone gastrin in the treatment of duodenal ulcer.

antrochoanal polyp nasal polyp arising from the maxillary antrum, presenting in the nasopharynx.

antrooral *adj* pertaining to the maxillary antrum and the mouth. *antrooral fistula* can occur after extraction of an upper molar tooth, the root of which has protruded into the floor of the antrum.

antrostomy *n* an artificial opening from nasal cavity to antrum* of Highmore (maxillary sinus) for the purpose of drainage.

antrum *n* a cavity, especially in bone—**antral** *adj. antrum of Highmore* a cavity in the superior maxillary bone.

anuria *n* absence of secretion of urine by the kidneys—**anuric** *adj.*

anus *n* the end of the alimentary canal, at the extreme termination of the rectum. It is formed of a sphincter muscle which relaxes to allow faecal matter to pass through—**anal** *adj. artificial anus* ⇒ colostomy. *imperforate anus* ⇒ imperforate.

anxiety *n* a normal reaction to stress or threat. 'Clinical' anxiety is said to be present if the threat is minimal or nonexistent. Anxiety may occur in discrete attacks ('panic' attacks) or as a persistent state (anxiety state). *Free-floating anxiety* psychological and physical symptoms occur, unrelated to any event or circumstance; generalized and pervasive feelings of fear may be present for most of the time.

anxiolytics *npl* agents which reduce anxiety.

aorta *n* the main artery arising out of the left ventricle of the heart.

aortic *adj* pertaining to the aorta. *aortic incompetence* regurgitation of blood from aorta back into the left ventricle. *aortic murmur* abnormal heart sound heard over aortic area; a systolic murmur alone is the murmur of aortic stenosis, a diastolic murmur denotes aortic incompetence. The combination of both systolic and diastolic murmurs causes the so-called 'to and fro' aortic murmur. *aortic stenosis* narrowing of aortic valve. This is usually due to rheumatic heart disease, a congenital bicuspid valve which predisposes to the deposit of calcium, or age-related valvular degeneration.

aortitis *n* inflammation of the aorta.

aortography *n* demonstration of the aorta after introduction of a contrast medium, either via a catheter passed along the femoral or brachial artery or by direct translumbar injection—**aortographic** *adj,* **aortograph** *n,* **aortographically** *adv.*

apathy *n* **1** abnormal listlessness and lack of activity. **2** attitude of indifference—**apathetic** *adj.*

aperients *npl* ⇒ laxatives.

aperistalsis *n* absence of peristaltic* movement in the bowel. Characterizes the condition of paralytic ileus—**aperistaltic** *adj.*

apex *n* the narrowest part of anything which is cone-shaped, e.g. the tip of the root of a tooth.—**apices** *pl,* **apical** *adj.* In a heart of normal size the *apex beat* (systolic impulse) can be seen or felt in the 5th left intercostal space in the midclavicular line. It is the lowest and most lateral point at which an impulse can be detected and provides a rough indication of the size of the heart.

Apgar score a measure used to evaluate the general condition of a newborn baby, developed by an American anaesthetist, Dr Virginia Apgar. A score of 0, 1, or 2 is given to each of the criteria—heart rate, respiratory effort, skin colour, muscle tone and reflex response to a nasal catheter. A score of between 8 and 10 would indicate a baby in excellent condition, whereas a score of below 7 would cause concern.

aphagia *n* inability to swallow—**aphagic** *adj.*

aphakia *n* absence of the crystalline lens. Describes the eye after removal of a cataract—**aphakic** *adj.*

aphasia *n* a disorder of language following brain damage, due primarily to impairment to the linguistic system. The term does not include disorders in language comprehension or expression that are primarily due to mental disorders including psychosis, dementia and confusion, or to hearing impairment or muscle weakness. There are several classification systems but the most commonly used terms are *expressive* aphasia* and *receptive* aphasia* although patients may exhibit difficulties in both language comprehension and expression.—**aphasic** *adj.* ⇒ dysarthria.

apheresis *n* the process whereby blood is drawn from a donor into a blood cell separator which collects the required components, plasma (plasmapheresis) or platelets (plateletpheresis), and returns the remainder to the donor. Plasmapheresis may be used in the treatment of some diseases caused by antibodies or immune complexes circulating in the patient's plasma.

aphonia *n* loss of voice. ⇒dysphonia—**aphonic** *adj.*

aphrodisiac *n* an agent which stimulates sexual excitement.

aphthae *npl* small ulcers of the oral mucosa surrounded by a ring of erythema—**aphtha** *sing,* **aphthous** *adj.*

aphthous stomatitis ⇒ stomatitis.

apicectomy *n* excision of the apex of the root of a tooth.

aplasia *n* incomplete development of tissue; absence of growth.

aplastic *adj* **1** without structure or form. **2** incapable of forming new tissue. *aplastic anaemia* ⇒ anaemia.

apnoea *n* cessation of breathing as seen, e.g. in Cheyne–Stokes respiration*. It is due to lack of the necessary CO_2 tension in the blood for stimulation of the respiratory centre—**apnoeic** *adj.* *apnoea mattress* a mattress which gives an auditory alarm signal when a baby has not breathed for a preset time, usually 15 to 20 seconds. The baby can then be stimulated to breathe before he or she becomes hypoxic. ⇒ sudden infant death syndrome. *apnoea of the newborn* ⇒ periodic breathing. *apnoea of prematurity* commonly occurs in preterm babies of less than 34 weeks' gestation: due to immaturity of both the respiratory centre and chemoreceptors. *sleep apnoea* breathing pauses (and near pauses as in hypopnoea) due to periodic upper airway closure during sleep. This results in awakenings, disturbing nocturnal sleep and also in daytime sleeping and risk of accidents.

apocrine glands modified sweat glands, especially in axillae, genital and perineal regions. Responsible, after puberty, for body odour; hormone dependent.

apodia *n* congenital absence of the feet.

aponeurosis *n* a broad glistening sheet of tendon-like tissue which serves to invest and attach muscles to each other, and also to the parts which they move—**aponeuroses** *pl,* **aponeurotic** *adj.*

aponeurositis *n* inflammation of an aponeurosis.

apophysis *n* a projection, protuberance or outgrowth. Usually used in connection with bone.

apoplexy *n* condition more commonly referred to as cerebrovascular* accident or stroke—**apoplectic, apoplectiform** *adj.*

appendicectomy *n* excision of the appendix* vermiformis. *laparoscopic appendicectomy* excision of the appendix via a laparoscope*, using a minimally invasive approach.

appendicitis *n* inflammation of the appendix* vermiformis.

appendix *n* an appendage. *appendix vermiformis* a worm-like appendage of the caecum about the thickness of the little finger and usually measuring from 50.8 to 152.4 mm in length. Its position is variable and it is apparently functionless in humans.—**appendices** *pl,* **appendicular** *adj.*

apperception *n* clear perception of a sensory stimulus, in particular where there is identification or recognition—**apperceptive** *adj.*

appetite *n* pleasant anticipation of taking food and fluid; it can become fickle in illness; offering small attractive portions will be helpful.

applicator *n* an instrument for local application of remedies.

apposition *n* the approximation or bringing together of two surfaces or edges.

apraxia *n* a disorder, resulting from brain damage, in the ability to control motor movements. Involuntary movements may be relatively normal but more deliberate or voluntary movements are affected ⇒ dyspraxia—**apraxic, apractic** *adj. constructional apraxia* inability to arrange objects to a plan.

aptitude *n* natural ability and facility in performing tasks, either mental or physical.

apyrexia *n* absence of fever—**apyrexial** *adj.*

aqueous *adj* watery. *aqueous humour* the fluid contained in the anterior and posterior chambers of the eye.

arachidonic acid one of the essential fatty acids. Found in most tissues of human and animal origin.

arachnodactyly *n* congenital abnormality resulting in spider fingers.

arachnoid *adj* resembling a spider's web. *arachnoid membrane* a delicate membrane enveloping the brain and spinal cord, lying between the pia mater internally and the dura mater externally; the middle serous membrane of the meninges.⇒ phobia.—**arachnoidal** *adj.*

arborization *n* an arrangement resembling the branching of a tree. Characterizes both ends of a neurone, i.e. the dendrons and the axon.

arboviruses *npl* an abbreviation for RNA viruses transmitted by arthropods. Members of the mosquito-borne group include those causing yellow fever, dengue and viruses causing infections of the CNS. Sandflies transmit the virus causing sandfly fever. The tickborne viruses can cause haemorrhagic fevers.

ARC *abbr* AIDS*-related complex.

arcus senilis an opaque ring round the edge of the cornea, seen in elderly people.

areola *n* the pigmented area round the nipple of the breast. A *secondary areola* surrounds the primary areola in pregnancy—**areolar** *adj.*

ARF *abbr* **1** acute renal failure ⇒ renal. **2** acute respiratory failure. ⇒ respiratory failure.

arginase *n* an enzyme found in the liver, kidney and spleen. It splits arginine into ornithine and urea.

arginine *n* one of the essential amino acids. Used in treatment of acute liver failure to tide patient over acute ammonia intoxication.

argininosuccinuria *n* the presence of arginine and succinic acid in urine. Currently associated with learning disability.

argon *n* a rare inert gas used in measurement. Less than 0.1% in atmospheric air.

Argyll Robertson pupil one which reacts to accommodation*, but not to light. Diagnostic sign in neurosyphilis*, but other important causes include multiple sclerosis and diabetes mellitus. In the nonsyphilitic group the pupil is not small, but often dilated and unequal and is called atypical.

ariboflavinosis *n* a deficiency state caused by lack of riboflavine* and other members of the vitamin B complex. Characterized by cheilosis, seborrhoea, angular stomatitis, glossitis and photophobia.

Arnold Chiari malformation a group of disorders affecting the base of the brain. Commonly occurs in hydrocephalus associated with meningocele and myelomeningocele. There are degrees of severity but usually there is some 'kinking' or 'buckling' of the brain stem with cerebellar tissue herniating through the foramen magnum at the base of the skull.

aromatherapy *n* a complementary therapy involving the therapeutic use of fragrances derived from essential oils. These may be inhaled or combined with a base oil and massaged into the skin.

arrectores pilorum internal, plain, involuntary muscles attached to hair follicles, which, by contraction, erect the follicles, causing 'gooseflesh'—**arrector pili** *sing.*

arrhenoblastoma *n* ⇒ androblastoma.

arrhythmia *n* any deviation from the normal rhythm, usually referring to the heart beat.⇒ sinus, extrasystole, fibrillation, heart, Stokes-Adams syndrome, tachycardia.

arsenic *n* a metal which, in some forms, is a potent toxin, causing malaise, anaemia, gastrointestinal and nervous symptoms.

artefact *n* any artificial product resulting from a physical or chemical agent; an unnatural change in a structure or tissue.

arteriography *n* demonstration of the arterial system after injection of a contrast medium—**arteriographic** *adj,* **arteriograph** *n,* **arteriographically** *adv.*

arteriole *n* a small artery, joining an artery to a capillary.

arteriopathy *n* disease of any artery—**arteriopathic** *adj.*

arterioplasty *n* plastic surgery applied to an artery—**arterioplastic** *adj.*

arteriosclerosis *n* degenerative arterial change associated with advancing age. Primarily a thickening of the tunica media and usually associated with some degree of atheroma*—**arteriosclerotic** *adj. cerebral arteriosclerosis* a syndrome characterized by progressive memory loss, confusion and childlike behaviour.

arteriotomy *n* incision or needle puncture of an artery.

arteriovenous *adj* pertaining to an artery and a vein, e.g. an arteriovenous aneurysm, fistula, anastomosis, or shunt for haemodialysis. *arteriovenous filtration* haemofiltration*.

arteritis *n* an inflammatory disease affecting the middle walls of the arteries. It may be due to an infection such as syphilis or it may be part of a collagen disease. The arteries may become swollen and tender and the blood may clot in them. *Giant cell arteritis* occurs in elderly people and mainly in the scalp arteries. Blindness can ensue if there is thrombosis of the ophthalmic vessels. Treatment with cortisone is effective—**arteritic** *adj.*

artery *n* a vessel carrying blood from the heart to the various tissues. The internal endothelial lining provides a smooth surface to prevent clotting of blood. The middle layer of plain muscle and elastic fibres allows for distension as blood is pumped from the heart. The outer, mainly connective tissue, layer prevents overdistension. The lumen is largest nearest to the heart; it gradually decreases in size—**arterial** *adj. artery forceps* forceps used to produce haemostasis*.

arthralgia *n* (*syn* articular neuralgia, arthrodynia) pain in a joint, used especially when there is no inflammation—**arthralgic** *adj. intermittent* or *periodic arthralgia* is the term used when there is pain, usually accompanied by swelling of the knee at regular intervals.

arthritis *n* inflammation of one or more joints which swell, become warm to touch, are painful and are restricted in movement. There are many causes and the treatment varies according to the cause. ⇒ arthropathy, osteoarthritis, rheumatoid arthritis.—**arthritic** *adj. arthritis deformans juvenilis* ⇒ Still's disease. *arthritis nodosa* gout*.

arthrodesis *n* the stiffening of a joint by operative means.

arthrodynia *n* ⇒ arthralgia—**arthrodynic** *adj.*

arthrography *n* a radiographic examination to determine the internal structure of a joint, outlined by contrast media—either a gas or a liquid contrast medium or both—**arthrographic** *adj,* **arthrograph** *n,* **arthrographically** *adv.*

arthrology *n* the science which studies the structure and function of joints, their diseases and treatment.

arthropathy *n* any joint disease—**arthropathies** *pl,* **arthropathic** *adj.* The condition is currently defined as: **enteropathic arthropathies** resulting from chronic diarrhoeal diseases; **psoriatic arthropathies** ⇒ psoriasis; *seronegative arthropathies* include all other instances of inflammatory arthritis other than rheumatoid arthritis; *seropositive arthropathies* include all instances of rheumatoid arthritis.

arthroplasty *n* surgical remodelling of a joint—**arthroplastic** *adj. cup arthroplasty* articular surface is reconstructed and covered with a vitallium cup. *excision arthroplasty* gap is filled with fibrous tissue as in Keller's* operation. *Girdlestone arthroplasty* excision arthroplasty of the hip. *replacement arthroplasty* insertion of an inert prosthesis of similar shape. *total replacement arthroplasty* replacement of the head of femur and the acetabulum, both being cemented into the bone.

arthroscope *n* an instrument used for the visualization of the interior of a joint cavity. ⇒ endoscope—**arthroscopic** *adj.*

arthroscopy *n* the act of visualizing the interior of a joint by the insertion of an optic device—**arthroscopic** *adj.*

arthrosis *n* degeneration in a joint.

arthrotomy *n* incision into a joint.

articular *adj* pertaining to a joint or articulation. Applied to cartilage, surface, capsule, etc. *articular neuralgia* ⇒ arthralgia.

articulation 1 the junction of two or more bones; a joint. **2** enunciation of speech—**articular** *adj.*

artificial feeding ⇒ enteral.

artificial insemination ⇒ insemination.

artificial limb ⇒ prosthesis.

artificial lung ⇒ respirator.

artificial pacemaker cardiac pacemaker. ⇒ cardiac.

artificial pneumothorax ⇒ pneumothorax.

artificial respiration ⇒ resuscitation.

art therapy the therapeutic use of painting, drawing, modelling or sculpture to express emotions and stimulate a mood. The use of certain colours is thought to promote particular emotions, affecting breathing and circulatory rhythms. Sculpture and modelling therapy may be used in certain psychiatric conditions involving loss of orientation in space, giddiness and lack of concentration.

asbestos *n* a fibrous, mineral substance which does not conduct heat and is incombustible. It has many uses, including brake linings, asbestos textiles and asbestos-cement sheeting. Inhalation of asbestos dust and fibre can lead to pneumoconiosis* and strict health and safety legislation controls its use or removal.

asbestosis *n* a form of pneumoconiosis* from inhalation of asbestos dust and fibre. ⇒ mesothelioma.

ascariasis *n* infestation by the ascarides* worm. The bowel is most commonly affected but, in the case of roundworm, infestation may spread to the stomach, liver and lungs.

ascaricide *n* a substance lethal to ascarides*—**ascaricidal** *adj.*

ascarides *n* nematode worms of the family Ascaridae, to which belong the roundworm (*Ascaris lumbricoides*) and the threadworm (*Oxyuris vermicularis*).

Aschoff's nodules nodules in the myocardium in rheumatism.

ascites *n* (*syn* hydroperitoneum) free fluid in the peritoneal cavity producing abdominal distension. May have benign or malignant causes, including cirrhosis of the liver and right-sided heart failure. Ascites in a cancer patient may result from metastatic breast, lung or gastrointestinal tumours—**ascitic** *adj.*

ascorbic acid vitamin* C. A water-soluble vitamin which is necessary for healthy connective tissue, particularly the collagen fibres and cell walls. It is present in fresh fruits and vegetables. It is destroyed by cooking in the presence of air and by plant enzymes released when cutting and grating food: it is also lost by storage. Deficiency causes scurvy.

ASD *abbr* atrial* septal defect.

asepsis *n* the state of being free from living pathogenic microorganisms—**aseptic** *adj.*

aseptic technique a precautionary method used in any procedure where there is a possibility of introducing organisms into the patient's body. Every article used must have been sterilized.

asparaginase *n* an enzyme used pharmacologically to treat cancers, e.g. acute lymphocytic leukaemia.

aspergillosis *n* opportunist infection, mainly of lungs, caused by any species of *Aspergillus.* ⇒ bronchomycosis.

Aspergillus *n* environmental fungi which produce spores. The spores are present in air and are therefore continuously inhaled. They are found in soil, manure and on various grains. Some species are pathogenic.

aspermia *n* lack of secretion or expulsion of semen—**aspermic** *adj.*

asphyxia *n* suffocation; cessation of breathing. The O_2 content of the air in the lungs falls while the CO_2 rises and similar changes follow rapidly in the arterial blood. *blue asphyxia, asphyxia livida* deep blue appearance of a newborn baby which otherwise has good muscle tone and is responsive to stimuli. *white (pale) asphyxia, asphyxia pallida* more severe condition of newborn: pale, flaccid, unresponsive to stimuli. ⇒ respiratory distress syndrome.

aspiration *n* (*syn* paracentesis, tapping) the withdrawal of fluids from a body cavity by means of suction or siphonage apparatus. Examples include aspiration of the lung to relieve pleural effusion or the aspiration of mucus from a newborn's oropharynx.—**aspirate** *vt. aspiration pneumonia* inflammation of lung from inhalation of foreign body, usually fluid or food particles.

aspirator *n* a negative pressure apparatus for withdrawing fluids from cavities.

aspirin *n* an effective analgesic for minor painful disorders, such as headache, toothache or muscle strain. It may be used as an antipyretic to lower the temperature of fevered patients. It also relieves pain and reduces inflammation in a variety of diseases affecting the joints, tendons, cartilages and muscles. Aspirin acts mainly by blocking the synthesis of prostaglandins; as very low concentrations inhibit platelet aggregation and prevent clotting, it can be used in the prevention of coronary thrombosis and strokes. Aspirin is usually well-tolerated but can cause nausea, indigestion and gastric irritation with blood loss. Some of the gastric side-effects can be reduced by taking the drug after meals or with an alkali. The use of aspirin for children under 12 years of age is no longer recommended as it may be a causative factor in Reye* syndrome; it may, however, be specifically indicated for conditions such as juvenile rheumatoid arthritis.

assertiveness training aims at developing self-confidence in personal relationships. It focuses on the honest expression of feelings, both negative and positive: the technique is learned by role playing in a therapeutic setting followed by practice in actual situations.

assessment *n* **1** the collection by the nurse of relevant data about a patient or client in order to enable individualized nursing. The most detailed information is usually ascertained at the initial interview. Assessment is an ongoing activity, however, and nursing interventions and the goals of patient care should constantly be reevaluated in the light of this. ⇒ biographical* and health data, interviewing. **2** the measurement of a candidate's level of competence in theoretical and practical nursing skills.

assimilation *n* the process whereby the already digested foodstuffs are absorbed and utilized by the tissues—**assimilable** *adj*, **assimilate** *vt, vi*.

assisted ventilation mechanical assistance with breathing. ⇒ ventilator.

association *n* a word used in psychology. *association of ideas* the principle by which ideas, emotions and movements are connected so that their succession in the mind occurs. *controlled association* ideas called up in consciousness in response to words spoken by the examiner. *free association* ideas arising spontaneously when censorship is removed: an important feature of psychoanalysis*.

astereognosis *n* loss of ability to recognize the shape and consistency of objects.

asthenia *n* lack of strength; weakness, debility—**asthenic** *adj*.

asthma *n* paroxysmal dyspnoea* characterized by wheezing and difficulty in expiration because of muscular spasm in the bronchi. Mast cells in bronchial walls produce immunoglobulin on encountering pollen grains; when another grain is inhaled, the alveolar mast cells burst producing an asthmatic attack. Antiasthmatic drugs can prevent this but the incidence is rising, especially in children, with traffic pollution and the increase in the house dust mite thought to be possible causes. ⇒ bronchial asthma, renal asthma—**asthmatic** *adj*.

astigmatism *n* defective vision caused by inequality of one or more refractive surfaces, usually the corneal, so that the light rays do not converge to a point on the retina. May be congenital or acquired—**astigmatic, astigmic** *adj*.

astringent *adj* describes an agent which contracts organic tissue, thus lessening secretion—**astringency, astringent** *n*.

astrocytoma *n* a slowly growing tumour of the glial tissue of brain and spinal cord. A glioma.

Astrup test estimates the degree of acidosis* by measuring the pressures of oxygen and carbon dioxide in arterial blood.

AST test aspartate aminotransferase (AST) is an enzyme normally present in liver, heart, muscles and kidneys. Values greater than 400 units per millilitre of serum are abnormal and are the commonest indication of liver disease. ⇒ serum* glutamic oxaloacetic transaminase (SGOT).

asymmetry *n* lack of similarity of the organs or parts on each side.

asymptomatic *adj* symptomless.

atavism *n* the reappearance of a hereditary trait which has skipped one or more generations—**atavic, atavistic** *adj*.

ataxia, ataxy *n* defective muscular control resulting in irregular and jerky movements: staggering—**ataxic** *adj*. *ataxic gait* ⇒ gait. *Friedreich's ataxia* ⇒ Friedreich's.

atelectasis *n* numbers of pulmonary alveoli do not contain air due to failure of expansion (congenital atelectasis) or resorption of air from the alveoli (collapse*)—**atelectatic** *adj*.

ATF *abbr* antihaemophilic factor.

atherogenic *adj* capable of producing atheroma—**atherogenesis** *n*.

atheroma *n* deposition of hard yellow plaques of lipoid material in the intimal layer of the arteries. May be related to high level of cholesterol in the blood or excessive consumption of refined sugar. Of great significance in the coronary arteries in predisposing to coronary thrombosis—**atheromatous** *adj.*

atherosclerosis *n* coexisting atheroma and arteriosclerosis—**atherosclerotic** *adj.*

athetosis *n* a condition marked by purposeless movements of the hands and feet and generally due to a brain lesion—**athetoid, athetotic** *adj.*

athlete's foot tinea pedis. ⇒ tinea.

atom *n* the smallest particle of an element capable of existing individually, or in combination with one or more atoms of the same or another element—**atomic** *adj. atomic weight* now known as *relative atomic mass* the relative average mass of an atom based on the mass of an atom of carbon-12.

atomizer *n* nebulizer*.

atonic *adj* without tone; weak—**atonia, atony, atonicity** *n.*

atonic bladder urinary bladder with no tone–the detrusor has lost its contractility, resulting in incomplete voiding or inability to void at all. It may be a temporary or permanent condition.

atopic syndrome a constitutional tendency to develop infantile eczema, asthma, hay fever or all three when there is a positive family history.

ATP *abbr* adenosine* triphosphate.

atresia *n* imperforation or closure of a normal body opening, duct or canal—**atresic, atretic** *adj.*

atrial fibrillation chaotic irregularity of atrial rhythm without any semblance of order. The ventricular rhythm, depending on conduction through the atrioventricular node, is irregular. Commonly associated with mitral stenosis or thyrotoxicosis.

atrial flutter rapid regular cardiac rhythm caused by irritable focus in atrial muscle and usually associated with organic heart disease. Speed of atrial beats between 260 and 340 per minute. Ventricles usually respond to every second beat, but may be slowed by carotid sinus pressure.

atrial septal defect (ASD) a communication between right and left atria, commonly due to nonclosure of foramen ovale at birth.

atrioventricular *adj* pertaining to the atria and the ventricles of the heart. Applied to a node, tract and valves.

atrium *n* cavity, entrance or passage. One of the two upper cavities of the heart—**atria** *pl,* **atrial** *adj.*

atrophic rhinitis (*syn* ozaena) an atrophic condition of the nasal mucous membrane with associated crusting and fetor.

atrophy *n* wasting, emaciation, diminution in size and function—**atrophied, atrophic** *adj. acute yellow atrophy* massive necrosis of liver associated with severe infection, pregnancy induced hypertension or ingested poisons. *progressive muscular atrophy (syn* motor neurone disease) disease of the motor neurones of unknown cause, characterized by loss of power and wasting in the upper limbs. May also have upper motor neurone involvement (spasticity) in lower limbs.

atropine *n* principal alkaloid of belladonna*. Has spasmolytic, mydriatic and central nervous system depressant properties. Given before anaesthetic to decrease secretion in bronchial and salivary systems and to prevent cardiac depression by depressing the vagus nerve thus quickening the heart beat. *atropine methonitrate* is used in pylorospasm and in spray preparations for asthma and bronchospasm.

ATS *abbr* antitetanus serum. Contains tetanus antibodies.

Produces artificial passive immunity. A test dose is given to ensure that the patient will not develop an anaphylactic* reaction.

ATT *abbr* antitetanus toxoid. Contains inactivated but antigenically intact tetanus toxins. Produces active immunity.

attempted suicide ⇒ parasuicide.

attenuation *n* the process by which pathogenic microorganisms are induced to develop or show less virulent characteristics. They can then be used in the preparation of vaccines—**attenuant, attenuated** *adj,* **attenuate** *vt, vi.*

attrition *n* erosion of the occlusal* surfaces of the teeth by use.

atypical *adj* not typical; unusual, irregular; not conforming to type, e.g. atypical pneumonia.

audiogram *n* a visual record of the acuity of hearing tested with an audiometer.

audiology *n* the scientific study of hearing—**audiological** *adj,* **audiologically** *adv.*

auditory *adj* pertaining to the sense of hearing. *auditory acuity* ⇒ acuity. *auditory area* that portion of the temporal lobe of the cerebral cortex which interprets sound. *auditory meatus* the canal between the pinna and eardrum. *auditory nerve* the eighth cranial nerve. *auditory ossicles* the three small bonesómalleus, incus and stapes–in the middle ear.

aura *n* a premonition; a peculiar sensation or warning of an impending attack, such as occurs in epilepsy*.

aural *adj* pertaining to the ear.

aural toilet removal of wax, debris or discharge from the external auditory canal.

auricle *n* **1** the pinna of the external ear. **2** an appendage to the cardiac atrium*. **3** commonly used mistakenly for atrium* (historical usage)—**auricular** *adj.*

auricular fibrillation atrial* fibrillation.

auricular flutter atrial* flutter.

auriculoventricular *adj* atrioventricular*.

auriscope *n* an instrument for examining the ear, usually incorporating both magnification and illumination.

auscultation *n* a method of listening to the body sounds, particularly the heart, lungs and fetal circulation for diagnostic purposes. It may be: (a) immediate, by placing the ear directly against the body (b) mediate, by the use of a stethoscope—**auscultatory** *adj,* **auscult, auscultate** *v.*

Australia antigen hepatitis* B surface antigen found in the serum of individuals with acute or chronic serum hepatitis, or who are carriers of that disease. Extremely dilute concentrations of the antigen can cause the disease and it is easily transmitted by blood, needles and other instruments. Blood for transfusion is routinely screened for this antigen.

Australian lift better described as shoulder lift. A method of lifting a heavy patient, whereby the weight is taken by the upper shoulder muscles of the two lifters, and the lift is achieved by straightening the lifters' flexed hips. ⇒ lifting, patient handling.

autism *n* a condition of self-absorption, usually first noted in childhood. There is retreat from reality into a private world of thought, fantasies and in extreme cases hallucinations.

autistic person a person who has lost or never achieved normal contact with other people and who is totally withdrawn and preoccupied with his or her own fantasies, thoughts, and stereotyped behaviour, such as rocking.

autoagglutination *n* the clumping together of the body's own red blood cells caused by autoantibodies: this occurs in acquired haemolytic anaemia, an autoimmune disease.

autoantibody *n* an antibody which can bind to normal constituents of the body, such as DNA, smooth muscle and parietal cells.

autoantigen *n* antigens in normal tissues which can bind to autoantibodies.

autoclave 1 *n* an apparatus for high-pressure steam sterilization. 2 *vt* sterilize in an autoclave.

autodigestion *n* self-digestion of tissues within the living body. ⇒ autolysis.

autoeroticism *n* self-gratification of the sex instinct. ⇒ masturbation—**autoerotic** *adj*.

autogenic therapy a complementary therapy which combines relaxation and self-hypnosis. The client is 'trained' to enter a relaxed, receptive state to which certain conditions such as indigestion or cardiac arrhythmias may be susceptible. Autogenic modification amplifies the training and directs it to certain areas.

autograft *n* tissue grafted from one part of the body to another.

autoimmune disease an illness caused by, or associated with, the development of an immune response to normal body tissues.

autoimmunization *n* the process which leads to an autoimmune disease.

autoinfection *n* ⇒ infection.

autointoxication *n* poisoning from faulty or excessive metabolic products elaborated within the body. Such products may be derived from infected or dead tissue.

autologous blood transfusion (ABT) donation of blood or blood products prior to elective surgery to be transfused postoperatively. Crossmatching and compatibility problems are avoided as is the risk of receiving infected blood or blood products.

autolysis *n* autodigestion* which occurs if digestive enzymes escape into surrounding tissues—**autolytic** *adj*.

automatic *adj* performed without the influence of the will; spontaneous; nonvolitional acts; involuntary acts.

automatism *n* organized behaviour which occurs without subsequent awareness of it. ⇒ epilepsy, somnambulism.

autonomic *adj* independent; self-governing. *autonomic nervous system (ANS)* is divided into parasympathetic and sympathetic portions. They are made up of nerve cells and fibres which cannot be controlled at will. They are concerned with reflex control of bodily functions.⇒ central nervous system.

autonomic dysreflexia syndrome occurring in people with spinal injuries as a result of a sympathetic response to noxious stimuli. Includes bladder or bowel distension, hypertension and exaggerated reflex.

autopsy *n* the examination of a dead body (cadaver) for diagnostic purposes.

autosome *n* a chromosome other than a sex chromosome (gonosome).

autosuggestion *n* self-suggestion; uncritical acceptance of ideas arising in the individual's own mind. Occurs in neurosis*.

autotransfusion *n* the infusion into a patient of the actual blood lost by haemorrhage, especially when haemorrhage occurs into the abdominal cavity.

avascular *adj* bloodless; not vascular, i.e. without blood supply. *avascular necrosis* death of bone from deficient blood supply following injury or possibly through disease, often a precursor of osteoarthritis—**avascularize** *vt, vi.*

aversion therapy a method of treatment by deconditioning. Effective in some forms of addiction and abnormal behaviour.

avian *adj* pertaining to birds. *avian tubercle bacillus (Mycobacterium avium)* resembles the other types of tubercle bacilli in its cultural requirements. Avian tuberculosis is also caused by *M. tuberculosis* and *M. xenopi;* both cause disease in man.

avidin *n* a high molecular weight protein with a high affinity for biotin* which can interfere with the absorption of biotin. Found in raw egg white.

avidity *n* a imprecise measure of the strength of antigen-antibody binding based on the rate at which the complex is formed.

avulsion *n* a forcible wrenching away, as of a limb, nerve or polypus.

axilla *n* the armpit.

axillary *adj* applied to nerves, blood and lymphatic vessels, of the armpit.

axis *n* **1** the second cervical vertebra. **2** an imaginary line passing through the centre; the median line of the body—**axial** *adj.*

axon *n* that process of a nerve cell conveying impulses away from the cell; a direct prolongation of the nerve cell—**axonal** *adj.*

axonotmesis *n* (*syn* neuronotmesis, neurotmesis) peripheral degeneration as a result of damage to the axons of a nerve. The internal architecture is preserved and recovery depends upon regeneration of the axons, and may take many months (about 25.4 mm a month is the usual speed of regeneration). Such a lesion may result from pinching, crushing or prolonged pressure.

azoospermia *n* sterility of the male through nonproduction of spermatozoa.

azoturia *n* pathological excretion of urea in the urine—**azoturic** *adj.*

azygos *adj* occurring singly, not paired. *azygos veins* three unpaired veins of the abdomen and thorax which empty into the inferior vena cava—**azygous** adj.

B

Babinski's reflex, or sign movement of the great toe upwards (dorsiflexion) instead of downwards (plantar flexion) on stroking the sole of the foot. It is indicative of disease or injury to upper motor neurones. Babies exhibit dorsiflexion, but after learning to walk they show the normal plantar flexion response.

Bacille-Calmette-Guérin *n* ⇒ BCG.

bacilluria *n* the presence of bacilli in the urine—**bacilluric** *adj.*

Bacillus *n* a genus of bacteria consisting of aerobic, Gram-positive, rod-shaped cells which produce endospores. The majority are motile by means of peritrichate flagella. These organisms are saprophytes and their spores are common in soil and dust of the air. Colloquially, the word is still used to describe any rod-shaped microorganism. *Bacillus anthracis* causes anthrax in man and in animals.

bacitracin *n* an antibiotic used mainly for external application in conditions resistant to other forms of treatment. It does not cause sensitivity reactions.

backache *n* describes a chronic low grade sensation of pain* usually in the lower back. It is estimated that 1 in 20 adults visiting their general practitioner each year do so because of low back pain; the most common causes are degenerative disease of the spine, prolapsed intervertebral disc and nerve entrapment syndrome. Nurses are at special risk and should avoid manual lifting of patients wherever possible. ⇒ prolapse, sciatica.

bacteraemia *n* the presence of bacteria in the blood—**bacteraemic** *adj.*

bacteria *npl* a group of microorganisms, also called the 'schizomycetes'. They are typically small cells of about 1 μm in transverse diameter. Structurally there is a protoplast, containing cytoplasmic and nuclear material (not seen by ordinary methods of microscopy) within a limiting cytoplasmic membrane, and a supporting cell wall. Other structures such as flagella, fimbriae and capsules may also be present. Individual cells may be spherical, straight or curved rods or spirals; they may form chains or masses and some show branching with mycelium formation. They may produce various pigments including chlorophyll. Some form endospores. Reproduction is chiefly by simple binary fission. They may be free living, saprophytic or parasitic; some are pathogenic to man, animals and plants—**bacterium** *sing,* **bacterial** *adj.*

bactericide *n* any agent which destroys bacteria—**bactericidal** *adj,* **bactericidally** *adv.*

bactericidin *n* an antibody which kills bacteria.

bacteriologist *n* a person who is an expert in bacteriology.

bacteriology *n* the scientific study of bacteria—**bacteriological** *adj,* **bacteriologically** *adv.*

bacteriolysin *n* a specific antibody formed in the blood which causes dissolution (break-up) of bacteria.

bacteriolysis *n* the disintegration and dissolution of bacteria—**bacteriolytic** *adj.*

bacteriophage *n* a virus parasitic on bacteria. Some of these are used in phage-typing staphylococci etc.

bacteriostasis *n* arrest or hindrance of bacterial growth—**bacteriostatic** *adj.*

bacteriuria *n* the presence of bacteria in the urine (100 000 or more pathogenic microorganisms per ml). Acute urinary tract infection may be preceded by, and active pyelonephritis may be associated with asymptomatic bacteriuria.⇒ perineal toilet.

baker's itch 1 contact dermatitis* resulting from flour or sugar. 2 itchy papules from the bite of the flour mite *Pyemotes.*

balanus *n* the glans of the penis or clitoris.

baldness *n* ⇒ alopecia.

Balkan beam overhead beam attached to a hospital bed that may hold suspension and traction pulleys.

balloon angioplasty ⇒ angioplasty.

ballottement *n* testing for a floating object, especially used to diagnose pregnancy. A finger is inserted into the vagina and the uterus is pushed forward; if a fetus is present it will fall back again, bouncing in its bath of fluid. External ballottement may be used to determine per abdomen whether the fetal presenting part has entered the pelvis—**ballottable** *adj.*

bandage *n* a piece of material applied to a wound or used to bind an injured part of the body. Available in strips or circular form in a range of different materials and applying varying levels of pressure. Compression bandages are widely used in the management of venous ulcers.

Bankart's operation capsular repair in the glenoid* cavity, for recurrent dislocation of shoulder joint.

Banti's disease ⇒ anaemia.

barany box noise making device used to mask one ear when testing hearing in the other.

Barbados leg (*syn* elephant leg) ⇒ elephantiasis.

barber's itch ⇒ sycosis barbae.

barbiturates *npl* a widely used group of sedative drugs derived from barbituric acid (a combination of malonic acid and urea). Small changes in the basic structure result in the formation of rapid-acting, medium or long-acting barbiturates. Only used to treat severe intractable insomnia; continual use may result in addiction. Action potentiated in presence of alcohol.

barbiturism *n* addiction to any of the barbiturates. Characterized by confusion, slurring of speech, yawning, sleepiness, depressed respiration, cyanosis and even coma.

barium enema the retrograde introduction of barium sulphate suspension, plus a quantity of air, into the large bowel via a rectal catheter, during fluoroscopy. Used for diagnostic purposes.

barium meal, swallow after swallowing a contrast agent, X-rays are taken of successive parts of the alimentary tract. ⇒ barium sulphate.

barium sulphate a heavy insoluble powder used, in an aqueous suspension, as a contrast agent in X-ray visualization of the alimentary tract.

Barlow's disease infantile scurvy*.

baroreceptors *npl* sensory nerve endings which respond to changes in pressure; they are present in the cardiac atria, venae cavae, aortic arch, carotid sinus and the internal ear.

barotrauma *n* injury due to a

change in atmospheric or water pressure, e.g. ruptured eardrum.

barrier nursing a method of preventing the spread of infection from an infectious patient to others. It is achieved by isolation* technique. *reverse barrier nursing* every attempt is made to prevent carrying infection to the patient.

bartholinitis *n* inflammation of Bartholin's* glands.

Bartholin's glands two small glands situated at each side of the external orifice of the vagina. Their ducts open just outside the hymen.

basal ganglia grey cells at the cerebral base concerned with modifying and coordinating voluntary muscle movement. Site of degeneration in Parkinson's disease.

basal metabolic rate (BMR) the amount of heat given off from the body at rest, indicating the rate of oxygen uptake.

basal narcosis the preanaesthetic administration of narcotic drugs which reduce fear and anxiety, induce sleep and thereby minimize postoperative shock. ⇒ premedication.

base *n* **1** the lowest part. **2** the main part of a compound. **3** in chemistry, the substance which combines with an acid to form a salt—**basal, basic** *adj.*

basic life support a term which describes maintenance of a clear airway and cardiopulmonary rescusitation.

basilar-vertebral insufficiency vertebrobasilar* insufficiency.

basilic *adj* prominent. *basilic vein* on the inner side of the arm. *median basilic* a vein at the bend of the elbow which is generally chosen for venepuncture.

basophil *n* **1** a cell which has an affinity for basic dyes. **2** a basophilic granulocyte (white blood cell) which takes up a particular dye: its cytoplasm contains blue-staining granules, which contain the important chemical mediators (e.g. histamine) of acute inflammation.

basophilia *n* **1** increase of basophils in the blood. **2** basophilic staining of red blood corpuscles.

Batchelor plaster a type of double abduction plaster, with the legs encased from groins to ankles, in full abduction and medial rotation. The feet are then attached to a wooden pole or 'broomstick'. Alternative to frog plaster, but the hips are free.

Bazin's disease (*syn* erythema induratum) a chronic recurrent disorder, involving the skin of the legs of women. There are deep-seated nodules which later ulcerate.

BBA *abbr* born before arrival (at hospital or of the midwife or doctor).

BCG *abbr* Bacille-Calmette-Guérin. An attenuated form of tubercle bacilli: it has lost its power to cause tuberculosis, but retains its antigenic function; it is the base of a vaccine used for immunization against tuberculosis.

BDI *abbr* Beck* Depression Inventory

bearing-down *n* **1** a pseudonym for the expulsive contractions in the second stage of labour. **2** a feeling of weight and descent in the pelvis associated with uterine prolapse or pelvic tumours.

beat *n* pulsation of the blood in the heart and blood vessels brought about by cardiac contraction *apex beat* ⇒ apex. *dropped beat* refers to the loss of an occasional ventricular beat as occurs in extrasystoles*, *premature beat* an extrasystole*.

Beck Depression Inventory (BDI) a self-scoring set of items to determine the presence and severity of clinical depression.

becquerel (Bq) *n* a unit of radioactivity. It equals the amount of a substance undergoing one disintegration per second. This unit has replaced the curie.

bedbug *n* a blood-sucking insect belonging to the genus *Cimex. Cimex lecturlarius* is the most common species in temperate and *C. hemipterus* in tropical zones. They live and lay eggs in cracks and crevices of furniture and walls. They are nocturnal in habit and their bites leave a route for secondary infection.

bedfast *n* confinement of a person to bed for most of each 24 hours. Patient can usually be lifted or helped out to a commode as research has shown that eliminating into a bedpan in bed uses more energy. For some patients, their treatment, e.g. traction, is the reason for being bedfast and it prevents use of a commode; for others, being bedfast is a means of providing bedrest*. ⇒ bedrest–complications of.

bedrest *n* confinement of a person to bed for most of each 24 hours with the prime objective of minimal functioning of all body systems. To avoid the complications* of bedrest, it is currently less frequently used; instead the patient is well supported in a comfortable chair during the day. ⇒ pressure sores–prevention of.

bedrest, complications of potential problems associated with confinement to bed. They include loss of interest, depression, loss of appetite, loss of weight, pulmonary infection due to stagnant secretions, kidney stones (renal calculi), pressure sores, bone thinning (osteoporosis), foot drop, deep vein thrombosis, cystitis from stagnation of urine in bladder, gaseous intestinal distension. ⇒ bedfast, bedrest.

bedsore a word previously used for a pressure* sore which is now the preferred term, as pressure is the main cause of the sore, and many surfaces other than beds can cause pressure.

bedwetting *n* ⇒ enuresis.

behaviour *n* the observable behavioural response of a person to an internal or external stimulus. *behaviour modification* in a general sense, an inevitable part of living, resulting from the consistent rewarding or punishing of response to a stimulus, whether that response is negative or positive. Some education systems deliberately employ a behaviour modification approach to maximize learning. *behaviour therapy* a kind of psychotherapy to modify observable, maladjusted patterns of behaviour by the substitution of a learned response or set of responses to a stimulus. The treatment is designed for a particular patient and not for the particular diagnostic label which has been attached to him. Such treatment includes assertiveness training, aversion therapy, conditioning and desensitization.

behaviourism *n* a word used in psychology to describe an approach which studies and interprets behaviour by objective observation of that behaviour without reference to the underlying subjective mental phenonema such as ideas, emotions and will. Behaviour is seen as a series of conditioned responses.

Behçet syndrome described by Behçet in 1937. Starts with ulceration of mouth and/or genitalia with eye changes such as conjunctivitis, keratitis or hypopyon iritis. One site may be affected months or years before others. There may also be skin nodules, thrombophlebitis and arthritis of one or more of the large joints. Pulmonary, gastrointestinal and neurological complications are being increasingly reported. Cause unknown; some favour virus, others an allergic vasculitis. No effective treatment apart from attempts to suppress worst phases with steroids. Blindness may result from ocular complications.

beliefs *npl* principles of living which are acquired from cumulative experience. Those pertinent to nursing include such subjects as the sanctity of life, abortion, euthanasia, health, illness and risk-taking.

belladonna *n* deadly nightshade *Atropa belladonna.* Powerful antispasmodic; preparations of belladonna are used as an anticholinergic* drug. The alkaloid from belladonna is poisonous but from it atropine* and hyoscine* are extracted.

'belle indifference' the incongruous lack of appropriate emotion in the presence of incapacitating symptoms commonly shown by patients with conversion hysteria. First noted by Janet in 1893.

Bell's palsy facial hemiparesis* from oedema of the seventh (facial) cranial nerve. Cause unknown.

Bence-Jones protein protein bodies appearing in the urine of some patients with myelomatosis*. On heating the urine they are precipitated out of solution at 50–60°C; they redissolve on further heating to boiling point and reprecipitate on cooling.

bends *npl* ⇒ caisson disease.

benchmarking *n* a quality* assurance initiative. It involves identifying examples of best practice from others engaged in similar practice. From this, best practice benchmark scores in agreed areas of care are identified, against which individual units can compare their own performance.

benign *adj* **1** noninvasive, noncancerous (of a growth). **2** describes a condition or illness which is not serious and does not usually have harmful consequences. *benign myalgic encephalomyelitis (BME)* a flu-like illness with symptoms including dizziness, muscle fatigue and spasm, headaches and other neurological pain. A high percentage of BME sufferers have a higher level of Coxsackie B antibodies in their blood than the rest of the population.

benign hypotonia term applied to babies who are initially floppy but otherwise healthy. Improvement occurs and the infant regains normal tone and motor development.

Bennett's fracture fracture of proximal end of first metacarpal involving the articular surface.

benzene *n* a colourless inflammable liquid obtained from coal tar. Extensively used as a solvent. Its chief importance in the medical sphere is in industrial toxicology. Continued exposure to it results in leucopenia, anaemia, purpura and, rarely, leukaemia.

benzodiazepines *npl* a group of minor tranquillizers which has similar pharmacological activities such as reducing anxiety, relaxing muscles, sedating and having hypnotic effects.

bereavement *n* a life event, not an illness. Includes that which happens to a person after the death of another person who has been important in his or her life.⇒ grieving. *bereavement counsellors* those who work in a professional capacity helping bereaved people to work through the emotions which they are experiencing during bereavement. Nurses need to be aware of the availability of skilled bereavement counsellors, yet at the same time they need to develop the necessary skills to help a person who is bereaved who may be encountered in both hospital and the community, as well as in school and at work. There are also various groups available to those whose loved one has died from a particular disease or in particular circumstances. Some are voluntary organisations; some are led by a professional person who enhances the skills of the volunteers.

beri-beri *n* a deficiency disease caused by lack of vitamin B_1. It occurs mainly in those countries where the staple diet is polished rice. The symptoms are pain from neuritis, paralysis, muscular wasting, progressive oedema, mental deterioration and, finally, heart failure.

berylliosis *n* an industrial disease: there is impaired lung function because of interstitial fibrosis from inhalation of beryllium. Steroids are used in treatment.

Besnier's prurigo an inherited flexural neurodermatitis with impaired peripheral circulation giving rise to dry, thickened epidermis and outbreaks of eczema in childhood. Old term for atopic* syndrome. ⇒ eczema.

beta blocker a drug which prevents stimulation of the beta-adrenergic receptors thus decreasing the heart's activity.

bibliotherapy *n* literally 'book therapy'. Extracts from books are used to help patients gain insight into their problems and promote communication with therapist. In a group situation, making a positive contribution helps to maintain self-esteem. Also used for encouraging elderly people to talk about their lives.

bicarbonate *n* a salt of carbonic acid. *blood bicarbonate* that in the blood indicating the alkali reserve. Also called 'plasma bicarbonate'.

biceps *n* the two-headed muscle on the front of the upper arm.

biconcave *adj* concave or hollow on both surfaces.

biconvex *adj* convex on both surfaces.

bicornuate *adj* having two horns, generally applied to a double uterus or a single uterus possessing two horns.

bicuspid *adj* having two cusps or points. *bicuspid teeth* the premolars. *bicuspid valve* the mitral valve between the left atrium and ventricle of the heart.

BID *abbr* brought* in (to hospital) dead.

bidet *n* low-set, trough-like basin in which the perineum can be immersed, whilst the legs are outside and the feet on the floor. Can have attachments for douching the vagina or rectum.

bifid *adj* divided into two parts. Cleft or forked.

bifurcation *n* division into two branches—**bifurcate** *adj, vt, vi.*

biguanides *npl* oral antidiabetic agents. They do not act on the islets of Langerhans but appear to stimulate the uptake of glucose by muscle tissue in diabetic subjects. Unwanted side-effects include lactic acidosis. Only used when some residual activity of the beta islets is apparent.

bilateral *adj* pertaining to both sides—**bilaterally** *adv.*

bile *n* a bitter, alkaline, viscid, greenish-yellow fluid secreted by the liver and stored in the gallbladder. It contains water, mucin, lecithin, cholesterol, bile salts and the pigments bilirubin and biliverdin. *bile ducts* the hepatic and cystic, which join to form the common bile duct. *bile salts* emulsifying agents, sodium glycocholate and taurocholate—**bilious, biliary** *adj.*

Bilharzia *n* ⇒ Schistosoma.

bilharziasis *n* ⇒ schistosomiasis.

biliary *adj* pertaining to bile. *biliary colic* pain in the right upper quadrant of abdomen, due to obstruction of the gallbladder or common bile duct, usually by a stone: it is severe and often occurs about an hour after a meal; it may last several hours and is usually steady which differentiates it from other forms of colic. Vomiting may occur. *biliary fistula* an abnormal track conveying bile to the surface or to some other organ.

bilious *adj* 1 a word usually used to signify vomit containing bile. 2 a nonmedical term, usually meaning 'suffering from indigestion'.

bilirubin *n* a pigment largely derived from the breakdown of haemoglobin from red blood cells destroyed in the spleen. When it is released it is fat-soluble, gives an indirect reaction with Van* den Bergh's test and is potentially harmful to metabolically active tissues in the body, particularly the basal nuclei of the immature brain. *indirect bilirubin* is transported to the blood attached to albumen to make it less likely to enter and damage brain cells. In the liver the enzyme glucuronyl tranferase conjugates indirect fat-soluble bilirubin with glucuronic acid to make it water-soluble, in which state it is relatively nontoxic, reacts directly with Van den Bergh's test and can be excreted in stools and urine. ⇒ phototherapy.

biliuria *n* (choluria) the presence of bile pigments in the urine—**biliuric** *adj.*

biliverdin *n* the green pigment of bile formed by oxidation of bilirubin.

Billroth's operation ⇒ gastrectomy.

bilobate *adj* having two lobes.

bilobular *adj* having two little lobes or lobules.

bimanual *adj* performed with both hands. A method of examination used in gynaecology whereby the internal genital organs are examined between one hand on the abdomen and the other hand or finger within the vagina.

binge-purge syndrome ⇒ bulimia* nervosa.

binocular vision the focusing of both eyes on one object at the same time, in such a way that only one image of the object is seen. It is not an inborn ability but is acquired in the first few months of life.

binovular *adj* derived from two separate ova. Binovular twins may be of different sexes. ⇒ uniovular *opp.*

biochemistry *n* the chemistry of life—**biochemical** *adj.*

bioengineering *n* manipulating living cells so as to promote their growth in a desired way.

bioethics *n* the application of ethics* to biological problems.

biofeedback *n* physiological activities such as excessive muscle tension, raised blood pressure and heart rate are measured graphically and presented to the patient. Either by trial and error or by operant conditioning a person can learn to repeat behaviour which relaxes muscles or lowers blood presssure, etc.

biographical and health data a term usually applied to information collected at the initial assessment of a patient after admission to the health care service whether in hospital or in the community. Most of the biographical data will not change but it will be helpful to nurses on succeeding shifts enabling them to individualize conversation with the person. The health data, particularly those about dependence/independence for carrying out everyday living activities, may well change during the patient's admission. All data will be useful when planning the person's discharge from the service. ⇒ boredom, prevention of.

biohazard *n* any hazard arising from inadvertent human biological processes. It includes accidental inoculation*, cadaver* bags, linen, needlestick injury and spills.

biological engineering provision of aids, electrical or electronic, to aid functioning of the body, e.g. hearing aids, pacemakers.

biology *n* the science of life, dealing with the structure, function and organization of all living things—**biological** *adj*, **biologically** *adv*.

bionursing *n* direct application of knowledge from the life sciences to the theory and practice of nursing.

biopsy *n* excision of tissue from a living body for microscopic examination to establish diagnosis.

biorhythm *n* any of the recurring cycles of physical, emotional and intellectual activity which affect people's lives—**biorhythmic** *adj*.

biosensors *npl* noninvasive instruments which measure the result of biological processes, e.g. local skin temperature and humidity; or biological response to, e.g. external pressure.

biotechnology *n* the use of biological knowledge in the scientific study of technology and vice versa—**biotechnical** *adj*, **biotechnically** *adv*.

biotin *n* a member of vitamin B complex; functions as a coenzyme. Synthesized by intestinal flora. Lack of it may cause scaly skin, fatigue and muscular pains.

bipolar *adj* having two poles.

bipolar affective disorder ⇒ depression, manic depression.

bipolar depression ⇒ depression, manic depression.

birth *n* the act of expelling the young from the mother's body; delivery; being born. *birth canal* the cavity or canal of the pelvis through which the baby passes during labour. *birth certificate* a legal document given on registration, within 42 days of a birth. *birth control* prevention or regulation of conception by any means; contraception. *birth injury* any injury occurring during parturition, e.g. fracture of a bone, subluxation of a joint, injury to peripheral nerve, intracranial haemorrhage. *birth mark* naevus*. *premature birth* one occurring after the 7th month of pregnancy, but before term.

bisexual *adj* **1** having some of the physical genital characteristics of both sexes; a hermaphrodite. When there is gonadal tissue of both sexes in the same person, that person is a true hermaphrodite. **2** describes a person who is sexually attracted to both men and women.

bistoury *n* a long narrow knife, straight or curved, used for cutting from within outwards in the opening of a hernial sac, an abscess, sinus or fistula.

Bitot's spots (*syn* xerosis conjunctivae) collections of dried epithelium, flaky masses and microorganisms at the sides of the cornea. A manifestation of vitamin A deficiency.

bivalve *adj* having two blades such as in the vaginal speculum. In orthopaedic work, the division of a plaster of Paris splint into two portions—an anterior and posterior half.

blackhead *n* ⇒ comedone.

blackwater fever a malignant form of malaria* occurring in the tropics, especially Africa. There is great destruction of red blood cells, and this causes a very dark coloured urine.

bladder *n* a membranous sac containing fluid or gas ⇒ atonic bladder, bladder retraining, neurogenic bladder, urinary bladder.

bladder retraining a nursing

intervention to prevent episodes of urinary incontinence and to reduce symptoms of frequency and urgency by gradually increasing the time interval between voiding. Time intervals may be mandatory or self scheduled. ⇒ habit retraining.

Blalock-Hanlon operation a surgical opening between the right and left atrium of the heart in patients with complete transposition.

Blalock's operation anastomosis of the pulmonary artery (distal to obstruction to the right ventricular outflow) to a branch of the aorta to increase pulmonary blood flow. Most often performed for Fallot's* tetralogy.

blanket bath an old term to denote bathing a patient in bed.

Blastomyces *n* a genus of pathogenic yeast-like organisms—**blastomycetic** *adj.*

blastomycosis *n* granulomatous condition caused by budding, yeast-like organisms called *Blastomyces dermatitidis*. May affect skin, viscera and bones—**blastomycotic** *adj.*

blastula *n* an early stage in development of the fertilized ovum when the morula* becomes cystic and infolds to become the gastrula.

bleb *n* a large blister*. ⇒ bulla, vesicle.

blennorrhagia *n* **1** a copious mucous discharge, particularly from the vagina or male urethra. **2** gonorrhoea.

blennorrhoea *n* blennorrhagia*.

blepharitis *n* inflammation of the eyelids, particularly the edges—**blepharitic** *adj.*

blepharon *n* the eyelid; palpebra—**blephara** *pl.*

blepharoplasty *n* (*syn* tarsoplasty) surgery to the eyelid.

blepharospasm *n* spasm of the muscles in the eyelid, causing rapid involuntary blinking—**blepharospastic** *adj.*

blind loop syndrome resulting from intestinal obstruction or surgical anastomosis; there is stasis in the small intestine which encourages bacterial growth thus producing diarrhoea and malabsorption.

blind spot the spot at which the optic nerve leaves the retina. It is insensitive to light.

blister *n* separation of the epidermis from the dermis by a collection of fluid, usually serum or blood.

blood *n* a complex liquid tissue, it consists of a colourless fluid, plasma, in which are suspended the red blood cells or erythrocytes, the white corpuscles (leucocytes) and the blood platelets or thrombocytes. The plasma contains a great many substances in solution, including factors which enable the blood to clot. The blood also contains nutrients, amino acids, glucose, minerals and proteins.

blood bank a special refrigerator in which blood is kept after withdrawal from donors until required for transfusion.

blood-brain barrier (BBB) the membranes between the circulating blood and the brain. Some drugs can pass from the blood through this barrier to the cerebrospinal fluid, others cannot, e.g. streptomycin.

blood casts casts of coagulated red blood corpuscles, formed in the renal tubules and found in the urine, usually indicating kidney disease.

blood clotting the process by which bleeding is arrested. Primary phase: the vessel closes itself off from circulation and a plug of tiny particles (platelets) collects to fill the gap, attracted by collagen present in the blood vessel walls. Collagen is normally separated from flowing blood by a thin layer of cells which line the vessel wall; blood only

The ABO system

Blood group	Antigen	Antibody
A	A	anti-B
B	B	anti-A
AB (universal recipient)	A & B	none
O (universal donor)	none	anti-A & anti-B

Fig. 1 Blood groupings and compatibility.

comes into contact with collagen when a break occurs in this lining and the first platelets stick to it. These two processes occur normally in haemophilia A and B. Secondary phase: involves coagulation over and through the platelet mass. Plasma coagulation factors are as follows: –

Factor No.	*Synonyms*
I	Fibrinogen
II	Prothrombin
III	Tissue thromboplastin
IV	Calcium ions
V	Proaccelerin
VII	Factor VII
VIII	Antihaemophilic factor (AHF)
IX	Christmas factor
X	Stuart factor (Power factor)
XI	Plasma thromboplastin antecedent (PTA)
XII	Hageman factor
XIII	Fibrin-stabilizing factor

Factor VIII is affected in haemophilia A; Factor IX is affected in haemophilia B (Christmas disease). In von Willebrand's disease there is a deficiency in both Factor VIII and in platelet function.

blood count calculation of the number of red or white cells per cubic millimetre of blood, using a haemocytometer or coulter counter. *differential blood count* the estimation of the relative proportions of the different white blood cells in the blood. The normal differential count is: neutrophils, 65–70%, lymphocytes, 20–25%, monocytes, 5%, eosinophils, 0–3%, basophils 0–0.5%. In childhood the proportion of lymphocytes is higher.

blood culture a venous blood sample is incubated in a suitable medium at an optimum temperature, so that any contained organisms can multiply and so be isolated and identified under the microscope. ⇒ septicaemia.

blood formation haemopoiesis*.

blood glucose profiles used to make rational adjustments to treatment of individual diabetic patients. They can show the peaks and troughs and the duration of action of a given insulin preparation, which can vary from patient to patient. Blood samples are taken on fasting, 2 h after breakfast, before lunch, 2 h after lunch, before the evening meal, at bedtime and possibly during the night. Some patients are independent for collecting these profiles and do so at home.

blood groups ABO system (see Fig. 1). There are four groups, A, B, AB and O. The cells of these groups contain the corresponding antigens, A, B, A and B, except group O cells, which contain neither antigen A nor B. For this reason group O blood can be given to any of the other groups and it is known as the 'universal donor'. In the plasma there are agglutinins* which will cause agglutination of any cell carrying the corresponding antigen, e.g. group A plasma contains anti-B agglutinins; group B plasma contains anti-A agglutinins; group O plasma contains both anti-A and anti-B agglutinins; group AB plasma contains no agglutinins. Group AB is therefore known as the 'universal recipient' and can receive A, B and O blood. Blood grouping is determined by (a) testing a suspension of red cells with anti-A and anti-B serum or (b) testing serum with known cells. Transfusion with an incompatible ABO group will cause a severe haemolytic reaction and death may occur unless the transfusion is promptly stopped. *Rhesus blood group* the red cells contain four pairs of antigens which are known by the letters Cc, Dd, Ee and Ff. The letters denote allelomorphic genes which are present in all cells except the sex cells where a chromosome can carry C or c, but not both. In this way the Rhesus genes and blood groups are derived equally from each parent. When the cells contain only the cde groups, then the blood is said to be Rhesus negative (Rh-); when the cells contain C, D or E singly or in combination with cde, then the blood is Rhesus positive (Rh+). These groups are antigenic and can, under suitable conditions, produce the corresponding antibody in the serum. These antibodies are then used to detect the presence of Rh groups in cells. Antibodies to the Rh group are produced by (a) transfusion with Rh incompatible blood (b) immunization during pregnancy by fetal cells containing the antigen entering the mother's circulation. This can cause erythroblastosis* fetalis. ⇒ Rhesus incompatibility.

blood-letting venesection*.

blood plasma ⇒ plasma.

blood pressure the pressure exerted by the blood on the blood vessel walls. Usually refers to the pressure within the arteries which may be measured in millimetres of mercury using a sphygmomanometer. The arterial blood pressure fluctuates with each heart beat, having a maximum value (the systolic pressure) which is related to the ejection of blood from the heart into the arteries and a minimum value (diastolic pressure) when the aortic and pulmonary valves are closed and the heart is relaxed. Usually values for both systolic and diastolic pressures are recorded (e.g. 120/70). ⇒ hypertension, hypotension.

blood sedimentation rate (BSR) ⇒ erythrocyte* sedimentation rate.

blood serum the fluid which exudes when blood clots; it is plasma minus the clotting agents.

blood sugar the amount of glucose in the circulating blood; varies within the normal limits. This level is controlled by various enzymes and hormones, the most important single factor being insulin*. ⇒ hyperglycaemia, hypoglycaemia.

blood transfusion ⇒ transfusion.

blood urea the amount of urea* (the end product of protein metabolism) in the blood; varies within the normal range. This is virtually unaffected by the amount of protein in the diet, when the kidneys which are the main organs of urea excretion are normal. When they are diseased the blood urea quickly rises. ⇒ uraemia.

BLS *abbr* basic* life support.

'blue baby' the appearance produced by some congenital heart defects. The appearance, by contrast, of a newborn child suffering from temporary anoxia is described as 'blue asphyxia'. ⇒ asphyxia.

blue pus bluish discharge from a wound infected with *Pseudomonas aeruginosa (pyocyanea).*

blues *n* a lay term for a low mood which lasts several days and occurs at a particular time, e.g. after discharge from hospital, postoperatively.⇒ postnatal.

bluxism *n* teeth clenching; it can cause headache from muscle fatigue.

BME *abbr* benign* myalgic encephalomyelitis.

BMI *abbr* body mass index.

BMR *abbr* basal* metabolic rate.

BM stix chemically impregnated 'stick' for estimating the capillary blood sugar by colour change.

BMT *abbr* bone marrow transplant/transplantation. ⇒ transplantation.

BNF *abbr* British National Formulary. ⇒ formulary.

body cavities central areas of the body, completely or partially protected by bone; they contain various organs; they are named cranial, thoracic, abdominal and pelvic cavity.

body defence mechanisms in a general sense the body's ability to defend itself; most commonly used in the context of immunity*. ⇒ antitoxin, fight or flight mechanism, mental defence mechanisms, immunoglobulins, lymphocyte, lysozyme.

body image the image in an individual's mind of his own body. Distortions of this occur in anorexia* nervosa. ⇒ disfigurement, mutilation.

body language nonverbal symbols that express a person's current physical and mental state. They include body movements, postures, gestures, facial expressions, spatial positions, clothes and other bodily adornments. *body language problems* apart from the individuality involved in expression of personality, problems can arise when a person consistently conveys the wrong message, e.g. a dour look may mask a pleasant personality in familiar circumstances. However, a person may temporarily or permanently lack control of some muscles used in body language, for instance after Bell's palsy*, cerebrovascular* accident, paraplegia*, and tetraplegia*. Communication has to be achieved in the context of the person's deprivation.

body lice ⇒ Pediculus.

body mass index (BMI) a measure achieved using the formula weight/height^2.

body temperature the balance between heat production and heat loss in the human body, maintained around 37°C throughout the 24 h. Metabolism, voluntary and involuntary muscular activities produce most of the heat, and heat is lost by conduction, convection, and evaporation of sweat from the skin; a small amount is lost at defaecation, urination and expiration. *core body temperature* that which registers in the central tissues of the body, e.g. it can be measured in the sublingual* sockets and the anal* canal. *shell body temperature* that which registers outwith the trunk, e.g. in the dried axilla or groin.

Boeck's disease a form of sarcoidosis*.

Bohn's nodules tiny white nodules on the palate of the newly born.

boil *n* (*syn* furuncle) an acute inflammatory condition, surrounding a hair follicle; caused by *Staphylococcus aureus.* Usually attended by suppuration; it has one opening for drainage in contrast to a carbuncle*.

bolus *n* **1** a soft, pulpy mass of masticated food. **2** a large dose of a drug given at the beginning of a treatment programme to raise the concentration in the blood rapidly to a therapeutic level.

bonding *n* the emotional tie one person forms with another, making an enduring and special emotional relationship. There is a fundamental biological need for this to occur between an infant and its parents. When newborn babies have to be nursed in an intensive care unit, special arrangements have to be made to encourage a relationship to form between the parents and their new baby by encouraging contact and touch despite possible physical barriers.

bone *n* connective tissue in which salts, such as calcium carbonate and calcium phosphate, are deposited to make it hard and dense. The separate bones make up the skeleton*.

bone graft the transplantation of a piece of bone from one part of the body to another, or from one person to another. Used to repair bone defects or to supply osteogenic tissue.

bone marrow the substance contained within bone cavities. At birth the cavities are filled with blood-forming *red marrow* but in later life, deposition of fat in the long bones converts the red into *yellow bone marrow. bone marrow puncture* an investigatory procedure whereby a sample of marrow is obtained by aspiration after piercing the sternum or iliac crest. *bone marrow transplant* ⇒ transplantation.

Bonnevie-Ullrich syndrome ⇒ Noonan syndrome.

borborygmi *n* rumbling noises caused by the movement of gas in the intestines.

Bordetella *n* a genus of Brucellaceae bacteria. *B. pertussis* causes whooping cough.

boredom, prevention of this element of nursing is considered essential in children's nursing but it is also necessary for adults. Information written at the patient's initial assessment about their occupation and hobbies, where they live, etc., helps nurses to achieve patient-focused conversation with the objective of helping patients to prevent boredom. ⇒ institutionalization.

boric acid *n* a mild antiseptic.

Bornholm disease (*syn* epidemic myalgia) a viral disease due to B group of coxsackie viruses named after the Danish island where it was described by Sylvest in 1934. 2–14 days' incubation. Symptoms include sudden onset of severe pain in lower chest or abdominal or lumbar muscles. Breathing may be difficult, because of the pain, and fever is common. May last up to one week. There is no specific treatment.

botulism *n* an intoxication with the preformed exotoxin of *Clostridium botulinum*. Vomiting, constipation, ocular and pharyngeal paralysis and sometimes aphonia manifest within 24–72 h of eating food contaminated with the spores, which require anaerobic conditions to produce the toxin. Hence the danger of home-tinned vegetables and meat.

bougie *n* a cylindrical instrument made of gum elastic, metal or other material. Used in varying sizes for dilating strictures, e.g. oesophageal or urethral.

bovine *adj* pertaining to the cow or ox. *bovine tuberculosis* ⇒ tuberculosis. *bovine spongiform encephalopathy (BSE)* infective, fatal neurological disease affecting cattle. There may be a link between BSE and Creutzfeldt-Jakob* disease in humans.

bowel *n* the large intestine. ⇒ intestine. *bowel movement* a lay term for the act of defaecation*. ⇒ faeces.

bowleg *n* varum genu*.

Bq *abbr* ⇒ becquerel.

brachial *adj* pertaining to the arm. Applied to vessels in this region and a nerve plexus at the root of the neck.

brachium *n* the arm (especially from shoulder to elbow), or any arm-like appendage—**brachia** *pl*, **brachial** *adj*.

brachytherapy *n* radiotherapy delivered from a small radioactive source which is implanted in or adjacent to the tumour. The technique is used to treat cancers of the cervix, tongue, anus, lung and oesophagus.

Bradford frame a stretcher type of bed used for: (a) immobilizing spine (b) resting trunk and back muscles (c) preventing deformity. It is a tubular steel frame fitted with two canvas slings allowing 100–150 mm gap to facilitate the use of a bedpan.

bradycardia *n* slow rate of heart contraction, resulting in a slow pulse rate. In febrile states, for each degree rise in body temperature the expected increase in pulse rate is ten beats per minute. When the latter does not occur, the term 'relative bradycardia' is used.

brain *n* the encephalon; the largest part of the central nervous system: it is contained in the cranial cavity and is surrounded by three membranes called meninges. The fluid inside the brain contained in the ventricles, and outside in the subarachnoid space, acts as a shock absorber to the delicate nerve tissue. *brain death* irreversible damage to the cerebrum, cerebellum and brain stem requiring artificial life support mechanisms if life is to be maintained. Brain death is confirmed when there is no evidence of cerebral or brain stem activity, according to strict criteria. Distinguishable from irreversible coma, when the brain stem and cerebellum remain functional so vital functions continue and patients can be kept alive by maintaining feeding and fluids. ⇒ death.

bran *n* the husk of grain. The coarse outer part of cereals, especially wheat, high in dietary* fibre and the vitamin* B complex.

branchial *adj* pertaining to the fissures or clefts which occur on each side of the neck of the human embryo and which are involved in the development of the nose, ears and mouth. *branchial cyst* a cyst* in the neck arising from abnormal development of the branchial* clefts.

Braun's frame a metal frame, bandaged for use, and equally useful for drying a lower leg plaster and for applying skeletal traction (Steinmann's* pin or Kirschner* wire inserted through the calcaneus) to a fractured tibia, after reduction.

break-bone fever ⇒ dengue.

breast *n* **1** the anterior upper part of the thorax. **2** the mammary gland. *breast bone* the sternum. *breast cancer* cancer* of the breast. One in 12 women is at risk of developing it, and it is responsible for one in five deaths from malignant disease in women.⇒ lumpectomy, mastectomy. *breast awareness* where a woman regularly examines her breasts, visually and manually, for signs of change. *breast feeding* breast milk, providing the mother is taking an adequate diet, provides nutrition in the form in which it is best suited to the baby. The required intimate skin and body contact helps to establish bonding*. *breast prosthesis* an artificial breast usually worn inside a brassière on the side from which the breast has been removed. *breast pump* a glass or plastic cup which encircles the tissue around the nipple; it is attached to a rubber or plastic bulb from which air is evacuated to provide suction which withdraws milk from the breast. *breast reconstruction* can be performed after mastectomy when the outer skin and nipple is preserved and a silicone implant put in place of the breast tissue. *breast reduction* an operation to reduce the tissue in painfully heavy or pendulous breasts. *breast shell* a device which can be used to protect the nipple of a lactating woman. For breast feeding the nipple protrudes through the centre of the shell.

breast, self-examination of a method of preventive screening*. A woman's familiarity with her breasts, gained from regular examination 7–10 days after the first day of the menstrual cycle, enables her to detect small abnormalities. A chart showing the method is available in most health centres. ⇒ breast cancer.

breath-H_2 (hydrogen) test for disaccharide intolerance. An indirect method for detecting lactase deficiency.

breech *n* the buttocks. ⇒ buttock.

breech presentation refers to the position of a baby in the uterus such that the buttocks would be born first: the normal position is head first.

bregma *n* the anterior fontanelle. ⇒ fontanelle.

Bright's disease inflammation of the kidneys. ⇒ nephritis.

Broadbent's sign visible retraction of the left side and back, in the region of the 11th and 12th ribs, synchronous with each heart beat and due to adhesions between the pericardium and diaphragm. ⇒ pericarditis.

broad ligaments lateral ligaments; double fold of parietal peritoneum which hangs over the uterus and outstretched uterine tubes, forming a lateral partition across the pelvic cavity.

broad thumb syndrome Rubenstein-Taybi* syndrome.

Broca's area often described as the motor centre for speech; situated at the third convolution in the precentral gyrus, in the left hemisphere of the cerebrum. Injury to this area can result in expressive aphasia*.

Brodie's abscess chronic abscess* in bone.

bromidrosis *n* a profuse, fetid perspiration, especially associated with the feet—**bromidrotic** *adj.*

bromism *n* chronic poisoning due to continued or excessive use of bromides (a sedative).

bromosulphthalein test used to assess liver function; 5 mg per kg of body weight of the blue dye are injected intravenously. If more than 5% of the dye is circulating in the blood 45 min after injection there is impaired hepatic function.

bronchi *npl* the two tubes into which the trachea* divides at its lower end—**bronchus** *sing,* **bronchial** *adj.*

bronchial asthma reversible airflow obstruction precipitated by intake of allergens or drugs, infection, vigorous exercise, temperature/weather changes or emotional stress. There is often a family history of asthma* and/or other allergic conditions.

bronchial carcinoma cancer* occurring in one or other bronchus; statistics support a strong link with smoking. In their role as health teachers, nurses are encouraged to be nonsmokers and to encourage patients to stop smoking. ⇒ oat cell carcinoma.

bronchial tubes *npl* subdivisions of the bronchi* after they enter the lungs.

bronchiectasis *n* dilatation of the bronchial tubes which, when localized, is usually the result of pneumonia or lobar collapse in childhood, but when more generalized is due to some inherent disorder of the bronchial mucous membrane as in cystic fibrosis. Associated with profuse, fetid, purulent expectoration. Characterized by recurrent respiratory infections and digital clubbing. May lead eventually to respiratory failure—**bronchiectatic** *adj.*

bronchiole *n* one of the minute subdivisions of the bronchi* which terminate in the alveoli or air sacs of the lungs—**bronchiolar** *adj.*

bronchiolitis *n* inflammation of the bronchioles*, caused in most cases by respiratory syncytial virus and most common in children in the 1st year of life, peaking in winter months. The younger the child, the more likely the symptoms are to be severe, often requiring hospitalization—**bronchiolitic** *adj.*

bronchitis *n* inflammation of the bronchi. *acute bronchitis* as an isolated incident is usually a primary viral infection as a complication of the common cold, influenza, whooping cough, measles or rubella. Secondary infection occurs with bacteria, commonly *Haemophilus influenzae* or *Streptococcus pneumoniae.* In *chronic bronchitis* the bronchial mucous glands are hypertrophied due to irritating cigarette smoke or atmospheric pollutants and the patient's only complaint is of cough productive of mucoid sputum most days for 3 consecutive months in 2 consecutive years—**bronchitic** *adj.*

bronchoconstrictor *n* any agent which constricts the bronchi.

bronchodilator *n* any agent which dilates the bronchi.

bronchogenic *adj* arising from one of the bronchi.

bronchography *n* radiological demonstration of the bronchial tree after introduction of a small amount of a liquid contrast medium—**bronchographic** *adj,* **bronchograph** *n,* **bronchographically** *adv.*

bronchomycosis *n* general term used to cover a variety of fungal infections of the bronchi and lungs, e.g. pulmonary candidiasis*, aspergillosis*—**bronchomycotic** *adj.*

bronchopleural fistula pathological communication between the pleural cavity and one of the bronchi.

bronchopneumonia *n* a term used to describe a form of pneumonia in which areas of consolidation are distributed widely around bronchi and not in a lobar pattern—**bronchopneumonic** *adj.*

bronchopulmonary *adj* pertaining to the bronchi and the lungs—**bronchopulmonic** *adj.*

bronchorrhoea *n* an excessive discharge of mucus from the bronchial mucous membrane—**bronchorrhoeal** *adj.*

bronchoscope *n* an endoscope* used for examining and taking biopsies from the interior of the bronchi. Also used for removal of inhaled foreign bodies. Traditional, surgical bronchoscopes are rigid tubes, are more widely available. Modern bronchoscopes are flexible fibreoptic instruments—**bronchoscopic** *adj,* **bronchoscopically** *adv.*

bronchospasm *n* sudden constriction of the bronchial tubes due to contraction of involuntary plain muscle in their walls—**bronchospastic** *adj.*

bronchostenosis *n* narrowing of one of the bronchi—**bronchostenotic** *adj.*

bronchotracheal *adj* pertaining to the bronchi and trachea.

bronchus ⇒ bronchi.

brought in dead (BID) describes a corpse when death has occurred prior to arrival at the hospital.

brow *n* the forehead; the region above the supraorbital ridge.

brown fat present in infant tissue. Contains enzymes which in the presence of oxygen rapidly produce energy and heat–a form of nonshivering thermogenesis. ⇒ fat.

Brucella *n* a genus of bacteria causing brucellosis* (undulant fever in man; contagious abortion in cattle). *Brucella abortus* is the bovine strain. *Brucella melitensis* the goat strain, both transmissible to man via infected milk.

brucellosis *n* (*syn* melitensis) an infective reticulosis. A generalized infection in man resulting from one of the species of *Brucella*. Transmitted to man from farm animals through contaminated milk or contact with the carcass of an infected animal. There are recurrent attacks of fever and mental depression. Other symptoms include headache, aches and pains, and anaemia. The condition may last for months. The condition is also called 'Malta fever', 'abortus fever', 'Mediterranean fever' and 'undulant fever'.

Brudzinski's sign immediate flexion of knees and hips on raising head from pillow. Seen in meningitis.

bruise *n* (*syn* contusion) a discolouration of the skin due to an extravasation of blood into the underlying tissues; there is no abrasion of the skin. ⇒ ecchymosis.

bruit *n* ⇒ murmur.

bruxism *n* abnormal grinding of teeth, often producing excessive wear or attrition.

Bryant's 'gallows' traction skin traction* is applied to the lower limbs, the legs are then suspended vertically (from an overhead beam), so that the buttocks are lifted just clear of the bed. Used for fractures of the femur in children up to 4 years.

BSE *abbr* bovine* spongiform encephalopathy.

bubo *n* enlargement of lymphatic glands, especially in the groin. A feature of soft sore (chancroid), lymphogranuloma inguinale and plague–**bubonic** *adj*.

buccal *adj* pertaining to the cheek or mouth (buccal cavity).

Buerger's disease (*syn* thromboangiitis obliterans) a chronic obliterative vascular disease of peripheral vessels which results in intermittent claudication*. In an investigation, the incidence of HLA-A9 and HLA-B5 was significantly greater in those with Buerger's disease than in the controls. *Buerger's exercises* were designed to treat this condition. The legs are placed alternately in elevation and dependence to assist perfusion of the extremities with blood.

buffer *n* **1** generally, a mixture of substances in solution with the ability to bind both hydrogen and hydroxyl ions and the property of resistance to pH change when acids or alkalis are added. **2** anything used to reduce shock or jarring due to contact.

bulbar *adj* pertaining to the medulla* oblongata. *bulbar palsy or paralysis* paralysis* which involves the labioglossopharyngeal (lips, tongue and pharynx) region and results from degeneration of the motor nuclei in the medulla oblongata. The patient is deprived of the safety reflexes and is in danger of choking and aspiration pneumonia. Associated with feeding difficulties in profoundly handicapped children.

bulbourethral *adj* applied to two racemose* glands which open into the bulb of the male urethra. Their secretion is part of seminal fluid.

bulimia nervosa *n* (*syn* binge-purge syndrome) an eating disorder involving repeated episodes of uncontrolled consumption of large quantities of food in a short time with self-induced vomiting thereafter. Many anorexics have a history of such episodes.

bulla *n* a large watery blister. In dermatology, bulla formation is characteristic of the pemphigus group of dermatoses, but occurs sometimes in other diseases of the skin, e.g. in impetigo, in dermatitis herpetiformis, etc.—**bullae** *pl,* **bullate, bullous** *adj.*

bundle of His mass of neuromuscular fibres across the atrioventricular septum of the heart. Branches into right and left segments into each ventricle, terminating in Purkinje's* fibres. Conducts the impulse of contraction from the atrioventricular node*.

bunion *n* (*syn* hallux valgus) a deformity on the head of the metatarsal bone at its junction with the great toe. Friction and pressure of shoes at this point cause a bursa to develop. The prominent bone, with its bursa, is known as a bunion.

buphthalmos *n* (oxeye) congenital glaucoma.

Burkitt's lymphoma a malignant lymphoma, principally affecting the jaw in children. Most common in areas of Africa and New Guinea where malaria is endemic. In western countries other sites can be affected.

burn *n* a lesion of the tissues due to chemicals, dry heat, electricity, flame, friction or radiation; classified as partial or full thickness according to the depth of skin destroyed: the latter requiring skin grafts. The prevention of shock, infection and malnutrition are important aspects of treatment.

burnout *n* term used to describe the process of physical and emotional exhaustion which it is thought can result from job-related stress factors. Spouse burnout can occur and support should be offered to all family carers.

burr *n* an attachment for a surgical drill which is used for cutting into tooth or bone.

bursa *n* a fibrous sac lined with synovial membrane and containing a small quantity of synovial fluid. Bursae are found be-tween (a) tendon and bone (b) skin and bone (c) muscle and muscle. Their function is to facilitate movement without friction between these surfaces—**bursae** *pl.*

bursitis *n* inflammation of a bursa. *olecranon bursitis* inflammation of the bursa over the point of the elbow. *prepatellar bursitis* (*syn* housemaid's knee) a fluid-filled swelling of the bursa in front of the kneecap (patella). It is frequently associated with excessive kneeling. A blow can result in bleeding into the bursa and there can be infection with pyogenic pathogens.

buttock *n* one of the two projections posterior to the hip joints. Formed mainly of the gluteal* muscles.

butyrophenones *npl* antipsychotic drugs used mainly in schizophrenia*.

byssinosis *n* a form of pneumoconiosis* caused by inhalation of cotton or linen dust.

C

cachexia *n* a term denoting a state of constitutional disorder, malnutrition and general ill-health. The chief signs of this condition are bodily emaciation, sallow unhealthy skin and heavy lustreless eyes—**cachectic** *adj.*

cadaver *n* a dead body. If the dead person had an infectious disease including hepatitis B, AIDS and HIV-antibody positive, the body is put in a cadaver bag bearing a biohazard* label.

cadmium *n* a metallic element present in zinc ores and used in several industries. Inhalation of fumes over time can cause serious lung damage. Food can be contaminated, e.g. by contact with cadmium-containing industrial waste.

caecostomy *n* a surgically established fistula between the caecum* and anterior abdominal wall, usually to achieve drainage and/or decompression of the caecum. It is usually created by inserting a wide-bore tube into the caecum at operation.

caecum *n* the blind, pouch-like commencement of the colon* in the right iliac fossa. To it is attached the vermiform appendix; it is separated from the ileum by the ileocaecal valve—**caecal** *adj.*

caesarean section delivery of the fetus through an adominal incision. It is said to be named after Caesar, who is supposed to have been born in this way. A low, horizontal 'lower segment caesarian section' is preferable to the 'classical' which involves a vertical incision in the body of the uterus.

caesium 137 (^{137}Cs) a radioactive substance which, when sealed in a container, can be used for beam therapy instead of cobalt; when sealed in needles or tubes it can be used for local application instead of radium.

caffeine *n* the central nervous system stimulant which is present in tea and coffee. It has been given as a diuretic, but its main use is in analgesic preparations.

caisson disease (*syn* the bends, decompression sickness) results from sudden reduction in atmospheric pressure, as experienced by divers on return to surface, airmen ascending to great heights. Caused by bubbles of nitrogen which are released from solution in the blood; symptoms vary according to the site of these. The condition is largely preventable by proper and gradual decompression technique.

calamine *n* zinc carbonate tinted pink with ferric oxide. Widely employed in lotions and creams for its mild astringent action on the skin. *calamine lotion* calamine dissolved in a weak solution of carbolic acid (phenol) for its anaesthetic effect in relieving itch.

calcareous *adj* pertaining to or containing lime or calcium; of a chalky nature.

calcification *n* the hardening of an organic substance by a deposit of calcium salts within it.

May be normal, as in bone, or pathological, as in arteries.

calcitonin *n* (*syn* thyrocalcitonin) hormone produced in the thyroid parafollicular or 'C' cells. It may play a role in regulating the blood calcium level. In therapeutic doses it lowers serum calcium and inhibits resorption of bone. It may be of benefit in Paget's* disease.

calcium a metallic element. An important constituent of the bones, teeth and blood and an essential dietary element. *calcium carbonate* a salt of calcium used in many antacid preparations. *calcium gluconate* a salt of calcium used to treat calcium deficiencies and disorders such as rickets.

calcium oxalate a salt which, if it occurs in high concentrations in the urine, may lead to the formation of urinary calculi.

calculus *n* abnormal deposits composed chiefly of mineral substances and formed in the passages which transmit secretions, or in the cavities which act as reservoirs for them. *dental calculus* mineralized dental plaque deposited on the tooth surface—**calculi** *pl,* **calculous** *adj.*

Caldwell-Luc operation (*syn* radical antrostomy*) an opening is made above the upper canine tooth into the anterior wall of the maxillary antrum for dependent drainage.

caliper *n* **1** a two-pronged instrument for measuring the diameter of a round body. **2** a two-pronged instrument with sharp points which are inserted into the lower end of a fractured long bone. A weight is attached to the other end of the caliper, which maintains a steady pull on the distal end of the bone. **3** *Thomas' walking caliper* is similar to the Thomas'* splint, but the W-shaped junction at the lower end is replaced by two small iron rods which slot into holes made in the heel of the boot. The ring should fit the groin perfectly, and all weight is then borne by the ischial tuberosity.

callosity *n* (*syn* keratoma) a local hardening of the skin caused by pressure or friction. The epidermis becomes hypertrophied. Most commonly seen on the feet and palms of the hands.

callus *n* **1** a callosity, hardened thickened skin on the bottom of the foot. **2** the partly calcified tissue which forms about the ends of a broken bone and ultimately accomplishes repair of the fracture—**callous** *adj.*

calor *n* heat; one of the four classic local signs of inflammation; the others are dolor*, rubor*, tumor*.

caloric test irrigation of the external ear canal with warm and/or cold fluid to assess vestibular function.

calorie *n* a unit of heat. In practice the calorie is too small a unit to be useful and the kilocalorie is the preferred unit in studies in metabolism. A kilocalorie (kcal) is the amount of heat required to raise the temperature of 1 kg of water by 1°C. In science generally, the calorie has been replaced by the joule as a unit of energy, work and heat; a joule is approximately ¼ calorie. ⇒ kilojoule.

calorific *adj* describes any phenomena which pertain to the production of heat.

camphor *n* carminative and expectorant internally, and used as a camphorated tincture of opium in cough mixtures. Applied externally in the form of camphorated oil as an analgesic and as a rubefacient—**camphorated** *adj.*

Campylobacter *n* a Gram-negative motile bacterium that may be curved rods or spiral-shaped.

It causes an acute diarrhoeal illness lasting several days. Associated with raw meat and poultry, raw milk and infected pets who excrete the bacteria in faeces, thereby contaminating their hair.

canaliculus *n* a minute capillary passage. Any small canal, such as the passage leading from the edge of the eyelid to the lacrimal sac or one of the numerous small canals leading from the Haversian canals and terminating in the lacunae of bone—**canaliculi** *pl*, **canaliculization** *n*.

cancellous *n* resembling latticework; light and spongy; like a honeycomb.

cancer *n* a general term which covers any malignant growth in any part of the body. The growth is purposeless, parasitic, and flourishes at the expense of the human host. Characteristics are the tendency to cause local destruction, to invade adjacent tissues and to spread by metastasis. Cancer develops from the loss of normal cellular regulation. Frequently recurs after removal. Carcinoma refers to malignant tumours of epithelial tissue, sarcoma to malignant tumours of connective tissue—**cancerous** *adj*.

cancerocidal *n* lethal to cancer.

cancerophobia *n* obsessive fear of cancer—**cancerophobic** *adj*.

Cancer Relief Macmillan Fund founded in 1911 by Douglas Macmillan to provide care and support for cancer patients, Macmillan* nurses work in hospices*, hospitals and patients' homes. Grants are given by the Fund to finance nurses, doctors, social workers, etc.; to train nurses and doctors in the skills of cancer and palliative care and to provide financial help to patients and their families. The Fund also provides capital for the development of hospices, day care and information centres, and funds educational projects.

cancrum oris *n* gangrenous stomatitis of cheek as a result of dental sepsis. Often called 'noma'. Commoner in children from developing countries and mostly associated with malnourishment.

Candida *n* (*syn* Monilia) a genus of dimorphic fungi. Yeast-like cells which form some filaments. They are widespread in nature. *Candida (Monilia) albicans* is a commensal of the gastrointestinal tract of man. It causes infections such as thrush, vulvovaginitis, balanoprosthitis and systemic disease in some physiological and pathological states. Disease can result from disturbed flora due to use of wide-spectrum antibiotics, steroids, immunosuppressive and/or cytotoxic drugs. Infection can also occur during pregnancy or secondary to debilitating general disease such as diabetes mellitus or Cushing's syndrome. Oral infection can be due to poor oral hygiene, including carious teeth and ill-fitting dentures.

candidiasis *n* (*syn* candidosis, moniliasis, thrush) disease caused by infection with a species of *Candida*.

canicola fever leptospirosis*.

canine *adj* of or resembling a dog. *canine teeth* four in all, two in each jaw, situated between the incisors and the premolars. Those in the upper jaw are popularly known as the 'eye teeth'.

cannabis indica (*syn* marihuana, pot, hashish) Indian hemp, a narcotic drug once used as a cerebral sedative in nervous disorders. Possession and use of cannabis is illegal in many countries. ⇒ soft drugs.

cannula *n* a hollow tube for the introduction or withdrawal of fluid from the body. In some types, e.g. intravenous, the lumen is fitted with a sharp-pointed trocar to facilitate insertion which is withdrawn when the cannula is in situ—**cannulae** *pl.*

cannulation *n* insertion of a cannula*.

canthus *n* the angle formed by the junction of the eyelids. The inner one is known as the *nasal canthus* and the outer as the *temporal canthus*—**canthi** *pl,* **canthal** *adj.*

CAPD *abbr* continuous* ambulatory peritoneal dialysis.

CAPE *abbr* Clifton* Assessment Procedures for the Elderly.

capeline bandage (divergent spica) a bandage applied in a circular fashion to the head or an amputated limb.

capillary *n* (literally, hair-like) any tiny thin-walled vessel forming part of a network which facilitates rapid exchange of substances between the contained fluid and the surrounding tissues. *bile capillary* begins in a space in the liver and joins others, eventually forming a bile duct. *blood capillary* unites an arteriole and a venule. *capillary fragility* an expression of the ease with which blood capillaries may rupture. *lymph capillary* begins in the tissue spaces throughout the body and joins others, eventually forming a lymphatic vessel.

capping *n* a process by which cell surface molecules are caused to aggregate (usually using antibody) on the cell membrane.

capsule *n* **1** the outer membranous covering of certain organs, such as the kidney, liver, spleen and adrenals. *joint capsule* the fibrous tissue, including the synovial membrane, surrounding a freely moveable joint. **2** a gelatinous or rice paper container enclosing noxious drugs for swallowing. **3** the slimy substance forming a protective envelope around certain bacteria—**capsular** *adj.*

capsulectomy *n* the surgical excision of a capsule. Refers to a joint or lens; less often to the kidney.

capsulitis *n* inflammation of a capsule. Sometimes used as a synonym for frozen* shoulder.

capsulotomy *n* incision of a capsule, usually referring to that surrounding the crystalline lens of the eye.

captopril *n* a drug which inhibits angiotensin-converting enzyme (ACE), thus preventing the formation of active angiotensin II. ⇒ angiotensin.

caput succedaneum an oedematous swelling of the baby's soft scalp tissue which is apparent at or shortly after birth. The swelling is diffuse, not delineated by scalp suture lines and usually disappears rapidly.

carbaminohaemoglobin *n* a compound formed between carbon dioxide and haemoglobin. Part of the carbon dioxide in the blood is carried in this form.

carbaryl *n* pesticide used for the treatment of head lice. Its availability in over-the-counter* preparations has been restricted because of a possible link with cancer.

carbohydrate *n* an organic compound containing carbon, hydrogen and oxygen. Formed in nature by photosynthesis in plants, they include starches, sugars and cellulose, and are classified in three groups: monosaccharides, disaccharides and polysaccharides. Carbohydrates are the principal energy source in humans. ⇒ kilojoule.

carboluria *n* green or dark-coloured urine due to excretion of carbolic acid, as occurs in carbolic acid poisoning—**carboluric** *adj.*

carbon *n* a nonmetallic tetrad element occurring in all living matter. *carbon dioxide* a gas; a waste product of many forms of combustion and metabolism, excreted via the lungs. Accumulates in respiratory insufficiency or respiratory failure and carbon dioxide tension in arterial blood (P_2CO_2) increases above the reference range of 36–44 mmHg (*c*5.0 kPa). *carbon monoxide* a poisonous gas which forms a stable compound with haemoglobin, thus blocking its normal reversible oxygen-carrying function and causing signs and symptoms of hypoxia to ensue. *carbon tetrachloride* colourless volatile liquid with an odour similar to chloroform.

carbonic anhydrase a zinc-containing enzyme which facilitates the transfer of carbon dioxide from tissues to blood and to alveolar air by catalysing the decomposition of carbonic acid into carbon dioxide and water.

carboxyhaemoglobin *n* a compound formed by the union of carbon monoxide and haemoglobin; the haemoglobin has a high affinity for CO_2 and is reluctant to give it up; hence, the haemoglobin becomes unavailable to carry oxygen.

carboxyhaemoglobinaemia *n* carboxyhaemoglobin* in the blood—**carboxyhaemoglobinaemic** *adj.*

carboxyhaemoglobinuria *n* carboxyhaemoglobin* in the urine—**carboxyhaemoglobinuric** *adj.*

carbuncle *n* an acute inflammation (usually caused by *Staphylococcus*) involving several hair follicles and surrounding subcutaneous tissue, forming an extensive slough with several discharging sinuses.

carcinogen *n* any cancer-producing substance or agent—**carcinogenic** *adj,* **carcinogenicity** *n.*

carcinogenesis *n* the production of cancer—**carcinogenetic** *adj.*

carcinoid syndrome the name given to a histologically malignant but clinically mostly benign tumour of the appendix or ileum that may secrete serotonin*, which stimulates smooth muscle causing diarrhoea, asthmatic spasm, flushing and other miserable symptoms. Methysergide may give prompt relief of the diarrhoea.

carcinoma *n* a cancerous growth of epithelial tissue (e.g. mucous membrane). *basal cell carcinoma* a localized, slow-growing tumour, usually occurring on the face. ⇒ rodent ulcer. *carcinoma-in-situ* a very early cancer that is asymptomatic and that has not invaded the basement membrane. Well described in uterus and prostate. Previously called preinvasive carcinoma. *squamous carcinoma* a malignant tumour arising from squamous* epithelium—**carcinomata** *pl,* **carcinomatous** *adj.*

carcinomatosis *n* a condition in which cancer is widespread throughout the body.

cardia *n* opening in the upper part of the stomach, adjacent to the oesophageal sphincter. *cardiac* pertaining to the cardia. *cardiac achalasia* food fails to pass normally into the stomach, though there is no obvious obstruction. The oesophagus does not demonstrate normal waves of contraction after swallowing: this prevents the normal relaxation of the cardiac sphincter. Associated with loss of ganglion cells within muscle layers of at least some areas of the affected oesophagus.

cardiac/cardio- *adj* pertaining to the heart. *cardiac arrest* complete cessation of the heart's activity. Failure of the heart action to maintain an adequate cerebral circulation in the absence of a causative and irreversible disease. The clinical picture of cessation of circulation in a patient who was not expected to die at the time. This naturally rules out the seriously ill patient who is dying slowly with an incurable disease. *cardiac asthma* nocturnal paroxysmal dyspnoea precipitated by pulmonary congestion resulting from left-sided heart failure. ⇒ asthma. *cardiac bed* one which can be manipulated so that the patient is supported in a sitting position. *cardiac bypass operation* the channelling of blood through an extracorporeal pump and oxygenator, to allow the surgeon to operate on the heart. *cardiac catheterization* ⇒ catheterization. *cardiac cycle* the series of movements through which the heart passes in performing one heart beat which corresponds to one pulse beat and takes about one second ⇒ diastole, systole. *cardiac oedema* gravitational oedema. Such patients excrete excessive aldosterone which increases excretion of potassium and conserves sodium and chloride. Antialdosterone drugs are useful, e.g. spironolactone, triamterene. Both act as diuretics. ⇒ oedema. *cardiac pacemaker* an electrical apparatus for maintaining myocardial contraction by stimulating the heart muscle. A pacemaker may be permanent, emitting the stimulus at a constant and fixed rate, or it may fire only on demand when the heart does not contract spontaneously at a minimum rate. *cardiac sphincter* the muscle dividing the oesophagus and the stomach. *cardiac tamponade* compression of heart. Can occur in surgery and penetrating wounds or rupture of the heart from haemopericardium.

cardialgia *n* literally, pain in the heart or cardia. Often used to mean heartburn (pyrosis*).

cardiogenic *adj* of cardiac origin, such as the shock in coronary thrombosis.

cardiograph *n* an instrument for recording graphically the force and form of the heart beat—**cardiographic** *adj*, **cardiographically** *adv*.

cardiologist *n* a person who specializes in diagnosing and treating diseases of the heart.

cardiology *n* study of the structure, function and diseases of the heart.

cardiomegaly *n* enlargement of the heart.

cardiomyopathy *n* an acute, subacute, or chronic disorder of heart muscle, of unknown aetiology or association, often with associated endocardial or sometimes with pericardial involvement (WHO definition)—**cardiomyopathic** *adj*.

cardiophone *n* a microphone strapped to patient which allows audible and visual signal of heart sounds. By channelling pulse through an electrocardiograph, a graphic record can be made. Can be used for the fetus.

cardioplegia *n* the induction of electromechanical cardiac arrest. *cold cardioplegia* cardioplegia combined with hypothermia to reduce the oxygen consumption of the myocardium during open heart surgery.

cardiopulmonary *adj* pertaining to the heart and lungs (see Fig. 2). *cardiopulmonary bypass* used in open heart surgery. The heart and lungs are excluded from the circulation and replaced by a pump oxygenator—**cardiopulmonic** *adj*.

cardiopulmonary resuscitation (CPR) means of artificially maintaining respiration and circulation after a cardiac arrest. It involves maintenance of a clear airway, ventilation of the person's lungs using mouth-mouth, mouth-nose, or oxygen with a bag and face mask, and

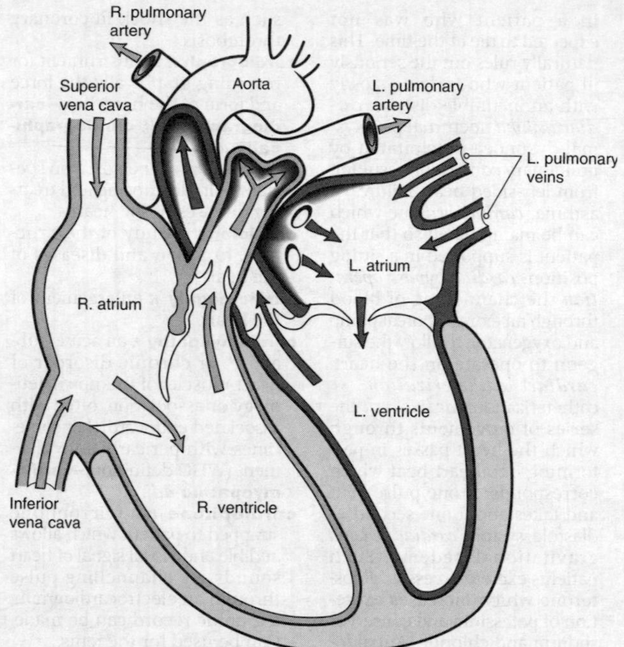

■ **Fig. 2** Cardiopulmonary circulation. The right side of the heart receives deoxygenated blood from the body via the inferior and superior venae cavae. This is pumped into the pulmonary artery and carried to the lungs. It returns as oxygenated blood into the left side of the heart via the pulmonary veins and is pumped into the body via the aorta.

maintenance of circulation by external chest compressions.

cardiorator *n* apparatus for visual recording of the heart beat.

cardiorenal *adj* pertaining to the heart and kidney.

cardiorespiratory *adj* pertaining to the heart and the respiratory system.

cardiorraphy *n* stitching of the heart wall: usually reserved for traumatic surgery.

cardioscope *n* an instrument fitted with a lens and illumination, for examining the inside of the heart—**cardioscopic** *adj,* **cardioscopically** *adv.*

cardiothoracic *adj* pertaining to the heart and thoracic cavity. A specialized branch of surgery.

cardiotocograph (CTG) *n* the instrument used in cardiotocography*.

cardiotocography *n* a procedure whereby the fetal heart rate is measured either by an external microphone or by the application of an electrode to the fetal scalp, recording the fetal ECG and from it the fetal heart rate. Using either an internal catheter which is passed into the amniotic cavity, or an external transducer placed on the mother's abdomen, the maternal contractions can also be measured. Both measurements are fed through a monitor in such a way that extraneous sounds are excluded and both measurements are recorded on heat-sensitive paper.

cardiotomy syndrome pyrexia, pericarditis and pleural effusion following heart surgery. It may develop weeks or months after the operation and is thought to be an autoimmune reaction.

cardiotoxic *adj* describes any agent which has an injurious effect on the heart.

cardiovascular *adj* pertaining to the heart and blood vessels.

cardioversion *n* use of electrical countershock for restoring the heart rhythm to normal.

carditis *n* inflammation of the heart. A word seldom used without the appropriate prefix, e.g. endo-, myo-, pan-, peri-.

care *n* is not the prerogative of nursing but it is one of its components; most commonly used to imply its psychological and social (psychosocial) dimensions. Each nurse/patient interaction* and nursing activity which involves touching the patient has a psychosocial aspect which can be perceived by the patient as negative, neutral or positive.

care plan the document on which nursing information is recorded. In some instances, it is used as a collective term which includes information from the initial patient assessment, statement of patient's actual and potential problems with everyday living activities which are amenable to nursing intervention; statement of the goals related to the problems to be achieved by the patient; and the plan of nursing interventions and their implementation, together with information from ongoing assessment and evaluation of whether or not the goals have been, or are being achieved.

carer *n* someone who takes the responsibility for caring for another (child, disabled or elderly person). The Association of Carers seeks to restrict the term to cover the 6 million unpaid family and friends of vulnerable people in the UK, and not to paid helpers such as nurses or social workers. They also oppose the term 'informal carer'.

caries *n* **1** inflammatory decay of bone, usually associated with pus formation. **2** a microbial disease of the calcified tissue of the teeth characterized by demineralization of the inorganic portion and destruction of the organic substance of the tooth. Potentiated by sugary substances—**carious** *adj*.

carina *n* a keel-like structure exemplified by the keel-shaped cartilage at the bifurcation of the trachea into two bronchi—**carinal** *adj*.

cariogenic *adj* any agent causing caries*, by custom referring to dental caries.

carminative *adj, n* having the power to relieve flatulence and associated colic. The chief carminatives administered orally are aromatics, e.g. cinnamon, cloves, ginger, nutmeg and peppermint.

carneous mole a fleshy mass in the uterus comprising blood clot and a dead fetus or parts thereof which have not been expelled with abortion.

carotenes *npl* a group of naturally occurring pigments within the larger group of carotenoids*. Carotene occurs in three forms alpha (α), beta (β) and gamma (γ). The β form is converted in the body to vitamin A; it is therefore a provitamin.

carotenoids *npl* a group of about 100 naturally occurring yellow to red pigments found mostly in plants, some of which are carotenes*.

carotid *n* the principal artery on each side of the neck. At the bifurcation of the common carotid into the internal and external carotids there are: (a) the *carotid bodies* a collection of chemoreceptors which, being sensitive to chemical changes in the blood, protect the body against lack of O_2 (b) the *carotid sinus* a collection of receptors (baroreceptors) sensitive to pressure changes; increased pressure causes slowing of the heart beat and lowering of blood pressure. *carotid angiogram* the inspection of the carotid arteries after injection of an opaque medium.

carpal tunnel syndrome nocturnal pain, numbness and tingling in the area of distribution of the median nerve in the hand. Due to compression as the nerve passes under the fascial band. Most common in middle-aged or pregnant women.

carphology *n* involuntary picking at the bedclothes, as seen in exhaustive or febrile delirium.

carpometacarpal *adj* pertaining to the carpal and metacarpal bones, the joints between them and the ligaments joining them.

carpopedal *adj* pertaining to the hands and feet. *carpopedal spasm* (*syn* Trousseau's sign) spasm of hands and feet in tetany*, provoked by constriction of the limb.

carrier *n* **1** a person who, without manifesting an infection, harbours the microorganism which can cause the overt infection, and who can transmit infection to others. **2** a person who carries a recessive (i.e. a nonmanifesting) gene at a specific chromosome location (locus).

cartilage *n* a dense connective tissue capable of withstanding pressure. There are several types according to the function it has to fulfil. There is relatively more cartilage in a child's skeleton but much of it has been converted into bone by adulthood.—**cartilaginous** *adj*.

cascara *n* purgative bark, used as the dry extract in tablets and as liquid extract and elixir for chronic constipation.

caseation *n* the formation of a soft, cheese-like mass, as occurs in tuberculosis—**caseous** *adj*.

casein *n* a protein produced when milk enters the stomach. Coagulation in children occurs due to the action of rennin* upon the caseinogen* in the milk, splitting it into two proteins, one being casein. The casein combines with calcium and a clot is formed. ⇒ caseinogen.

caseinogen *n* the principal protein in milk. It is not soluble in water but is kept in solution in milk by inorganic salts. The proportion to lactalbumin* is much higher in cows' milk than in human milk. In the presence of rennin* it is converted into insoluble casein.

case manager senior member of social services community care team whose role is to assess elderly or disabled clients living in their own homes, for the amount and type of home care and support they require to live as independently as possible. Each assessment leads to the construction of an individualized 'package of care' for that client, one that may involve intervention by a home* carer, district nurse, occupational therapist and physiotherapist. The case manager's role is that of assessor, coordinator, and evaluator of care.

caseous degeneration cheese-like tissue resulting from atrophy in a tuberculoma or gumma*.

cast *n* **1** fibrous material and exudate which has been moulded to the form of the cavity or tube in which it has collected; this can be identified under the microscope. 2 a rigid casing made with plaster of Paris and applied to a part of the body. Additional materials such as fibreglass and plastics may be used instead of plaster of Paris.

castor oil a vegetable oil which has a purgative action when taken orally. Also used with zinc ointment for napkin rash and pressure sores.

castration *n* surgical removal of the testicles in the male, or of the ovaries in the female. Castration can be part of the treatment for a hormone-dependent cancer—**castrated** *adj,* **castrate** *n, vt.*

CAT *abbr* computed* axial tomography.

catabolism *n* the series of chemical reactions in the living body in which complex substances are broken down into simpler ones—**catabolic** *adj.*

catalase *n* an enzyme present in most human cells to catalyse the breakdown of hydrogen peroxide.

catalysis *n* an increase in the rate at which a chemical action proceeds to equilibrium through the medium of a catalyst or catalyser. If there is retardation it is negative catalysis—**catalytic** *adj.*

catalyst *n* (*syn* catalyser, enzyme, ferment) an agent which produces catalysis*. It does not undergo any change during the process.

cataplexy *n* a condition of muscular rigidity induced by severe mental shock or fear. The patient remains conscious—**cataplectic** *adj.*

cataract *n* an opacity of the crystalline lens or its capsule. It may be congenital, senile, traumatic or due to metabolic defects, in particular diabetes mellitus. *hard cataract* contains a hard nucleus, tends to be dark in colour and occurs in older people. *soft cataract* one without a hard nucleus, occurs at any age, but particularly in the young. Cataract usually develops slowly and when mature is called a *ripe cataract*—**cataractous** *adj.*

catarrh *n* chronic inflammation of a mucous membrane with constant flow of a thick sticky mucus—**catarrhal** *adj.*

catatonic schizophrenia ⇒ schizophrenia.

catchment area a geographical area which is serviced by e.g. a health centre, a district general hospital, a specialist service such as an oncology unit.

cat cry syndrome 'cri* du chat' syndrome.

catecholamines *npl* any of a group of amines which are secreted in the human body to act as neurotransmitters; adrenaline (epinephrine in USA), noradrenaline (norepinephrine in USA) and dopamine are examples. Some of them have been synthesized and they can be prescribed as treatment.

catgut *n* a form of ligature and suture of varying thickness, strength and absorbability, prepared from sheep's intestines. After sterilization it is hermetically sealed in a container. The 'plain' variety is usually absorbed in 5–10 days. 'Chromicized' catgut and 'iodized' catgut will hold for 20–40 days.

catharsis *n* in psychology, the outpouring from the patient's mind—**cathartic** *adj.*

catheter *n* a hollow tube of variable length and bore, usually having one fluted end and a tip of varying size and shape according to function. Catheters are made of many substances including soft and hard rubber, gum elastic, glass, silver, other metals and plastic materials, which may be radiopaque. They

CATS (CREDIT ACCUMULATION AND TRANSFER SCHEME) POINTS

Credit Accumulation and Transfer Scheme points are a different type of currency to CEPs and are used for a different purpose (*see* RCN CEPs, p. 315). CATS points are an academic currency, accumulated by studying and being assessed in units or modules of academic work, usually in an institution of higher education. Once they have been accumulated then they can be transferred towards an academic award or qualification.

In general, CATS points are not worth having in 'chunks' smaller than about 15–20 points. That usually represents a module or unit of study of about 120–160 hours of total 'student effort'. For the purposes of professional updating, and meeting the UKCC's PREP* requirements, this is clearly in excess of what is needed, which is why RCN advocates the use of CEPs for this purpose.

In England, Wales and Northern Ireland, to gain an Honours degree a student has to accumulate 360 CATS points. Of these, 120 must be at CATS Level 1(equal in challenge to the first year of a degree course, often termed Certificate Level). A further 120 points must be at CATS Level 2 (equal in challenge to the second year of a degree course, often called diploma level). Finally, 120 points must be gained at CATS Level 3 (equal in challenge to the final year of an Honours degree).

From this you can see that if a nurse qualifies having completed a Project 2000 (Diploma in Higher Education) preparation, he or she will already have gained 240 CATS points as a result of having completed a diploma course. The nurse will need to 'top-up' a final 120 Level 3 CATS points in an appropriate and acceptable subject area to gain a degree.

In Scotland a currency called SCOTCATS is used, and to gain an Honours degree a student has to accumulate 480 SCOTCATS points (120 at Levels 1, 2, 3 and 4).

The idea of being able to accumulate and transfer these points is to avoid repetitious learning and to promote mobility, when necessary, between institutions of higher education. (Note that you do not necessarily have to *attend* at an institution to gain CATS points: increasingly they are available using distance learning.)

As an example, suppose you undertook two modules, each worth 20 CATS points at Level 3 at University X. You then changed your job before completing your degree. You could take the 40 CATS points you had already gained at Level 3 to University Y and ask them if the 40 points could be transferred into the degree programme that they offer in a similar subject area. If they felt that the points you had gained 'matched' points they would award for similar modules then they would allow you to enter their programme without having to repeat modules.

If University Y felt that there wasn't sufficient equivalence between what you had studied at University X and what they required you to study, then they might allow you to transfer only 20 of your Level 3 points, or even none at all.

What is APL?
APL refers to Accreditation of Prior Learning, and this is where the student provides an institution of higher education with evidence of prior learning (usually in the form of assessments, certificates or awards of CATS points previously completed at another institution) and asks the institution to assign a value to it in terms of CATS points. It is up to the student to convince the authorities of his or her achievements, and it is then up to the institution to assign a value to it. This value may differ between institutions, as each has their own established 'tariff'.

Is APL different to APEL?
Yes. In general APL refers to the accreditation of prior *certificated* learning, whereas APEL refers to the accreditation of prior *experiential* learning, which is not certificated. Such learning can be acquired through life and work experiences, and it is again up to the potential student to persuade an institution of higher education that such experiences resulted in learning that is worth CATS points at a particular level. It is then up to the institution to examine evidence of this learning and to decide how many points should be awarded, and at what level.

Clearly your Personal Professional Portfolio* can be useful here in identifying learning that occurs in practice, and it will obviously be a useful tool in helping you to prepare an APEL claim, should you wish to do so. Institutions of higher education usually supply guidelines to help you with this.

have many uses, from insufflation of hollow tubes to introduction and withdrawal of fluid from body cavities. *catheter valve* a valve inserted into the end of the indwelling catheter–instead of a urine drainage bag–which normally remains closed, but which can be opened to allow urine to drain through it into a suitable receptacle. Can be left open at night with a 2 litre drainage bag attached. One valve can be left in situ for a week, or longer, according to the manufacturer's instructions. *self-retaining catheter* a deflated 'collar' around a catheter tip has its own tube alongside the catheter tube enabling a specific amount of air or water to be inserted after aseptic insertion of the catheter into the urinary bladder. The balloon so formed holds the catheter in the bladder. The balloon is deflated before removal. ⇒ Foley catheter.

catheterization *n* insertion of a catheter, most usually into the urinary bladder. *cardiac catheterization* a long plastic catheter or tubing is inserted into an arm vein and passed along to the right atrium, ventricle and pulmonary artery for (a) recording pressure in these areas (b) introducing contrast medium prior to X-ray and high speed photography. Especially useful in the diagnosis of congenital heart defects–**catheterize** *vt.*

CATS points ⇒ CATS box.

cat scratch fever a viral infection resulting from a scratch by a cat. There is fever and glandular swelling about a week after

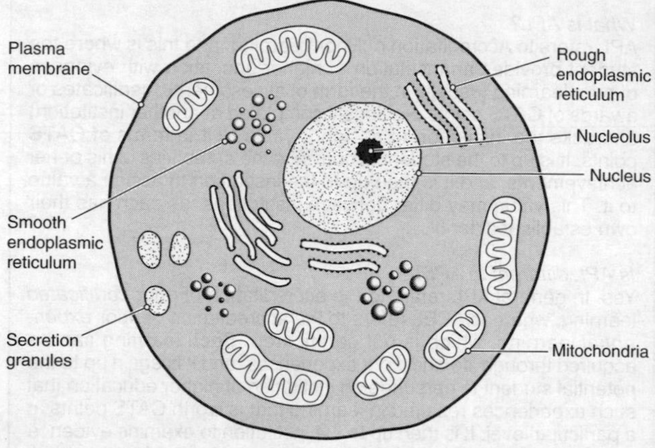

■ **Fig. 3** A typical cell.

the incident. Recovery is usually complete, although there may be some abscesses.

cauda *n* a tail or tail-like appendage—**caudal, caudate** *adj.*

caudal anaesthetic an anaesthetic administered by means of an approach to the epidural space through the caudal canal in the sacrum.

caul *n* the amnion, instead of rupturing as is usual to allow the baby through, persists and covers the baby's head at birth.

causalgia *n* excruciating neuralgic pain, resulting from physical trauma to a cutaneous nerve. Also known as reflex sympathetic dystrophy.

caustic *adj, n* corrosive or destructive to organic tissue; the agents which produce such results. Used to destroy overgrowths of granulation tissue, warts or polypi. Carbolic acid, carbon dioxide snow and silver nitrate (lunar caustic) are most commonly employed.

cauterize *vt* to cause the destruction of tissue by applying a heated instrument, a cautery*—**cauterization** *n.*

cautery *n* ⇒ cauterize.

cavernous *adj* having hollow spaces. *cavernous sinus* a channel for venous blood, on either side of the sphenoid bone. It drains blood from the lips, nose and orbits. Sepsis in these areas can cause cavernous sinus thrombosis.

cavitation *n* the formation of a cavity, as in pulmonary tuberculosis.

Cavitron *n* proprietary name for an ultrasonic surgical aspirator.

cavity *n*

CCU *abbr* coronary care unit. ⇒ intensive therapy unit.

CDH *abbr* congenital* dislocation of the hip.

cell *n* a histological term for a minute mass of protoplasm containing a nucleus (see Fig. 3). Some cells, e.g. the erythrocytes, are nonnucleated and others, e.g. in striated muscle, may be multinucleated—**cellular** *adj.*

cell mediated immunity ⇒ immunity.

cellulitis *n* a diffuse inflammation of connective tissue, especially the loose subcutaneous tissue. When it involves the pelvic tissues in the female it is called parametritis. When it occurs in the floor of the mouth it is called Ludwig's angina.

cellulose *n* a carbohydrate forming the outer walls of plant and vegetable cells. A polysaccharide which cannot be digested by man but supplies fibre.

Celsius ⇒ centigrade.

censor *n* term employed by Freud to define the resistance which prevents repressed material from readily reentering the conscious mind from the subconscious (unconscious) mind.

centigrade *n* having one hundred divisions or degrees. Usually applied to the thermometric scale in which the freezing point of water is fixed at 0° and the boiling point at 100°. The centigrade thermometer was first constructed by Celsius (1701–1744).

central cyanosis ⇒ cyanosis.

central nervous system (CNS) includes the brain and 12 pairs of cranial nerves plus the spinal cord and 31 pairs of spinal nerves.

Central Sterile Supplies Department (CSSD) an area in which packets are prepared containing the equipment and/or swabs and dressings necessary to carry out particular activities requiring aseptic* technique. It functions under the surveillance of the Control of Infection Committee. ⇒ hospital sterilization and disinfection unit.

central venous line a special catheter is skin-tunnelled along the chest to enter the cephalic vein, along which it is guided so that the tip rests in the right atrium. It is inserted under general anaesthesia and can stay in situ for a year or longer. Drugs, blood, other fluids and parenteral nutrition can be administered via this route and blood samples can be taken. ⇒ Broviac catheter, Hickman line, Portacath.

central venous pressure (CVP) *n* the pressure of the blood within the right atrium. It is measured by an indwelling catheter and a pressure manometer.

centrifugal *adj* efferent. Having a tendency to move outwards from the centre, as the rash in smallpox.

centripetal *adj* afferent. Having a tendency to move towards the centre, as the rash in chickenpox.

CEPs ⇒ RCN Continuing Education Points (CEPs) box, p. 315.

cephalalgia *n* pain in the head; headache.

cephalhaematoma *n* a collection of blood in the subperiosteal tissues of the scalp, delineated by suture lines. May resolve slowly.

cephalic *adj* pertaining to the head; near the head. *cephalic version* ⇒ version.

cephalocele *n* hernia of the brain; protrusion of part of the brain through the skull.

cephalohaematoma cephalhaematoma*.

cephalometry *n* measurement of the living human head.

cephalosporin *n* a large group of antibiotics, similar to the penicillins, with a wide spectrum of antibacterial activity. Previously only available by injection, oral preparations are now available.

cerebellar gait ⇒ gait.

cerebellum *n* that part of the brain which lies behind and below the cerebrum. Its chief functions are the coordination of fine voluntary movements and the control of posture—**cerebellar** *adj.*

cerebral *adj* pertaining to the cerebrum. *cerebral compression* arises from any space-occupying intracranial lesion. *cerebral palsy* nonprogressive brain damage before the completion of brain development, resulting in a range of mainly motor conditions ranging from clumsiness to severe spasticity.

cerebration *n* mental activity.

cerebrospinal *adj* pertaining to the brain and spinal cord. *cerebrospinal fluid* the clear fluid filling the ventricles of the brain and central canal of the spinal cord. Also found beneath the cranial and spinal meninges in the pia-arachnoid space.

cerebrovascular *adj* pertaining to the blood vessels of the brain. *cerebrovascular accident (CVA)* interference with the cerebral blood flow due to embolism, haemorrhage or thrombosis. Signs and symptoms vary according to the duration, extent and site of tissue damage; there may only be a passing, even momentary inability to move a hand or foot; weakness or tingling in a limb; stertorous breathing, incontinence of urine and faeces, coma; paralysis of a limb or limbs and speech deficiency (aphasia).

cerebrum *n* the largest and uppermost part of the brain; it does not include the cerebellum, pons and medulla. The longitudinal fissure divides it into two hemispheres, each containing a lateral ventricle. The internal substance is white, the outer convoluted cortex is grey—**cerebral** *adj*.

certified *adj* now a historical term used in relation to insanity, prior to the Mental Health Act, 1959. Those patients who cannot leave a mental hospital of their own accord (once described as 'certified') are now referred to as 'detained' or 'sectioned' patients.

cerumen *n* ear wax—**ceruminous** *adj*.

cervical *adj* **1** pertaining to the neck. **2** pertaining to the cervix (neck) of an organ. *cervical amnioscopy* ⇒ amnioscopy. *cervical canal* the lumen of the cervix uteri, from the internal to the external os. *cervical rib* (*syn* thoracic inlet syndrome) a supernumerary rib in the cervical region, which may present no symptoms or it may press on nerves of the brachial plexus. *cervical smear* ⇒ Pap test. *cervical vertebrae* the seven spinal vertebrae in the neck region.

cervical intraepithelial neoplasia (CIN) cellular change in the cervix uteri. CIN1—mild dysplasia. CIN2—moderate dysplasia. CIN3—severe dysplasia, carcinoma-in-situ.

cervicectomy *n* amputation of the uterine cervix usually for cancer. Rarely performed.

cervicitis *n* inflammation of the uterine cervix.

cervix *n* a neck. *cervix uteri, uterine cervix* the neck of the uterus.

cestode *n* tapeworm ⇒ Taenia.

CF *abbr* cystic* fibrosis.

CFT *abbr* complement* fixation test.

chalazion *n* a cyst on the edge of the eyelid from retained secretion of the Meibomian* glands.

chalone *n* a substance which inhibits rather than stimulates, e.g. enterogastrone inhibits gastric secretions and motility.

chancre *n* the primary syphilitic ulcer, associated with swelling of local lymph glands. The picture of chancre with regional adenitis constitutes 'primary syphilis'. The chancre is painless, indurated, solitary and highly infectious.

chancroid *n* (*syn* soft sore) a type of venereal disease prevalent in warmer climates. Causes multiple, painful, ragged ulcers on the penis and vulva, often associated with bubo* formation. Infection is by *Haemophilus ducreyi*.

character *n* the sum total of the known and predictable mental characteristics of an individual. *character change* denotes change in the form of conduct, to one foreign to the patient's natural disposition, e.g. indecent behaviour in a hitherto respectable person. Common in the psychoses.

charcoal *n* the residue after burning organic substances at a high temperature in an enclosed vessel. Used in medicine for its adsorptive and deodorant properties.

Charcot's joint complete disorganization of a joint associated with syringomyelia or advanced cases of tabes dorsalis (locomotor ataxia). The condition is painless. *Charcot's triad* manifestation of disseminated sclerosisnystagmus, intention tremor and staccato speech.

charts *npl* documents on which diverse data such as TPR (temperature*, pulse* and respiration*); blood* pressure; intake* and output; relief of pressure, and medications* are recorded: accepted as part of nursing documentation.

cheilitis *n* inflammation of the lip. *angular cheilitis* the term used when the inflammation is confined to the two angles of the lips.

cheiloplasty *n* plastic surgery repair of a defect to the lip.

cheilosis *n* maceration at the angles of the mouth; fissures occur later. May be due to riboflavine* deficiency.

cheiropompholyx *n* symmetrical eruption of skin of hands (especially fingers) characterized by the formation of tiny vesicles and associated with itching or burning. On the feet the condition is called 'podopompholyx'.

chelating agents soluble organic compounds that can fix certain metallic ions into their molecular structure. When given in cases of poisoning the new complex so formed is excreted in the urine.

chemonucleolysis *n* injection of an enzyme, usually into an invertebral disc, for dissolution of same—**chemonucleolytic** *adj.*

chemopallidectomy *n* the destruction of a predetermined section of globus* pallidus by chemicals.

chemoreceptor *n* **1** a chemical linkage in a living cell having an affinity for, and capable of combining with, certain other chemical substances. **2** afferent nerve endings sensitive to concentrations of certain chemicals, such as carbon dioxide and lactic acid. Affects sympathetic and parasympathetic activity of the autonomic nervous system.

chemosis *n* an oedema or swelling of the bulbar conjunctiva*—**chemotic** *adj.*

chemotaxis *n* movements of a cell (e.g. leucocyte) or an organism in response to chemical stimuli; attraction towards a chemical is *positive chemotaxis,* repulsion is *negative chemotaxis*—**chemotactic** *adj.*

chemotherapy *n* use of a specific chemical agent to arrest the progress of, or eradicate, disease in the body without causing irreversible injury to healthy tissues. Chemotherapeutic agents are administered mainly by oral, intramuscular and intravenous routes, and are distributed usually by the bloodstream. The term is used mainly in relation to the treatment of cancer.

Cheyne-Stokes respiration cyclical waxing and waning of breathing, characterized at one extreme by deep fast breaths and at the other by apnoea: it generally indicates that death is imminent.

CHF *abbr* congestive* heart failure.

chiasma *n* an X-shaped crossing or decussation. *optic chiasma* the meeting of the optic nerves;

where the fibres from the medial or nasal half of each retina cross the middle line to join the optic tract of the opposite side—**chiasmata** *pl.*

chickenpox *n* (*syn* varicella) a mild, specific infection with varicella zoster virus. Successive crops of vesicles appear first on the trunk; they scab and heal without leaving scars.

chikungunya *n* one of the mosquito*-transmitted haemorrhagic fevers occurring in the tropics.

chilblain *n* (*syn* erythema pernio) congestion and swelling attended with severe itching and burning sensation in reaction to cold.

child abuse deliberate harm caused to a child by either physical, sexual or emotional abuse*, or by maternal deprivation, i.e. failure to feed or clothe a child.

childbirth *n* the act of giving birth. *natural childbirth* giving birth without medical intervention.

child mishandling ⇒ abuse, nonaccidental injury.

chimney sweep's cancer scrotal epithelioma ⇒ epithelioma.

chiropodist *n* a person who is qualified in chiropody*, also known as a podiatrist*.

chiropody *n* the theory and practice relating to the maintenance of feet in healthy condition and the treatment of disabilities. Synonymous with podiatry.

chiropractic *n* technique of manipulation of the spine, based on the principle that disorders are caused by aberrations in the functioning of the nervous system.

chiropractor *n* a person who practises chiropractic*. The practitioner believes that many diseases are due to interference with nerve flow, is skilled in vertebral manipulation and does not use drugs or surgery.

Chlamydia *n* a genus of spiral-shaped microorganisms, smaller than bacteria but larger than viruses, which can cause disease in man and birds. Some *Chlamydia* infections of birds can be transmitted to man. *Chlamydia trachomatis* causes trachoma*. Sexual transmission of chlamydial infection is common. The population most at risk are sexually active young people who may be asymptomatic; the organism is difficult and costly to culture so routine tests are not done. Erythromycin and tetracycline cure the condition. Untreated it can lead to inflammatory disease. There is an increasing number of babies who acquire neonatal chlamydial ophthalmia. ⇒ ornithosis, psittacosis.

chloasma *n* patchy brown discolouration of the skin, especially the face. Can appear during pregnancy.

chloral hydrate *n* rapid acting sedative and hypnotic of value in nervous insomnia.

chlorhexidine *n* a bactericidal solution which is effective against a wide range of bacteria. Used as 1:2000 solution as a general antiseptic, 1:5000 for douches and irrigation. Hand cream (1%) is effective in reducing cross infection.

chlorine *n* a greenish-yellow, irritating gaseous element. Powerful germicide, bleaching and deodorizing agent in the presence of moisture when nascent oxygen is liberated. Used chiefly as hypochlorites (eusol*, Milton*) or other compounds which slowly liberate active chlorine.

chloroform *n* a heavy liquid, once used extensively as a general anaesthetic. Much used in the form of chloroform water as a flavouring and preservative in aqueous mixtures.

chloroma *n* a condition in which multiple greenish-yellow growths grow on the periosteum of facial and cranial bones, and on vertebrae, in association with acute* myeloblastic leukaemia.

chlorpromazine *n* a drug of exceptional pharmacological action, as it is a sedative, antiemetic, antispasmodic and hypotensive. It increases the effectiveness of hypnotics, anaesthetics, alcohol and analgesics. Valuable in psychiatric conditions and management of senile patients. May cause skin sensitization, leucopenia, parkinsonism, jaundice and hypothermia.

choanae *npl* funnel-shaped openings. ⇒ nares*—**choana** *sing*, **choanal** *adj*.

chocolate cyst an endometrial cyst* containing altered blood. The ovaries are the most usual site.

choanal atresia congenital abnormality where there is no communication between the nose and the nasopharynx. Bilateral atresia presents as a respiratory emergency at birth.

choked disc ⇒ papilloedema.

choking *n* when the airway is blocked by a foreign body, swelling or external pressure. The face becomes purple, the eyes protrude, as the distressed person tries to cough, to dislodge the foreign body, usually food. Cyanosis can occur, with dizziness and unconsciousness. A less dramatic choking can occur from oedema of the lower pharynx and larynx, or outside pressure on the respiratory tube as from a solid tumour. ⇒ Heimlich manoeuvre.

cholaemia *n* the presence of bile* in the blood—**cholaemic** *adj*.

cholagogue *n* a drug which causes an increased flow of bile into the intestine.

cholangiography *n* the radiographic examination of hepatic, cystic and bile ducts. Can be performed: (a) after oral or intravenous administration of contrast medium (b) by direct injection at operation to detect any further stones in the ducts (c) during or after operation by way of a T-tube in the common bile duct (d) by means of an injection via the skin on the anterior abdominal wall and the liver when it is called percutaneous transhepatic cholangiography. ⇒ endoscopic retrograde cholangiopancreatography—**cholangiographic** *adj*, **cholangiograph** *n*, **cholangiographically** *adv*.

cholangiohepatitis *n* inflammation of the liver and bile ducts.

cholangitis *n* inflammation of the bile ducts.

cholecalciferol *n* one of a group of fat-soluble compounds which can be produced artificially. This, or natural vitamin D_3, is essential for the uptake and utilization of calcium. Given in rickets and to prevent hypocalcaemia in coeliac disease, in parathyroid deficiency and lupus vulgaris.

cholecystectomy *n* surgical removal of the gallbladder. Usually advised for stones, inflammation and occasionally for growths. *laparoscopic cholecystectomy* surgical removal of the gallbladder via the minimally invasive transperitoneal approach, using specially designed instruments, diathermy and laser, usually under video control.

cholecystenterostomy *n* literally, the establishment of an artificial opening (anastomosis) between the gallbladder and the small intestine.

cholecystitis *n* inflammation of the gallbladder.

cholecystoduodenal *adj* pertaining to the gallbladder and duodenum as an anastomosis between them.

cholecystoduodenostomy *n* the establishment of an anastomosis between the gallbladder and the duodenum. Usually necessary in cases of stricture of common bile duct, which may be congenital, or due to previous inflammation or operation.

cholecystography *n* radiographic examination of the gallbladder after administration of contrast medium—**cholecystographic** *adj,* **cholecystograph** *n,* **cholecystographically** *adv.*

cholecystojejunostomy *n* an anastomosis between the gallbladder and the jejunum. Performed for obstructive jaundice due to growth in head of pancreas.

cholecystokinin *n* a hormone which contracts the gallbladder. Secreted by the upper intestinal mucosa.

cholecystolithiasis *n* the presence of stone or stones in the gallbladder.

cholecystostomy *n* a surgically established fistula between the gallbladder and the abdominal surface; used to provide drainage, in empyema of the gallbladder or after the removal of stones.

cholecystotomy *n* incision into the gallbladder.

choledochoduodenal *adj* pertaining to the bile ducts and duodenum, e.g. *choledochoduodenal fistula.*

choledochography *n* cholangiography*.

choledocholithiasis *n* the presence of a stone or stones in the bile ducts.

choledocholithotomy *n* surgical removal of a stone from the common bile duct.

choledochostomy *n* drainage of the common bile duct using a T-tube, usually after exploration for a stone.

choledochotomy *n* incision into the common bile duct.

cholelithiasis *n* the presence of stones in the gallbladder or bile ducts.

cholera *n* an acute epidemic disease, caused by *Vibrio comma,* occurring in the East. The main symptoms are the evacuation of copious 'rice-water' stools accompanied by agonizing cramp and severe collapse. Spread mainly by contaminated water, overcrowding and insanitary conditions. Mortality is reduced with prompt treatment with adequate fluid and electrolyte therapy.

choleric temperament *n* one of the four classical types of temperament*, hasty and prone to emotional outbursts.

cholestasis *n* diminution or arrest of the flow of bile. *intrahepatic cholestasis* a syndrome comprising jaundice of an obstructive type, itching, pale stools and dark urine, but in which the main bile ducts outside the liver are patent—**cholestatic** *adj.*

cholesteatoma *n* collection of squamous epithelium. *acquired cholesteatoma* usually seen in a chronically diseased ear. If untreated, erodes bone and may lead to complications, such as cerebral abscess or facial nerve palsy. Treated by surgical removal, e.g. modified radical mastoidectomy. *congenital cholesteatoma* squamous epithelial cysts that can arise anywhere within the temporal bone. Aetologically this has no relationship with acquired cholesteatoma—**cholesteatomatous** *adj.*

cholesterol *n* a crystalline substance of a fatty nature found in the brain, nerves, liver, blood, bile and plasma membrane. It is not easily soluble and may crystallize in the gallbladder and along arterial walls. Precursor molecule of glucocorticoid steroids, mineralocorticosteroids and sex hormones.

cholesterosis *n* abnormal deposition of cholesterol*.

choline *n* a chemical moiety of phosphoglycerides. Found in most cell membranes of humans.

cholinergic *adj* applied to nerves which liberate acetylcholine* at their termination. Includes nerves which cause voluntary muscle to contract and all parasympathetic nerves.⇒ adrenergic *opp. cholinergic crisis* respiratory failure resulting from overtreatment with anticholinesterase* drugs. It is distinguished from myasthenic* crisis by giving 10 mg edrophonium chloride intravenously. If there is no improvement cholinergic crisis is confirmed and 1 mg atropine sulphate is given intravenously together with immediate mechanical respiration. ⇒ edrophonium test.

cholinesterase *n* an enzyme which hydrolyses acetylcholine into choline and acetic acid at nerve endings.

choluria *n* biliuria*–**choluric** *adj.*

chondritis *n* inflammation of cartilage.

chondrocostal *adj* pertaining to the costal cartilages and ribs.

chondrodynia *n* pain in a cartilage.

chondrolysis *n* dissolution of cartilage–**chondrolytic** *adj.*

chondroma *n* a benign, slow-growing tumour of cartilage; tends to recur after removal. *enchondroma* grows within cartilage.

chondromalacia *n* softening of cartilage.

chondrosarcoma *n* malignant neoplasm of cartilage–**chondrosarcomata** *pl,* **chondrosarcomatous** *adj.*

chondrosternal *adj* pertaining to the rib cartilages and sternum.

chorda tympani nerve supplying anterior two-thirds of the tongue, which may be damaged during middle ear surgery.

chordee *n* painful erection of the penis associated with urethritis.

chorditis *n* inflammation of the spermatic or vocal cords.

chordotomy ⇒ cordotomy.

chorea *n* a disease manifested by irregular and spasmodic movements, beyond the patient's control. Even voluntary movements are rendered jerky and ungainly. The childhood disease is often called rheumatic chorea or 'St Vitus' Dance'; the adult form is part of a cerebral degenerative process called Huntington's* chorea–**choreal, choreic** *adj.*

choreiform *n* resembling chorea*.

choriocarcinoma *n* chorionepithelioma*.

chorion *n* the outer membrane forming the embryonic or fetal sac. *chorion frondosum* the part of the chorion covered by villi in the early weeks of embryonic development before the placenta is formed.–**chorial, chorionic** *adj. chorion biopsy* ⇒ chorionic villus biopsy.

chorionepithelioma *n* a highly malignant tumour arising from chorionic cells, usually after a hydatidiform* mole although it may follow abortion or even normal pregnancy, quickly metastasizing especially to the lungs. Cytotoxic drugs have improved the prognosis.

chorionic villi projections from the chorion* from which the fetal part of the placenta is formed. Through the chorionic villi diffusion of gases, nutrient and waste products from the maternal to the fetal blood and vice versa occurs.

chorionic villus biopsy also known as chorionic villus sampling (CVS). Tissue is removed from the gestational sac early in pregnancy for the detection of chromosomal and other inherited disorders. Because this can be done as early as 8 weeks' gestation, termination (if indicated) can be undertaken before 12 weeks, which is not possible with amniocentesis*.

chorioretinitis *n* (*syn* choroidoretinitis) inflammation of the choroid and retina.

choroid *n* the middle pigmented, vascular coat of the posterior five-sixths of the eyeball, continuous with the iris in front. It lies between the sclera* externally and the retina* internally, and prevents the passage of light rays—**choroidal** *adj*.
choroiditis *n* inflammation of the choroid. *Tay's choroiditis* degenerative change affecting the retina around the macula* lutea.
choroidocyclitis *n* inflammation of the choroid and ciliary body.
choroidoretinal *adj* pertaining to the choroid and the retina.
choroidoretinitis *n* ⇒ chorioretinitis.
Christmas disease deficiency in blood clotting factor IX.
chromatogram *n* any recording of the results of chromatography.
chromosome *n* thread-like body which can be seen within the cell nucleus as a cell prepares to divide and during cell division (e.g. by mitosis). Chromosomes split longitudinally in that process. They carry hereditary factors (genes). The chromosomes are made essentially of DNA*, of which the genes are made, and the chromosome number is constant for each species. In man, there are 46 in each cell, except in the mature ovum and sperm in which the number is halved as a result of reduction division (meiosis). A set of 23 chromosomes is inherited from each parent. The human male produces two types of sperm, with the Y chromosome to generate males and with the X chromosome to generate females—**chromosomal** *adj*.
chronic *adj* lingering, lasting, opposed to acute*. The word does not imply anything about the severity of the condition. *chronic heart failure* ⇒ congestive heart failure. *chronic lymphocytic leukaemia* a proliferation of lymphocytes in the blood, which occurs mainly in the elderly. Little active treatment is necessary and patients may live comfortably for many years. *chronic myelocytic leukaemia* proliferation of myelocytes in the blood. The condition may run a static course over several years but eventually an acute phase supervenes (blast crisis). *chronic obstructive airways disease* chronic obstructive bronchitis*.
chronological age a person's actual age in years.
Chvostek's sign excessive twitching of the face on tapping the facial nerve: a sign of tetany*.
chyle *n* digested fats which as an alkaline, milky fluid pass from the small intestine via the lymphatics to the bloodstream—**chylous** *adj*.
chylothorax *n* leakage of chyle from the thoracic duct into the pleural cavity.
chyluria *n* chyle* in the urine, which can occur in some nematode* infestations, either when a fistulous communication is established between a lymphatic vessel and the urinary tract or when the distension of the urinary lymphatics causes them to rupture—**chyluric** *adj*.
chyme *n* partially digested food which as an acid, creamy-yellow, thick fluid passes from the stomach to the duodenum. Its acidity controls the pylorus so that chyme is ejected at frequent intervals—**chymous** *adj*.
chymotrypsin *n* a protein-digesting enzyme secreted by the pancreas: it is activated by trypsin. Used in the treatment of intracapsular cataract extraction.
cicatrix *n* ⇒ scar.
cilia *npl* 1 the eyelashes. 2 microscopic hair-like projections from certain epithelial cells. Membranes containing such cells, e.g. those lining the trachea and uterine tubes, are known as

ciliated membranes—**cilium** *sing.* **ciliary, ciliated, cilial** *adj.*

ciliary *adj* hair-like. *ciliary body* a specialized structure in the eye connecting the anterior part of the choroid to the circumference of the iris; it is composed of the ciliary muscles and processes. *ciliary muscles* fine hair-like muscle fibres arranged in a circular manner to form a greyish-white ring immediately behind the corneoscleral junction. *ciliary processes* about 70 in number, are projections on the undersurface of the choroid which are attached to the ciliary muscles.

Cimex *n* a genus of insects of the family Cimicidae. *Cimex lectlarius* is the common bedbug, parasitic to man and bloodsucking.

CIN *abbr* ⇒ cervical intraepithelial neoplasia.

circadian rhythm rhythm with a periodicity of approximately 24 h. May refer to hormone secretion, urine production, etc.

circinata *n* ⇒ tinea.

circinate *adj* in the form of a circle or segment of a circle, e.g. the skin eruptions of late syphilis, ringworm, etc.

circulation *n* passage in a circle. Usually means circulation of the blood, i.e. the passage of blood from heart to arteries to capillaries to veins and back to heart.—**circulatory** *adj.* **circulate** *vi, vt. circulation of bile* the passage of bile from the liver cells, where it is formed, via the gallbladder and bile ducts to the small intestine, where its constituents are partly reabsorbed into the blood and then return to the liver. *circulation of cerebrospinal fluid* takes place from the ventricles of the brain to the cisterna magna, from where the fluid surrounds the surface of the brain and the spinal cord, including its central canal. It is absorbed into the blood in the cerebral venous sinuses. *collateral circulation* ⇒ collateral. *coronary circulation* the system of vessels which supply blood to the heart muscle. *extracorporeal circulation* ⇒ extracorporeal. *fetal circulation* ⇒ fetal. *lymph circulation* lymph is collected from the tissue spaces and passed in the lymphatic capillaries, vessels, glands and ducts to be poured back into the blood stream. *portal circulation* venous blood, collected from the intestines, pancreas, spleen and stomach, passes through the liver before returning to the heart. *pulmonary circulation* passage of deoxygenated blood from right ventricle to pulmonary* artery, to lungs and, oxygenated, back to left atrium of the heart (see Fig. 2, p. 62). *systemic circulation* passage of oxygenated blood from left ventricle to aorta, to tissue and, deoxygenated, back to right atrium of the heart (i.e. flows throughout the body).

circumcision *n* excision of the prepuce or foreskin of the penis, usually for religious or ethnic reasons. The operation is sometimes required for phimosis* or paraphimosis*. *female circumcision* excision of the clitoris, labia minora and labia majora. The extent of cutting varies from country to country. The simplest form is clitoridectomy*; the next form entails excision of the prepuce, clitoris and all or part of the labia minora. The most extensive form, infibulation, involves excision of clitoris, labia minora and labia majora. The vulval lips are sutured together but total obliteration of the vaginal introitus is prevented by inserting a piece of wood or reed to preserve a small passage for urine and menstrual fluid.

circumcorneal *adj* around the cornea.

circumoral *adj* surrounding the

mouth. *circumoral pallor* a pale appearance of the skin around the mouth, in contrast to the flushed cheeks. A characteristic of scarlet fever*—**circumorally** *adv.*

circumvallate *adj* surrounded by a raised ring, as the large circumvallate papillae at the base of the tongue.

cirrhosis *n* hardening of an organ. There are degenerative changes in the tissues with resulting fibrosis. *cirrhosis of liver* increasing in prosperous countries. Damage to liver cells can be from virus, microorganisms or toxic substances and dietary deficiencies interfering with the nutrition of liver cells. Often the result of alcoholism. Associated developments include ascites*, obstruction of the circulation through the portal vein with haematemesis*, jaundice and enlargement of the spleen—**cirrhotic** *adj.*

cirsoid *adj* resembling a tortuous, dilated vein (varix*). *cirsoid aneurysm* a tangled mass of pulsating blood vessels appearing as a subcutaneous tumour, usually on the scalp.

cisplatin *n* a platinum compound used in the treatment of malignant conditions.

cisterna *n* any closed space serving as a reservoir for a body fluid. *cisterna magna* is a subarachnoid space in the cleft between the cerebellum and medulla oblongata—**cisternal** *adj.*

cisternal puncture ⇒ puncture.

citrus fruit includes lemons, limes, oranges and grapefruit. An important source of vitamin* C in the prevention of scurvy.

CJD *abbr* Creutzfeldt-Jakob* disease.

clam cystoplasty a surgical procedure to augment the size of the bladder. The bladder is dissected like a 'clam' and a piece of intestinal tissue is inserted.

clap *n* a slang term for gonorrhoea*.

claudication *n* limping caused by interference with the blood supply to the legs. The cause may be spasm or disease of the vessels themselves. In *intermittent claudication* the patient experiences severe pain in the calves when walking but is able to continue after a short rest. A symptom of arterial insufficiency.

claustrophobia *n* a form of mental disturbance in which there is an irrational fear of enclosed spaces—**claustrophobic** *adj.*

clavicle *n* the collar-bone—**clavicular** *adj.*

clavus *n* a corn*.

claw-foot *adj, n* (*syn* pes cavus) a deformity where the longitudinal arch of the foot is increased in height and associated with clawing of the toes. It may be acquired or congenital in origin.

claw-hand *n* the hand is flexed and contracted giving a claw-like appearance; the condition may be due to injury or disease.

cleanser *n, adj* (describes) a cleansing agent. Term often applied to drugs of the cetrimide type, which have both antiseptic and cleaning properties, and so are valuable in removing grease, dirt, etc. from skin and wounds, and scabs and crusts from skin lesions.

cleft lip a congenital defect in the lip; a fissure extending from the margin of the lip to the nostril; may be single or double, and is often associated with cleft* palate.

cleft palate congenital failure of fusion between the right and left palatal processes. Often associated with cleft lip*, but a variety of types of defect can occur.

client *n* the person to whom a (nursing) service is supplied. Community nurses in particular prefer this word, as it does not have the illness connotation of the word patient*.

CLINICAL SUPERVISION

Clinical supervision was proposed by the Department of Health in 1993, in the Chief Nursing Officer's strategy document *A Vision for the Future*.

It is a formal process of providing professional support, learning and supervision for individual practitioners in the clinical setting. It is aimed at allowing nurses to extend their practical skills and professional competence, thus encouraging autonomous and accountable practice and enlarging the scope of professional practice.

Clinical supervision can be provided in a variety of ways and on a group or individual basis. It can include formal and informal mentorship schemes; preceptorship, which is specifically aimed at newly qualified practitioners, and appraisal, whereby plans for the development of an individual's clinical practice are agreed and monitored. It encourages techniques such as reflection, critical incident analysis and critical debate.

See also: reflective practice.

Clifton Assessment Procedures for the Elderly a series of tests which measure cognitive function as well as behaviour.

climacteric *n* in the female, the menopause*. A corresponding period occurs in men and is called the *male climacteric*.

clinical *adj* pertaining to a clinic. In nursing, it is used to describe the practical observation, treatment and care of sick persons as opposed to theoretical study.

clinical audit a quality assurance programme. It involves defining the expected level of quality in a specific area of care, measuring and comparing actual practice against the expected level, and taking action to improve any deficiencies identified.

clinical effectiveness a drive to ensure that clinical interventions and practice are based on evidence of their effectiveness, through the use of clinical guidelines* and the systematic assessment of health outcomes.

clinical guidelines systematically developed statements which assist the clinical practitioner and patient in making decisions about a specific aspect of care. ⇒ clinical effectiveness, evidence based practice.

clinical nurse specialist a nurse who develops skills in relation to a particular group of patients, e.g. those with a stoma or with diabetes; or a particular area of nursing, e.g. infection control or intravenous therapy. ⇒ specialist* nursing practice.

clinical supervision ⇒ Clinical supervision box.

clinical thermometer traditionally the glass and mercury thermometer. The one used to take the core 'rectal' temperature has a short thick mercury bulb to prevent injury; that used to measure oral core temperature and skin shell temperature in the dried axilla or groin has a longer, thinner mercury bulb. ⇒ anal, body temperature, clinical thermometry, sublingual socket.

clinical thermometry traditionally measuring the body* temperature was accomplished by using a clinical* thermometer; research supports a placement time of 3 minutes. There are now electronic thermometers which use a probe in the same way as a clinical thermometer; many of them register in as short a time as 3 seconds, without sacrificing accuracy. Chemical crystals, made into a band, can be applied to the skin of the forehead, and change colour as they register the temperature. These are especially useful for babies, children and the elderly. Tempadot is a chemical dot thermometer placed in the sublingual* socket. It takes only seconds to register and since it can only be used once it cannot contribute to hospital-acquired infection*. The flexibility of the stem can help with efficient sublingual placing, even in the presence of dentures.

clinician *n* in a nursing context, the word is used to designate those nurses who work with patients/clients as opposed to those who indirectly serve patients, e.g. nurse managers and nurse educators. ⇒ practitioners.

clitoridectomy *n* the surgical removal of the clitoris. ⇒ female circumcision.

clitoriditis *n* inflammation of the clitoris.

clitoris *n* a small erectile organ situated just below the mons veneris at the junction anteriorly of the labia minora, homologous to the penis.

cloaca *n* in osteomyelitis*, the opening through the involucrum* which discharges pus—**cloacal** *adj.*

clofazimine a red dye, given orally to control symptoms of erythema nodosum leprosum reaction in lepromatous leprosy.

clonic *adj* ⇒ clonus.

clonus *n* a series of intermittent muscular contractions and relaxations. ⇒ tonic *opp.*—**clonic** *adj,* **clonicity** *n.*

closed urinary drainage system a means of draining urine via a self-retaining catheter into a drainage bag which has a non-return valve at the inlet and may have a drainage tap as an outlet. The capacity of the bag may be 2 litres, for those patients who are in bed and/or are prescribed bladder irrigation. There are also a variety of body-worn bags with a capacity of 350–750 ml to which a 2 litre bag may be attached at night 'piggy back'. The 2 litre bag is discarded in the morning. The leg bag may be worn for up to 7 days without disconnection from the catheter.

Clostridium *n* a bacterial genus. Clostridia are large Gram-positive anaerobic bacilli found as commensals of the gut of animals and man and as saprophytes in the soil. Endospores* are produced which are widely distributed. Many species are pathogenic because of the exotoxins produced, e.g. *Clostridium tetani* (tetanus), *C. botulinum* (botulism); *C. perfringens (welchii)* (gas gangrene), *C. difficile* (pseudomembranous colitis).

clothing, modification of may be required by people with a physical or learning disability, frail and elderly people and those who are incontinent, in order to promote independent living. The Disabled Living Foundation's Clothing Advisory Service will answer letters or telephone enquiries about clothing and dressing.

clubbed fingers a thickening and broadening of the bulbous fleshy portion of the fingers under the nails. The cause is not known but it occurs in people who have heart and/or lung disease.

club-foot *n* (*syn* congenital talipes equinovarus) a congenital malformation, either unilateral or bilateral. The components include forefoot adduction with medial displacement of the talus, ankle equinus and heel varus. ⇒ talipes.

clumping *n* agglutination*.

Clutton's joints joints which show symmetrical swelling, usually painless. The knees are often involved. Associated with congenital syphilis.

CMV *abbr* cytomegalovirus*.

CNS *abbr* central nervous* system.

COAD *abbr* chronic obstructive airways disease. ⇒ chronic bronchitis and emphysema, usually the consequence of chronic cigarette smoking.

coagulase *n* an enzyme produced by some bacteria of the genus *Staphylococcus:* it coagulates plasma and is used to classify staphylococci as coagulase-negative or coagulase-positive.

coalesce *vi* to grow together; to unite into a mass. Often used to describe the development of a skin eruption, when discrete areas of affected skin coalesce to form sheets of a similar appearance—**coalescence** *n,* **coalescent** *adj.*

coal tar the black substance obtained by the distillation of coal. It is used in an ointment for psoriasis and eczema. Liq. picis. carb. is an alcoholic solution of the soluble constituents used for similar purposes.

coarctation *n* contraction, stricture, narrowing; applied to a vessel (as in coarction of the aorta) or canal.

coarse tremor violent trembling.

cobalamin *n* a generic term for the vitamin B_{12} group. ⇒ cyanocobalamin.

cobalt *n* a mineral element considered nutritionally essential in minute traces; a constituent of vitamin B_{12} (cobalamin) the antipernicious anaemia factor. It is therefore linked with iron and copper in the prevention of anaemia.

cocaine *n* a powerful local anaesthetic obtained from the leaves of the coca plant *Erythroxylon coca.* Toxic, especially to the brain; may cause agitation, disorientation, convulsions and can induce addiction. It has vasoconstrictor properties, hence the blanching which occurs when it is applied to mucous membranes. It can be obtained illegally as purified uncut cocaine, which is ground to a white powder and sniffed in small doses ('cocaine abuse/addiction').

cocainism *n* mental and physical degeneracy caused by a morbid craving for, and excessive use of, cocaine*.

coccus *n* a spherical or nearly spherical bacterium—**cocci** *pl,* **coccal, coccoid** *adj.*

coccyalgia *n* pain in the region of the coccyx.

coccygectomy *n* surgical removal of the coccyx.

coccyx *n* the last bone of the vertebral column. It is triangular in shape and curved slightly forward. It is composed of four rudimentary vertebrae, cartilaginous at birth, ossification being completed at about the 30th year—**coccygeal** *adj.*

cochlea *n* a spiral canal resembling the interior of a snail shell, in the anterior part of the bony labyrinth of the ear—**cochlear** *adj.*

codeine *n* an alkaloid of opium*. It has mild analgesic properties, and is often combined with aspirin*. Valuable as a cough sedative (linctus codeine) in dry and useless cough.

cod liver oil contains vitamins A and D and is used on that account as a dietary supplement in mild deficiency.

coeliac *adj* relating to the abdominal cavity; applied to arteries, veins, nerves and a plexus. *coeliac disease* (*syn* gluten-induced enteropathy) due to intolerance to the protein gluten* in wheat and rye, it being the gliadin fraction that is the harmful substance. Sensitivity occurs in the villi of the small intestine, and produces the malabsorption syndrome. Symptoms become apparent at 3–6 months, soon after the child is weaned on to cereals, as up to this time the digestion is not interfered with. On weaning the absorption of fats is impaired, and large amounts of split fats may be excreted in the stools (steatorrhoea*).

coenzyme *n* an enzyme activator.

coffee ground vomit vomit containing blood, which in its partially digested state resembles coffee grounds. Indicative of slow upper gastrointestinal bleeding ⇒ haematemesis.

cognition *n* a general term used to describe all the psychological processes by which people become aware of and gain knowledge about the world in which they live.

cognitive therapy an approach to the psychological treatment of depression, anxiety and anxiety-related disorders, eating disorders and schizophrenia. It focuses on, and is effective through, correcting the patient's cognitive dysfunctions such as errors in thinking and poor problem-solving.

coitus *n* insertion of the erect penis into the vagina; the act of sexual intercourse or copulation. *coitus interruptus* removal from the vagina of the penis before ejaculation of semen as a means of contraception. The method is considered unsatisfactory as it is not only unreliable but can lead to sexual disharmony—**coital** *adj.*

cold abscess ⇒ abscess.

cold sore oral herpes*.

colectomy *n* excision of part or the whole of the colon.

colic *n* severe pain resulting from periodic spasm in an abdominal organ. *biliary colic* ⇒ biliary. *intestinal colic* abnormal peristaltic movement of an irritated gut. *painter's (lead) colic* spasm of intestine and constriction of mesenteric vessels, resulting from lead poisoning. *renal colic* spasm of ureter due to a stone. *uterine colic* ⇒ dysmenorrhoea*—**colicky** *adj.*

coliform *adj* a word used to describe any bacterium of faecal origin which is morphologically similar to *Escherichia coli.*

colitis *n* inflammation of the colon. May be acute or chronic, and may be accompanied by ulcerative lesions. *ulcerative colitis* an inflammatory and ulcerative condition of the colon. There may be an immunological basis for the condition rather than (or as well as) a psychosomatic one. Characteristically it affects young and early middle-aged adults, producing periodic bouts of diarrhoeal stools containing mucus and blood, and it may vary in severity from a mild form with little constitutional upset to a severe, dangerous and prostrating illness.

collagen *n* the main protein constituent of white fibrous tissue (skin, tendon, bone, cartilage and all connective tissue). It is composed of bundles of tropocollagen molecules, which contain three intertwined polypeptide chains. The *collagen diseases* are characterized by an inflammatory lesion of unknown aetiology affecting collagen and small blood vessels. Said to be due to development of a hypersensitivity state, they include dermatomyositis, lupus erythematosus, polyarteritis (periarteritis) nodosa, purpura, rheumatic fever, rheumatoid arthritis and scleroderma—**collagenic, collagenous** *adj.*

collapse *n* **1** the 'falling in' of a hollow organ or vessel, e.g. collapse of lung from change of air pressure inside or outside the organ. **2** physical or nervous prostration.

collapsing pulse the water-hammer pulse of aortic incompetence with high initial upthrust which quickly falls away.

collar-bone *n* the clavicle.

collateral *adj* accessory or secondary. *collateral circulation* an alternative route provided for the blood by secondary blood vessels when a primary vessel is blocked.

Colles' fracture a break at the lower end of the radius following a fall on the outstretched hand. The backward displacement of the hand produces the 'dinner fork' deformity.

collodion *n* a solution of pyroxylin with resin* and castor* oil. It forms a flexible film on the skin, and is used mainly as a protective dressing.

colloid *n* a glue-like noncrystalline substance; diffusible but not soluble in water; unable to pass through an animal membrane. Some drugs can be prepared in their colloidal form. *colloid degeneration* mucoid degeneration of tumours. *colloid goitre* abnormal enlargement of the thyroid gland, due to the accumulation in it of viscid, iodine-containing colloid.

colloidal gold test carried out on cerebrospinal fluid to assist the diagnosis of neurosyphilis.

coloboma *n* a congenital fissure or gap in the eyeball or one of its parts, particularly the uvea—**colobomata** *pl.*

colon *n* the large bowel extending from the caecum* to the rectum*. In its various parts it has appropriate names: ascending, transverse, descending and sigmoid colon. ⇒ flexure. *spasmodic colon* megacolon*—**colonic** *adj.*

colonic washout with the patient in the left lateral position, fluid—usually water at body temperature (37°C)—is introduced via a funnel, tubing and a large bore catheter inserted per rectum. Each funnelful is returned into a bucket on the floor by inverting the funnel over it. The procedure is repeated until the fluid returns clear and free from faecal stain. It is carried out before operations on, or investigations of the large bowel.

colonize *vt* when commensal* microorganisms establish a presence on or in the human body. Soon after birth commensals form a natural flora and do not usually cause infection*. Tissue can therefore be 'colonized' but not infected. Infection results when there is imbalance between the commensals and defence mechanisms.

colonoscopy *n* use of a fibreoptic colonoscope to view the inner membrane of the colon. One of medium length, approximately 110 cm, permits viewing as far as the splenic flexure and occasionally beyond; one of 180 cm views the total colon to the caecum and views of the terminal ileum are sometimes possible—**colonoscopic** *adj,* **colonoscopically** *adv.*

colony *n* a mass of bacteria which is the result of multiplication of one or more organisms. A colony may contain many millions of individual organisms and may become macroscopic*; its physical features are often characteristic of the species.

colorectal *adj* pertaining to the colon and the rectum.

colostomy *n* a surgically established fistula between the colon and the surface of the abdomen; this acts as an artificial anus.

colostrum *n* the relatively clear fluid secreted in the breasts in late pregnancy and during the first 3 days after parturition, before the formation of true milk is established. A source of proteins, fats and antibodies.

colotomy *n* incision into the colon.

colour blindness applies to various conditions in which certain colours are confused with one another. Inability to distinguish between reds and greens is called daltonism.

colpitis *n* inflammation of the vagina.

colpocele *n* protrusion of prolapse of either the bladder or rectum so that it presses on the vaginal wall.

colpocentesis *n* withdrawal of fluid from the vagina, as in haematocolpos*.

colpohysterectomy *n* removal of the uterus through the vagina.

colpoperineorrhaphy *n* the surgical repair of an injured vagina and deficient perineum.

colpophotography *n* a photograph of the cervix taken in women who have had an abnormal smear result. ⇒ colposcopy.

colporrhaphy *n* surgical repair of the vagina. An anterior colporrhaphy repairs a cystocele* and a posterior colporrhaphy repairs a rectocele*.

colposcope *n* an endoscopic instrument that magnifies cells of the vagina and cervix to allow direct observation. The cervix may be painted with acetic acid and iodine to highlight abnormal cells—**colposcopy** *n*, **colposcopically** *adv.*

Colposuspension operation the vagina is suspended from the ileopectineal ligament. Carried out for severe stress incontinence of urine.

colpotomy *n* incision of the vaginal wall. A posterior colpotomy drains an abscess in the pouch* of Douglas through the vagina.

coma *n* a state of unrousable unconsciousness, the severity of which can be assessed by cranial nerve activity. ⇒ Glasgow coma scale.

comatose *adj* in a state of coma*.

combined oral contraceptive commonly referred to as 'the pill'. Many different brands are available: each contains varying concentrations of the two hormones oestrogen and progestogen. ⇒ contraceptive.

comedone, comedo *n* a worm-like cast formed of sebum* which occupies the outlet of a hair follicle in the skin, a feature of acne* vulgaris. Comedones have a black colour because of pigmentation (blackheads).

commensals *npl* parasitic microorganisms adapted to grow on the skin and mucous surfaces of the host, forming part of the normal flora. Some commensals are potentially pathogenic.

communicable *adj* transmissible directly or indirectly from one person to another.

communicating *v* the exchange of information between at least two people. It is usually accomplished by using language*; verbal, which can be spoken, written, typed, printed or tapped on to a video screen; or nonverbal, which transmits attitudes, values and beliefs relevant to the information exchanged. When two people do not speak the same language, miming can be used to exchange information. Some profoundly deaf people communicate by a sign language. People with a partial hearing loss are usually helped to continue communicating by the use of a hearing aid and lip reading. After, e.g. a stroke or head injury, the person may have language difficulties. ⇒ aphasia, dysarthria, dysphasia, nonverbal communication.

community a social group determined by geographical boundaries and/or common values and interests. Community has also come to imply shared relationships, lifestyles and a greater frequency and intimacy of contact among those who live in a community. *community care* term

COMMUNITY CARE

The care of people in the community is organized under the terms of the NHS and Community Care Act of 1990, which also introduced the purchaser-provider model into health care in the UK.

The Act was based on a Government White Paper, *Caring for People*, published in 1989, which was itself developed from a 1988 report by Sir Roy Griffiths. Griffiths suggested that individualized 'packages of care' could be organized for those who required care in the community, based on people's individual needs and circumstances. The aim was that, wherever possible, people could be cared for at home, with whatever support was required to make that feasible.

Under the NHS and Community Care Act, local authorities assumed full responsibility for coordinating and funding community care from April 1, 1993. Despite Griffiths' recommendation that community care should be funded by central government, the policy is financed from the standard revenue support grant to local authorities, and since its implementation there have been persistent claims from local authorities that funding is not adequate.

applied to the care of people in the community, now extended to include those to be cared for in hospitals or institutions. ⇒ Community care box.

community nurse generic term which describes those nurses based in the community and concerned with caring for people in their homes and with the provision of health education and the prevention of illness and disability. Community nurses may be, e.g. health visitors, public health nurses, district nurses, community psychiatric or learning disability nurses, family planning nurses or school nurses.

compartment syndrome compromise of circulation and function of tissue within a closed space (usually a muscle compartment) due to increased pressure, leading to muscle necrosis.

compatibility *n* suitability; congruity. The power of a substance to mix with another without unfavourable results, e.g. two medicines, blood plasma and cells, similar blood groups in blood transfusions—**compatible** *adj.*

compensation *n* **1** a mental mechanism, employed by a person to cover up a weakness, by exaggerating a more socially acceptable quality. **2** In psychiatry the term *compensation neurosis* denotes symptoms motivated by a wish for monetary compensation for accident or injury. In many cases it is difficult to decide whether or not an element of malingering is involved or if the mechanism is entirely unconscious. **3** The state of counterbalancing a functional or structural defect, e.g. cardiac compensation.

Complan *n* a proprietary powder, which may be given when a normal diet cannot be tolerated or supplements are required. 100 g contains approximately 31 g protein, 16 g fat, 44 g carbohydrate and sufficient mineral salts and vitamins to maintain health. Can be taken orally or as liquid by nasogastric or gastrostomy tube.

complement *n* a normal constituent of plasma which is of

COMPLEMENTARY THERAPIES

Complementary, or alternative, therapies are currently undergoing a huge expansion in Western health care as people look for complements or alternatives to conventional medicine.

There is a wide range of complementary therapies available, including osteopathy*, homeopathy*, acupuncture*, reflexology*, massage*, aromatherapy*, hypnotherapy*, chiropractic* and herbalism*. Such therapies traditionally use a more holistic* approach than conventional medicine, for example, questioning a person carefully about diet and lifestyle before applying any treatment or remedy. A growing number of nurses are employing the techniques of complementary therapies such as massage, aromatherapy, and reflexology alongside traditional nursing care, attracted by the holistic principles of the therapies and by the opportunity for autonomous practice.

Many people who use complementary therapies do so when they feel conventional medicine has no more to offer them, often in the case of a chronic or even terminal condition. Others continue to use conventional medicine but will seek other forms of therapy in addition. The nurse must respect the patient's right to choose.

great importance in immunity mechanisms, as it combines with antigen-antibody complex (complement fixation), and this leads to the completion of a reaction like bacteriolysis. *complement fixation test* measures the amount of complement fixed by any given antigen-antibody complex. It can confirm infection with a specific microorganism.

complemental air the extra air that can be drawn into the lungs by deep inspiration.

complementary feed a bottle feed given to an infant to complement breast milk, if this is an insufficient amount. Now generally accepted to interfere with the establishment of lactation.

complementary medicine the term currently in use for such diverse techniques as acupuncture, chiropractic, homeopathy, massage, reflexology, relaxation and yoga. They may be used as an adjunct to conventional techniques and medical treatments. ⇒ Complementary therapies box.

complete abortion ⇒ abortion.

complex *n* a series of emotionally charged ideas, repressed because they conflict with ideas acceptable to the individual, e.g. *Oedipus* complex,* Electra* complex.

complication *n* in medicine, an accident or second disease arising in the course of a primary disease; it can be fatal.

compos mentis of sound mind.

compound *n* a substance composed of two or more elements, chemically combined in a definitive proportion to form a new substance with new properties.

comprehension *n* mental grasp of meaning and relationships.

compress *n* usually refers to a wet dressing of several layers of lint. A cold compress on the forehead may relieve headache.

compression *n* the state of being compressed. The act of pressing or squeezing together. ⇒ hand, intermittent pneumatic compression. *compression bandage* used in the management of venous leg ulcers to increase venous return and reduce venous hypertension. Compression stockings are used to prevent venous leg ulcers occurring where there is venous insufficiency or to reduce the risk of deep vein thrombosis following surgery. *compression fracture* ⇒ fracture.

compromise *n* in psychiatry, a mental mechanism whereby a conflict* is evaded by disguising the repressed wish to make it acceptable in consciousness.

compulsion *n* in psychiatry, an urge to carry out an act, recognized to be irrational. Resisting the urge leads to increasing tension which is only relieved by carrying out the act.

computed axial tomography computed* tomography.

computed tomography (CT) computer-constructed imaging technique of a thin slice through the body, derived from X-ray absorption data collected during a circular scanning motion.

conation *n* willing or desiring. The conscious tendency to action. One of the three aspects of mind, the others being cognition (awareness, understanding) and affection (feeling or emotion).

concept *n* an abstract generalization resulting from the mental process of abstracting and recombining certain qualities or characteristics of a number of ideas, to produce, e.g. a nurse's concept of client, doctor, doctoring, nurse, nursing and patient.

conception *n* **1** the creation of a state of pregnancy: impregnation of the ovum by the spermatozoon. **2** an abstract mental idea—**conceptive** *adj*.

conceptual framework for nursing a group of concepts which are defined and organised in such a way that they describe the author's interpretation of the highly complex activity called nursing. The framework provides the matrix in which the selected concepts are related to each other, thus providing a way of 'thinking about nursing'.

conceptualising *n* the mental processes involved in developing and continually refining a concept.

concretion *n* a deposit of hard material; a calculus*.

concussion *n* a condition resulting from a violent jar or shock. *cerebral concussion* characterized by loss of consciousness, pallor, coldness and usually an increase in the pulse rate. There may be incontinence of urine and faeces.

conditioned reflex a reflex in which the response occurs, not to the sensory stimulus which caused it originally, but to another stimulus which the subject has learned to associate with the original stimulus: it can be acquired by training and repetition. In Pavlov's classic experiments, dogs learned to associate the sound of a bell with the sight and smell of food: even when food was not presented, salivation occurred at the sound of a bell.

conditioning *n* the encouragement of new (desirable) behaviour by modifying the stimulus/response associations. *operant conditioning* the term used when there is a programme to reward (or withold a reward) a response each time it occurs, so that given time, it occurs more (or less) frequently. ⇒ deconditioning.

condom *n* a latex sheath used as a male contraceptive*. It protects both partners against sexually transmitted disease.

condom urinary drainage used for males suffering urinary incontinence. It comprises application to the penis of a modified condom which has a tube attached to its base, via which urine escapes into a body-worn drainage bag which has a clamped outlet at its base to facilitate emptying. ⇒ closed urinary drainage system.

conduction *n* the transmission of heat, light, or sound waves through suitable media; also the passage of electrical currents and nerve impulses through body tissues—**conductivity** *n*.

conductor *n* a substance or medium which transmits heat, light, sound, electric current, etc. The words bad, good or non-conductor designate the degree of conductivity.

condyloma *n* papilloma*. *Condylomata acuminata* are acuminate (pointed) dry warts found under prepuce (male), on the vulva and vestibule (female) or on the skin of the perianal region (both sexes). *Condylomata lata* are highly infectious, moist, warty excrescences found in moist areas of the body (vulva, anus, axilla, etc.) as a manifestation of late secondary syphilis*—**condylomata** *pl,* **condylomatous** *adj*.

confabulation *n* a symptom common in confusional states when there is impairment of memory for recent events. The gaps in the patient's memory are filled in with fabrications of his own invention, which nevertheless he appears to accept as fact. Occurs in senile and toxic confusional states, cerebral trauma and Korsakoff* syndrome.

confidentiality *n* under the UKCC* Code of Professional Conduct, nurses are required to 'protect all confidential information concerning patients and clients obtained in the course of professional practice and make disclosures only with consent, where required by the order of a court or where [they] can justify disclosure in the wider public interest'. ⇒ Ethics box, p. 134.

conflict *n* in psychiatry, presence of two incompatible and contrasting wishes or emotions. When the conflict becomes intolerable, repression* of the wishes may occur. Mental conflict and repression form the basic causes of many neuroses.

confluence *n* becoming merged; flowing together; a uniting, as of neighbouring pustules.

confusion *n* a mental state which is out of touch with reality and associated with a clouding of consciousness. Can occur in many illnesses but particularly associated with postepileptic fits, cerebral arteriosclerosis, dementia, infection, trauma and severe toxaemia. *acute confusional state, (ACS),* sudden and acute onset of confusion which, when seen in older people, may be mistaken for dementia. It usually has an acute medical cause, such as anaemia, cerebral vascular accident or chest or urinary tract infection, but may be due to incorrect medication or recent bereavement or loss. *chronic confusional state* has a slow onset and may be due to a chronic, unnoticed condition such as thyroid gland deficiency.

congenital *adj* of abnormal conditions, present at birth, often genetically determined. ⇒ genetic. Existing before or at birth, usually associated with a defect or disease, e.g. congenital dislocation of the hip, congenital heart disease.

congestion *n* hyperaemia*. Passive congestion results from obstruction or slowing down of venous return, as in the lower limbs or the lungs—**congestive** *adj,* **congest** *vi, vt.*

congestive heart failure a chronic inability of the heart to maintain an adequate output of blood from one or both ventricles resulting in manifest congestion and overdistension of certain veins and organs with blood, and an inadequate blood supply to the body tissues.

conization *n* removal of a cone-shaped part of the cervix by the knife or cautery. May be referred to as a cone biopsy.

conjugate *n* a measurement of the bony pelvis used to assess its adequacy for childbirth.

conjunctiva *n* the delicate transparent membrane which lines the inner surface of the eyelids (palpebral conjunctiva) and reflects over the front of the eyeball (bulbar or ocular conjunctiva)—**conjunctival** *adj.*

conjunctivitis *n* inflammation of the conjunctiva ⇒ pink-eye, TRIC. *inclusion conjunctivitis* (*syn* inclusion blennorrhoea) occurs in countries with low standards of hygiene. The reservoir of infection is the urogenital tract.

Conn syndrome hyperplasia or adenoma of the adrenal cortex producing increased aldosterone*. Results in hypertension*, hypokalaemia* and muscular weakness.

Conradi-Hünermann syndrome a skeletal dysplasia which is genetically transmitted as an autosomal dominant trait. Skeletal abnormalities are variable; they are present at birth. After the first few weeks, life expectancy is normal. Mental development is not retarded.

consanguinity *n* blood relationship. This varies in degree from close (as between siblings) to less close (as between cousins etc.)—**consanguineous** *adj.*

consciousness *n* a complex concept which implies that a person is consciously perceiving the environment via the five senses and responding to the perceptions. ⇒ anaesthesia, sleep.

consent form patients are legally required to consent to surgery preoperatively. It is the doctor's responsibility to explain to the patient in advance of surgery what the procedure will involve and any additional measures that may be required and to obtain written consent. If the patient is a minor, or incapable of giving informed* consent, the next-of-kin must sign the consent form.

conservative treatment aims at preventing a condition from becoming worse without using radical measures.

consolidation *n* becoming solid, as, for instance, the state of the lung due to exudation and organization in lobar pneumonia.

constipation *n* an implied chronic condition of infrequent and often difficult evacuation of faeces due to insufficient food or fluid intake, or to sluggish or disordered action of the bowel musculature or nerve supply, or to habitual failure to empty the rectum *acute constipation* signifies obstruction or paralysis of the gut of sudden onset. ⇒ faeces.

consumption *n* **1** act of consuming or using up. **2** a once popular term for pulmonary tuberculosis* (which 'consumed' the body)—**consumptive** *adj.*

contact *n* **1** direct or indirect exposure to infection. **2** a person who has been so exposed. *contact lens* of glass or plastic, worn under the eyelids in direct contact with conjunctiva (in place of spectacles) for therapeutic or cosmetic purposes. *contact tracer* a person, usually a nurse, who works from a genitourinary* clinic, and visits the people with whom the patient has had a sexual relationship (male or female) to encourage them to attend the clinic in an attempt to prevent the spread of sexually transmitted disease.

contagious *adj* capable of transmitting infection or of being transmitted.

containment isolation separation of a patient with any sort of

CONTINUING PROFESSIONAL DEVELOPMENT (CPD)

This is also referred to as Continuing Education (CE), and it can be thought of as lifelong learning, which embraces the acceptance of education occurring at all points in the lifespan. This implies, of course, that teaching methods appropriate to adult learners must be used, focusing on learning derived from experience, using a student-centred, needs-based approach. This approach allows the learner to set his or her own agenda and assess its success. It stresses active, rather than passive learning, frequently using peers as a source of knowledge.

It also embraces the linkage of education and work—the application of learning to practice and the notion that practice itself is not static. Alongside this is the acceptance that theory not only informs practice, but also that knowledge can be embedded in, and emerge from, practice.

Dynamic, changing practice is underpinned by education that is work-focused. The nature of work changes rapidly these days. The education that fits a practitioner for practice now will not be relevant in 5 years, let alone in 15. Practitioners need to be able to access knowledge and skills, and to develop attitudes to upgrade, consciously, systematically and continuously, their existing repertoire. CPD is a way of meeting this need for education 'on the job', and the UKCC, in *The Future of Professional Practice—the Council's Standards for Education and Practice following Registration*, has acknowledged that practitioners should be encouraged to undertake professional development additional to the statutory 5 days of study every 3 years.

infection to prevent spread of the condition to others. ⇒ exclusion isolation.

continuous ambulatory peritoneal dialysis (CAPD) the patient remains ambulant while on peritoneal dialysis*.

continuous positive airways pressure (CPAP) a method of assisted ventilation which applies a constant pressure of humidified gas to the airway during spontaneous inspiration; short term as ventilatory support, long term nocturnal domicillary as pneumatic splinting of upper airway to prevent closure on sleep apnoea*. It may be used as a means of weaning babies from ventilators, or as a way of treating babies with respiratory distress syndrome* who have a tendency to alveolar collapse.

Continuing Professional Development (CPD) ⇒ CPD box.

continuous subcutaneous insulin infusion (CSII) the use of a pump to deliver a continuous controlled dose of insulin subcutaneously to achieve almost physiological control of diabetes mellitus.

contraceptive *n, adj* describes an agent used to prevent conception, e.g. male or female condom, spermicidal vaginal pessary or cream, sponge, rubber cervical cap or diaphragm, intrauterine* device or emergency contraceptive. ⇒ coitus, combined oral contraceptive, postcoital—**contraception** *n.*

contract *vb* 1 draw together; shorten; decrease in size. 2 acquire by contagion or infection.

contractile *adj* possessing the ability to shorten usually when stimulated, special property of muscle tissue—**contractility** *n*.

contraction *n* shortening, especially applied to muscle fibres.

contracture *n* shortening of muscle or scar tissue, producing deformity ⇒ Dupuytren's contracture, Volkmann's ischaemic contracture.

contraindication *n* a sign or symptom suggesting that a certain line of treatment (usually used for that disease) should be discontinued or avoided.

contralateral *adj* on the opposite side—**contralaterally** *adv*.

contrecoup *n* injury or damage at a point opposite the impact, resulting from transmitted force. It can occur in an organ or part containing fluid, such as the skull.

controlled cord traction withdrawal of the placenta and membranes after birth by holding back the contracted uterus while applying traction to the umbilical cord. Forms part of the active management of the third stage of labour. May lead to acute uterine inversion if improperly performed.

controlled-dose transdermal absorption of drugs application of a drug patch to the skin: gradual absorption gives a constant level in the blood.

controlled drugs drugs which are defined in the UK Misuse of Drugs Act 1971.

control of infection use of domestic cleanliness, disinfection and sterilization to prevent the spread of infection. The most important contribution is by adequate handwashing before and/or after particular nursing activities. ⇒ barrier nursing, Infection Control Committee, Infection Control Nurse.

contusion *n* ⇒ bruise—**contuse** *vt*.

convalescence *n* the period after an illness before achievement of previous health status, or coping with a changed health status. ⇒ rehabilitation.

conversion *n* a psychological conflict* manifesting as a physical symptom.

conversion disorder a psychological disorder in which conflict is converted into physical symptoms, e.g. loss of sensation or blindness.

convolutions *npl* folds, twists or coils as found in the intestine, renal tubules and the surface of the brain—**convoluted** *adj*.

convulsions *npl* involuntary contractions of muscles resulting from abnormal cerebral stimulation: there are many causes. They occur with or without loss of consciousness. *tonic-clonic convulsions*, previously called grand mal convulsions or seizures, show alternating contraction and relaxation of muscle groups. Person becomes rigid, falls to the ground and jerks all over. *tonic convulsions* reveal sustained rigidity—**convulsive** *adj*.

convulsive therapy electroconvulsive* therapy.

Cooley's anaemia β thalassaemia major.

Coombs' test a highly sensitive test designed to detect antibodies to red blood cells: the 'direct' method detects those bound to the red cells; the 'indirect' method detects those circulating unbound in the serum. The 'direct' method is especially useful in the diagnosis of haemolytic syndromes.

coordination *n* moving in harmony. *muscular coordination* is the harmonious action of muscles, permitting free, smooth and efficient movements under perfect control.

coping the way in which a person deals with a circumstance which can be either negative or positive. The coping response can be negative, e.g. foregoing social activities because of increased frequency of micturition; or it can be positive, e.g. increasing one's level of physical exercise although confined to a wheelchair.

copper *n* essential trace element in all animal tissues, being a component of certain proteins and enzymes.

coprolalia *n* filthy or obscene speech. Occurs as a symptom most commonly in cerebral deterioration or trauma affecting frontal lobes of the brain.

coprolith *n* faecalith*.

coproporphyrin *n* naturally occurring porphyrin* in the faeces, formed in the intestine from bilirubin.

copulation *n* coitus*.

cord *n* a thread-like structure. *spermatic cord* that which suspends the testicles in the scrotum. *spinal cord* a cord-like structure which lies in the spinal column, reaching from the foramen magnum to the first or second lumbar vertebra. It is a direct continuation of the medulla oblongata and is about 45 cm long in the adult. *umbilical cord* the navel-string, attaching the fetus to the placenta. *vocal cord* the membranous bands in the larynx, vibrations of which produce the voice.

cordectomy *n* surgical excision of a cord, usually reserved for a vocal cord.

cordotomy *n* (*syn* chordotomy) division of the anterolateral nerves in the spinal cord to relieve intractable pain in the pelvis or lower limbs.

core *n* central portion, usually applied to the slough in the centre of a boil.

corn *n* a painful, cone-shaped overgrowth and hardening of the epidermis, with the point of the cone in the deeper layers; it is produced by friction or pressure. A *hard corn* usually occurs over a toe joint; a *soft corn* occurs between the toes.

cornea *n* the outwardly convex transparent membrane forming part of the anterior outer coat of the eye. It is situated in front of the iris and pupil and merges backwards into the sclera—**corneal** *adj*.

corneal graft (*syn* corneoplasty, keratoplasty) a corneal opacity is excised and replaced by healthy, transparent, human cornea from a donor.

corneoplasty *n* corneal* graft.

corneoscleral *adj* pertaining to the cornea and sclera, as the circular junction of these structures.

coronary *adj* crown-like; encircling, as of a vessel or nerve. *coronary arteries* those supplying the heart, the first pair to be given off by the aorta as it leaves the left ventricle. Spasm or narrowing of these vessels produces angina pectoris. *coronary sinus* channel receiving most cardiac veins and opening into the right atrium. *coronary thrombosis* occlusion of a coronary vessel by a clot of blood. The area deprived of blood becomes necrotic and is called an infarct*. ⇒ ischaemic heart disease, myocardial infarction.

coronaviruses *npl* a group of viruses that can cause acute respiratory illnesses.

coroner *n* in England and Wales, an officer of the Crown, usually a solicitor, barrister or doctor, who presides over the Coroner's Court responsible for determining the cause of unexpected or suspicious death. When doubt exists a doctor is advised to consult the Coroner and act on his advice. He must be notified if a patient is admitted to hospital and dies within 24 h. Likewise all theatre/anaesthetic deaths must be reported to the coroner. Any death, where the deceased has not consulted a doctor recently means that a coroner's postmortem will be ordered. In Scotland, reports about such deaths are submitted to the Procurator Fiscal but a postmortem is normally only ordered if foul play is suspected. The Scottish equivalent of the Coroner's Inquest is the Fatal Accident Enquiry, presided over by the Sheriff.

cor pulmonale heart disease following on disease of lung (emphysema*, silicosis*, etc.) which strains the right ventricle.

corpus *n* any mass of tissue which is easily distinguishable from its surroundings—**corpora** *pl. corpus luteum* ⇒ luteum.

corpuscle *n* a microscopic mass of protoplasm. There are many varieties but the word generally refers to the red and white blood cells—**corpuscular** *adj.* ⇒ erythrocytes, leucocytes.

corrective *adj, n* (something) which changes, counteracts or modifies something harmful.

cortex *n* **1** the outer bark or covering of a plant. **2** the outer layer of an organ beneath its capsule or membrane, as in the kidney or adrenal glands. *cerebral cortex* the grey matter covering the cerebrum. *renal cortex* the outer tissue of the kidney, underneath the renal capsule—**cortices** *pl*, **cortical** *adj.*

corticosteroids *npl* hormones produced by the adrenal cortex. The word is also used for synthetic steroids such as prednisolone* and dexamethasone*.

corticotrophin *n* the hormone of the anterior pituitary gland which specifically stimulates the adrenal cortex to produce corticosteroids. Synthetic 1–34 corticotrophin is available as tetracosactrin*, given by injection, usually for test purposes.

cortisol *n* hydrocortisone, one of the principal adrenal cortical steroids. It is increased in Cushing's disease and syndrome and decreased in Addison's disease. It is essential to life. It is given as physiological replacement treatment in Addison's disease and hypopituitarism. Synthetic steroids such as prednisolone* and dexamethasone* are usually used when larger doses are required for antiinflammatory or immunosuppressive purposes, e.g. in asthma, some skin conditions or following transplant surgery.

cortisone *n* one of the hormones of the adrenal gland. It is converted into cortisol* before use by the body. *cortisone suppression test* differentiates primary from secondary hypercalcaemia*. Sarcoidosis* causes secondary hypercalcaemia: primary hyperparathyroidism causes primary hypercalcaemia.

Corynebacterium *n* a bacterial genus: Gram-positive, rod-shaped bacteria averaging 3 μm in length, showing irregular staining in segments (metachromatic granules). Many strains are parasitic and some are pathogenic, e.g. *Corynebacterium diphtheriae,* producing a powerful exotoxin.

coryza *n* another name for the common cold. An acute upper respiratory infection of short duration; highly contagious; causative viruses include rhinoviruses, coronaviruses and adenoviruses. Since antibiotics are not antiviral, it is recommended that they are not prescribed.

cosmetic *adj, n* (that which is) done to improve the appearance or prevent disfigurement.

costal *adj* pertaining to the ribs. *costal cartilages* those which attach the ribs to the sternum.

cost effectiveness a measurement of the quantitative effectiveness of such things as surveillance programmes to detect breast cancer, cervical cancer, high blood pressure and testicular cancer in the early treatable stages. ⇒ clinical audit, Performance Indicators, quality assurance.

costive *adj* lay term for constipated. ⇒ constipation—**costiveness** *n.*

costochondral *adj* pertaining to a rib and its cartilage.

costochondritis *n* inflammation of the costochondral cartilage. ⇒ Tietze syndrome.

costoclavicular *adj* pertaining to the ribs and the clavicle. *costoclavicular syndrome* is a syonym for cervical rib syndrome ⇒ cervical.

cot death ⇒ sudden infant death syndrome.

cotyledon *n* one of the subdivisions of the uterine surface of the placenta*.

cough *n* explosive expulsion of air from the lungs as a voluntary or reflex action to expel a foreign body such as a crumb, mucus or sputum. A cough which achieves expulsion of sputum is said to be moist/productive. Patients who are at risk of chest infection postoperatively are taught to cough productively while supporting an abdominal wound with the palms of both hands. ⇒ postural drainage.

counselling *n* a professional helping relationship with a client who is experiencing psychological problems. The counsellor listens actively and helps the client to identify and clarify the problems and supports him as he makes a positive attempt to overcome them.

counterirritant *n* an agent which, when applied to the skin, produces a mild inflammatory reaction (hyperaemia) and relief of pain and congestion associated with a more deep-seated inflammatory process—**counterirritation** *n.*

countertraction *n* traction upon the proximal extremity of a fractured limb opposing the pull of the traction, necessary to prevent the whole body being pulled in the direction of the traction.

couvade *n* a custom in some cultures whereby a father exhibits the symptoms of his partner's pregnancy and childbirth.

Cowper's glands bulbourethral* glands.

coxa *n* the hip joint—**coxae** *pl. coxa valga* an increase in the normal angle between neck and shaft of femur. *coxa vara* a decrease in the normal angle plus torsion of the neck, e.g. slipped femoral epiphysis.

Coxiella *n* a genus closely related to *Rickettsia* including *Coxiella burneti* which causes Q fever.

coxitis *n* inflammation of the hip joint.

coxsackie viruses first isolated at Coxsackie, NY. One of the three groups included in the family of enteroviruses. Divided into groups A and B. Many in group A appear to be nonpathogenic. Others cause aseptic meningitis and herpangina. Those in group B also cause aseptic meningitis, Bornholm* disease and myocarditis.

CPAP *abbr* continuous* positive airways pressure.

CPK *abbr* creatinephosphokinase ⇒ creatine kinase.

CPN *abbr* Community Psychiatric Nurse.

CPR *abbr* cardiopulmonary resuscitation.

crab louse Pediculus* pubis.

cradle cap scaling of the scalp of infants, often due to atopic dermatitis* or seborrhoeic dermatitis.

cramp *n* spasmodic contraction of a muscle or group of muscles; involuntary and painful: may result from fatigue. Occurs in tetany, food poisoning and cholera. *occupational cramp* is such as occurs amongst certain groups of workers, e.g. miners.

cranial *adj* pertaining to the cranium*.

craniofacial *adj* pertaining to the cranium and the face. *craniofacial resection* a procedure which can be used in all age groups for the removal of paranasal sinus tumours, particularly those inaccessible through a usual nasal approach. It avoids the need for a total neurosurgical approach.

craniometry *n* the science which deals with the measurement of skulls.

craniopharyngioma *n* a tumour which develops between the brain and the pituitary gland.

cranioplasty *n* operative repair of a skull defect—**cranioplastic** *adj.*

craniosacral *adj* pertaining to the skull and sacrum. Applied to the parasympathetic nervous system.

craniostenosis *n* a condition in infancy in which the skull sutures fuse too early and the fontanelles close. It may cause increased intracranial pressure requiring surgery.

craniotabes *n* condition in which parts of the vortex of the skull are unusually soft and can be indented. May be found in newborn (usually preterm) infants, caused by delayed calcification; also associated with rickets*. Infants are otherwise normal—**craniotabetic** *adj.*

craniotomy *n* a surgical opening of the skull in order to remove a growth, relieve pressure, evacuate blood clot or arrest haemorrhage.

cranium *n* the part of the skull enclosing the brain. It is composed of eight bones: the occipital, two parietals, frontal, two temporals, sphenoid and ethmoid—**cranial** *adj.*

c-reactive protein test (CRP) c-reactive protein is a normal constituent of plasma: it is raised in bacterial meningitis.

creatinase *n* ⇒ creatine kinase.

creatine *n* a nitrogenous compound synthesized in vitro. *Phosphorylated creatine* is an important storage form of high-energy phosphate. *creatine kinase* (*syn* ATP: creatine phosphotransferase) occurs as three isoenzymes each having two components labelled M and B: the form in brain tissue is BB, in skeletal muscle and serum MM and in myocardial tissue both MM and MB. *creatine kinase test* the MB isoenzyme is raised in serum only in acute myocardial infarction and not in other cardiopathies.

creatinine *n* an anhydride of creatine*, a waste product of protein (endogenous) metabolism found in muscle and blood and excreted in normal urine.

creatinuria *n* an excess of the nitrogenous compound creatine* in the urine. Occurs in conditions in which muscle is rapidly broken down, e.g. acute fevers, starvation.

creatorrhoea *n* the presence of excessive nitrogen in the faeces. It occurs particularly in pancreatic dysfunction.

creosote *n* a phenolic antiseptic obtained from beechwood. Occasionally used as an antiseptic deodorant and expectorant.

crepitation *n* **1** (crepitus) grating of bone ends in fracture. **2** crackling sound in joints, e.g. in osteoarthritis. **3** crackling sound heard via stethoscope. **4** crackling sound elicited by pressure on tissue containing air (surgical emphysema).

cresol *n* chemically related to phenol* but it is a more powerful germicide. Cresol and/or related phenols are present in a wide range of general disinfectants.

cretinism *n* due to congenital thyroid deficiency; results in a dull-looking child, underdeveloped mentally and physically, dwarfed, large head, thick legs, pug nose, dry skin, scanty hair, swollen eyelids, short neck, short thick limbs, clumsy uncoordinated gait—**cretin** *n*.

Creutzfeldt-Jakob disease (CJD) form of progressive dementia transmissable through prion protein. Possibly linked with bovine prion of spongiform encephalopathy.

CRF *abbr* chronic renal failure. ⇒ renal.

cribriform *adj* perforated, like a sieve. *cribriform plate* that portion of the ethmoid bone allowing passage of fibres of olfactory nerve.

cricoid *adj* ring-shaped. Applied to the cartilage forming the inferior posterior part of larynx.

'cri du chat' syndrome produced by partial loss of one of the number 5 chromosomes leading to learning disability. There are certain physical abnormalities and a curious flat, toneless, catlike cry in infancy.

criminal abortion ⇒ abortion.

crisis *n* the turning point of a disease such as the point of defervescence in fever or the arrest of an anaemia. ⇒ lysis *opp*—**crises** *pl. crisis intervention* a problem-solving method to correct, or prevent the continuance of a crisis such as poisoning or suicide. *Dietl's crisis* severe kidney pain (nephralgia) caused by obstruction of the ureter.

Crohn's disease ⇒ regional ileitis.

Crosby capsule a special tube which is passed through the mouth to the small intestine; manoeuvre of the tube selects tissue for biopsy.

cross infection ⇒ infection.

croup *n* laryngeal obstruction. Croupy breathing in a child is often called 'stridulous', meaning noisy or harsh-sounding. Narrowing of the airway which gives rise to the typical attack with crowing inspiration may be the result of oedema or spasm, or both.

CRP *abbr* ⇒ c-reactive protein test.

cruciate *adj* shaped like a cross.

'crush' syndrome traumatic uraemia. Following an extensive trauma to muscle, there is a period of delay before the effects of renal damage manifest themselves. There is an increase of nonprotein nitrogen in the blood, with oliguria, proteinuria and urinary excretion of myohaemoglobin. Loss of blood plasma to damaged area is marked. Where hypotension has occurred the renal failure will be exacerbated by tubular* necrosis.

crutch palsy paralysis* of extensor muscles of wrist, fingers and thumb from repeated pressure of a crutch upon the radial nerve in the axilla.

cryaesthesia *n* **1** the sensation of coldness. **2** exceptional sensitivity to a low temperature.

cryoanalgesia *n* relief of pain achieved by use of a cryosurgical probe to block peripheral nerve function.

cryoextractor *n* a type of cryoprobe* used for removal of a cataractous lens.

cryogenic *adj, n* (anything) produced by low temperature. Also used to describe any means or apparatus involved in the production of low temperature.

cryoglobulins *npl* serum protein immunoglobulins which precipitate at low temperatures and are associated with diseases.

cryopexy *n* surgical fixation by freezing, as replacement of a detached retina.

cryophake *n* cataract extraction using freezing.

cryoprecipitate therapy use of factor VIII to prevent or treat bleeding in haemophilia. The term refers to the preparation of factor VIII for injection. Subarctic temperatures make it separate from plasma. ⇒ blood clotting.

cryoprobe *n* freezing probe. Can be used for biopsy. A flexible metal tube attached to liquid nitrogen equipment. The cryoprobe has tips of various sizes which can be cooled to a temperature of −180°C. Causes less tissue trauma and 'seeding' of malignant cells.

cryosurgery *n* the use of intense, controlled cold to remove or destroy diseased tissue. Instead of a knife or guillotine a cryoprobe* is used.

cryothalamectomy *n* freezing applied to destroy groups of neurones within the thalamus in the treatment of Parkinson's disease and other hyperkinetic conditions.

cryotherapy *n* the use of cold for the treatment of disease.

cryptococcosis *n* the disease resulting from infection with the yeast *Cryptococcus neoformans,* which occurs in soil and pigeon droppings. It affects the lungs, skin, bones and meninges. Meningitis is the most frequent manifestation.

Cryptococcus *n* a genus of fungi. *Cryptococcus neoformans* is pathogenic to man.

cryptogenic *adj* of unknown or obscure cause.

cryptomenorrhoea *n* retention of the menses due to a congenital obstruction, such as an imperforate hymen or atresia of the vagina. ⇒ haematocolpos.

cryptorchism *n* a developmental defect whereby the testes do not descend into the scrotum; they are retained within the abdomen or inguinal canal—**cryptorchid, cryptorchis** *n.*

crystallin *n* a globulin*, principal constituent of the lens of the eye.

crystalline *adj* like a crystal; transparent. Applied to various structures. *crystalline lens* a biconvex body, oval in shape, which is suspended just behind the iris of the eye, and separates the aqueous from the vitreous humor. It is slightly less convex on its anterior surface and it refracts the light rays so that they focus directly on to the retina.

CSF *abbr* cerebrospinal* fluid.

crystal violet *n* (*syn* gentian violet) a brilliant, violet-coloured, antiseptic aniline dye, used as 0.5% solution for ulcers and skin infections and also as a stain.

CSII *abbr* continuous* subcutaneous insulin infusion.

CSSD *abbr* central* sterile supplies department.

CSSU *abbr* central sterile supply unit. ⇒ Central Sterile Supplies Department, hospital sterilization and disinfection unit.

CT *abbr* computed* tomography.

CTG *abbr* cardiotocograph*.

cubital tunnel external compression syndrome ulnar paralysis* resulting from compression of the ulnar nerve within the cubital tunnel situated on the inner and posterior aspects of the elbow sometimes referred to as the 'funny bone'.

cubitus *n* the forearm; elbow—**cubital** *adj.*

cue *n* in the context of communicating, a verbal or nonverbal signal from another person which is perceived by the observer to warrant sensitive exploration (by prompting or reflection) as to its meaning for the person exhibiting it.

cuirass *n* a now rare mechanical breast plate-like apparatus fitted to the chest for artificial negative pressure respiration.

culdocentesis *n* aspiration of the pouch* of Douglas via the posterior vaginal wall.

culdoscope *n* an endoscope* used via the vaginal route.

culdoscopy *n* passage of an endoscope* through the posterior vaginal fornix, behind the uterus to enter the peritoneal cavity, for viewing of the rectovaginal pouch—**culdoscopic** *adj,* **culdoscopically** *adv.*

culture *n* 1 the growth of micro-organisms on artificial media under ideal conditions. 2 the attitudes, beliefs, ideas, knowledge, practices and values which members of different groups hold about themselves, and which inform the total behaviour of a group.

cumulative action if the dose of a slowly excreted drug is repeated too frequently, an increasing action is obtained. This can be dangerous as, if the drug accumulates in the system, toxic symptoms may occur, sometimes quite suddenly. Long acting barbiturates, strychnine, mercurial salts and digitalis are examples of drugs with a cumulative action.

cupping *n* a method of counter-irritation. A small bell-shaped glass (in which the air is expanded by heating, or exhausted by compression of an attached rubber bulb) is applied to the skin, resultant suction producing hyperaemia *dry cupping.* When the skin is scarified before application of the cup it is termed *wet cupping.*

curettage *n* the scraping of unhealthy or exuberant tissue from a cavity. This may be as treatment or to establish a diagnosis through laboratory analysis of the scrapings.

curette *n* a spoon-shaped instrument or a metal loop which may have sharp and/or blunt edges for scraping out (curetting) cavities.

curettings *npl* the material obtained by scraping or curetting and usually sent for examination in the pathology department.

curie *n* a measure of the radioactivity of a substance. Now replaced by the becquerel*.

Curling's ulcer an ulcer* which occurs either in the stomach or duodenum as a complication of extensive burns or scalds.

CUSA *abbr* Cavitron* ultrasonic surgical aspirator.

cushingoid *adj* used to describe the moon face and central obesity common in people with elevated levels of plasma corticosteroid from whatever cause.

Cushing's disease a rare disorder, mainly of females, characterized principally by functional obesity, hyperglycaemia, glycosuria, hypertension and hirsutism. Due to excessive cortisol production by hyperplastic adrenal glands as a result of increased corticotrophin secretion by a tumour or hyperplasia of the anterior pituitary gland.

Cushing's reflex a rise in blood pressure and a fall in pulse rate; occurs in cerebral space-occupying lesions.

Cushing's syndrome a disorder clinically similar to Cushing's* disease and also due to elevated levels of plasma corticosteroid, but where the primary pathology is not in the pituitary gland. It can be due to adenoma or carcinoma of the adrenal cortex and to the secretion of ACTH* by nonendocrine tumours such as bronchial carcinoma. It can also be iatrogenic* due to excessive administration of corticosteroids.

cusp *n* a projecting point, such as the edge of a tooth or the segment of a heart valve. The cardiac tricuspid valve has three, the mitral valve two cusps.

cutaneous *adj* relating to the skin. *cutaneous ureterostomy* the ureters are transplanted so that they open on to the skin of the abdominal wall.

cuticle *n* the epidermis* or dead epidermis, as that which surrounds a nail—**cuticular** *adj.*

CVA *abbr* cerebrovascular* accident.

CVP *abbr* central* venous pressure.
CVS *abbr* ⇒ chorionic villus biopsy.
cyanocobalamin *n* vitamin* B_{12} (antianaemic factor), found in liver, fish, meat and eggs. Needed for maturation of erythrocytes. It can only be absorbed in the presence of the intrinsic* factor secreted in the gastric juice. ⇒ cobalamin.
cyanosis *n* a bluish or purple colouration of the skin and mucous membranes due to insufficient oxygen and excess carbon dioxide in the blood—**cyanosed, cyanotic** *adj.*
cyclical syndrome some people prefer this term to that of premenstrual* syndrome.
cyclical vomiting periodic attacks of vomiting in children, usually associated with ketosis and usually with no demonstrable pathological cause. Occurs mainly in highly-strung children Recovery is usually spontaneous; in some cases, dehydration can occur.
cyclitis *n* inflammation of the ciliary body of the eye, shown by deposition of small collections of white cells on the posterior cornea called 'keratitic precipitates' (KP). Often coexistent with inflammation of the iris. ⇒ iridocyclitis.
cycloplegia *n* paralysis of the ciliary muscle of the eye—**cycloplegic** *adj.*
cycloplegics *npl* drugs which cause paralysis of the ciliary muscle, e.g. atropine, homatropine, scopolamine and lachesine.
cyclothymia *n* a tendency to alternating but relatively mild mood swings between elation and depression—**cyclothymic** *adj.*
cyclotron *n* an apparatus in which radioactive isotopes can be prepared.
cyesis *n* pregnancy. When there are signs and symptoms of pregnancy in a woman who believes she is pregnant, and this is not so, it is called pseudocyesis. ⇒ phantom pregnancy.
cyst *n* a sac with membranous wall, enclosing fluid or semisolid matter—**cystic** *adj.*
cystadenoma *n* a cystic growth of glandular epithelium. Liable to occur in the female breast or ovary.
cystathioninuria *n* inherited disorder of cystathionine metabolism marked by excessive excretion of cystathionine in the urine, an intermediate product in conversion of methionine to cysteine. Associated with learning disabilities, Marfan-like syndrome and thrombotic episodes.
cystectomy *n* usually refers to the removal of part or the whole of the urinary bladder. This necessitates urinary diversion. The ureters may then be implanted into an isolated ileal segment (ileal conduit) or into the sigmoid colon.
cysteine *n* a sulphur-containing amino acid produced by the breaking down of proteins during the digestive process. Easily oxidized to cystine*.
cysticercosis *n* infection of man with cysticercus*.
cysticercus *n* the larval form of Taenia*. After ingestion, the ova do not develop beyond this form in man, but form 'cysts' in subcutaneous tissues, skeletal muscles and the brain where they provoke epilepsy.
cystic fibrosis (CF) (*syn* fibrocystic disease of the pancreas, mucoviscidosis) the commonest genetically-determined disease in Caucasian populations; there is abnormality of secretion of the exocrine glands. Thick mucus can block the intestinal glands and cause meconium ileus in a baby; later it can cause steatorrhoea, creatorrhoea and malabsorption. Thick mucus in the

respiratory glands predisposes to repeated infections and bronchiectasis. Improved treatment involving intensive antibiotic therapy and nutritional support means many children with CF now survive into early adulthood and beyond. Abnormality of the sweat glands increases the chloride content of sweat which is a diagnostic tool. ⇒ sweat test.

cystine *n* a sulphur-containing amino acid, produced by the breakdown of proteins during the digestive process. It is readily reduced to two molecules of cysteine*.

cystinosis *n* a recessively inherited metabolic disorder in which crystalline cystine* is deposited in the body. Cystine and other amino acids are excreted in the urine.

cystinuria *n* metabolic disorder in which cystine* and other amino acids appear in the urine. A cause of renal stones—**cystinuric** *adj.*

cystitis *n* inflammation of the urinary bladder; the cause is usually bacterial. The condition may be acute or chronic, primary or secondary to stones, etc. More frequent in females.

cystocele *n* prolapse of the posterior wall of the urinary bladder into the anterior vaginal wall. ⇒ colporrhaphy.

cystodiathermy *n* the application of a cauterizing electrical current to the walls of the urinary bladder through a cystoscope, or by open operation.

cystography *n* radiographic examination of the urinary bladder, after it has been filled with a contrast medium. ⇒ micturating cystogram.—**cystographic** *adj,* **cystogram** *n,* **cystographically** *adv.*

cystolithiasis *n* the presence of a stone or stones in the urinary bladder.

cystometrogram *n* a record of the changes in pressure within the urinary bladder under various conditions; used in the study of bladder dysfunction.

cystometry *n* the study of pressure changes within the urinary bladder—**cystometric** *adj.*

cystoplasty *n* surgical repair of the urinary bladder—**cystoplastic** *adj.*

cystoscope *n* an endoscope* used in diagnosis and treatment of bladder, ureter and kidney conditions—**cystoscopic** *adj,* **cystoscopically** *adv.*

cystoscopy *n* use of a cystoscope* to view the internal surface of the urinary bladder. It can also incorporate a biopsy or fulguration of a bladder tumour.

cystostomy *n* (*syn* vesicostomy) an operation whereby a fistulous opening is made into the urinary bladder via the abdominal wall. Usually the fistula can be allowed to heal when its purpose has been achieved.

cystotomy *n* incision into the urinary bladder via the abdominal wall; often done to remove a large stone or tumour or to gain access to the prostate gland in the operation of transvesical prostatectomy*.

cystourethritis *n* inflammation of the urinary bladder and urethra.

cystourethrography *n* radiographic examination of the urinary bladder and urethra, after the introduction of a contrast medium—**cystourethrographic** *adj,* **cystourethrograph** *n,* **cystourethrographically** *adv.*

cystourethropexy *n* forward fixation of the urinary bladder and upper urethra in an attempt to combat incontinence of urine.

cytodiagnosis *n* diagnosis by the microscopic study of cells—**cytodiagnostic** *adj.*

cytogenetics *n* The science concerned with the study of normal and abnormal chromosomes, and of their behaviour. In man a person's chromosomes can be studied by culture techniques, using either lymphocytes or a piece of tissue such as skin, or cells such as those of the amniotic fluid (fetal cells). Chromosome abnormalities of either number or make-up (structure) can be associated with physical and mental disorder or with spontaneous abortion or stillbirth—**cytogenesis** *n.*

cytology *n* the microscopic study of cells. The term *exfoliative cytology* is used when the cells studied have been shed, or exfoliated, from the surface of an organ or lesion—**cytological** *adj.*

cytolysis *n* the degeneration, destruction, disintegration or dissolution of cells—**cytolytic** *adj.*

cytomegalovirus *n* belongs to the same group of viruses as herpes simplex. Can cause latent and symptomless infection. Virus excreted in urine and saliva. Congenital infection is the most severe form of *cytomegalovirus infection.* Can infect the fetus in utero, sometimes causing microcephaly, intracranial calcification and mental defect, or an illness at birth characterized by hepatosplenomegaly and thrombocytopenia. Infection can also be transmitted by blood transfusion, especially in patients with impaired immunity, in whom it causes a glandular fever-like illness and pneumonia.

cytopathic *adj* pertaining to abnormality of the living cell.

cytoplasm *n* (*syn* protoplasm) the protoplasm* of a cell surrounding the nucleus—**cytoplasmic** *adj.*

cytostasis *n* arrest or hindrance of cell development—**cytostatic** *adj.*

cytotoxic *adj* any substance which is toxic to cells. Applied to the drugs used for the treatment of carcinomas and the reticuloses. Two main groups: (a) antimetabolites which block action of an enzyme system, e.g. methotrexate, fluorouracil, mercaptopurine (b) alkylating agents which poison cells directly, e.g. cyclophosphamide, mustine. There are known and potential dangers while handling cytotoxic drugs: dermatitis, nasal sores, pigmentation of the skin, blisters and excessive lacrimation have been reported.

cytotoxins *npl* antibodies which are toxic to cells.

D

D and C *abbr* dilatation* and curettage.

Da Costa syndrome cardiac neurosis. An anxiety* state in which palpitations and left-sided chest pain are the most prominent symptoms.

dacry(o)adenitis *n* inflammation of a lacrimal gland. It is a rare condition which may be acute or chronic. May occur in mumps*.

dacryocyst *n* an old term for the lacrimal sac (tear sac). The word is still used in its compound forms.

dacryocystectomy *n* excision of any part of the lacrimal sac.

dacryocystitis *n* inflammation of the lacrimal sac, which usually results in abscess formation and obliteration of the tear duct, giving rise to epiphora*.

dacryocystography *n* radiographic examination of the tear drainage apparatus after it has been rendered radiopaque—**dacryocystographic** *adj*, **dacryocystographically** *adv*.

dacryocystorhinostomy *n* (*syn* Toti's operation) an operation to establish drainage from the lacrimal sac into the nose when there is obstruction of the nasolacrimal duct.

dacryolith *n* a concretion in the lacrimal passages.

dactyl *n* a digit, finger or toe—**dactylar, dactylate** *adj*.

dactylitis *n* inflammation of finger or toe. The digit becomes swollen due to periostitis. Met with in congenital syphilis, tuberculosis, etc.

dactylology *n* finger spelling. A form of communication used with people with hearing impairment. Can be used in conjunction with British Sign Language.

daltonism *n* red/green colour* blindness.

dandruff *n* (*syn* scurf) the common scaly condition of the scalp. May be the forerunner of skin diseases of the seborrhoeic type, such as flexural dermatitis.

dandy fever dengue*.

data *npl* pieces of information, usually collected for a specific purpose. In clinical nursing, data which are requested on the patient assessment form are collected at an initial interview with the patient. Other data are collected by ongoing assessment and evaluation.—**datum** *sing*.

data analysis data collected at the initial interview are analysed, with the patient when possible, to identify the patient* problems (actual or potential) which are being experienced in everyday living that are amenable to nursing intervention. The cause may or may not be the medical diagnosis.

data base the term is used in two ways in nursing. The data collected at the initial interview is referred to as base data in that nurses record the patient's status on the day of admission, against which evaluation can reveal whether there is improvement/no change/deterioration; increased, decreased, or no change in dependence/independence and so on. In a wider context, all patients' nursing data, or those collected about a specific group of patients, can be analysed retrospectively to identify further knowledge about nursing.

data collection data can be collected by interviewing, during which a structured form such as a patient assessment form may be used. In some circumstances an unstructured interview might be appropriate. The data are referred to as subjective or soft data. The nurse as a skilled interviewer prompts and reflects so that the patient describes his condition as factually as possible. The nurse records the information as factually as possible to decrease bias. Other data are the result of measurement, e.g. the amount of urine passed in 24 h; and yet others are the result of testing, e.g. urine, and these are called objective or hard data.

dawn phenomenon early morning hyperglycaemia; it does not result from the waning of subcutaneously injected insulin and has been found in nondiabetic subjects, as well as those with insulin dependent diabetes mellitus, and noninsulin dependent diabetes mellitus. Large surges of growth hormone (GH) secretion have been implicated in the pathogenesis of the phenomenon. ⇒ Somogyi phenomenon.

day centre a centre which people attend for 1, 2 or more days weekly. Recreational and occupational therapy and physiotherapy or other services as appropriate are provided. Greatest use is in the psychiatric and geriatric fields.

day surgery patients are admitted for surgery but discharged home the same day. The practice is increasingly common, especially with children. Ideally, patients are admitted to a specialized day surgery unit but some day admissions are cared for on a general ward.

DBH *abbr* dopamine*-8-hydroxylase.

deafness *n* a partial or complete loss of hearing. *conductive deafness* is due to an obstruction which prevents the conduction of sound waves from the atmosphere to the inner ear. *perceptive* or *nerve deafness* is due to a lesion in the inner ear, the auditory nerve or the auditory centres in the brain. *congenital deafness* can be caused by the mother contracting rubella in early pregnancy. ⇒ body language, finger spelling, sign language.

deamination *n* removal of the amino group from organic compounds such as amino acids.

death *n* cessation of the body's vital functions usually assessed by the absence of a pulse and breathing. Death may be immediate and unexpected as when a child is killed in an accident; it can be sudden and unexpected, e.g. a person collapses and within 24 hours is dead: death can be expected because of the medical diagnosis, but in the end it can occur suddenly, or a person can be terminally ill for a period varying from a few days to several weeks or months. Nowadays mechanical ventilation can maintain vital functions despite brain stem damage; consequently stringent tests are necessary to diagnose death. ⇒ coroner. *biological death* death of tissues. ⇒ gangrene. *brain death* a new concept used when the brain stem is fatally and irreversibly damaged. In different countries, different criteria are used to diagnose brain death. *clinical death* death of the person. *neonatal death* the baby is born alive but dies within 28 days.

debility *n* a condition of weakness with lack of muscle tone.

debridement *n* the removal of foreign matter and injured or infected tissue from a wound. *chemical/medical debridement* is accomplished by the external application of a substance to the wound. *surgical debridement* is accomplished by using surgical instruments and aseptic technique.

decalcification *n* the removal of mineral salts, as from teeth in dental caries, or bone in disorders of calcium metabolism.

decannulation *n* the removal of a cannula, especially a tracheostomy tube. May need to be done on a controlled and gradual basis if the patient has difficulty in adjusting to normal breathing.

decapsulation *n* the surgical removal of a capsule.

decerebrate *adj* without cerebral function; a state of deep unconsciousness. *decerebrate posture* a condition of the unconscious patient in which all four limbs are spastic and which indicates severe damage to the cerebrum.

decidua *n* the endometrial lining of the uterus thickened and altered for the reception of the fertilized ovum. It is shed when pregnancy terminates. *decidua basalis* that part which lies under the embedded ovum and forms the maternal part of the placenta. *decidua capsularis* that part that lies over the developing ovum. *decidua vera* the decidua lining the rest of the uterus—**decidual** *adj.*

deciduous *adj* by custom refers to the primary (or milk) teeth which on shedding are normally replaced by permanent teeth.

decision-making *n* in nursing decision-making by both nurses and patients is becoming increasingly overt as patient participation in care and care planning is increasingly encouraged. The concept of informed* consent acknowledges the patient's right to make decisions.

decompensation *n* a failure of compensation usually referring to heart disease.

decompression *n* removal of pressure or a compressing force. *decompression of brain* achieved by trephining the skull. *decompression of bladder* in cases of chronic urinary retention, by continuous or intermittent drainage via catheter inserted per urethra. *decompression chamber* used when returning deep-sea divers to the surface. ⇒ caisson disease.

deconditioning eliminating an unwanted particular response to a particular stimulus ⇒ aversion therapy, conditioning.

decongestants *npl* agents which reduce or eliminate congestion, usually referring to nasal congestion. They can be taken by mouth, or they can be applied locally as drops or sprays.

decongestion *n* relief of congestion—**decongestive** *adj.*

decortication *n* surgical removal of cortex or outer covering of an organ. *decortication of lung* carried out when thickening of the visceral pleura prevents reexpansion of lung as may occur in chronic empyema. The visceral pleura is peeled off the lung, which is then reexpanded by positive pressure through an anaesthetic apparatus.

decubitus *n* the recumbent position; lying down. *decubitus ulcer* ⇒ pressure sore—**decubiti** *pl,* **decubital** *adj.*

decussation *n* intersection; crossing of nerve fibres at a point beyond their origin, as in the optic and pyramidal tracts.

deep vein thrombosis (DVT) phlebothrombosis* ⇒ intermittent pneumatic compression, pulmonary.

defaecation *n* voluntary intermittent voiding per anus of faeces previously stored in the rectum.

defaecatory system comprises the large bowel, rectum, anal canal and anus.

defence mechanisms ⇒ body defence mechanisms.

defervescence *n* the time during which a fever is declining. If the body temperature falls rapidly it is spoken of as 'crisis'; if it falls slowly the term 'lysis' is used.

defibrillation *n* the arrest of fibrillation* of the cardiac muscle (atrial or ventricular), and restoration of normal cycle, usually by electrical countershock—**defibrillate** *vt.*

defibrillator *n* any agent, e.g. an electric shock, which arrests ventricular fibrillation* and restores normal rhythm.

defibrinated *adj* rendered free from fibrin*. A necessary process in the preparation of serum from whole blood. ⇒ blood—**defibrinate** *v.*

deficiency disease disease resulting from dietary deficiency of any substance essential for good health, especially the vitamins.

degeneration *n* deterioration in quality or function. Regression from more specialized to less specialized type of tissue—**degenerative** *adj,* **degenerate** *vi.*

deglutition *n* the process of swallowing, partly voluntary, partly involuntary.

dehiscence *n* the process of splitting or bursting open, as of a wound.

dehydration *n* loss or removal of fluid. In the body this condition arises when the fluid intake fails to replace fluid loss. This is liable to occur when there is bleeding, diarrhoea, excessive exudation from a raw area, excessive sweating, polyuria or vomiting, and usually upsets the body's electrolyte balance. If suitable fluid replacement cannot be achieved orally then parenteral administration must be instituted ⇒ oral—**dehydrate** *vt, vi.*

deja vu phenomenon occurs in epilepsy involving temporal lobes of the brain and in certain epileptic dream states. An intense feeling of familiarity as if everything had happened before.

Delhi boil ⇒ oriental sore.

deliberate self-harm (DSH) ⇒ parasuicide.

delirium *n* abnormal mental condition based on hallucinations or illusion. May occur in high fever, in mental disease, or be toxic in origin. *delirium tremens* results from alcoholic intoxication and is represented by a picture of confusion, terror, restlessness and hallucinations—**delirious** *adj.*

delta agent a deadly virus which has been found in people who carry the virus of hepatitis B. It can be spread by sharing an infected needle, sexual contact, kissing or spitting.

deltoid *adj* triangular. *deltoid muscle* covers the shoulder joint and is inserted into the mid-humerus.

delusion *n* a false belief, inconsistent with the individual's culture, use and level of intelligence, which cannot be altered by argument or reasoning. Found as a psychotic symptom in several types of mental illness, notably schizophrenia, paraphrenia, paranoia, senile psychoses, mania and depressive states.

demarcation *n* an outlining of the junction of diseased and healthy tissue, often used when referring to gangrene.

dementia *n* (*syn* organic brain syndrome, OBS) an irreversible organic brain disease causing memory and personality disorders, deterioration in personal care, impaired cognitive ability and disorientation. ⇒ Creutzfeldt-Jakob disease. *presenile dementia* signs and symptoms of dementia occurring in people between 40 and 60 years of age due to early hyaline degeneration of both the medium and small cerebral blood vessels. ⇒ Alzheimer's disease, Pick's disease.

demography *n* the study of population.

demulcent *n* a slippery, mucilaginous fluid which allays irritation and soothes inflammation, especially of mucous membranes.

demyelinization *n* destruction of the myelin* sheaths surrounding nerve fibres; occurs in multiple sclerosis.

dendrite *n* (*syn* dendron) one of the branched filaments which are given off from the body of a nerve cell. That part of a neurone which transmits an impulse to the nerve cell—**dendritic** *adj.*

dendritic ulcer a linear corneal ulcer that sends out tree-like branches. Caused by herpes simplex. Treated with idoxuridine.

dendron *n* ⇒ dendrite.

denervation *n* the means by which a nerve supply is cut off. Usually refers to incision, excision or blocking of a nerve.

dengue *n* (*syn* 'break-bone fever') one of the mosquito*-transmitted haemorrhagic fevers, a disease of the tropics. Causative agent is an arbovirus conveyed by a mosquito. Characterized by rheumatic pains, fever and a skin eruption. The haemorrhagic form has a high mortality.

denial *n* a complex unconscious mental* defence mechanism in which anxiety and emotional conflict are avoided by refusing to acknowledge the changed circumstances, e.g. sudden incapacitating illness, impending loss of part of the body, or terminal illness. Psychological support provided by nurses can help the patient gradually to bear the reality in consciousness, and begin planning to cope. Recognized as one of the phases of the grieving* process.

Denis Browne splints splints used to correct congenital talipes equinovarus (club*-foot). The splints are of metal padded with felt, with a joining bar to which the baby's feet are strapped.

dental amalgam ⇒ amalgam.

dental plaque *n* noncalcified deposit on the surface of a tooth composed of a soft mass of bacteria and cellular debris which accumulates rapidly in the absence of oral hygiene.

dentate *adj* having own teeth present.

dentine *n* the calcified tissue forming the body of the tooth beneath the enamel and cementum enclosing the pulp chamber and root canals.

dentition *n* refers to the teeth. In man the primary or deciduous* teeth are called *primary dentition* and are normally 20 in number. The adult, permanent teeth are called the *secondary dentition,* and are normally 32 in number.

denture *n* a removable dental prosthesis* containing one or several teeth, or maybe a complete upper or lower denture.

DEO *abbr* Disability* Employment Officer.

deodorants *npl* in a medical context, substances which are used to reduce malodour in infected wounds: describes diverse substances such as calcium alginate; icing sugar which prevents the invasion of bacteria; lactic acid bacilli contained in natural live yoghurt; metronidazole and Neutradol. ⇒ Lyofoam C.

deoxycortone acetate (DOCA) an important hormone of the adrenal cortex, controlling the metabolism of sodium and potassium. Previously used mainly in the management of Addison's disease.

deoxygenation *n* the removal of oxygen—**deoxygenated** *adj.*

deoxyribonucleic acid (DNA) a nucleic acid molecule found in the chromosomes of all organisms (except some viruses) which carries genetic information. It consists of two polynucleotide chains containing phosphate and deoxyribose (a sugar), and linked by hydrogen bonds between the complementary bases (adenine and thymine, or cytosine and guanine).

dependence *n* **1** the level of reliance a person has on others for activities* of daily living. ⇒ dependency. **2** on a drug or chemical substance. Characterized by a compulsion to continue taking the substance and often the presence of specific symptoms if the drug is withdrawn.

dependency *n* a measure of the level of nursing care a patient will require. Used to calculate how many nursing staff will be required for a particular group of patients. *high dependency unit* where patients who need a high level of nursing care, but not necessarily in an intensive* therapy unit, may be nursed.

depersonalization *n* a subjective feeling of having lost one's personality, sometimes that one no longer exists. Occurs in schizophrenia and more rarely in depressive states.

depilate *vt* to remove hair from—**depilatory** *adj, n,* **depilation** *n.*

depilatories *npl* substances usually made in pastes (e.g. barium sulphide) which temporarily remove excess hair; they do not act on the papillae, consequently the hair grows again. ⇒ epilation—**depilatory** *sing. preoperative depilation* lessens the risk of wound infection because it is nonabrasive.

depot *n* a body area in which a substance, usually a drug, can be deposited or stored, and from which it can be distributed. *depot injections* preparations given by deep intramuscular injection, usually of a psychotrophic drug, used when clients fail to take their medications regularly.

depression *n* **1** a hollow place or indentation. **2** diminution of power or activity. **3** a common psychiatric disorder. It may be described as *reactive,* usually occurring in response to loss or some other stressful event; or *endogenous,* which is more severe and occurs without apparent cause. Depression is diagnosed when lowered mood, loss of interest and pleasure and four or more of the following symptoms are present: feelings of worthlessness or guilt, impaired concentration, loss of energy and fatigue, suicidal thoughts, loss (or increase) of appetite and weight, sleep disturbances, general slowing down or agitation. *unipolar (UP) depression* is characterized only by feelings of depression. *bipolar (BP) depression* (manic depression) coexists with episodes of hypomania*, possibly accompanied by hostility, irritability and, in extreme cases, delusions and hallucinations. The main methods of management of depression are with drugs ⇒ antidepressants, and, in severe cases, electroconvulsive* therapy. ⇒ seasonal affective disorder (SAD).

Derbyshire neck goitre*.

derealization *n* feelings that people, events or surroundings have changed and are unreal. Similar sensations may occur in normal people during dreams. May sometimes be found in schizophrenia and depressive states.

dereistic *adj* of thinking, not adapted to reality. Describes autistic thinking.

dermabrasion *n* ⇒ abrasion.

dermatitis *n* inflammation of the skin (by custom limited to an eczematous reaction). ⇒ eczema. *atopic dermatitis* that variety of infantile eczema which may be associated with asthma or hay fever. *dermatitis herpetiformis* (*syn* hydroa) an intensely itchy skin eruption of unknown cause, most commonly characterized by vesicles, bullae and pustules on urticarial plaques, which remit and relapse. Associated with gluten-sensitive enteropathy. *juvenile dermatitis herpetiformis* recurrent bullous eruption on the genitalia, lower abdomen, buttocks and face, mainly in children under 5 years, boys being affected more than girls. *occupational dermatitis* occurs as a result of handling some sensitizing agent while at work.

dermatoglyphics *n* study of the ridge patterns of the skin of the fingertips, palms and soles to discover developmental anomalies.

dermatographia *n* ⇒ dermographia.

dermatologist *n* one who studies skin diseases and is skilled in their treatment. A skin specialist.

dermatology *n* the study of the skin, its structure, functions, diseases and their treatment—**dermatological** *adj*, **dermatologically** *adv*.

dermatome *n* an instrument for cutting slices of skin of varying thickness, usually for grafting.

dermatomycosis *n* a fungal infection of the skin—**dermatomycotic** *adj*.

dermatomyositis *n* an acute inflammation of the skin and muscles which presents with oedema and muscle weakness. May result in the atrophic changes of scleroderma*. ⇒ collagen.

dermatophytes *npl* a group of fungi which invade the superficial skin.

dermatophytosis *n* infection of the skin with dermatophyte species.

dermatosis *n* generic term for skin disease—**dermatoses** *pl*.

dermis *n* the true skin; the cutis vera; the layer below the epidermis—**dermal** *adj*.

dermographia *n* (*syn* dermatographia, factitial urticaria) a condition in which weals occur on the skin after a blunt instrument or fingernail has been lightly drawn over it. Seen in vasomotor instability and urticaria—**dermographic** *adj*.

dermoid *adj* pertaining to or resembling skin. *dermoid cyst* a cyst* which is congenital in origin and usually occurs in the ovary. It contains elements of hair, nails, skin, teeth, etc.

desensitization *n* **1** injection of antigens* to diminish or cancel out hypersensitivity to insect venoms, drugs, pollen and other causes of acute hypersensitivity reactions. **2** of phobic patients, using intravenous methohexitone sodium to achieve psychological relaxation. In this state the phobic situation is imagined without fear and the patient 'unlearns' his irrational fear—**desensitize** *vt*.

desferrioxamine *n* an iron chelating agent which can be used in iron poisoning, including that resulting from repeated blood transfusions for thalassaemia, and in haemochromatosis.

desiccation *n* drying out. There can be desiccation of the nucleus* pulposus, thus diminishing the 'water cushion' effect of a healthy intervertebral disc.

desloughing the process of removing slough* from a wound.

desquamation *n* shedding; flaking off; casting off—**desquamate** *vi, vt*.

detached retina separation of the neuroretina from the pigment epithelium, usually accompanied by retinal tears or holes. Exudative retinal detachment is separation of the combined neuroretina and pigment epithelium from the choroid. Treatment aims to produce scar tissue between all layers of the retina and choroid.

deterioration *n* progressive impairment of function: worsening of the patient's condition.

detoxication *n* the process of removing the poisonous property of a substance—**detoxicant** *adj, n,* **detoxicate** *vt.*

detritus *n* waste matter from disintegration.

detrusor *n* the smooth muscle of the urinary bladder. *detrusor instability* failure to inhibit a reflex contraction of the detrusor.

detrusor/sphincter dyssynergia a loss of the normal balance between detrusor contraction and sphincter relaxation to allow normal micturition to occur. The sphincter remains contracted although the detrusor contracts, and the result is incomplete voiding and an increase in the residual volume of urine.

detumescence *n* subsidence of a swelling.

deviance *n* a variation from normal.

dexamethasone *n* 30 times as active as cortisone* in suppressing inflammation. Less likely to precipitate diabetes than the other steroids. Sometimes used to prevent cerebral oedema.

dextran *n* a blood plasma substitute, obtained by the action of a specific bacterium on sugar solutions. Used as a 6% or 10% solution in haemorrhage, shock, etc.

dextranase *n* an enzyme that reduces the formation of dextran* from sucrose and has been used to prevent the formation of dental plaque.

dextrin *n* a soluble polysaccharide formed during the hydrolysis of starch.

dextrocardia *n* transposition of the heart to the right side of the thorax—**dextrocardial** *adj.*

dextrose *n* (*syn* glucose) a soluble carbohydrate (monosaccharide) widely used as intravenous infusion in dehydration, shock and postoperatively. Also given orally as a readily absorbed sugar in fluid and electrolyte imbalance, hypoglycaemia and other nutritional disturbances.

dextroxylase test xylose* test.

dhobie itch *n* tinea* cruris. Name derived from belief that ringworm of the groin originated from infection of the Indian laundryman (dhobie).

DI *abbr* donor* insemination.

diabetes *n* a disease characterized by polyuria*. Used without qualification it means diabetes mellitus. *diabetes insipidus* polyuria and polydipsia caused by deficiency of ADH. Usually due to trauma or tumour involving posterior pituitary but may be idiopathic. Treated with desmopressin. *nephrogenic diabetes insipidus* polyuria resulting from abnormality or disease rendering renal tubules insensitive to ADH. *diabetes mellitus* a condition characterized by hyperglycaemia due to deficiency or diminished effectiveness of insulin. The hyperglycaemia leads to glycosuria, which in turn causes polyuria and polydipsia. Impaired utilization of carbohydrate is associated with increased secretion of antistorage hormones such as glucagon and growth hormone in an attempt to provide alternative metabolic substrate. Glycogenolysis, gluconeogenesis and lipolysis are all increased. The latter results in excessive formation of ketone bodies which in turn leads to acidosis. If untreated this will eventually cause coma (ketoacidotic diabetic coma) and death. Diabetic patients are either *insulin* *dependent* (Type I) or *noninsulin dependent* (Type II), irrespective of the patient's age at the onset of the condition. *Potential diabetics* have a normal glucose tolerance test but are at increased risk of developing diabetes for genetic reasons. *Latent diabetics* have a normal glucose tolerance test but are known to have had an abnormal test under conditions imposing a burden on the pancreatic beta cells, e.g. during infection or pregnancy. In the latter instance the term *gestational diabetes* is commonly used. Gestational diabetes can only be accurately diagnosed in retrospect, as pregnancy onset diabetes can clear up or develop into the disease. ⇒ hyperosmolar diabetic coma—**diabetic** *adj, n.*

diabetogenic *adj* **1** causing diabetes*. **2** applied to an anterior pituitary hormone.

diagnosis *n* the art or act of determining the nature of a condition or disease. *differential diagnosis* the act of distinguishing one condition from another from similar symptoms. *nursing diagnosis* a statement of actual problems with everyday living activities as they are experienced by the patient. The nurse may perceive potential problems for which there is a nurse-initiated intervention to prevent them becoming actual ones.

diagnostic *adj* **1** pertaining to diagnosis. **2** serving as evidence in diagnosis—**diagnostician** *n.*

dialysate *n* the type of fluid used in dialysis*.

dialyser *n* used for dialysis*. Contains two compartments, one for blood and the other for dialysate: these are separated by a semipermeable membrane. ⇒ haemodialysis.

dialysis *n* separation of substances in solution by taking advantage of their differing diffusability through a porous membrane as in the artificial kidney. ⇒ haemodialysis—**dialyses** *pl,* **dialyse** *vt. peritoneal dialysis* the peritoneum is used as the porous membrane in achieving dialysis for the removal of urea and other waste products into the irrigation fluid which is then withdrawn from the abdominal cavity. Peritoneal dialysis can be used intermittently or continuously ⇒ continuous ambulatory peritoneal dialysis (CAPD).

diamorphine *n* (*syn* heroin) a derivative of morphine*, but has a more rapid action. Liable to cause addiction. Valuable in severe pain, and as a cough depressant in useless cough.

diapedesis *n* the passage of cells, e.g. neutrophils, from within blood vessels through the intact vessel walls into the tissues—**diapedetic** *adj.*

diaphoresis *n* perspiration.

diaphragm *n* **1** the dome-shaped muscular partition between the thorax above and the abdomen below. **2** any partitioning membrane or septum. **3** a rubber cap which encircles the cervix to act as a contraceptive. It should be used with a spermicidal jelly—**diaphragmatic** *adj.*

diaphragmatic hernia ⇒ hernia.

diaphysis *n* the shaft of a long bone—**diaphyses** *pl,* **diaphyseal** *adj.*

diarrhoea *n* deviation from established bowel rhythm characterized by an increase in frequency and fluidity of the stools. ⇒ arthropathy, spurious diarrhoea.

diarthrosis *n* a synovial, freely movable joint—**diarthroses** *pl,* **diarthrodial** *adj.*

diastasis *n* a separation of bones without fracture.

diastole *n* the relaxation period of the cardiac cycle, as opposed to systole*—**diastolic** *adj.*

diastolic murmur an abnormal sound heard during diastole;

occurs in valvular diseases of the heart.

diathermy *n* the passage of a high frequency electric current through the tissues whereby heat is produced. When both electrodes are large, the heat is diffused over a wide area according to the electrical resistance of the tissues. In this form it is widely used in the treatment of inflammation, especially when deeply seated (e.g. sinusitis, pelvic cellulitis). When one electrode is very small the heat is concentrated in this area and becomes great enough to destroy tissue. In this form (surgical diathermy) it is used to stop bleeding at operation by coagulation of blood, or to cut through tissue in operation for malignant disease.

diazepam *n* tranquillosedative with muscle relaxant properties. Useful in intravenous infusion or as rectal preparation for status epilepticus and tetanus, and as a premedicant.

DIC *abbr* disseminated* intravascular coagulation.

dicephalous *adj* two-headed.

dichuchwa *n* word for nonvenereal syphilis used in Botswana.

dicrotic *adj, n* (pertaining to, or having,) a double beat, as indicated by a second expansion of the artery during diastole. *dicrotic wave* the second rise in the tracing of a dicrotic pulse.

dietary fibre ⇒ nonstarch polysacchrides.

dietetics *n* the interpretation and application of the scientific principles of nutrition to feeding in health and disease.

dietitian *n* one who applies the principles of nutrition* to the feeding of an individual or a group of individuals in a heterogeneous setting of economics or health, e.g. in schools, hospitals, institutions, restaurants, hotels and food manufacturing factories.

Dietl's crisis ⇒ crisis.

differential blood count ⇒ blood count.

differential diagnosis ⇒ diagnosis.

diffusion *n* the process whereby gases and liquids of different concentrations intermingle when brought into contact, until their concentration is equal throughout (see Fig. 8, p. 265) ⇒ dialysis.

digestion *n* the process by which food is rendered absorbable—**digestible, digestive** *adj,* **digest** *vt.*

digit *n* a finger or toe—**digital** *adj.*

digital compression pressure applied by the fingers, usually to an artery to stop bleeding.

digitalis *n* leaf of the common foxglove. Powerful cardiac tonic, used in congestive heart failure and atrial fibrillation. The active principle of the Austrian fox glove, digoxin, is now preferred as the action is more consistent and reliable.

dilatation *n* stretching or enlargement. May occur physiologically, pathologically or be induced artificially. *dilatation and curettage* by custom refers to artificial stretching of the cervical os to procure scrapings of the uterine epithelium.

dimercaprol (BAL) *n* an organic compound used as an antidote for poisoning by arsenic or gold. Also useful in mercury poisoning if treatment is prompt, but it is not suitable for lead poisoning. It forms soluble compounds with the metals, which are then rapidly excreted.

Diogenes syndrome gross self-neglect.

dioptre *n* a unit of measurement in refraction. A lens of one dioptre has a focal length of 1 metre.

dioxide *n* oxide with two atoms of oxygen in each molecule.

diphtheria *n* an acute, specific, infectious notifiable disease caused by *Corynebacterium diphtheriae*. Characterized by a grey, adherent, false membrane growing on a mucous surface, usually that of the upper respiratory tract. Locally there is pain, swelling and may be suffocation. Systemically the toxins attack the heart muscle and nerves—**diphtheritic** *adj*.

diphtheroid *adj* any bacterium morphologically and culturally resembling *Corynebacterium diphtheriae*.

diplegia *n* symmetrical paralysis of legs, usually associated with cerebral damage—**diplegic** *adj*.

diplococcus *n* a coccal bacterium characteristically occurring in pairs. *Diplococcus* may be used in a binomial to describe a characteristically paired coccus, e.g. *Diplococcus pneumoniae (Streptococcus pneumoniae)* = pneumococcus.

diploid *adj* refers to the chromosome complement of organisms, like man, in which each chromosome exists in duplicate form, one member of each pair being derived from the mother, the other from the father. The two sets are united at fertilization. Man has a diploid number of 46 chromosomes, 23 pairs.

diplopia *n* the word used alone implies the seeing of two objects when only one exists (double vision). There are several binomials which locate or describe the disability in more detail.

dipsomania *n* alcoholism* in which the drinking occurs in bouts, often with long periods of sobriety between—**dipsomaniac** *adj, n*.

disability *n* any restriction or lack of ability (resulting from an impairment*) to perform an activity in the manner or within the range considered normal for a human being. It is likely to result in social disadvantage in a society geared towards the nonimpaired majority, e.g. when a person in a wheelchair is faced with an unramped flight of steps or a deaf person is interviewed by a nurse unable to use sign language.

Disability Employment Officer (DEO) part of Placing, Assessment and Counselling Teams (PACTs). Their work is coordinated by the Employment Service, an agency within the Department for Education and Employment. PACTs provide employers with practical help and advice on the employment of people with disabilities, e.g. equipment and adaptations.

disaccharide *n* a sugar (i.e. carbohydrate) e.g. lactose, maltose, sucrose, which yields two molecules of monosaccharide on hydrolysis.

disarticulation *n* amputation at a joint.

discectomy *n* surgical removal of a disc, usually an intervertebral disc.

discharge *n* **1** used to designate a person's exit from treatment in the health service, e.g. from a community nursing service, health centre, outpatients' clinic, ward, or special unit. **2** the exudate from an infected wound. **3** excessive secretion from a mucous membrane (usually inflamed), e.g. vaginal and urethral.

disciplinary action ⇒ professional disciplinary process.

disclosing tablet *n* contains erythrosine*; when chewed, it identifies dental* plaque, by staining it red.

discogenic *adj* arising in or produced by a disc, usually an intervertebral disc.

discrete *adj* distinct, separate, not merging.

discrimination *n* attitude to, and treatment of, a person solely on the grounds of prejudice towards a characteristic of the group to which the person belongs, e.g.

gender, sexual preference or skin colour.

disease *n* any deviation from or interruption of the normal structure and function of any part of the body. It is manifested by a characteristic set of signs and symptoms and in most instances the aetiology, pathology and prognosis are known. It can be of an acute or chronic nature.

disfigurement *n* disfigurement occurs after, e.g. removal of any part of the body, or formation of a scar with consequent disruption of body* image. It usually takes longer to come to terms with visible disfigurement but all need to go through a psychological process of incorporating the change into the body image.

disimpaction *n* separation of the broken ends of a bone which have been driven into each other during the impact which caused the fracture. Traction may then be applied to maintain the bone ends separate and in good alignment.

disinfectants *npl* a word usually reserved for germicides which are too corrosive or toxic to be applied to tissues, but which are suitable for application to inanimate objects.

disinfection *n* the removal or destruction of harmful microbes but not usually bacterial spores. It is commonly achieved by using heat or chemicals.

disinfestation *n* extermination of infesting agents, especially lice (delousing).

dislocation *n* a displacement of organs or articular surfaces, so that all apposition between them is lost. It may be congenital, spontaneous, traumatic, or recurrent—**dislocated** *adj,* **dislocate** *vt.*

disobliteration *n* rebore. Removal of that which blocks a vessel, most often intimal plaques in an artery, when it is called endarterectomy*.

disorientation *n* loss of orientation*.

displacement *n* an unconscious mental* defence mechanism whereby, e.g. a person who is dissatisfied with the information being offered by nurses, displaces the object of dissatisfaction to the type of bed or the menu provided by the hospital.

dissection *n* separation of tissues by cutting.

disseminated *adj* widely spread or scattered. *disseminated intravascular coagulation (DIC)* a condition in which there is overstimulation of the body's clotting and anticlotting process in response to disease or injury. *disseminated sclerosis*⇒ multiple sclerosis.

dissociation *n* in psychiatry, an abnormal mental process by which the mind achieves nonrecognition and isolation of certain unpalatable facts. This involves the actual splitting off from consciousness of all the unpalatable ideas so that the individual is no longer aware of them. It is seen in its most exaggerated form in delusional psychoses, e.g. a woman who, being deluded, believes she is the Queen cheerfully scrubbing the ward floor. Her royal status and her actions are completely separated or dissociated in her mind and she does not recognize the incongruity.

dissociative state conflict converted into psychological symptoms, e.g. amnesia.

distal *adj* farthest from the head or source—**distally** *adv.*

distichiasis *n* an extra row of eyelashes at the inner lid border, which is turned inward against the eye.

distractibility *n* in psychiatry, a disorder of the power of attention, which can only be applied momentarily.

distraction therapy a term preferred by some nurses for diversional* therapy.

district nurses registered nurses holding a District Nursing Certificate who are employed to provide skilled nursing for patients in the community. They are qualified and accountable for assessing, prescribing and evaluating the nursing plan for such patients.

diuresis *n* secretion of urine.

diuretics *npl* drugs which increase the flow of urine. Those which enhance the excretion of sodium and other ions thereby increasing urinary output are called *saluretic diuretics* and comprise the thiazide group of drugs. Those which act on the loop of Henle are called *loop diuretics;* they produce a rapid diuresis, onset of action being 5–10 min when given parenterally or 20–30 min if given orally; the duration of action is 4–6 h.

divarication separation of two points on a straight line.

diversional therapy the conscious use of diverting the focus of attention from one activity, object or person to another. It can be used to prevent boredom, institutionalisation and pain. Especially useful in children. ⇒ distraction therapy.

diver's paralysis caisson* disease.

diverticulitis *n* inflammation of a diverticulum*.

diverticulosis *n* a condition in which there are many diverticula, especially in the intestines.

diverticulum *n* a pouch or sac protruding from the wall of a tube or hollow organ, most commonly the large bowel. May be congenital or acquired. ⇒ diverticulitis, diverticulosis.—**diverticula** *pl.*

DNA *abbr* deoxyribonucleic* acid. *DNA probe* blood from a finger prick is applied to a radioactively labelled probe.

documentation of nursing documentation usually reflects the phases of the process of nursing—assessing, planning, implementing and evaluating. Nursing records and documentation may be required when there is litigation in a court of law.

Döderlein's bacillus a non-pathogenic Gram-positive rod which normally lives in the vagina and by its action provides an acid medium.

Dogger Bank itch sensitization dermatitis due to *Alcyonidium* (seaweed family). Clinical features include a papular and vesicular rash on hands and forearms with facial erythema and oedema.

dolor *n* pain; usually used in the context of being one of the four classical signs of inflammation—the others being calor*, rubor*, tumor*.

dominant *adj* describes a character possessed by one parent which, in the offspring, overrides the corresponding alternative character derived from the other parent. The words, and concepts, of dominance and recessivity are now extended to the genes themselves which control the respective characters. ⇒ recessive *opp*, Mendel's law.

dominant hemisphere on the opposite side of the brain to that of the preferred hand. The dominant hemisphere for language is the left in 90% of right-handed and 30% of left-handed people.

donor *n* 'to give a gift', such as blood for transfusion, semen or eggs for fertility treatment, or an organ for transplantation.

donor insemination (DI) insemination* of a female with donor sperm, either by direct insertion into the cervical canal or combined with IVF* techniques. HIV screening is now expected of the donor.

Donovan bodies Leishman-Donovan* bodies.

dopa *n* dihydroxyphenylalanine—an important compound formed in the intermediate stage in the synthesis of catecholamines* from tyrosine*.

dopamine *n* a catecholamine neurotransmitter, closely related to adrenaline* and noradrenaline*. Increases cardiac output and renal blood flow but does not produce peripheral vasoconstriction. Most valuable in hypotension and shock of cardiac origin. Normally present in high concentration in those regions of the brain which are selectively damaged in parkinsonism. *dopamine-β-hydroxylase* an enzyme present in blood; it is increased in high blood pressure.

Doppler technique used to measure the velocity of blood flow through a vein to determine the degree of occlusion or stenosis of artery. *Doppler ultrasound technique* uses ultrasonagraphy. *Doppler scanning* combines ultrasonography with pulse echo.

Doptone a trade name for an instrument using echo-sound principles to detect the fetal heart at a very early stage.

Dornier lithotriptor a piece of equipment which can destroy certain types of kidney stones by shock waves thereby rendering invasive surgery unnecessary. The technique is called extracorporeal shock-wave lithotripsy (ESWL).

dorsal *adj* pertaining to the back, or the posterior part of an organ. *dorsal position* lying on the back with the head supported on a pillow.

dorsiflexion *n* bending backwards. In the case of the great toe upwards ⇒ Babinski's reflex.

dorsolumbar *adj* pertaining to the lumbar region of the back.

dosimeter, dosemeter *n* an instrument worn by personnel or placed within equipment to measure incident X-rays or gamma rays. Commonly a small photographic film in a special filter holder.

double vision ⇒ diplopia.

douche *n* a stream of fluid directed against the body externally or into a body cavity.

down-regulation process, used in assisted conception, of temporarily 'switching off' the pituitary gland, preventing ovulation and therefore making easier the management of superovulation*.

Down syndrome (*syn* mongolism) a congenital condition in which there is generally severe mental subnormality and facial characteristics vaguely resembling the Mongoloid races: stigmata include oval tilted eyes, squint and a flattened occiput. The chromosome abnormality is of two types: (a) primary trisomy, caused by abnormal division of chromosome 21 (atmeiosis). This results in an extra chromosome instead of the normal pair: the infant has 47 chromosomes and is often born of an elderly mother (b) structural abnormality involving chromosome 21, with a total number of 46 chromosomes, one of which has an abnormal structure as the result of a special translocation. Such infants are usually born of younger mothers and there is a higher risk of recurrence in subsequent pregnancies.

doxapram hydrochloride *n* a respiratory stimulant; can be given intravenously.

dracontiasis *n* infestation with *Dracunculus* medinensis* common in India and Africa.

Dracunculus medinensis (*syn* Guinea worm) a nematode parasite which infests man from contaminated drinking water. From the patient's intestine the adult female migrates to the skin surface to deposit her larvae, producing a cord-like thickening which ulcerates.

drain *n* ⇒ wound drains.

drainage of wounds ⇒ wound drains.

drama therapy the promotion of personal growth by using games and improvisation to encourage spontaneity and positive ways of relating to self and others by means of verbal and non-verbal techniques. Incorporates many of the ideas of psychodrama* but is more of an art therapy than a psychotherapy.

dressings *npl* ⇒ wound dressings.

drip *n* ⇒ intravenous.

drop attacks periodic falling because of sudden loss of postural control of the lower limbs, without vertigo or loss of consciousness. Usually followed by sudden return of normal muscle tone, allowing the person to rise, if uninjured.⇒ vertebrobasilar insufficiency.

dropsy *n* ⇒ oedema–**dropsical** *adj.*

drug *n* the generic name for any substance used for the prevention, diagnosis and treatment of diagnosed disease and also for the relief of symptoms. The term 'prescribed drug' describes such usage. The word medicine is usually preferred for therapeutic drugs to distinguish them from the addictive drugs which are used illegally. For alleviating unpleasant symptoms of self-limiting illnesses, any remedy which does not require a medical prescription is termed an 'over-the-counter' medicine. ⇒ noncompliance, noncomprehension. *drug abuse* the term used by many lay and professional people for the illegal use of 'hard' drugs. The term substance* abuse includes other substances as well as hard and soft* drugs. *drug dependence* a state arising from repeated administration of a drug on a periodic or continuous basis (WHO, 1964). Now a preferable term to drug addiction and drug habituation. *drug-fast* a term used to describe resistance of microbial cells to the action of antimicrobial drugs. *drug interaction* occurs when the pharmacological action of one drug is affected by another drug taken previously or simultaneously.

dry eye syndrome ⇒ Sjögren syndrome.

DSA *abbr* digital subtraction angiography*.

DSH *abbr* deliberate self-harm ⇒ parasuicide.

Dubowitz score assesses gestational age.

Duchenne muscular dystrophy an X-linked recessive disorder affecting only boys. The disorder usually begins to show between 3 and 5 years and is characterized by progressive muscle weakness and loss of locomotor skills. Death usually occurs during the teens or early twenties from respiratory or cardiac failure.

Ducrey's bacillus *Haemophilus* ducreyi.*

duct *n* a tube or duct for carrying away the secretions from a gland.

ductless glands endocrine* glands.

ductus arteriosus a blood vessel connecting the left pulmonary artery to the aorta, to bypass the lungs in the fetal circulation. At birth the duct closes, but if it remains open it is called *persistent ductus arteriosus* a congenital heart defect.

Duhamel's operation a surgical operation for Hirschsprung's* disease.

dumbness *n* ⇒mutism.

'dumping syndrome' the name given to the symptoms which sometimes follow a partial gastrectomy–epigastric fullness and a feeling of faintness and sweating after meals.

duodenal intubation ⇒ intubation.

duodenal ulcer an ulcer* which occurs in the duodenal lining caused by the action of acid and pepsin. Pain(s) occur several hours after meals, so they are described as hunger pains, relieved by food. The ulcer can bleed, leading to occult blood in the stools, or it can perforate, constituting an abdominal emergency. Severe scarring following chronic ulceration may produce pyloric stenosis.

duodenitis *n* inflammation of the duodenum.

duodenojejunal *adj* pertaining to the duodenum and jejunum.

duodenopancreatectomy *n* surgical excision of the duodenum and part of the pancreas, carried out in cases of cancer arising in the region of the head of the pancreas.

duodenoscope *n* a side-viewing flexible fibreoptic endoscope*—**duodenoscopic** *adj*, **duodenoscopy** *n*.

duodenostomy *n* a surgically made fistula between the duodenum and another cavity, e.g. cholecystoduodenostomy, a fistula between the gallbladder and duodenum made to relieve jaundice in inoperable cancer of the head of the pancreas.

duodenum *n* the fixed, curved, first portion of the small intestine, connecting the stomach* above to the jejunum* below—**duodenal** *adj*.

Dupuytren's contracture painless, chronic flexion of the digits of the hand, especially the third and fourth, towards the palm. The aetiology is uncertain but some cases are associated with hepatic cirrhosis.

DVT *abbr* deep vein thrombosis ⇒ phlebothrombosis.

dwarf *n* person of stunted growth. May be due to growth hormone deficiency. Also occurs in untreated congenital hypothyroidism (cretinism*) and juvenile hypothyroidism, achondroplasia and other conditions.

dwarfism *n* arrested growth and development as occurs in cretinism*, and in some chronic diseases such as intestinal malabsorption, renal failure and rickets.

dying *adj* a word which describes a person before the event of death*. At first there may be a period of denial and isolation, followed by anger when the person asks 'Why me? What have I done to deserve this?' This may be followed by bargaining and, as the inevitability dawns, depression may manifest. There is evidence that if people are helped and supported to live a day at a time, a positive approach to life and death can be achieved. ➡ bereavement, death, grieving.

dynamic psychology a psychological approach which stresses the importance of (typically unconscious) energy or motives, as in Freudian or psychoanalytic theory.

dynamometer *n* apparatus to test the strength of grip.

dysaesthesia *n* impairment of touch sensation.

dysarthria *n* a speech disorder resulting from disturbance in muscular control of the speech mechanism due to damage to the central and/or peripheral nervous system. The loss of muscular control may involve weakness, slowness and/or incoordination. Disturbance may involve respiration, phonation, resonance and prosody*—**dysarthric** *adj*.

dyscalculia *n* impairment of numeral ability.

dyschezia *n* difficult or painful defaecation.

dyschondroplasia *n* an hereditary disorder of bone growth resulting in normal trunk, short arms and legs.

dysentery *n* inflammation of the bowel with evacuation of blood and mucus, accompanied by tenesmus and colic—**dysenteric** *adj*. *amoebic dysentery* is caused by the protozoon *Entamoeba histolytica*. ⇒ amoebiasis. *bacillary dysentery* is caused by *Shigella shigae, S. flexneri* or *S. sonnei*. Disease results from poor sanitation and the house-fly carries the infection from faeces to food.

dysfunction *n* abnormal functioning of any organ or part.

dysgammaglobulinaemia *n* (*syn* antibody deficiency syndrome) disturbance of gammaglobulin production. Can be transient, congenital or acquired. Normally there is transfer of IgG from mother to baby before birth; the level gradually falls after birth. This can lead to transient hypogammaglobulinaemia with repeated respiratory infections. Injections of gammaglobulin are given until normal blood levels occur.

dysgenesis *n* malformation during embryonic development—**dysgenetic** *adj*, **dysgenetically** *adv*.

dysgerminoma *n* a tumour of the ovary of low grade malignancy. It is not hormone secreting, as it is developed from cells which date back to the undifferentiated state of gonadal development, i.e. before the cells have either male or female attributes.

dysgraphia *n* an acquired disorder of written language due to brain injury. The ability to spell familiar and/or unfamiliar words is affected in one or many modalities (handwriting, typing, etc.). A number of different types of dysgraphia are recognized—**dysgraphic** *adj*.

dyshidrosis *n* a vesicular skin eruption, formerly thought to be caused by blockage of the sweat ducts at their orifice, histologically an eczematous process.

dyskaryosis *n* abnormal cellular change (dysplasia). Applied to results of a cervical smear. Follow-up tests may revert to normal, but some may become positive and demand biopsy.

dyskinesia *n* (clumsy child syndrome) a long recognized but only recently diagnosed condition. There is inability to coordinate and programme voluntary movement, so that the child appears to be clumsy, writes badly, cannot tie shoelaces and so on. Responds to a special system of behavioural training—**dyskinetic** *adj*. *tardive dyskinesia* occurs as a side-effect of antipsychotic medication. At initial assessment patient is asked to put out tongue and hold it out which he or she cannot do voluntarily: it starts to withdraw into the mouth. Repeated at weekly intervals there will be cumulative data for the set date for evaluation of reduction of the side-effect.

dyslexia *n* a disorder of reading. A number of different types of dyslexia are recognized, e.g. deep dyslexia and surface dyslexia. Many patients with dyslexia may also present with dysgraphia*—**dyslexic** *adj*.

dysmaturity *n* signs and symptoms of growth retardation at birth. ⇒ low birthweight.

dysmelia *n* malformation in the development of the limbs.

dysmenorrhoea *n* painful menstruation, which in some women responds to an oral antiprostaglandin and in others to an oral contraceptive. *spasmodic dysmenorrhoea* comes on during the first day of a period, often within an hour or two of the start of bleeding. It comes in spasms of acute colicky pain in the lower part of the abdomen, and sometimes in the back and inner parts of the thighs. The spasms can be bad enough to cause fainting and vomiting. *congestive dysmenorrhoea* sufferers know several days in advance that their period is coming, because they have a dull aching pain in the lower abdomen, increasing heaviness, perhaps constipation, nausea and lack of appetite. There may also be breast tenderness, headache and backache. Fluid retention at this time leads to typical oedema and weight gain; this can be helped by the use of diuretics.

dysmorphogenic *adj* now preferred to teratogenic when applied to drugs taken during pregnancy. ⇒ teratogen.

dyspareunia *n* painful or difficult coitus, experienced by the woman.

dyspepsia *n* indigestion—**dyspeptic** *adj.*

dysphagia *n* a disorder of swallowing characterized by difficulty in oral preparation and/or in moving a bolus from the mouth to the stomach. May arise due to neurological, structural, surgical, developmental or cognitive causes—**dysphagic** *adj.*

dysphasia *n* ⇒ aphasia.

dysphonia *n* a disorder of voice due to organic, neurological, behavioural or psychogenic causes—**dysphonic** *adj.*

dysplasia *n* formation of abnormal tissue—**dysplastic** *adj.*

dyspnoea *n* difficulty in, or laboured, breathing; can be mainly of an inspiratory nature as in choking*, or expiratory as in asthma*.—**dysponoeic** *adj.*

dyspraxia *n* lack of voluntary control over muscles, particularly the orofacial ones. A range of different dyspraxias can occur, e.g. limb dyspraxia, dressing dyspraxia and ideometer dyspraxia. Articulatory dyspraxia affects the ability to control the positioning of speech muscles and the sequencing of speech movements. Developmental dyspraxias may be found in children. ⇒ apraxia—**dyspraxic** *adj.*

dysreflexia *n* ⇒ autonomic dysreflexia.

dysrhythmia *n* disordered rhythm, usually of heart, e.g. atrial fibrillation*—**dysrhythmic** *adj.*

dystaxia *n* difficulty in controlling voluntary movements—**dystaxic** *adj.*

dystocia *n* difficult or slow labour.

dystrophy *n* defective nutrition of an organ or tissue, usually muscle. ⇒ muscular dystrophy, Duchenne muscular dystrophy.

dysuria *n* painful micturition*—**dysuric** adj.

E

EAB *abbr* ⇒ extraanatomic bypass.

ear *n*–the sensory organ for hearing and balance. Composed of the pinna* and the external auditory meatus along which sound waves pass to vibrate the tympanic membrane, and in turn the three tiny bones (auditory ossicles) in the middle ear. The last of these communicates with the internal ear (cochlea*) which contains the sensory mechanisms for hearing and balance.

eardrum *n* a membrane at the end of the external auditory canal. To its inner surface is attached the first of the auditory ossicles. ⇒ ear.

EBM *abbr* expressed breast milk.

Ebola *n* one of the viral* haemorrhagic fevers, usually transmitted by ticks.

EBV *abbr* Epstein*-Barr virus.

ecbolic *adj* describes any agent which stimulates contraction of the gravid uterus and hastens expulsion of its contents ⇒ oxytocic.

ecchondroma *n* a benign tumour composed of cartilage which protrudes from the surface of the bone in which it arises–**ecchondromata** *pl.*

ecchymosis *n* an extravasation of blood under the skin. ⇒ bruise–**ecchymoses** *pl.*

ECG *abbr* electrocardiogram ⇒ electrocardiograph. Also electrocorticography*.

Echinococcus *n* a genus of tapeworms, the adults infesting a primary host, e.g. a dog. In man (secondary host) the encysted larvae cause 'hydatid* disease'.

echocardiography *n* the use of ultrasound as a diagnostic tool for studying the structure and motion of the heart.

echoencephalography *n* passage of ultrasound waves across the head. Can detect abscess, blood clot, injury or tumour within brain.

echolalia *n* repetition, almost automatically of words or phrases heard. Occurs most commonly in schizophrenia and dementia; sometimes in toxic delirious states. A characteristic of all infants' speech–**echolalic** *adj.*

echopraxia *n* involuntary mimicking of another's movements.

echoviruses *npl* the name derives from Enteric Cytopathic Human Orphan. It was given because these viruses were originally found in the stools of diseaseless children. Echoviruses have caused meningitis and mild respiratory infection in children. At least 30 types have been identified.

eclampsia *n* **1** a severe manifestation of pregnancy-induced hypertension*, associated with fits and coma ⇒ preeclampsia. **2** a sudden convulsive attack–**eclamptic** *adj.*

ecmnesia *n* impaired memory for recent events with normal memory of remote ones. Common in old age and in early cerebral deterioration.

Ecstasy *n* colloquial name for an amphetamine which acts as a stimulant and can produce hallucinations.

ECT *abbr* ⇒ electroconvulsive therapy.

ecthyma *n* a crusted eruption of impetigo* contagiosa on the legs, producing necrosis of the skin, which heals with scarring. A similar condition occurs in syphilis.

ectoderm *n* the external primitive germ layer of the embryo. From it are developed the skin structures, nervous system, organs of special senses, pineal gland and part of the pituitary and adrenal glands, and mucous membrane of the mouth and anus–**ectodermal** *adj.*

ectodermosis *n* disease of any organ or tissue derived from the ectoderm.

ectogenesis *n* the growth of the embryo outside the uterus (in* vitro fertilization).

ectogenous *adj* –originating outside an organism. ⇒ endogenous *opp.*

ectoparasite *n* a parasite that lives on the exterior surface of its host–**ectoparasitic** *adj.*

ectopia *n* malposition of an organ or structure, usually congenital. *ectopia vesicae* an abnormally placed urinary bladder which protrudes through or opens on to the abdominal wall–**ectopic** *adj.*

ectopic beat ⇒ extrasystole.

ectopic pregnancy (*syn* tubal pregnancy) extrauterine gestation, the uterine tube being the most common site. At about the 6th week the tube ruptures, constituting a 'surgical emergency'.

ectozoa *npl* external parasites.

ectrodactyly, ectrodactylia *n* congenital absence of one or more fingers or toes or parts of them.

ectropion *n* an eversion or turning outward, especially of the lower eyelid or of the pupil margin–*ectropion uveae.*

ECV *abbr* external cephalic version*.

eczema *n* an inflammatory skin condition accompanied by intense itching of the affected area. The eczema skin reaction begins with erythema, then vesicles appear. These rupture, forming crusts or leaving pits which ooze serum. This is the exudative or weeping stage. In the process of healing, the area becomes scaly. Some authorities limit the word 'eczema' to the cases with internal (endogenous) causes while those caused by external (exogenous) contact factors are called dermatitis or eczematous dermatitis. The lesions may be colonized or infected with hospital strains of *Staphylococcus aureus*. Due to the exfoliative nature of eczema, modification of patient management is required to protect others from infection. ⇒ dermatitis–**eczematous** *adj.*

eczema-asthma syndrome affected infants begin with infantile eczema and in childhood develop asthma as the eczema remits; frequently the asthma remits at puberty.

EDD *abbr* ⇒ expected date of delivery.

edentulous *adj* without natural teeth.

edrophonium test in patients with myasthenia* gravis, a small intramuscular dose of edrophonium chloride will immediately relieve symptoms, albeit temporarily, while quinine sulphate will increase the muscular weakness.

Edward syndrome an autosomal trisomy* associated with mental subnormality. The cells have 47 chromosomes. Sometimes called trisomy E.

EEG *abbr* electroencephalogram* ⇒ electroencephalograph.

EFAs *abbr* ⇒ essential fatty acids.

effector *n* a motor or secretory nerve ending in a muscle, gland or organ.

efferent *adj* carrying, conveying, conducting away from a centre. ⇒ afferent *opp.*

effleurage *n* a massage technique of using long, whole-hand strokes in one direction only, with the aim of assisting the venous return of blood which then increases arterial blood supply: oedematous swelling can be reduced by this method. Alternatively, circular, finger-only movements can be applied, as in the Lamaze method of natural childbirth.

effort syndrome a form of anxiety neurosis, manifesting itself in a variety of cardiac symptoms including precordial pain, for which no pathological explanation can be discovered.

effusion *n* extravasation of fluid into body tissues or cavities. ⇒ pleural effusion.

ego *n* refers to the conscious self, the 'I' which, according to Freud, deals with reality, is influenced by social forces and controls unconscious instinctual urges (the id*).

EIA *abbr* exercise induced asthma. ⇒ asthma.

ejaculation *n* the sudden emission of semen from the erect penis at the moment of male orgasm.

elder abuse physical, sexual, psychological or financial abuse of older people, usually carried out in the domestic setting by those relatives responsible for their care. ⇒ abuse, nonaccidental injury.

elderly mentally ill (EMI) applies to older people suffering mental illness. The term is now preferred to psychogeriatric. The mental disorders most commonly associated with older people are acute or chronic confusional* states, depression* and dementia*.

Electra complex excessive emotional attachment of daughter to father. The name is derived from Greek mythology.

electroacupuncture *n* originated in Europe but widely used in China. An electric current is applied to inserted acupuncture needles in order to intensify the sensory stimulation and extend the effect.

electrocardiogram (ECG) *n* a recording of the electrical activity of the heart on a moving paper strip, made by an electrocardiograph*.

electrocardiograph *n* an instrument which records the electrical activity of the heart from electrodes on the limbs and chest—**electrocardiographic** *adj,* **electrocardiographically** *adv.*

electrocoagulation *n* technique of surgical diathermy*. Coagulation, especially of bleeding points, by means of electrodes.

electrocochleography (ECoG) *n* direct recording of the action potential generated following stimulation of the cochlear nerve.

electroconvulsive therapy (ECT) a form of physical treatment still frequently used by psychiatrists mainly in the treatment of severe depression. An apparatus is used which delivers a definite voltage for a precise fraction of a second to electrodes placed on the head, producing a convulsion. *modified ECT* the convulsion is modified with an intravenous anaesthetic and a muscle relaxant, thus reducing the risk of unpleasant sequelae. ECT is currently invariably modified. *unilateral ECT* avoids the sequela of amnesia for recent events. The mechanism for memory of recent events is probably in the dominant cerebral hemisphere which is the left in practically all people. ECT is therefore applied to the right hemisphere to minimize memory disturbance.

electrocorticography *n* direct recording from the cerebral cortex during operation—

electrocorticographic *adj*, **electrocorticograph** *n*, **electrocorticographically** *adv*.

electrode *n* in medicine, a conductor in the form of a pad or plate, whereby electricity enters or leaves the body in electrotherapy.

electrodesiccation *n* a technique of surgical diathermy*. There is drying and subsequent removal of tissue, e.g. papillomata.

electroencephalogram *n* (EEG) a recording of the electrical activity of the brain on a moving paper strip, made by an electroencephalograph*.

electroencephalograph *n* an instrument by which electrical impulses derived from the brain can be amplified and recorded on paper, in a fashion similar to that of the electrocardiograph—**electroencephalographic** *adj*, **electroencephalographically** *adv*.

electrolysis *n* **1** chemical decomposition by electricity, with migration of ions shown by changes at the electrodes. **2** term used for the destruction of individual hairs (epilation), eradication of moles, spider naevi, etc. using electricity.

electrolyte *n* a liquid or solution of a substance which is capable of conducting electricity because it dissociates into ions. In medical usage it refers to the ion itself, e.g. sodium, potassium, chloride and potassium ions in the serum. Various diseases can cause serum electrolyte imbalance; deficient ones can be replaced orally or by intravenous drip; those in excess can be removed by dialysis or by resins which can be taken by mouth or given by enema—**electrolytic** *adj*.

electromyography *n* the use of an instrument which records electric currents generated in active muscle—**electromyographical** *adj*, **electromyograph** *n*, **electromyographically** *adv*.

electrooculography *n* the use of an instrument which records eye position and movement, and potential difference between front and back of the eyeball using electrodes placed on skin near socket. Can be used as an electrodiagnostic test—**electrooculographical** *adj*, **electrooculograph** *n*, **electrooculographically** *adv*.

electroretinogram (ERG) *n* graphic record of electrical currents generated in active retina.

element *n* one of the constituents of a compound. The elements are the primary substances which in pure form, or combined into compounds, constitute all matter.

elephantiasis *n* the swelling of a limb, usually a leg, as a result of lymphatic obstruction (lymphoedema), followed by thickening of the skin (pachydermia) and subcutaneous tissues. A complication of filariasis in tropical countries, but also seen in UK as a result of syphilis or recurring streptococcal infection (elephantiasis nostras).

elimination *n* the passage of waste from the body, usually reserved for urine and faeces—**eliminate** *vt*.

ELISA *abbr* ⇒ enzyme-linked immunosorbent assay.

elixir *n* a sweetened, aromatic solution of a drug, often containing an appreciable amount of alcohol. Elixirs differ from syrups in containing very little sugar and in requiring dilution before use.

elliptocytosis *n* anaemia in which the red blood cells are oval. Seen in autosomal dominant disorder hereditary elliptocytosis and in varying amounts in anaemias.

emaciation *n* excessive leanness, or wasting of body tissue—**emaciate** *vt*.

emasculation *n* castration* in the male.

embolectomy *n* surgical removal of an embolus*. Usually a fine balloon (Fogarty) catheter is used to extract the embolus.

embolic *adj* pertaining to an embolism or an embolus.

embolism *n* the condition in which there is obstruction of an artery by the impaction of a solid body (e.g. thrombi, fat globules, tumour cells) or an air bubble. Distal tissue, deprived of blood, may become gangrenous. ⇒ pulmonary embolism.

embologenic *adj* capable of producing an embolus*.

embolus *n* solid body or air bubble transported in the circulation. ⇒ embolism—**emboli** *pl.*

embrocation *n* a liquid which is applied topically by rubbing.

embryo *n* the word applied to the developing ovum (zygote*) from the time of fertilization of the ovum until the beginning of the 3rd month of pregnancy—**embryonic** *adj.*

embryology *n* study of the development of an organism from fertilization to extrauterine life—**embryological** *adj,* **embryologically** *adv.*

embryoma *n* ⇒ teratoma.

embryopathy *n* disease or abnormality in the embryo. More serious if it occurs in the first 3 months. Includes the 'rubella* syndrome'—**embryopathic** *adj,* **embryopathically** *adv.*

embryotomy *n* mutilation of the fetus to facilitate removal from the womb, when natural birth is impossible.

emesis *n* vomiting.

emetic *n* any agent used to produce vomiting. ⇒ antiemetic *opp.*

emission *n* an ejaculation or sending forth, especially an involuntary ejaculation of semen.

EMLA *abbr* eutetic* mixture of local anaesthetics.

emmetropia *n* normal or perfect vision—**emmetropic** *adj.*

emollient *adj, n* (an agent) which softens and soothes skin or mucous membrane, e.g. used to soften the scaly skin that occurs with eczema*.

emotion *n* the tone of feeling recognized in ourselves by certain bodily changes, and in others by tendencies to certain characteristic behaviour. Aroused usually by ideas or concepts.

emotional *adj* characteristic of or caused by emotion. *emotional bias* tendency of emotional attitude to affect logical judgement. *emotional lability* ⇒ lability. *emotional state* effect of emotions on normal mood, e.g. agitation.

empathy *n* identifying with another person or the actions of another person—**empathic** *adj.*

emphysema *n* gaseous distension of the tissues. ⇒ crepitation, pulmonary, surgical emphysema—**emphysematous** *adj.*

empirical *adj* based on observation and experience and not on scientific reasoning.

empowerment *n* philosophy underpinning the care of chronically sick, elderly or disabled people usually, though not necessarily, living in their own homes. Emphasizes the active role played by the client in stating own preferences about care, rather than simply being passive recipient of care organized elsewhere. Professionals (including nurses) try to motivate the client to make decisions for himself or herself, and provide the necessary information on which the client can make appropriate decisions. A disabled client may advertise for, interview, hire, and pay the helpers he or she needs, rather than accepting those chosen for him or her by local social services. Nurses may initially feel uncomfortable working with a client who exercises control over his or her own life and treatment.

empyema *n* a collection of pus in a cavity, hollow organ or space.

emulsion *n* a uniform suspension of fat or oil particles in an aqueous continuous phase *(O/W emulsion)* or aqueous droplets in an oily continuous phase *(W/O emulsion)*.

enamel *n* the hard, acellular external covering of the crown of a tooth.

encapsulation *n* enclosure within a capsule.

encephalins, enkephalins *npl* two pentapeptides which are neuroleptic and relieve pain. They are *methionine-encephalin* and *isoleucine encephalin*. Researchers have isolated them in the brain, gastrointestinal tract and the pituitary gland ⇒ endorphins.

encephalitis *n* inflammation of the brain.

encephalocele *n* protrusion of brain substance through the skull. Often associated with hydrocephalus when the protrusion occurs at a suture line.

encephalography *n* a technique to examine the brain, to produce a printed or visible record of the investigation. ⇒ echoencephalography, electroencephalograph, pneumoencephalography—**encephalogram** *n*.

encephalomalacia *n* softening of the brain.

encephalomyelitis *n* inflammation of the brain and spinal cord.

encephalomyelopathy *n* disease affecting both brain and spinal cord—**encephalomyelopathic** *adj*.

encephalon *n* the brain.

encephalopathy *n* any disease of the brain—**encephalopathic** *adj*.

enchondroma *n* ⇒ chondroma—**enchondromata** *pl*.

encopresis *n* involuntary passage of faeces at an age by which faecal continence is normally achieved. May be associated with mental illness—**encopretic** *adj, n*.

encounter group a form of psychotherapy. Members of a small group focus on becoming aware of their feelings and developing the ability to express them openly, honestly and clearly. The objective is to increase self-awareness, promote personal growth and improve interpersonal communication.

Endamoeba ⇒ Entamoeba.

endarterectomy *n* the surgical removal of an atheromatous core from an artery, sometimes called disobliteration or 'rebore'. Carbon dioxide gas can be used to separate the occlusive core.

endarteritis *n* inflammation of the intima or inner lining coat of an artery. *endarteritis obliterans* the new intimal connective tissue obliterates the lumen.

endaural *adj* incision of external meatus, extending in front of the ear, used in ear surgery.

endemic *adj* recurring in an area ⇒ epidemic *opp*.

endemiology *n* the special study of endemic diseases.

endocardial mapping the recording of electrical potentials from various sites on the endocardium to determine the site of origin of cardiac arrhythmia.

endocardial resection surgical removal of that part of the endocardium causing cardiac arrhythmia.

endocarditis *n* inflammation of the inner lining of the heart (endocardium*), particularly of the valves, due to infection by microorganisms (bacteria, fungi or *Rickettsia*), or to rheumatic fever. There may be temporary or permanent damage to the heart valves.

endocardium *n* the lining membrane of the heart, which covers the valves.

endocervical *adj* pertaining to the inside of the cervix uteri*.

endocervicitis *n* inflammation of the mucous membrane lining the cervix uteri.

endocrine *adj* secreting internally. Describes glands whose secretions flow directly into the blood stream; ductless glands. ⇒ exocrine *opp*—**endocrinal** *adj. endocrine glands* the ductless glands of the body; those which make an internal secretion or hormone which passes into the blood stream and has an important influence on general metabolic processes: e.g. the pineal, pituitary, thyroid, parathyroids, adrenals, ovaries, testes and pancreas. The pancreas, stomach, liver, ovaries and testes have both internal and external secretions.

endocrinology *n* the study of the ductless glands and their internal secretions.

endocrinopathy *n* abnormality of one or more of the endocrine glands or their secretions.

endoderm *n* innermost layer of the three primitive germ layers of the embryo. From it are derived the epithelium of the pharynx, respiratory tract, digestive tract, bladder and urethra.

endogenous *adj* originating within the organism. ⇒ ectogenous, exogenous *opp*.

endolymph *n* the fluid contained in the membranous labyrinth of the internal ear.

endolysin *n* an intracellular, leucocytic substance which destroys engulfed bacteria.

endometrioma *n* a tumour of misplaced endometrium ⇒ chocolate cyst—**endometriomata** *pl*.

endometriosis *n* the presence of endometrium in abnormal sites, e.g. the uterine tubes where it can cause infertility. ⇒ chocolate cyst.

endometritis *n* inflammation of the endometrium*.

endometrium *n* the lining mucosa of the uterus—**endometrial** *adj*.

endomyocardium *n* relating to the endocardium and myocardium—**endomyocardial** *adj*.

endoneurium *n* the delicate, inner connective tissue surrounding the nerve fibres.

endoparasite *n* any parasite living within its host—**endoparasitic** *adj*.

endophthalmitis *n* internal infection of the eye, usually bacterial.

endorphins *n* a group of opiate-like neuropeptides activated by the pituitary gland, which have an analgesic effect. Involved in both central and peripheral nervous functions, their role is to modulate pain interpretation and to induce a euphoric after-effect.

endoscope *n* an instrument for visualization of body cavities or organs. The older ones are rigid, tubular and made of metal. If of the fibreoptic variety, light is transmitted by means of very fine glass fibres along a flexible tube. It can permit examination, photography, biopsy and surgery of the cavities or organs, with or without a general anaesthetic—**endoscopic** *adj*, **endoscopy** *n*.

endoscopic retrograde cholangiopancreatography (ERCP) introduction of a contrast medium into the pancreatic and bile ducts via a catheter from an endoscope located in the duodenum.

endospore *n* a bacterial spore which has a purely vegetative function. It is formed by the loss of water and probably rearrangement of the protein of the cell, so that metabolism is minimal and resistance to environmental conditions, especially high temperature, desiccation and antibacterial drugs, is high. The only genera which include pathogenic species that form spores are Bacillus and Clostridium.

endothelioid *adj* resembling endothelium*.

endothelioma *n* a malignant tumour derived from endothelial cells.

endothelium *n* the lining membrane of serous cavities, heart, blood and lymph vessels—**endothelial** *adj.*

endotoxin *n* a toxic product of bacteria which is associated with the bacterial cell wall, and can only be obtained by destruction of the cell. Endotoxins are not antigenic and do not stimulate antibody production. ⇒ exotoxin *opp.*—**endotoxic** *adj.*

endotracheal *adj* within the trachea. *endotracheal anaesthesia* the administration of an anaesthetic through an endotracheal tube passed into the trachea.

enema *n* the introduction of a liquid into the bowel via the rectum, to be returned or retained. The word is usually preceded by the name of the liquid used. It can be further designated according to the function of the fluid. The evacuant enemas are usually prepared commercially in small bulk as a disposable enema: the chemicals attract water into the bowel promoting cleansing and peristaltic contractions of the lower bowel. The enemas to be retained are usually drugs, the most common being cortisone. ⇒ barium enema—**enemas, enemata** *pl.*

enflurane *n* halogenated ether, a volatile liquid anaesthetic agent.

enkephalins *n* ⇒ encephalins.

enophthalmos *n* abnormal retraction of an eyeball within its orbit.

enrolled nurse (EN) one who has undergone a 2-year nursing programme in the UK. These education programmes have now been discontinued and enrolled nurses enabled where possible to undertake conversion courses to attain registered status.

ensiform *adj* sword-shaped; xiphoid.

ENT *abbr* ear, nose and throat.

Entamoeba *n* (*syn* Endamoeba) a genus of protozoon parasites, three species infesting man: *Entamoeba coli,* nonpathogenic, infesting intestinal tract; *E. gingivalis,* nonpathogenic, infesting mouth; *E. hystolytica,* pathogenic causing amoebic dysentery*.

enteral *adj* within the gastrointestinal tract. *enteral diets* those which are taken by mouth or through a nasogastric* tube: low residue enteral diets can be whole protein/polymeric, or amino acid/peptide. *enteral feeding* includes the introduction of nutrients into the gastrointestinal tract by modes other than eating ⇒ gastrostomy, nasogastric.

enteric *adj* pertaining to the small intestine. *enteric fever* includes typhoid* and paratyphoid* fever.

enteritis *n* inflammation of the intestines. The term 'regional enteritis' is currently preferred for Crohn's* disease.

enteroanastomosis *n* intestinal anastomosis.

Enterobacter *n* a genus of aerobic, nonspore-bearing, Gram-negative bacilli of the family Enterobacteriaceae. Includes two species, *Enterobacter aerogenes* and *Enterobacter cloacae.*

enterobiasis *n* infestation with *Enterobius vermicularis* (threadworms).

Enterobius vermicularis (threadworm) a nematode which infests the small and large intestine. Because of the autoinfective lifecycle, treatment aims at complete elimination. Each member of household given three single dose treatments at weekly intervals of piperazine citrate, 75 mg/kg. Hygiene measures necessary to prevent reinfestation during treatment.

enterocele *n* prolapse* of intestine. Can be into the upper third of vagina.

enteroclysis *n* (*syn* proctoclysis) the introduction of fluid into the rectum.

Enterococcus *n* a Gram-positive coccus which occurs in short chains and is relatively resistant to heat. Enterococci belong to Lancefield's group D, and occur as commensals in human and warm-blooded animal intestines, and sometimes as pathogens in infections of the urinary tract, ear, wounds and, more rarely, in endocarditis.

enterocolitis *n* inflammation of the small intestine and colon ⇒ necrotizing enterocolitis.

enterocutaneous fashioning of one of the abdominal organs lined with mucous membrane so that it is raised above the surface of the skin. ⇒ colostomy, ileostomy, ileoureterostomy.

enterokinase *n* (*syn* enteropeptidase) an enzyme in intestinal juice secreted by the duodenal lining cells. A proteolytic enzyme of the pancreatic juice which converts inactive trypsinogen into active trypsin.

enterolith *n* an intestinal concretion.

enterolithiasis *n* the presence of intestinal concretions.

enteron *n* the gut.

enteropeptidase *n* ⇒ enterokinase.

enterostomy *n* a surgically established fistula between the small intestine and some other surface. ⇒ gastroenterostomy, ileostomy, jejunostomy—**enterostomal** *adj*.

enterotomy *n* an incision into the small intestine.

enterotoxin *n* a toxin which has its effect on the gastrointestinal tract, causing vomiting, diarrhoea and abdominal pain.

enterotribe *n* a metal clamp which causes necrosis of the spur of a double-barrelled colostomy, as a preliminary to its closure.

enteroviruses *npl* viruses which enter the body by the alimentary tract. Comprise the poliomyelitisvirus, coxsackieviruses and echoviruses, which tend to invade the central nervous system. Enteroviruses, together with rhinoviruses*, are now called picornaviruses.

enterozoa *npl* any animal parasites infesting the intestines—**enterozoon** *sing*.

entropion *n* inversion of an eyelid so that the lashes are in contact with the globe of the eye.

enucleation *n* the removal of an organ or tumour in its entirety, as of an eyeball from its socket.

enuresis *n* incontinence of urine, especially bedwetting. *nocturnal enuresis* incontinence during sleep.

environment *n* external surroundings. Environmental factors are conditions influencing an individual from without—**environmental** *adj*.

enzyme *n* a soluble protein produced by living cells; it acts as a catalyst* without being destroyed or altered, and the substrate is often specific—**enzymatic** *adj*. *enzyme tests* since abnormal levels of particular enzymes can indicate specific underlying disease, tests for various enzymes can be a diagnostic tool.

enzyme-linked immunosorbent assay (ELISA) a method of testing for HIV antibodies. The test is not highly specific for HIV. If positive, it is usually followed by a second ELISA test and then by the more specific Western* blot test before HIV infection is confirmed.

enzymology *n* the science dealing with the structure and function of enzymes*—**enzymological** *adj*.

eosin *n* a red staining agent used in histology and laboratory diagnostic procedures.

eosinophil *n* 1 cells having an affinity for eosin. White blood cell concerned with immune responses. 2 a type of polymorphonuclear leucocyte containing eosin-staining granules—**eosinophilic** *adj.*

eosinophilia *n* increased eosinophils in the blood. Often seen in allergic disorders.

ependymoma *n* neoplasm arising in the lining of the cerebral ventricles or central canal of spinal cord. Can occur in all age groups.

ephedrine *n* a drug widely used in asthma and bronchial spasm for its relaxant action on bronchioles; raises blood pressure by peripheral vasoconstriction. Useful in hay fever.

ephelides *npl* freckles, an increase in pigment granules with a normal number of pigment cells ⇒ lentigo—**ephelis** *sing.*

EPI *abbr* ⇒ Eysenck Personality Inventory.

epicanthus *n* the congenital occurrence of a fold of skin obscuring the inner canthus of the eye—**epicanthal** *adj.*

epicardium *n* the visceral layer of the pericardium*—**epicardial** *adj.*

epicritic *adj* describes cutaneous nerve fibres which are sensitive to fine variations of touch or temperature. ⇒ protopathic *opp.*

epidemic *n* simultaneously affecting many people in an area ⇒ endemic *opp.*

epidemiology *n* the scientific study of the distribution of diseases—**epidemiological** *adj,* **epidemiologically** *adv.*

epidermis *n* the external nonvascular layer of the skin; the cuticle—**epidermal** *adj.*

Epidermophyton *n* a genus of fungi which affects the skin and nails.

epidermophytosis *n* infection with fungi of the genus *Epidermophyton.*

epididymectomy *n* surgical removal of the epididymis*.

epididymis *n* a small oblong body attached to the posterior surface of the testes. It consists of the seminiferous tubules which convey the spermatozoa from the testes to the vas deferens.

epididymitis *n* inflammation of the epididymis*.

epididymoorchitis *n* inflammation of the epididymis* and the testis*.

epidural *adj* upon or external to the dura. *epidural block* single injection or intermittent injection through a catheter of local anaesthetic for maternal analgesia during delivery or for surgical operations. *epidural space* the region through which spinal nerves leave the spinal cord. It can be approached at any level of the spine, but the administering of anaesthetic is commonly done at the lumbar level or through the sacral cornua for caudal epidural block.

epigastrium *n* the abdominal region lying directly over the stomach—**epigastric** *adj.*

epiglottis *n* the thin, leaf-shaped flap of cartilage behind the tongue which, during the act of swallowing, protects the opening leading into the larynx.

epiglottitis *n* inflammation of the epiglottis*.

epilation *n* extraction or destruction of hair roots, e.g. by coagulation necrosis, electrolysis or forceps. ⇒ depilation—**epilate** *vt.*

epilatory *adj, n* (describes) an agent which produces epilation*.

epilepsy *n* correctly called the epilepsies, a group of conditions resulting from disordered electrical activity of brain and manifesting as epileptic seizures or 'fits'. The seizure is caused by an abnormal electrical discharge that disturbs cerebration and results in a generalized or partial seizure, depending on the area of the brain in which the discharge originates. *Generalized seizures* may be: *tonic-clonic,* formerly called *grand mal* seizures and the commonest type of epileptic seizure with loss of consciousness and generalized convulsions; *tonic,* in which there is a sudden stiffening of muscles; *atonic,* with a sudden loss of muscle tone (also called a drop attack); *absences,* also known as *petit mal,* where there is a brief interruption of consciousness. *Partial seizures* occur when the electrical disturbance is limited to a particular focus of the brain and are manifested in a variety of ways, including limb twitching and paraesthesia or altered behavior patterns. *Secondary generalized seizures* partial seizures resulting from the spread of a focus of electrical disturbance to the whole brain. *status epilepticus* continuous convulsions where the person does not regain consciousness in between seizures.

epileptic 1 *adj* pertaining to epilepsy. **2** *n* a person with epilepsy. *epileptic aura* premonitory subjective phenomena (tingling in the hand or visual or auditory sensations) which precede an attack of major epilepsy. ⇒ aura. *epileptic cry* the croak or shout heard from the epileptic person as he falls unconscious.

epileptiform *adj* resembling epilepsy.

epileptogenic *adj* capable of causing epilepsy.

epiloia *n* ⇒ tuberous sclerosis.

epimenorrhoea *n* reduction of the length of the menstrual cycle.

epiphora *n* pathological overflow of tears on to the cheek.

epiphysis *n* the end of a growing bone. Separated from the shaft by a plate of cartilage (epiphyseal plate) which disappears due to ossification when growth ceases—**epiphyses** *pl,* **epiphyseal** *adj.*

epiphysitis *n* inflammation of an epiphysis*.

episclera *n* loose connective tissue between the sclera and conjunctiva—**episcleral** *adj.*

episcleritis *n* inflammation of the episclera*.

episiorrhaphy *n* surgical repair of a lacerated perineum.

episiotomy *n* a perineal incision made during the birth of a child when the vaginal orifice does not stretch sufficiently.

epispadias *n* a congenital opening of the urethra on the anterior (upper side) of the penis, often associated with ectopia* vesicae. ⇒ hypospadias.

epispastic *n* a blistering agent.

epistaxis *n* bleeding from the nose—**epistaxes** *pl.*

epithelialization *n* the growth of epithelium over a raw area; the final stage of healing.

epithelioma *n* a malignant growth arising from squamous or transitional epithelium, usually of the skin, oesophagus or external genital organs.

epithelium *n* the surface layer of cells covering cutaneous, mucous and serous surfaces. It is classified according to the arrangement and shape of the cells it contains—**epithelial** *adj.*

Epstein-Barr virus (EBV) causative agent of infectious* mononucleosis. A versatile herpes virus which infects many people throughout the world; does not always produce symptoms. Cancer research workers have discovered EBV genome in the malignant cells of Burkitt's lymphoma and nasopharyngeal carcinoma.

epulis *n* a tumour growing on or from the gums.

Erb's palsy paralysis* involving the shoulder and arm muscles from a lesion of the fifth and sixth cervical nerve roots. The arm hangs loosely at the side with the forearm pronated ('waiter's tip position'). Most commonly a birth injury.

ERCP *abbr* endoscopic* retrograde cholangiopancreatography.

erectile *adj* upright; capable of being elevated. *erectile tissue* highly vascular tissue, which, under stimulus, becomes rigid and erect from hyperaemia.

erection *n* the state achieved when erectile tissue is hyperaemic. The enlarged state of the penis during sexual arousal and coitus.

erector *n* a muscle which achieves erection of a part, as in erectori pili muscles which cause goose pimples and make the skin hairs stand erect.

ERG *abbr* ⇒ electroretinogram.

ergometrine *n* main alkaloid of ergot*. Widely used in obstetrics to reduce haemorrhage and improve contraction of uterus.

ergometry *n* measurement of work done by muscles—**ergometric** *adj.*

ergonomics *n* the application of various biological disciplines in relation to man and his working environment.

ergosterol *n* a provitamin present in the subcutaneous fat of man and animals. On irradiation* it is converted into vitamin D_2. Target site for some antifungal preparations.

ergot *n* the food storage body of a fungus, *Claviceps purpurea,* which infects rye. Widely used as ergometrine* for postpartum haemorrhage.

eroticism *n* arousal of sexual desire or instinct through suggestive or symbolic means, or as foreplay before the act of sexual intercourse.

eructation *n* belching: the act of noisily bringing up gas from the stomach and expelling it orally.

eruption *n* the process by which a tooth emerges through the alveolar bone or gingiva. *skin eruption* furuncle or skin rash.

erysipelas *n* an acute, specific infectious disease, in which there is a spreading, streptococcal inflammation of the skin and subcutaneous tissues, accompanied by fever and constitutional disturbances.

erysipeloid *n* a skin condition resembling erysipelas*. It occurs in butchers, fishmongers or cooks. The infecting organism is the *Erysipelothrix* of swine erysipelas.

erythema *n* reddening of the skin—**erythematous** *adj. erythema induratum* Bazin's* disease. *erythema multiforme* a form of toxic or allergic skin eruption which breaks out suddenly and lasts for days; the lesions are in the form of violet pink papules or plaques and suggest urticarial weals. Severe form called Stevens-Johnson syndrome. *erythema nodosum* an eruption of painful red nodules on the front of the legs. It occurs in young women, and is generally accompanied by rheumaticky pains. It may be a symptom of many diseases including tuberculosis, acute rheumatism and gonococcal septicaemia. *erythema pernio* ⇒ chilblain.

erythroblast *n* a nucleated red blood cell found in the red bone marrow from which the erythrocytes* are derived—**erythroblastic** *adj.*

erythroblastosis fetalis haemolytic* disease of the newborn.

erythrocyanosis frigida vasospastic disease with hypertrophy of arteriolar muscular coat—**erythrocyanotic** *adj.*

erythrocytes *npl* the normal non-nucleated red cells of the circulating blood; the red blood corpuscles—**erythrocytic** *adj.*

erythrocyte sedimentation rate (ESR) citrated blood is placed in a narrow tube. The red cells fall, leaving a column of clear supernatant serum, which is measured at the end of an hour and reported in millimetres. Tissue destruction and inflammatory conditions cause an increase in the ESR.

erythrocythaemia *n* overproduction of red cells. This may be due to: (a) a physiological response to a low atmospheric oxygen tension (high altitudes), or to the need for greater oxygenation of the tissues (congenital heart disease), in which case it is referred to as erythrocytosis; or (b) an idiopathic condition, polycythaemia* vera.

erythrocytopenia *n* deficiency in the number of red blood cells—**erythrocytopenic** *adj.*

erythrocytosis *n* ⇒ erythrocythaemia.

erythroderma *n* excessive redness of the skin.

erythrogenic *adj* **1** producing or causing a rash. **2** producing red blood cells.

erythromycin *n* an orally active antibiotic, similar to penicillin* in its range of action. Best reserved for use against organisms resistant to other antibiotics. Risk of jaundice, particularly with erythromycin estolate.

erythropoiesis *n* the production of red blood cells ⇒ haemopoiesis.

erythropoietin *n* a hormone secreted by certain cells in the kidney in response to a lowered oxygen content in the blood. It acts on the bone marrow, stimulating erythropoiesis*.

erythrosine *n* a red dye used in dental disclosing tablets.

eschar *n* a slough, as results from a burn, application of caustics, diathermy, etc.

escharotic *adj* describes any agent capable of producing a slough.

Escherichia *n* a genus of bacteria. Motile, Gram-negative rods (bacilli) which are widely distributed in nature, especially in the intestinal tract of vertebrates. Some strains are pathogenic to man, causing enteritis, peritonitis, pyelitis, cystitis and wound infections. The type species is *Escherichia coli.*

Esmarch's bandage a rubber roller bandage used to procure a bloodless operative field in the limbs.

ESR *abbr* erythrocyte* sedimentation rate.

ESRD *abbr* end stage renal disease ⇒ renal.

essence *n* a solution of a volatile oil in rectified spirit.

essential amino acids ⇒ amino acids.

essential fatty acids (EFAs) (arachidonic, tinoleic and linolenic acids). Polyunsaturated acids which cannot be synthesized in the body. They have diverse functions, the most important being that they are precursors of prostaglandins. They fulfil an important role in fat metabolism and form part of the plasma membrane. They are present in natural vegetable oils and fish oils. Research suggests that deficiency of some EFAs contributes to premenstrual* syndrome.

estradiol *n Am* ⇒ oestradiol.

estrogen *n Am* ⇒ oestrogen.

ESWL *abbr* extracorporeal shockwave lithotripsy. ⇒ Dornier lithotriptor.

ethanol *n* alcohol*.

ether *n* an inflammable liquid; one of the oldest volatile anaesthetics and less toxic than chloroform. Rarely used today in the Western world as a general anaesthetic.

ethics *n* a code of moral principles derived from a system of values and beliefs and concerned with rights and obligations. The study of nursing ethics as a discipline distinct from bioethics and medical ethics, has developed strongly in recent years ⇒ Ethics box.

ethmoid *n* a spongy bone forming the lateral walls of the nose and the upper portion of the bony nasal septum.

ethmoidectomy *n* surgical removal of a part of the ethmoid bone, usually that forming the lateral nasal walls.

ethnic *adj* pertaining to racial or cultural groups.

ethnology *n* a branch of anthropology which has implications for health care; it studies mainly the cultural differences between groups, particularly the attitudes, values and beliefs relating to such life events as birth, contraception, abortion, marriage, diet, health care and death—**ethnological** *adj*, **ethnologically** *adv*.

ethyl chloride *n* a volatile general anaesthetic for short operations, and a local anaesthetic by reason of the intense cold produced when applied to the skin; useful in sprains.

ethyl pyrophosphate (TEPP) organophosphorous compound used as insecticide in agriculture. Powerful and irreversible anticholinesterase action. Potentially dangerous to man for this reason.

etiology *n Am* ⇒ aetiology.

EUA *abbr* examination (of the uterus) under anaesthetic.

eucalyptus oil has mild antiseptic properties and is sometimes used in nasal drops for catarrh.

eugenics *n* the study of agencies and measures aimed at improving the hereditary qualities of human generations—**eugenic** *adj*.

eunuch *n* a human male from whom the testes have been removed; a castrated male.

EU nursing directives since 1979 attempts have been made to ensure that nurses in the different European countries have been exposed to a similar education programme to facilitate free movement of nursing personnel throughout the countries.

eupepsia *n* normal digestion.

euphoria *n* in psychiatry, an exaggerated sense of well-being—**euphoric** *adj*.

eusol *n* acronym for Edinburgh University Solution of Lime, an antiseptic solution prepared from chloride of lime and boric* acid.

eustachian tube (*syn* pharyngotympanic tube) a canal, partly bony, partly cartilaginous, measuring 40–50 mm in length, connecting the pharynx with the tympanic cavity. It allows air to pass into the middle ear, so that the air pressure is kept even on both sides of the eardrum. *eustachian catheter* an instrument used for insufflating the eustachian tube when it becomes blocked.

eutetic mixture of local anaesthetics a cream for anaesthetizing skin by applying it to the site 1 hour before, e.g. venepuncture* of a child.

euthanasia *n* literally an 'easy death'; the act of relieving a person's extreme suffering from an incurable disease by bringing about their death, e.g. with opiate overdose. Presently illegal in UK and opposed by many professional groups, it is practised in some European countries, including the Netherlands ⇒ Ethics box, p. 134.

euthyroid state denoting normal thyroid function.

eutocia *n* a natural and normal labour and childbirth without any complications.

evacuant *n* an agent which causes an evacuation, particularly of the bowel ⇒ enema.

evacuation *n* the act of emptying

ETHICS AND RELATED TOPICS

Ethics* is the theoretical pursuit of moral knowledge, where the type of knowledge sought refers to aspects of moral conduct, moral issues in society and moral analysis of the fundamental questions of life:

moral conduct is conduct or behaviour that has a moral component to it because it involves the way we either prefer to treat or interact with ourselves or others. It is behaviour that reflects our values, virtues, moral development and/or personal convictions.

moral issues are social, legal, cultural, religious or personal issues that have a moral aspect to them because they demand a moral as well as a sociocultural response, e.g. the relationship between the amount of health care tax paid by individuals, free access to health care as needed, and the standard of health care provided, is a moral issue. Some moral issues are very private, e.g. abortion.

moral analysis is analysis of events, concepts and behaviours from the perspective of moral philosophy/ethics, e.g. whistle-blowing may demand moral courage; a philosophical analysis of good or bad moral conduct, like lying, stealing or caring, is moral analysis, and so is analysing fundamental questions about life, such as whether to undergo life-prolonging treatment.

Abortion*

The product of an abortion may be a previable fetus,a premature but nonviable infant or, occasionally, a viable premature infant. The product of an abortion is granted no civil rights, e.g. to a burial or a name under the age of 24 weeks. A planned abortion is a medical intervention that requires the consent of two physicians. At present, planned abortions are legal within most of the countries of the European Union, but many individuals have ethical and religious objections to the planned interruption of a pregnancy.

Confidentiality*

All health care workers have a moral obligation to maintain confidential all information about a patient, particularly his or her private affairs and diagnosis. However, health care workers also maintain a clause that allows them to disclose to other professionals medical and relevant details on a 'need-to-know' basis, in order to promote the welfare of the patient, and/or protect the public, e.g. in the case of contagious diseases or violent behaviour. Confidentiality is not an absolute imperative but needless disclosure of information can lead to serious legal and professional consequences.

Euthanasia*

Euthanasia is the planned death of an individual who would not otherwise die at that time. Death is the result of a series of medical interventions by health care workers specifically undertaken at the request of the patient/individual to bring about a quick, controlled, reasonably pain-free end to that person's life.

Euthanasia, as it is presented for discussion among health care workers and society, involves the request of sentient adults to have their lives terminated by physicians because they are now, or may one day be, in pain or suffering, have a degenerative disease or be terminally ill, or are in a state between true living and death, e.g. PVS. In the UK, euthanasia is not permissable and, at present, the BMA and the RCN are opposed to any moves towards legalizing euthanasia. It is a highly emotive subject and many individuals are extremely uncomfortable with even the prospect of legalized euthanasia.

A *living will*, or advance directive, is a statement of intent by a patient or any individual about the treatment options and level of intervention they would wish for themselves should they become so incapacitated that they are unable to make their wishes known to health care providers. A living will is not legally binding but to violate a patient's known expressed wishes may be a legal matter.

a cavity; generally refers to the discharge of faecal matter from the rectum. *manual evacuation* digital removal of faeces from the rectum.

evacuator *n* an instrument for procuring evacuation, e.g. the removal from the bladder of a stone, crushed by a lithotrite.

evaluating *v* commonly accepted as the fourth phase of the nursing process. Care is evaluated to assess whether the stated patient goals* have been or are being achieved. Although it is the final step in the nursing process, it should occur continuously from the first assessment to the patient's discharge from the health care system—**evaluation** *n*.

evaporate *vt, vi* to convert from the liquid to the gaseous state by means of heat.

evaporating lotion one which, applied as a compress, absorbs heat in order to evaporate and so cools the skin.

eversion *n* a turning outwards, as of the upper eyelid to expose the conjunctival sac.

evidence based practice clinical practice that is based on the findings of good quality research. ⇒ clinical effectiveness, clinical guidelines.

evisceration *n* removal of internal organs.

evulsion *n* forcible tearing away of a structure.

Ewing's tumour (*syn* reticulocytoma sarcoma). A sarcoma usually involving the long bone in a child or young person.

exacerbation *n* increased severity, as of symptoms.

exanthema *n* a skin eruption—**exanthemata** *pl,* **exanthematous** *adj*.

excision *n* removal of a part by cutting—**excise** *vt*.

excitability *n* rapid response to stimuli; a state of being easily irritated—**excitable** *adj*.

excitation *n* the act of stimulating an organ or tissue.

exclusion isolation separation of a patient so that he can be protected from infection. This may be necessary when the patient is immunodeficient (immunocompromised*, immunosuppressed) most commonly from taking such things as steroids and cytotoxic drugs for whatever reason. ⇒ containment isolation, reverse barrier nursing.

excoriation *n* ⇒ abrasion.

excrement *n* faeces*.

excresence *n* an abnormal protuberance or growth of the tissues.

excreta *n* the waste matter which is normally discharged from the body, particularly urine and faeces.

excretion *n* the elimination of waste material from the body, and also the matter so discharged—**excretory** *adj,* **excrete** *vt*.

exenteration *n* removal of the viscera from its containing cavity, e.g. the eye from its socket, the pelvic organs from the pelvis.

exfoliation *n* **1** the scaling off of tissues in layers. **2** the shedding of the primary teeth—**exfoliative** *adj.*

exfoliative cytology ⇒ cytology.

exhibitionism *n* **1** any kind of 'showing off'; extravagant behaviour to attract attention. **2** a psychosexual disorder confined to males and consisting of repeated exposure of the genitals to a stranger. No further contact is sought with the victim, who is usually a female adult or a child—**exhibitionist** *n.*

Eximer laser laser used to perform photorefractive* keratectomy (PRK).

exocrine *adj* describes glands from which the secretion passes via a duct; secreting externally. ⇒ endocrine *opp*—**exocrinal** *adj.*

exogenous *adj* of external origin. ⇒ endogenous *opp.*

exomphalos *n* a condition present at birth and due to failure of the gut to return to the abdominal cavity during fetal development. The intestines protrude through a gap in the abdominal wall, still enclosed in peritoneum.

exophthalmos *n* protrusion of the eyeball—**exophthalmic** *adj.*

exostosis *n* an overgrowth of bone tissue forming a benign tumour.

exotoxin *n* a toxic product of bacteria which is synthesized and secreted by living bacteria. Exotoxins are antigenic proteins and can thus be neutralized by antibodies produced during the immune response. ⇒ endotoxin *opp.*—**exotoxic** *adj.*

expected date of delivery (EDD) usually calculated from the first day of the last normal menstrual period, even though for the next 14 days there is no pregnancy.

expectorant *n* a drug which promotes or increases expectoration*.

expectoration *n* **1** the elimination of secretion from the respiratory tract by coughing. **2** sputum*—**expectorate** *vt.*

expiration *n* the act of breathing out air from the lungs—**expiratory** *adj,* **expire** *vt, vi.*

expression *n* **1** expulsion by force as of the placenta from the uterus; milk from the breast, etc. **2** facial disclosure of feelings, mood, etc.

expressive aphasia a type of aphasia* characterized by difficulty in language production. Word finding difficulties and problems in producing sentence structures may occur. May occur with receptive* aphasia.

exsanguination *n* the process of rendering bloodless—**exsanguinate** *vt.*

extended family a term currently used to mean the wider group of family relations including aunts, uncles, cousins, grandparents, etc. It is used mainly in a comparative sense when considering the concept 'nuclear* family'.

extended role of the nurse nurses are increasingly taking on additional roles and responsibilities, traditionally regarded as belonging to doctors. These include specific skills, such as intravenous cannulation and venepuncture, and roles, such as nurse-led clinics. The UKCC* has set out the professional framework in which such practice may develop in its document 'The Scope of Professional Practice'.

extension *n* **1** traction upon a fractured or dislocated limb. **2** the increasing of the angle at a joint.

extensor *n* a muscle which, on contraction, extends or straightens a part ⇒ flexor *opp.*

external cephalic version (ECV) ⇒ version.

extirpation *n* complete removal or destruction of a part.

extraanatomic bypass (EAB) a prosthetic vascular graft is threaded subcutaneously to carry a limb-preserving blood supply from an efficient proximal part of an artery to a distal one, thus bypassing the inefficient part of the artery.

extraarticular *adj* outside a joint.

extracapsular *adj* outside a capsule. → intracapsular *opp.*

extracardiac *adj* outside the heart.

extracellular *adj* outside the cell membrane. ⇒ intracellular *opp.*

extracorporeal *adj* outside the body. *extracorporeal circulation* blood is taken from the body, directed through a machine ('heart-lung' or 'artificial kidney') and returned to the general circulation.

extracorporeal shock-wave lithotripsy ⇒ Dornier lithotriptor.

extract *n* a preparation obtained by evaporating a solution of a drug.

extraction *n* the removal of a tooth. *extraction of lens* surgical removal of the lens. *extracapsular extraction* the capsule is ruptured prior to delivery of the lens and preserved in part. *intracapsular extraction* the lens is removed within its capsule.

extradural *adj* external to the dura mater.

extragenital *adj* on areas of the body apart from genital organs. *extragenital chancre* is the primary ulcer of syphilis when it occurs on the finger, the lip, the breast, etc.

extrahepatic *adj* outside the liver.

extramural *adj* outside the wall of a vessel or organ—**extramurally** *adv.*

extraperitoneal *adj* outside the peritoneum.

extrapleural *adj* outside the pleura, i.e. between the parietal pleura and the chest wall. ⇒ plombage—**extrapleurally** *adv.*

extrapyramidal tracts transmit the motor neurones from the brain to the spinal cord except for the fibres in the pyramidal* tracts. They are functional rather than anatomical units; they control and coordinate the postural, static mechanisms which cause contractions of muscle groups in sequence or simultaneously.

extrarenal *n* outside the kidney—**extrarenally** *adv.*

extrasystole *n* premature beats (ectopic beats) in the pulse rhythm: the cardiac impulse is initiated in some focus apart from the sinoatrial node.

extrathoracic *adj* outside the thoracic cavity.

extrauterine *n* outside the uterus. *extrauterine pregnancy* ⇒ ectopic pregnancy.

extravasation *n* an escape of fluid from its normal enclosure into the surrounding tissues.

extravenous *adj* outside a vein.

extrinsic *adj* developing or having its origin from without; not internal. *extrinsic factor* vitamin B_{12}, essential for the maturation of erythrocytes, cannot be synthesized in the body but must be supplied in the diet, hence it is called the extrinsic factor. It is absorbed in the presence of the intrinsic factor secreted by the stomach.

extrinsic allergic alveolitis (Farmer's lung) an occupational asthma resulting from exposure to moulds, fungal spores or heterologous proteins when working in agriculture, forestry, handling birds or animals.

extroversion *n* turning inside out. *extroversion of the bladder* ectopia* vesicae. In psychology, the direction of thoughts to the external world.

extrovert *adj* Jungian description of an individual whose characteristic interests and modes of behaviour are directed outwards to other people and the physical environment. ⇒ introvert *opp.*

extubation *n* removal of a tube from a hollow organ, e.g. removal of endotracheal tube following assisted ventilation. ⇒ intubation *opp.*

exudate *n* the product of exudation*. Discharge from a wound.

exudation *n* the oozing out of fluid through the capillary walls, of sweat through the pores of the skin—**exudate** *n,* **exude** *vt, vi.*

eye contact looking at the face of the person to whom one is talking. In many instances it is a reciprocal activity and is such an important part of most cultures' nonverbal language that blind people are advised to turn their faces in the direction of the voice being heard. In some cultures, however, it is considered inappropriate to make or maintain eye contact during conversation, or when acknowledging a person on the street. *same-level eye contact* a term increasingly being used in nursing to remind nurses that sitting when talking to a bedfast patient or a person in a wheelchair is good nursing practice.

eye-teeth the canine teeth* in the upper jaw.

Eysenck Personality Inventory a self-scoring set of items which measure two independent dimensions of personality; neuroticism, and extroversion versus introversion.

F

facet *n* a small, smooth, flat surface of a bone or a calculus. *facet syndrome* dislocation of some of the gliding joints between vertebrae causing pain and muscle spasm.

facial *adj* pertaining to the face. *facial expression* part of nonverbal body language by which current mood can be conveyed. Paralysis of any of the facial muscles and an abnormality such as a keloid* can distort facial expression. ⇒ Bell's palsy, hemiparesis, ptosis. *facial gesture* part of nonverbal body language usually used to reinforce spoken language. Some people, such as those with cerebral* palsy, do not have control of the voluntary muscles involved, consequently nurses assessing a person with spasticities may have difficulty in interpreting facial gestures because of unfamiliarity with them. *facial nerve* seventh pair of the 12 pairs of cranial nerves which arise directly from the brain. *facial paralysis* paralysis of muscles supplied by the facial nerve.

facies *n* the appearance of the face, used especially of the subject of congenital syphilis with saddle nose, prominent brow and chin. *adenoid facies* open mouthed, vacant expression due to deafness from enlarged adenoids. *facies hippocratica* the drawn, pale, pinched appearance indicative of approaching death. *Parkinson facies* a mask-like appearance; saliva may trickle from the corners of the mouth.

factor P one component of the complement* system.

faecal fat collection the laboratory requires a whole stool, not a specimen from it, to estimate the amount of fat per weight of faeces.

faecal impaction the presence of a large amount of dried hardened faeces in the rectum and lower bowel. After taking medication to soften the faeces, an evacuant enema* is introduced into the rectum via the anus. ⇒ impacted, manual evacuation of the bowel, spurious diarrhoea.

faecalith *n* a concretion formed in the bowel from faecal matter: it can cause obstruction and/or inflammation.

faecal-oral route a term that describes the ingestion of microorganisms from faeces which can be transmitted directly or indirectly by hands.

faeces *n* the waste matter excreted from the bowel, consisting mainly of indigestible cellulose, unabsorbed food, intestinal secretions, water and bacteria. It is recommended that sufficient dietary fibre should be taken to produce 150–250 g of faeces daily—**faecal** *adj.*

Fahrenheit *n* a thermometric scale; the freezing point of water is 32° and its boiling point 212°.

failure to thrive failure to grow and develop at the expected rate, ascertained by consistent measurement of weight and height plotted on a growth chart. The syndrome may be the result of an organic disorder or have nonorganic causes, such as inadequate feeding, maternal* deprivation, or psychosocial problems. Systematic investigation is required to establish the cause.

faint *n* syncope*–**faint** *vi.*

falciform *adj* sickle-shaped.

fallopian tubes ⇒ uterine tubes.

Fallot's tetralogy a form of cyanotic congenital heart disease which comprizes four abnormalities: a large septal defect between the ventricles; stenosis of the pulmonary valve; overriding of the aorta; right ventricular hypertrophy. Increasingly, total surgical correction is being used.

falx *n* a sickle-shaped structure. *falx cerebri* that portion of the dura mater separating the two cerebral hemispheres.

familial *adj* pertaining to the family, as of a disease affecting several members of the same family.

family-centred care a philosophy of nursing usually applied to children which takes into account the needs and circumstances of the whole family, not just the child.

family planning the use of contraceptives to space or limit the number of children born to a couple.

Fanconi syndrome an inherited or acquired dysfunction of the proximal kidney tubules. Large amounts of amino acids, glucose and phosphates are excreted in the urine, yet the blood levels of these substances are normal. Symptoms may include thirst, polyuria, bone abnormalities and muscular weakness ⇒ aminoaciduria, cystinosis.

fantasy, phantasy *n* a 'day dream' in which the thinker's conscious or unconscious desires and impulses are fulfilled. May be accompanied by a feeling of unreality. Occurs pathologically in schizophrenia.

farinaceous *adj* pertaining to cereal substances, i.e. made of flour or grain. Starchy.

farmer's lung a form of alveolitis due to allergy to certain spores (e.g. *Micropolyspora faeni*) that occur in the dust of mouldy hay or other mouldy vegetable produce. Recognized as an industrial disease.

FAS *abbr* fetal* alcohol syndrome.

fascia *n* a connective tissue sheath consisting of fibrous tissue and fat which unites the skin to the underlying tissues. It also surrounds and separates many of the muscles, and, in some cases, holds them together–**fascial** *adj.*

fasciculation *n* visible flickering of muscle; can occur in the upper and lower eyelids.

fasciculus *n* a little bundle, as of muscle or nerve–**fascicular** *adj,* **fasciculi** *pl.*

fasciotomy *n* incision of a fascia*.

fastigium *n* the highest point of a fever; the period of full development of a disease.

fat *n* **1** a compound of glycerol with fatty acids which may be of animal or vegetable origin, and may be either solid or liquid. Vitamins A, D, E and K are fat-soluble. **2** adipose tissue, which acts as a reserve supply of energy and smooths out body contours–**fatty** *adj.* ⇒ brown fat, kilojoule.

Fatal Accident Enquiry ⇒ coroner.

fatigue *n* weariness. Term used in physiological experiments on muscle to denote diminishing reaction to stimulus applied–**fatigability** *n.*

fatty degeneration degeneration* of tissues which results in appearance of fatty droplets in the cytoplasm: found especially in diseases of liver, kidney and heart.

fauces *n* the opening from the mouth into the pharynx,

bounded above by the soft palate, below by the tongue. Pillars of the fauces, anterior and posterior, lie laterally and enclose the tonsil—**faucial** *adj.*

favism *n* describes the acute haemolytic anaemia resulting from eating or being in contact with the fava bean in people with the sex-linked disorder G6PD deficiency, in which there is a reduced amount of enzyme G6PD (glucose-6-phosphate dehydrogenase) in red blood cells.

favus *n* a type of ringworm not common in Britain; caused by *Trichophyton schoenleini.* Yellow cup-shaped crusts (scutula) develop especially on the scalp.

fear *n* an intense emotional state involving a feeling of unpleasant tension, and a strong impulse to escape, which is natural in response to a threat of danger but is unnatural as a continuous state ⇒ anxiety.

febrile *adj* feverish; accompanied by fever. *febrile convulsions* occur in children who have an increased body temperature; they do not usually result in permanent brain damage. Most common between the ages of 6 months and 5 years. ⇒ convulsions.

fecundation *n* impregnation. Fertilization.

fecundity *n* the power of reproduction; fertility.

feedback treatment ⇒ biofeedback.

Felty syndrome enlargement of the liver, spleen and lymph nodes as a complication of rheumatoid* arthritis.

femoral hernia ⇒ hernia

femur *n* the thigh bone; the longest and strongest bone in the body—**femora** *pl,* **femoral** *adj.*

fenestra *n* a window-like opening. *fenestra ovalis* an oval opening between the middle and internal ear. Below it lies the *fenestra rotunda* a round opening.

fenestration *n* the surgical creation of an opening (or fenestra) in the inner ear for the relief of deafness in otosclerosis.

ferment ⇒ catalyst.

fermentation *n* the glycolysis of carbohydrates to produce ATP in which simple organic compounds (not molecular oxygen) act as the terminal electron acceptors (e.g. alcohol). Excellent examples are the making of bread, cheese and wine.

ferrous *adj* pertaining to divalent iron, as of its salts and compounds. *Ferrous carbonate, ferrous fumarate, ferrous gluconate,* ferrous succinate and *ferrous sulphate* are oral preparations for iron-deficiency anaemias.

fertilization *n* the impregnation of an ovum by a spermatozoon.

FESS functional endoscopic sinus surgery.

fester *vi* to become inflamed; to suppurate.

festination *n* ⇒ fenestration.

fetal alcohol syndrome (FAS) stillbirth and fetal abnormality due to prenatal growth retardation caused by the mother's consumption of alcohol during pregnancy.

fetishism *n* a condition in which a particular material object is regarded with irrational awe or has a strong emotional attachment. Can have a psychosexual dimension in which such an object is repeatedly or exclusively used in achieving sexual excitement.

fetor *n* offensive odour, stench. *fetor oris* bad breath.

fetoscopy *n* direct visual examination of the fetus by using a suitable fibreglass endoscope.

fetus *n* the internationally preferred spelling. An unborn child. *fetus papyraceous* a dead fetus, one of twins which has become flattened and mummified—**fetal** *adj. fetal circulation* circulation of blood through the fetus, umbilical cord and placenta.

FEV *abbr* forced* expiratory volume. ⇒ respiratory function tests.

fever *n* (*syn* pyrexia) an elevation of body temperature above normal. Designates some infectious conditions, e.g. *paratyphoid fever, scarlet fever, typhoid fever*, etc. ⇒ pyrexia.

fibre *n* a thread-like structure—**fibrous** *adj.*

fibreoptics *n* the transmission of light through flexible glass fibres. The incorporation of fibreoptics into endoscopes* enables the user to visualize internal organs, aiding reliable and less traumatic diagnosis of pathological conditions.

fibril *n* a component filament of a fibre; a small fibre.

fibrillation *n* uncoordinated quivering contraction of muscle; referring usually to atrial* or ventricular* fibrillation in the myocardium wherein the atria or ventricles beat very rapidly and do not produce a synchronized beat.

fibrin *n* the matrix on which a blood clot is formed. The substance is formed from soluble fibrinogen* of the blood by the catalytic (enzymatic) action of thrombin*—**fibrinous** *adj. fibrin foam* a white, dry, spongy material made from fibrinogen. It is used in conjunction with thrombin as a haemostatic in brain and lung surgery.

fibrinogen *n* a soluble protein of the blood from which is produced the insoluble protein called fibrin* which is essential to blood coagulation.

fibrinogenopenia *n* (*syn* fibrinopenia) lack of blood plasma fibrinogen*. Can be congenital or due to liver disease.

fibrinolysin *n* enzyme in the blood stream which dissolves fibrin*. Sometimes administered intravenously in thrombosis.

fibrinolysis *n* the dissolution of fibrin* which can precede haemorrhage. There is normally a balance between blood coagulation and fibrinolysis in the body—**fibrinolytic** *adj.*

fibrinopenia *n* ⇒ fibrinogenopenia.

fibroadenoma *n* a benign tumour containing fibrous and glandular tissue.

fibroblast *n* (*syn* fibrocyte) a cell which produces collagen, a major constituent of the connective tissues—**fibroblastic** *adj.*

fibrocartilage *n* cartilage containing fibrous tissue—**fibrocartilaginous** *adj.*

fibrocaseous *adj* a soft, cheesy mass infiltrated by fibrous tissue, formed by fibroblasts.

fibrochondritis *n* inflammation of fibrocartilage.

fibrocyst *n* a fibroma which has undergone cystic degeneration, i.e. cystic fibroma.

fibrocystic *adj* pertaining to a fibrocyst*. *fibrocystic disease of bone* cysts may be solitary or—characterized by an overgrowth of fibrous tissue and development of cystic spaces, especially in a gland—generalized. If generalized and accompanied by decalcification of bone, it is symptomatic of hyperparathyroidism. *fibrocystic disease of breast* the breast feels lumpy due to the presence of cysts, usually caused by hormone imbalance. *fibrocystic disease of pancreas* cystic fibrosis*.

fibrocyte *n* ⇒ fibroblast—**fibrocytic** *adj.*

fibroid *n* a fibromuscular benign tumour usually found in the uterus, more commonly in women approaching menopause. Frequently asymptomatic but may cause abnormal bleeding.

Classified according to location: *interstitial (intramural) uterine fibroid* is embedded in the wall of the uterus. *subperitoneal (subserous) fibroid* extends to the outer wall. *submucous fibroid* extends to the inner or endometrial surface.

fibroma *n* a benign tumour composed of fibrous tissue—**fibromata** *pl,* **fibromatous** *adj.*

fibromuscular *adj* pertaining to fibrous and muscle tissue.

fibromyoma *n* a benign tumour consisting of fibrous and muscle tissue—**fibromyomata** *pl,* **fibromyomatous** *adj.*

fibroplasia *n* the production of fibrous tissue which is a normal part of healing. *retrolental fibroplasia* older term for retinopathy* of prematurity. Describes the final stages of more severe cases. The presence of fibrous tissue in the vitreous humor and retina extending in an area from the ciliary body to the optic disc, causing blindness. Noticed shortly after birth, more commonly in premature babies who have had continuous oxygen therapy.

fibrosarcoma *n* a form of sarcoma. A malignant tumour derived from fibroblastic cells—**fibrosarcomata** *pl,* **fibrosarcomatous** *adj.*

fibrosis *n* the formation of excessive fibrous tissues in a structure—**fibrotic** *adj.*

fibrositis *n* (*syn* muscular rheumatism) pain of uncertain origin which affects the soft tissues of the limbs and trunk. It is generally associated with muscular stiffness and local tender points—fibrositic nodules. Cause unknown; some disturbance in immunity may be a factor, as may be gout. Nonspecific factors include chill, postural trauma, muscular strain and psychological stress especially in tense, anxious people.

fibrovascular *adj* pertaining to fibrous tissue which is well supplied with blood vessels.

fibula *n* one of the longest and thinnest bones of the body, situated on the outer side of the leg and articulating at the upper end with the lateral condyle of the tibia and at the lower end with the lateral surface of the talus (astragalus) and tibia—**fibular** *adj.*

field of vision the area in which objects can be seen by the fixed eye.

fight or flight mechanism a body's extreme response to an immediate stressor such as perceived danger. Extra adrenaline is released, stimulating the heart, lungs and skeletal muscles to deal with the stressor or remove the body from it.

FIGO staging a system devised by the International Federation of Gynaecology and Obstetrics to classify tumours of the ovary, cervix and uterus according to the extent of spread.

Filaria *n* a genus of parasitic, thread-like worms, found mainly in the tropics and subtropics. The adults of *Filaria bancrofti* and *Brugia malayi* live in the lymphatics, connective tissues or mesentery, where they may cause obstruction, but the embryos migrate to the blood stream. Completion of the lifecycle is dependent upon passage through a mosquito. ⇒ loiasis—**filarial** *adj.*

filariasis *n* infestation with *Filaria* ⇒ elephantiasis.

filaricide *n* an agent which destroys *Filaria.*

filiform *adj* threadlike. *filiform papillae* small projections ending in several minute processes; found on the tongue.

filipuncture *n* insertion of wire thread etc. into an aneurysm to produce coagulation of contained blood.

filtrate *n* that part of a substance which passes through the filter.

filtration *n* the process of straining through a filter under gravity, pressure or vacuum. The act of passing fluid through a porous medium. *filtration under pressure* occurs in the kidneys, due to the pressure of blood in the glomeruli.

filum *n* any filamentous or thread-like structure. *filum terminale* a strong, fine cord blending with the spinal cord above, and the periosteum of the sacral canal below.

fimbria *n* a fringe or frond; resembling the fronds of a fern; e.g. the fimbriae of the uterine tubes—**fimbriae** *pl,* **fimbrial, fimbriated** *adj.*

fine tremor *n* slight trembling as seen in the outstretched hands or tongue of a patient suffering from thyrotoxicosis.

finger *n* a digit. *clubbed finger* swelling of terminal phalanx which occurs in many lung and heart diseases.

finger spelling a means of communicating by spelling words using the fingers of either one hand (in one-handed finger spelling) or two hands (in two-handed finger spelling) to make the letters of the alphabet.

fission *n* a method of reproduction common among the bacteria and protozoa.

fissure *n* a split or cleft. *palpebral fissure* the opening between the eyelids.

fistula *n* an abnormal communication between two body surfaces or cavities, e.g. gastrocolic fistula between the stomach and colon—**fistulae** *pl,* **fistular, fistulous** *adj.*

fistula-in-ano an abnormal track communicating with the skin around the anus. The base is usually an abscess in the deeper tissues.

fistulogram *n* X-ray of a fistula after injection into it of a contrast medium.

fixation *n* **1** in optics, the direct focusing of one or both eyes on an object so that the image falls on the retinal disc. **2** as a psychoanalytical term, an emotional attachment, generally sexual, to a parent, which may cause difficulty in forming new attachments later in life.

flaccid *adj* soft, flabby, not firm—**flaccidity** *n. flaccid paralysis* results mainly from lower motor neurone lesions. There are diminished or absent tendon reflexes.

flagellation *n* **1** the act of whipping oneself or others to gain sexual pleasure, or as a form of masochism or sadism. **2** a form of massage in which the skin is rhythmically tapped by either the outstretched hand or the little-finger side of the hand.

flagellum *n* a fine, hair-like appendage capable of lashing movement. Characteristic of spermatozoa, certain bacteria and protozoa—**flagella** *pl.*

flail chest unstable thoracic cage due to multiple rib fractures. ⇒ respiration.

flap *n* partially-removed tissue, retaining its blood supply, used to repair defects in an adjacent or distant part of the body. *cross leg flap* a flap with vascular attachment raised from one leg to cover defect on other leg. *free flap* an island flap detached from the body and reattached at the distant recipient site by microvascular surgery. *myocutaneous flap* a compound flap of skin and muscle with vascular attachment to permit sufficient tissue to be transferred to recipient site, e.g. delta pectoral flap used for breast reconstruction following mastectomy. *pedicle flap* a full thickness flap attached by a pedicle; used frequently by Sir Archibald McIndoe for facial reconstructive surgery on airmen injured in the Second World War. *rotation flap* pedicle flap whose width is increased by transforming the edge of the flap distal to the defect into a curved line; the flap is then rotated. *skin flap* a full thickness mass of tissue containing epidermis, dermis and subcutaneous tissue.

flat-foot *n* (*syn* pes planus) a congenital or acquired deformity marked by depression of the longitudinal arches of the foot.

flat pelvis a pelvis in which the anteroposterior diameter of the brim is reduced.

flatulence *n* gastric and intestinal distension with gas—**flatulent** *adj*.

flatus *n* gas in the stomach or intestines.

flatus tube used to relieve flatulent abdominal distension. It is a long open-ended tube which is passed along the bowel while the free end is immersed under water through which flatus (air) bubbles.

flea *n* a blood-sucking wingless insect of the order Siphonaptera; it acts as a host and can transmit disease. Its bite leaves a portal of entry for infection. *human flea Pulex irritans. rat flea Xenopsylla cheopis,* transmitter of plague*.

flex *vi, vt* bend.

flexibilitas cerea literally waxy flexibility. A condition of generalized hypertonia of muscles found in catatonic schizophrenia*. When fully developed, the patient's limbs retain positions in which they are placed, remaining immobile for hours at a time.

flexion *n* the reduction of the angle at a joint. ⇒ extension.

Flexner's bacillus *Shigella* flexneri*.

flexor *n* a muscle which on contraction flexes or bends a part ⇒ extensor *opp*.

flexure *n* a bend, as in a tube-like structure, or a fold, as on the skin—it can be obliterated by extension or increased by flexion in the locomotor system—**flexural** *adj*. *left colic (splenic) flexure* is situated at the junction of the transverse and descending parts of the colon. It lies at a higher level than the *right colic* or *hepatic flexure* the bend between the ascending and transverse colon, beneath the liver. *sigmoid flexure* the S-shaped bend at the lower end of the descending colon. It is continuous with the rectum below.

flight of ideas succession of thoughts with no rational connection. A feature of manic disorders.

floaters *npl* floating bodies in the vitreous humor (of the eye) which are visible to the person.

floating kidney abnormally mobile kidney.

flocculation *n* the coalescence of colloidal particles in suspension resulting in their aggregation into larger discrete masses which are often visible to the naked eye as cloudiness. *flocculation test* serum is set up against various salts such as gold, thymol, cephalin or cholesterol. When the presence of abnormal serum proteins results in cloudiness, abnormal forms of albumin and globulin are produced by diseased liver cells.

flooding *n* a popular term to describe excessive bleeding from the uterus.

floppy baby syndrome may be due to true muscle or nervous system disorder as opposed to benign* hypotonia.

flora *n* in medicine the word is used to describe the colonization of various parts of the body by microorganisms which in most instances are non-pathogenic but which in particular circumstances can become pathogenic. Colonization is referred to as natural or resident flora, as compared to transient flora found mainly on the hands and removed by effective handwashing*.

florid *adj* flushed, high coloured.

flowmeter *n* a measuring instrument for flowing gas or liquid.

flucloxacillin *n* an isoxazole penicillin, active against penicillinase-producing strains of *Staphylococcus aureus.* Well absorbed in man after oral and intramuscular administration. The chlorine of cloxacillin has been replaced with fluorine.

fluctuation *n* a wave-like motion felt on digital examination of a fluid-containing tumour, e.g. abscess—**fluctuant** *adj.*

fluke *n* a trematode worm of the order Digenea. The *European* or *sheep fluke (Fasciola hepatica)* usually ingested from watercress. There is fever, malaise, a large tender liver and eosinophilia. The *Chinese fluke (Clonorchis sinensis)* is usually ingested with raw fish. The adult fluke lives in the bile ducts and, while it may produce cholangitis, hepatitis and jaundice, it may be asymptomatic or be blamed for vague digestive symptoms. *lung fluke (Paragonimus)* usually ingested with raw crab in China and Far East. The symptoms are those of chronic bronchitis, including blood in the sputum.

fluorescein *n* red substance which forms a green fluorescent solution. Used as eye drops to detect corneal lesions, which stain green. It can be used in retinal angiography by injection into a vein, followed by viewing and photographing its passage through the retinal blood vessels. *fluorescein string test* used to detect the site of obscure upper gastrointestinal bleeding. The patient swallows a radio-paque knotted string. Fluorescein is injected intravenously and after a few minutes the string is withdrawn. If staining has occurred the site of bleeding can be determined.

fluorescent treponemal antibody test (FTA) carried out for syphilis: virulent *Treponema pallidum* is used as the antigen.

fluoridation *n* ⇒ fluoride.

fluoride *n* an ion sometimes present in drinking water. It can be incorporated into the structure of bone and provides protection against dental caries but in gross excess it causes mottling of the teeth. As a preventive measure it can be added to a water supply in a strength of 1 part fluoride in a million parts of water (fluoridation).

fluoroscopy *n* X-ray examination of movement in the body, observed by means of fluorescent screen and TV system.

foetus *n* fetus* is the internationally preferred spelling.

Foley catheter a self-retaining urinary catheter*.

folic acid (*syn* pteroylglutamic acid) a member of the vitamin* B complex which is abundant in green vegetables, yeast and liver. It is absorbed from the small intestine and is an essential factor for normal haemopoiesis and cell division generally. Used in the treatment of megaloblastic anaemias other than those due to vitamin B_{12} deficiency. Research suggests that taken before and in the first weeks after conception, it can help reduce the risk of neural tube defects in the fetus. Women who are pregnant or are planning to become pregnant are advised to supplement their intake.

follicle *n* **1** a small secreting sac. **2** an epidermal invagination enclosing a hair. **3** a simple tubular gland. *follicle stimulating hormone.(FSH)* secreted by the anterior pituitary gland; it acts on the ovaries in the female, where it develops the ovum-containing (Graafian) follicles; and on the testes in the male, where it is responsible for sperm production–**follicular** *adj.*

folliculitis *n* inflammation of follicles, such as the hair follicles. ⇒ alopecia.

fomentation *n* a hot, wet application to produce hyperaemia. When the skin is intact, strict cleanliness is observed (medical fomentation); when the skin is broken, aseptic technique is used (surgical fomentation).

fomite *n* any article which has been in contact with infection and is capable of transmitting same.

fontanelle *n* a membranous space between the cranial bones. The diamond-shaped anterior fontanelle (bregma) is at the junction of the frontal and two parietal bones. It usually closes in the second year of life. The triangular posterior fontanelle (lambda) is at the junction of the occipital and two parietal bones. It closes within a few weeks of birth.

food poisoning vomiting, with or without diarrhoea, resulting from eating food contaminated with chemical poison, preformed bacterial toxin or live bacteria or poisonous natural vegetation, e.g. berries, toadstools (fungi). ⇒ Campylobacter, Salmonella.

foot *n* that portion of the lower limb below the ankle. *foot drop* inability to dorsiflex foot, as in severe sciatica and nervous disease affecting lower lumbar regions of the cord. Can be a complication of being bedfast.

foramen *n* a hole or opening. Generally used with reference to bones–**foramina** *pl. foramen magnum* the opening in the occipital bone through which the spinal cord passes. *foramen ovale* a fetal cardiac interatrial communication which normally closes at birth.

forced expiratory volume (FEV) ⇒ respiratory function tests.

forced vital capacity (FVC) the maximum gas volume that can be expelled from the lungs in a forced expiration. ⇒ respiratory function tests.

forceps *n* surgical instruments with two opposing blades which are used to grasp or compress tissues, swabs, needles and many other surgical appliances. The two blades are controlled by direct pressure on them (tong-like), or by handles (scissor-like).

forensic medicine (*syn* medical jurisprudence) also called 'legal medicine'. The application of medical knowledge to questions of law.

foreskin *n* the prepuce or skin covering the glans* penis.

formaldehyde *n* powerful germicide. Formalin is a 40% solution; used mainly for room disinfection and the preservation of pathological specimens.

formication *n* a sensation as of ants running over the skin. Occurs in nerve lesions, particularly in the regenerative phase.

formula *n* a prescription. A series of symbols denoting the chemical composition of a substance–**formulae, formulas** *pl.*

formulary *n* a collection of formulas. The *British National Formulary* is an index of licensed pharmaceutical preparations, produced annually by the Joint Formulary Committee of the British Medical Association and the Royal Pharmaceutical Society.

fornix *n* an arch; particularly referred to the vagina, i.e. the space between the vaginal wall and the cervix of the uterus–**fornices** *pl.*

fossa *n* a depression or furrow–**fossae** *pl.*

fostering *n* placing a child in the

care of a compatible family as a short or long term measure. The aims are (a) to provide a child in need of care with the security of a home environment (b) to reunite child and natural family as soon as practical. Long term fosterings can be 'with a view to adoption'.

Fothergill's operation (*syn* Manchester Repair) anterior colporrhaphy*, amputation of part of the cervix and posterior colpoperineorrhaphy, performed for genital prolapse.

fourchette *n* a membranous fold connecting the posterior ends of the labia minora.

'fourth-day blues' emotional lability experienced by many women after childbirth. ⇒ puerperal psychosis.

fovea *n* a small depression or fossa; particularly the fovea centralis retinae, the site of most distinct vision.

fractionation *n* a method of dividing the total required dose of radiotherapy. Smaller doses given repeatedly allow normal cell recovery.

fracture *n* breach in continuity of a bone as a result of injury. *Bennett's* fracture. closed fracture* there is no communication with external air. *Colles' fracture* ⇒ Colles'. *comminuted fracture* a breach in the continuity of a bone which is broken into more than two pieces. *complicated fracture* a breach in the continuity of a bone when there is injury to surrounding organs and structures. *compression fracture* usually of lumbar or dorsal region due to hyperflexion of spine; the anterior vertebral bodies are crushed together. *depressed fracture* the broken bone presses on an underlying structure, such as brain or lung. *impacted fracture* one end of the broken bone is driven into the other. *incomplete fracture* the bone is only cracked or fissured – called *'greenstick fracture'* when it occurs in children. *open (compound) fracture* there is a wound permitting communication of broken bone end with air. *pathological fracture* occurring in abnormal bone as a result of force which would not break a normal bone. *spontaneous fracture* one occurring without appreciable violence; may be synonymous with pathological fracture.

fraenotomy *n* ⇒ frenotomy.

fraenum *n* the internationally preferred spelling is frenum*.

fragilitas *n* brittleness. *fragilitas ossium* congenital disease characterized by abnormal fragility of bone, multiple fractures and a china-blue colouring of the sclera.

framboesia *n* yaws*.

Freiberg's infarction an aseptic necrosis of bone tissue which most commonly occurs in the head of the second metatarsal bone.

Frei test an intradermal test for the diagnosis of lymphogranuloma venereum, using antigen from those infected and a control. A positive skin reaction to the killed antigen confirms diagnosis.

French chalk talc*.

Frenkel's exercises special exercises for tabes* dorsalis to teach muscle and joint sense.

frenotomy *n* surgical severance of a frenum*, particularly for tongue-tie.

frenum *n* a fold of membrane which checks or limits the movement of an organ. *frenulum linguae* from the undersurface of the tongue to the floor of the mouth.

frequency *n* the need to pass urine more often than is acceptable to the patient, usually more often than was experienced in the past.

Freyer's operation suprapubic transvesical type of prostatectomy*.

friable *adj* easily crumbled.

friction *n* rubbing. Can cause abrasion of skin, leading to superficial pressure sore; the adhesive property of friction, increased in the presence of moisture, can contribute to a shearing force which can cause a deep pressure sore. *friction massage* a form of massage in which strong circular manipulation of deep tissue is followed by centripetal stroking. The friction applied in drying after bathing can be therapeutic. *friction murmur* heard through the stethoscope when two rough or dry surfaces rub together, as in pleurisy and pericarditis.

Friedreich's ataxia a hereditary, degenerative disease of the spinocerebellar and pyramidal tracts and the posterior columns of the spinal cord, with onset in early childhood. Ataxia* and muscular weakness occurs; the heart may also be affected. The disease progresses slowly, with patients becoming increasingly handicapped and often using a wheelchair by early adult life.

frigidity *n* lack of normal sexual desire. Used mainly in relation to the female.

frog plaster conservative treatment of a congenital dislocation of the hip, whereby the dislocation is reduced by gentle manipulation and both hips are immobilized in plaster of Paris, the hips being abducted to 80 degrees and externally rotated.

frontal *adj* **1** pertaining to the front of a structure. **2** the forehead bone. *frontal sinus* a cavity at the inner aspect of each orbital ridge on the frontal bone.

frostbite *n* freezing of the skin and superficial tissues resulting from exposure to extreme cold. The lesion is similar to a burn and may become gangrenous. ⇒ trench foot.

frozen shoulder colloquial term for a kind of synovitis* in which there is initial pain followed by stiffness, lasting several months. As pain subsides, exercises are intensified until full recovery is gained. Cause unknown.

fructose *n* fruit sugar, a monosaccharide found in many sweet fruits. It is the sugar in honey and, combined with glucose, is the major constituent of cane sugar. Sweeter and more easily digested than ordinary sugar; it is useful for diabetics. *laevulose test* for hepatic function. A measured amount of laevulose does not normally increase the level of blood sugar, except in hepatic damage.

frusemide *n* produces prompt and effective diuresis. Lasts approximately 4 h after oral administration, and 2 h after parenteral administration. Valuable in pulmonary and cerebral oedema, and in congestive heart failure when the response to other diuretics is inadequate. Acts by inhibition of active chloride transport in the thick limb of the loop of Henle. It has been reported to cause a fall in glomerular filtration rate during diuresis. In consequence, handling of drugs which are removed from the body predominantly by glomerular filtration may be altered by coincidental frusemide therapy. Potassium supplements are given routinely in prolonged frusemide therapy. ⇒ diuretics.

FSH *abbr* follicle* stimulating hormone.

FTA *abbr* fluorescent* treponemal antibody.

fugue *n* a period of loss of memory in which a journey takes place. The behaviour of the person involved may appear normal or unspectacular to the casual observer. May occur in some forms of epilepsy.

fulguration *n* destruction of tissue by diathermy*.

full-term *adj* when pregnancy has lasted 40 weeks.

fulminant *adj* developing quickly and with an equally rapid termination.

fumigation *n* disinfection by exposure to the fumes of a vaporized disinfectant.

function *n* the special work performed by an organ or structure in its normal state.

functional *adj* **1** in a general sense, pertaining to function. **2** of a disorder, of the function but not the structure of an organ. **3** as a psychiatric term, of neurotic origin, i.e. psychogenic, without primary organic disease.

fundoplication *n* surgical folding of the gastric fundus to prevent reflux of gastric contents into the oesophagus.

fundus *n* the basal portion of a hollow structure, e.g. the uterus; the part which is distal to the opening—**fundi** *pl,* **fundal** *adj.*

fungicide *n* an agent which is lethal to fungi—**fungicidal** *adj.*

fungiform *adj* resembling a mushroom, like the fungiform papillae found chiefly in the dorsocentral area of the tongue.

fungistatic *adj* describes an agent which inhibits the growth of fungi.

fungus *n* a low form of vegetable life, including many microscopic organisms capable of producing superficial and systemic disease in man, such as actinomycosis* or ringworm*—**fungi** *pl,* **fungal** *adj.*

funiculitis *n* inflammation of the spermatic cord.

funiculus *n* a cord-like structure.

funnel chest (*syn* pectus excavatum) a congenital deformity in which the breast-bone is depressed towards the spine.

furor *n* a sudden outburst of uncontrolled fury or rage during which an irrational act of violence may be committed.

furuncle *n* ⇒ boil.

furunuculosis *n* an affliction due to boils.

furunculus orientalis oriental* sore.

fusidic acid has been shown to have anti-HIV activity. Taken orally it can cross the blood-brain barrier. It is relatively cheap and is not associated with any significant side-effects. ⇒ acquired immune deficiency syndrome.

fusiform *adj* resembling a spindle.

FVC *abbr* forced* vital capacity. ⇒ respiratory function tests.

G

gag *n* an instrument placed between the teeth to keep the mouth open.

gait *n* a manner or style of walking. *ataxic gait* an incoordinate or abnormal gait. *cerebellar gait* reeling, staggering, lurching. *scissors gait* one in which the legs cross each other in progressing. *spastic gait* stiff, shuffling, the legs being held together. *tabetic gait* the foot is raised high then brought down suddenly, the whole foot striking the ground.

galactagogue *n* an agent inducing or increasing the flow of milk.

galactocele *n* a cyst containing milk, or fluid resembling milk.

galactorrhoea *n* excessive flow of milk. Usually reserved for abnormal or inappropriate secretion of milk.

galactosaemia *n* excess of galactose in the blood and other tissues. Normally lactase in the small intestine converts lactose into glucose and galactose. In the liver another enzyme system converts galactose into glucose. Galactosaemia is the result of a congenital enzyme deficiency in this system (two types) and is one cause of mental subnormality—**galactosaemic** *adj.*

galactose *n* a monosaccharide found with glucose in lactose or milk sugar.

gall *n* bile*.

gallbladder *n* a pear-shaped bag on the undersurface of the liver. It concentrates and stores bile.

Gallie's operation the use of strips of fascia from the thigh for radical cure after reduction of a hernia.

gallipot *n* a small vessel for lotions.

gallows traction ⇒ Bryant's traction.

gallstones *n* concretions formed within the gallbladder or bile ducts; they are often multiple and faceted.

galvanocauterization *n* the use of a wire heated by galvanic current to destroy tissue.

galvanometer *n* an instrument for measuring an electrical current.

Gamblers Anonymous an organization which exists to help compulsive gamblers to resist the compulsion.

gamete *n* a male or female reproductive cell ⇒ ova, spermatazoon.

Gamete Intrafallopian Transfer (GIFT) a method of assisted fertilization. One patent uterine tube has to be identified. Oocytes* and spermatozoa are transferred to the distal end: fertilization takes place in vivo in the normal way, as opposed to in vitro when oocytes are fertilized outside the body and resultant embryos transferred into the uterus via the cervix.

gamma-encephalography a small dose of isotope is given. It is concentrated in many cerebral tumours. The pattern of radioactivity is then measured.

gamma rays short wavelength, penetrating rays of the electromagnetic spectrum produced by disintegration of the atomic nuclei of radioactive elements.

ganglion *n* **1** a mass of nerve tissue forming a subsidiary nerve centre which receives and sends out nerve fibres, e.g. the ganglionic masses forming the sympathetic nervous system. **2** localized cyst-like swelling near a tendon, sheath or joint. Contains a clear, transparent, gelatinous or colloid substance; sometimes occurs on the back of the wrist due to strain such as excessive use of the piano or word processor. **3** an enlargement on the course of a nerve such as is found on the receptor nerves before they enter the spinal cord—**ganglia** *pl,* **ganglionic** *adj. Gasserian ganglion* deeply situated within the skull, on the sensory root of the fifth cranial nerve. It is involved in trigeminal neuralgia.

ganglionectomy *n* surgical excision of a ganglion.

gangliosidosis ⇒ Tay-Sachs' disease.

gangrene *n* death of part of the tissues of the body. Usually the result of inadequate blood supply, but occasionally due to direct injury (traumatic gangrene) or infection (e.g. gas* gangrene). Deficient blood supply may result from pressure on blood vessels (e.g. tourniquets, tight bandages and swelling of a limb); from obstruction within healthy vessels (e.g. arterial embolism, frostbite where the capillaries become blocked); from spasm of the vessel wall (e.g. ergot poisoning); or from thrombosis due to disease of the vessel wall (e.g. arteriosclerosis in arteries, phlebitis in veins)—**gangrenous** *adj. dry gangrene* blood supply is inadequate and the affected part is dry and shrivelled. Arteries are obstructed but veins are not. *wet gangrene* inadequate blood supply gives rise to tissue necrosis associated with bacterial infection. The ischaemic area is moist.

gangrenous stomatitis ⇒ cancrum oris.

Ganser syndrome a condition characterized by inappropriate actions, absurd answers to questions, hallucinations, disturbances of consciousness, and amnesia. Also known as 'prison psychosis' or 'hallucinatory mania'.

gargoylism *n* (*syn* Hunter-Hurler syndrome) congenital disorder of mucopolysaccharide metabolism with recessive or sex-linked inheritance. The polysaccarides chondroitin sulphate 'B' and heparitin sulphate are excreted in the urine. Characterized by skeletal abnormalities, coarse features, enlarged liver and spleen, mental subnormality. ACTH is useful.

Gartner's bacillus Salmonella* enteritidis.

gas *n* one of the three states of matter, the others being solid and liquid. A gas retains neither shape nor volume when released—**gaseous** *adj. gas gangrene* a wound infection caused by anaerobic organisms of the genus clostridium, especially *Clostridium perfringens (welchii),* a soil microbe often harboured in the intestine of man and animals; consequently there are many sources from which infection can arise. ⇒ gangrene.

gasserectomy *n* surgical excision of the Gasserian ganglion*.

gastralgia *n* pain in the stomach.

gastrectomy *n* removal of a part or the whole of the stomach. *Billroth I gastrectomy* is a partial gastrectomy least commonly performed and usually reserved for ulcer on the lesser curvature. *Polya partial gastrectomy* (known in America as *Billroth II gastrectomy*) is the most commonly performed gastrectomy. Used for duodenal ulcer and as a palliative procedure for gastric cancer. Transverse colon and its mesentery intervene between stomach and jejunum. A hole can be made in the mesentery so that the anastomosis lies behind the transverse colon (retrocolic gastrectomy); or the loop of jejunum can be lifted up anterior to the transverse colon (antecolic gastrectomy). *total gastrectomy* is carried out only for cancer of the stomach . ⇒ Roux-en-Y operation.

gastric *adj* pertaining to the stomach. *gastric crisis* ⇒ crisis. *gastric aspiration* ⇒ aspiration. gastric influenza a term used when gastrointestinal symptoms predominate. *gastric juice* is acid in reaction and contains two proteolytic enzymes. *gastric suction* may be intermittent or continuous to keep the stomach empty after some abdominal operations. *gastric ulcer* an ulcer in the gastric mucous membrane. Characteristically there is pain shortly after eating food which may be so severe that the person fails to eat adequately and loses weight. H_2 antagonists are the drugs of choice. Can be complicated by haematemesis or perforation constituting a surgical abdominal emergency.

gastrin *n* a hormone secreted by the gastrin secreting cells of the gastric mucosa on entry of food, which causes a further flow of gastric juice.

gastritis *n* inflammation of the stomach, especially the mucous membrane lining.

gastrocnemius *n* the large two-headed muscle of the calf.

gastrocolic *adj* pertaining to the stomach and the colon. *gastrocolic reflex* sensory stimulus arising on entry of food into stomach, resulting in strong peristaltic waves in the colon.

gastroduodenal *adj* pertaining to the stomach and the duodenum.

gastroduodenostomy a surgical anastomosis between the stomach and the duodenum.

gastrodynia *n* pain in the stomach.

gastroenteritis *n* inflammation of mucous membranes of the stomach and the small intestine; although sometimes the result of dietetic error, the cause is usually a microbiological one. Infant gastroenteritis is usually caused by viruses, particularly the rotavirus although enteropathic *Escherichia coli* is still a common cause. Infection is spread by the faecal-oral route, either directly or indirectly.

gastroenterology *n* study of the digestive tract, including the liver, biliary tract and pancreas and the accompanying diseases—**gastroenterological** *adj,* **gastroenterologically** *adv.*

gastroenteropathy *n* disease of the stomach and intestine—**gastroenteropathic** *adj.*

gastroenteroscope *n* an endoscope* for visualization of stomach and intestine—**gastroenteroscopic** *adj,* **gastroenteroscopically** *adv.*

gastroenterostomy *n* a surgical anastomosis between the stomach and small intestine.

gastrointestinal *adj* pertaining to the stomach and intestine.

gastrojejunostomy *n* a surgical anastomosis between the stomach and the jejunum.

gastrooesophageal *adj* pertaining to the stomach and oesophagus, as gastric reflux in heartburn.

gastrooesophagostomy *n* a surgical operation in which the oesophagus is joined to the stomach to bypass the natural junction.

gastropathy *n* any disease of the stomach.

gastropexy *n* surgical fixation of a displaced stomach.

gastrophrenic *adj* pertaining to the stomach and diaphragm.

gastroplasty *n* any plastic operation on the stomach. Currently used for reconstruction of the cardiac orifice of the stomach, where fibrosis prevents replacement of the stomach below the diaphragm in cases of hiatus hernia.

gastroptosis *n* downward displacement of the stomach.

gastroschisis *n* a congenital incomplete closure of the abdominal wall to the right of a normal umbilical cord, with consequent protrusion of the viscera uncovered by peritoneum.

gastroscope *n* ⇒ endoscope—**gastroscopic** *adj*, **gastroscopy** *n*.

gastrostomy *n* a surgically established fistula between the stomach and the exterior abdominal wall; usually for artificial feeding.

gastrotomy *n* incision into the stomach during an abdominal operation for such purposes as removing a foreign body, securing a bleeding blood vessel, approaching the oesophagus from below to pull down a tube through a constricting growth.

gastrula *n* the next stage after blastula* in embryonic development.

Gaucher's disease a rare familial disorder, found mainly in Jewish children, characterized by a disordered lipoid metabolism (lipid reticulosis) and usually accompanied by very marked enlargement of the spleen. Diagnosis follows sternal marrow puncture and the finding of typical Gaucher cells (distended with lipoid).

gauze *n* a thin open-meshed absorbent material used in operations to dry the operative field and facilitate the procedure.

Geiger counter a device for detecting and registering radioactivity.

gelatin(e) *n* the protein-containing, glue-like substance obtained by boiling bones, skins and other animal tissues. Used as a base for pessaries, as the adhesive constituent of Unna's paste and in jellies and pastilles—**gelatinous** *adj*.

gene *n* a specific unit, located at a specific place (locus) of a specific chromosome. Genes are responsible for determining specific characteristics or traits. According to how they influence these characteristics, different forms of genes (alleles) may act as dominant (i.e. they manifest their presence in single doses of such alleles as are required). It is now known that each gene is a special and discrete coiled segment of the chemical DNA*, which is the principal and essential component of chromosomes. ⇒ Mendel's law.

general anaesthetic ⇒ anaesthesia.

general practitioner a doctor who, as part of the primary health care team, provides personal, primary and continuing medical care including prevention which is accessible to individuals and families irrespective of age, sex and illness and which is easily available at times of need. He or she will make initial decisions, give continuing medical care and refer patients for specialist advice and treatment.

generative *adj* pertaining to reproduction.

genetic *adj* that which pertains to heredity, e.g. disorders the basis of which resides in abnormalities of the genetic material, genes and chromosomes. ⇒ congenital.

genetic code the name given to arrangement of genetic material stored in the DNA molecule of the chromosome. It is in this coded form that the information contained in the genes is transmitted to the cells to determine their activity.

genetics *n* the science of heredity and variation, namely the study of the genetic material, its transmission (from cell to cell and generation to generation) and its changes (mutations). *biochemical genetics* the science concerned with the chemical and physical nature of genes, and with the mechanism by which they control the development and maintenance of the organism. *clinical genetics* the study of the possible genetic factors influencing the occurrence of a pathological condition. ⇒ immunogenesis.

genital *adj* pertaining to the organs of generation i.e. reproductive organs. *genital herpes* ⇒ herpes.

genitalia *n* the external, i.e. visible, parts of the reproductive system.

genitocrural *adj* pertaining to the genital area and the leg.

genitourinary *adj* pertaining to the reproductive and urinary organs. *genitourinary medicine* a term currently preferred to that of venereal* disease.

genome *n* the basic set of chromosomes*, with the genes contained therein, equivalent to the sum total of gene types possessed by different organisms of a species.

genotype *n* the total genetic information encoded in the chromosomes* of an individual. Also, the genetic constitution of an individual at a particular locus, namely the alleles* present at that locus.

gentamicin *n* an antibiotic produced by *Micromonospora purpurea.* Antibacterial, especially against *Pseudomonas* and staphylococci resistant to other antibiotics. Given intramuscularly and as eye and ear drops. Ototoxic and dangerous in renal failure.

gentian violet ⇒ crystal violet.

genu *n* the knee.

genupectoral position the knee-chest position, i.e. the weight is taken by the knees, and by the upper chest, while the shoulder girdle and head are supported on a pillow in front.

genus *n* a classification ranking between the family (higher) and the species (lower).

genu valgum (knock knee) abnormal incurving of the legs so that there is a gap between the feet when the knees are in contact.

genu varum (bow legs) abnormal outward curving of the legs resulting in separation of the knees.

geophagia *n* the habit of eating clay or earth.

geriatrician *n* one who specializes in old age and its diseases.

geriatrics *n* the branch of medical science dealing with old age and its diseases together with the medical care and nursing required by 'geriatric' patients. The nursing care of elderly people is the term now preferred in nursing. ⇒ ageism.

germ *n* a unicellular microorganism, especially used for a pathogen.

German measles ⇒ rubella.

germicide *n* an agent which kills germs—**germicidal** *adj.*

gerontology *n* the scientific study of ageing—**gerontological** *adj.*

gestation *n* ⇒ pregnancy—**gestational** *adj.*

GFR *abbr* glomerular* filtration rate.

GH *abbr* growth* hormone.

Ghon focus ⇒ primary complex.

giardiasis *n* (*syn* lambliasis) infection with the flagellate *Giardia intestinalis.* Often symptomless, especially in adults. Can cause diarrhoea with steatorrhoea. Treatment is mepacrine or metronidazole orally.

GIFT *abbr* ⇒ Gamete Intrafallopian Transfer.

gigantism *n* an abnormal condition characterized by excessive growth and height. Often associated with excessive secretion of growth hormone (GH).

gingiva *n* the gum; the vascular

tissue surrounding the necks of the erupted teeth–**gingival** *adj.*

gingival sulcus the invagination* made by the gingiva as it joins with the tooth surface.

gingivectomy *n* excision of a portion of the gum, usually for pyorrhoea.

gingivitis *n* inflammation of the gum or gingiva usually caused by irritation from dental plaque and calculus. Can occur with the systemic use of some drugs, e.g. dilantin sodium, or mercury, and may be associated with pregnancy, due to hormone changes.

girdle *n* usually a bony structure of oval shape such as the shoulder and pelvic girdles.

gland *n* an organ or structure capable of making an internal or external secretion. *lymphatic gland* (node) does not secrete, but is concerned with filtration of the lymph. ⇒ endocrine, exocrine–**glandular** *adj.*

glanders *n* a contagious, febrile, ulcerative disease communicable from horses, mules and asses to man.

glandular fever ⇒ infectious mononucleosis.

glans *n* the bulbous termination of the clitoris and penis.

Glasgow coma scale a standardized tool for evaluating responsiveness. It assesses eye opening according to four criteria; motor response using six criteria, and verbal response against five criteria. A score of 7 or less qualifies 'coma', that is, no response and no eye opening.

glaucoma *n* a condition where the intraocular pressure is raised. In the acute stage the pain is severe–**glaucomatous** *adj.*

glenohumeral *adj* pertaining to the glenoid cavity of scapula and the humerus.

glenoid *adj* a cavity on the scapula* into which the head of the humerus* fits to form the shoulder joint.

glia *n* ⇒ neuroglia–**glial** *adj.*

glioblastoma multiforme a highly malignant brain tumour.

glioma *n* a malignant growth which does not give rise to secondary deposits. It arises from neuroglia. One form, occurring in the retina, is hereditary–**gliomata** *pl.*

gliomyoma *n* a tumour of nerve and muscle tissue–**gliomyomata** *pl.*

globin *n* a protein which combines with haem to form haemoglobin.

globulin *n* the fraction of serum or plasma which contains the immunoglobulins* A, D, E, G and M.

globus hystericus a subjective feeling of neurotic origin of a lump in the throat. Can also include difficulty in swallowing due to tension of muscles of deglutition. May accompany acute anxiety and emotional conflict. Sometimes follows slight trauma to throat, e.g. scratch by foreign body.

globus pallidus literally pale globe; situated deep within the cerebral hemispheres, lateral to the thalamus.

glomerular filtration rate (GFR) the rate of filtration from blood in the glomerulus of renal capillaries to the fluid in Bowman's capsule. It is usually 120 ml per min and is an accurate index of renal function.

glomerulitis *n* inflammation of the glomeruli, usually of the kidney. The use of electron microscopes, and fluorescent staining of biopsy specimens have improved diagnosis and knowledge of the condition.

glomerulonephritis *n* a term which covers several diseases which have as their common denominator damage to the glomeruli of the renal cortex mediated through the immune mechanisms of the body and the immunoglobulins of the blood.

Proteinuria and microscopic haematuria are features but no bacteria appear in the urine.

glomerulosclerosis *n* fibrosis of the glomeruli of the kidney, usually the result of inflammation. *intercapillary glomerulosclerosis* a common pathological finding in diabetics—**glomerulosclerotic** *adj.*

glomerulus *n* a coil of minute arterial capillaries held together by scanty connective tissue. It invaginates the entrance of the uriniferous tubules in the kidney cortex—**glomerular** *adj,* **glomeruli** *pl.*

glomus *n* vascular tumour in middle ear.

glossa *n* the tongue—**glossal** *adj.*

glossectomy *n* excision of the tongue.

glossitis *n* inflammation of the tongue.

glossodynia *n* a name used for a painful tongue when there is no visible change.

glossopharyngeal *adj* pertaining to the tongue and pharynx. The ninth pair of the 12 pairs of cranial nerves arising directly from the brain.

glossoplegia *n* paralysis of the tongue.

glottis *n* the space between the vocal folds of the larynx, when they are abducted. Associated with voice production—**glottic** *adj.*

glucagon *n* hormone produced in alpha cells of pancreatic islets of Langerhans. Causes breakdown of glycogen into glucose thus preventing blood sugar from falling too low during fasting. Can now be obtained commercially from the pancreas of animals. Given to accelerate breakdown of glycogen in the liver and raise blood sugar rapidly. As it is a polypeptide hormone, it must be given by injection.

glucocorticoid *n* any steroid hormone which promotes gluconeogenesis (i.e. the formation of glucose and glycogen from protein) and which antagonizes the action of insulin. Occurring naturally in the adrenal cortex as cortisone and hydrocortisone, and produced synthetically as, e.g. prednisone and prednisolone.

glucogenesis *n* synthesis of glucose.

glucometer *n* an electronic meter to enable diabetics, both insulin dependent and noninsulin dependent, to carry out home blood glucose monitoring (HBGM). A drop of blood is obtained from the pulp of a finger tip. There is a variety of makes available.

gluconeogenesis *n* (*syn* glyconeogenesis) the formation of sugar from noncarbohydrate sources, e.g. protein or fat.

glucose *n* dextrose or grape sugar. A monosaccharide. The form in which carbohydrates are absorbed through the intestinal tract and circulated in the blood. It is stored as glycogen* in the liver. *glucose tolerance test* after a period of fasting, a measured quantity of glucose is taken orally; thereafter blood and urine samples are tested for glucose at intervals. Higher than normal levels are indicative of diabetes mellitus.

glucuronic acid an acid which acts on bilirubin* to form conjugated bilirubin; one of the main conjugating agents required for the metabolism of foreign compounds.

glue ear an accumulation of a glue-like substance in the middle ear which bulges the eardrum and impairs hearing. ⇒ grommet.

glue sniffing ⇒ solvent abuse.

glutamic oxaloacetic transaminase an enzyme present in serum and body tissues, especially the heart and liver. It is released into the serum following tissue damage such as myocardial infarction or acute damage to liver cells.

glutamic pyruvic transaminase an enzyme present in serum and body tissues, especially the liver. Acute damage to hepatic cells causes an increase in serum concentration.

glutaminase *n* an amino acid-degrading enzyme, used in the treatment of cancer.

gluteal *adj* pertaining to the buttocks*.

gluten *n* a protein constituent of wheat flour. Insoluble in water but an essential component of the elastic 'dough'. It is not tolerated in coeliac* disease.

glycerin(e) *n* a clear, syrupy liquid prepared synthetically or obtained as a by-product in soap manufacture. It has a hygroscopic action. *glycerine and borax* useful for softening sordes. *glycerine and honey* useful as a softening agent for oral toilet. *glycerine and ichthyol* applied as a compress to relieve inflammation. *glycerine and magnesium sulphate* useful for boils etc. *glycerine suppository* a suppository* incorporating glycerine, which, by its hygroscopic action, attracts fluid to soften hardened faeces in the rectum. The effectiveness of subsequent bowel evacuation is dependent on how long it has been retained.

glyceryl trinitrate (GTN) a vasodilator used mainly in angina pectoris. Given mainly as tablets which should be chewed, or dissolved under the tongue; transdermally by application as a gel to the skin; or sublingually as a spray.

glycine *n* a nonessential amino* acid.

glycogen *n* the main carbohydrate storage compound in animals, in which glucose molecules are linked in branched chains. The liver and muscle are the main sites of production. *glycogen storage disease* a metabolic recessive inherited condition caused by various enzyme deficiencies types 1–13 are now recognized. The liver becomes large and fatty due to the excessive glycogen deposits. Hypoglycaemia is a major problem. The body tends to metabolise fat rather than glucose and ketosis and acidosis are prevalent.

glycogenesis *n* formation of glycogen from blood glucose ⇒ glycogenolysis *opp*.

glycogenolysis *n* hydrolysis of glycogen stores to glucose within the liver ⇒ glycogenesis *opp*.

glycogenosis *n* a metabolic disorder leading to increased storage of glycogen*. Leads to glycogen myopathy.

glycolysis *n* the hydrolysis of glucose in the body—**glycolytic** *adj*.

glyconeogenesis *n* ⇒ gluconeogenesis*.

glycosides *npl* natural substances composed of a sugar with another compound. The non-sugar fragment is termed an 'aglycone', and is sometimes of therapeutic value. Digoxin is a familiar example of a glycoside.

glycosuria *n* the presence of large amounts of sugar in the urine.

gnathalgia *n* pain in the jaw.

gnathoplasty *n* plastic surgery of the jaw.

goal *n* a goal is set for each actual problem experienced by a patient which is amenable to nurse-initiated intervention. For each identified potential problem, the goal of the nurse-initiated intervention will be preventing it from becoming an actual problem. Goals may be short-, medium- or long-term.

goal setting an essential part of the process of nursing, which occurs after identification of the patient's actual and potential problems that are amenable to nurse-initiated intervention.

Whenever possible, the patient/client and/or family participate in goal setting.

goals, patient the desired outcomes of care, planned by the nurse, with the patient and/or family where possible, as part of the nursing* process. They form the basis for the later evaluating* of care.

goblet cells special mucus secreting cells, shaped like a goblet, found in the mucous membranes.

Goeckerman régime a method of treatment for psoriasis; exposure to ultraviolet light alternating with the application of a tar paste.

goitre *n* an enlargement of the thyroid gland. In *simple goitre* the patient does not show any signs of excessive thyroid activity. In *toxic goitre* the enlarged gland secretes an excessive amount of thyroid hormone. The patient is nervous, loses weight and often has palpitations and exophthalmos. ⇒ colloid.

goitrogens *npl* agents causing goitre. Some occur in plants, e.g. turnip, cabbage, brussels sprouts and peanuts.

Goldthwait belt wide belt with steel support for back injuries.

Golgi apparatus complex cellular organelle consisting mainly of membranous sacs. Involved in the synthesis of glycoproteins and lipoproteins.

gonad *n* a male or female sex gland. ⇒ ovary, testis—**gonadal** *adj*.

gonadotrophic *adj* having an affinity for, or influence on the gonads.

gonadotrophin *n* any gonad-stimulating hormone. ⇒ follicle stimulating hormone, human chorionic gonadotrophin test, luteotrophin.

gonioscopy *n* measuring angle of anterior chamber of eye with a gonioscope.

goniotomy *n* operation for glaucoma. Incision through the anterior chamber angle to the canal of Schlemm, typically used in treating congenital glaucoma.

gonococcal complement fixation test a specific serological test for the diagnosis of gonorrhoea*. ⇒VDRL test.

Gonococcus *n* a Gram-negative diplococcus (*Neisseria gonorrhoea*), the causative organism of gonorrhoea. It is a strict parasite. Occurs characteristically inside polymorphonuclear leucocytes in the tissues—**gonococci** *pl*, **gonococcal** *adj*.

gonorrhoea *n* a sexually-transmitted disease in adults. In children infection is accidental, e.g. gonococcal ophthalmia of the newborn, gonococcal vulvovaginitis of girls before puberty. Chief manifestations of the disease in the male are a purulent urethritis with dysuria; in the female, urethritis, endocervicitis and salpingitis which may be symptomless but can lead to pelvic* inflammatory disease. Incubation period is usually 2–5 days—**gonorrhoeal** *adj*.

gonorrhoeal *adj* resulting from gonorrhoea. *gonorrhoeal arthritis* is a metastatic manifestation of gonorrhoea. *gonorrhoeal ophthalmia* is one form of ophthalmia neonatorum.

good neighbourhood scheme a scheme which involves social service departments recruiting and supplying volunteers to visit and support elderly people at home who may not require a home help. The volunteers have no set tasks to perform.

Goodpasture syndrome a haemorrhagic lung disorder associated with glomerulonephritis.

goose flesh contraction of the tiny muscles attached to the sheath of the hair follicles causes the hair to stand on end: it is a reaction to either cold or fear and occurs in the early stages of increasing core body temperature.

Gordh needle an intravenous needle with a rubber diaphragm. Through it repeated injections can be given.

gouge *n* a chisel with a grooved blade for removing bone.

gout *n* a form of metabolic disorder in which sodium biurate is deposited in the cartilages of the joints, the ears, and elsewhere. The big toe is characteristically involved and becomes acutely painful and swollen. There are now drugs which increase the excretion of urates; these have largely controlled the disease.

GPI *abbr* general paralysis of the insane (paralytic dementia occurring in tertiary syphilis).

Graafian follicle minute vesicles contained in the stroma of an ovary*, each containing a single ovum. When an ovum is extruded from a Graafian follicle each month the corpus luteum is formed under the influence of luteotrophin from the anterior pituitary gland. If fertilization occurs, the corpus luteum persists for 12 weeks; if not, it only persists for 12–14 days. Degenerates to become the corpus albicans.

graft *n* any tisssue or organ for implantation or transplantation; to implant or transplant such tissues. *autograft* a tissue or organ which is transplanted to another part of the same person or animal. *allograft or homograft* tissue or organs which are transplanted between humans or animals of the same species. *heterograft or zenograft* tissue or organs which are transplanted between animals of different species. ⇒ transplantation.

graft versus host disease/reaction (GVHD) a pathological reaction between the host and the organ/tissue grafted. Rejection of the tissue/organ is due to inadequacy of the host's immunological response because of immunosuppression. ⇒ immunocompromized patients.

Gram's stain a bacteriological stain for differentiation of microorganisms. Those retaining the blue dye are Gram-positive (+), those unaffected by it are Gram-negative (–).

grand mal ⇒ epilepsy.

granulation *n* the outgrowth of new capillaries and connective tissue cells from the surface of an open wound. *granulation tissue* the young, soft tissue so formed—**granulate** *vi.*

granulocyte *n* white blood cell which contains granules in its cytoplasm. These may be neutrophils, eosinophils or basophils.

granuloma *n* a tumour formed of granulation tissue. *granuloma venereum* lymphogranuloma* inguinale.

Graves' disease ⇒ thyrotoxicosis.

gravid *adj* pregnant; carrying fertilized eggs or a fetus.

gravitational *adj* being attracted by force of gravity. *gravitational ulcer* ⇒ varicose ulcer.

gravity *n* weight. The weight of a substance compared with that of an equal volume of water is termed *specific gravity.*

Grawitz tumour ⇒ hypernephroma.

gray *n* a unit of measurement of the absorbed dose of radiation. The unit has replaced the rad.

green monkey disease ⇒ Marburg disease.

greenstick fracture ⇒ fracture.

gregarious *adj* showing a preference for living in a group, liking to mix. The gregrarious or herd instinct is an inborn tendency on the part of various species, including man.

grieving process the word 'process' has been added to what was traditionally known as grieving to signify increased knowledge about the phases which a person experiences in relation to bereavement* and dying*. Grieving is not only associated with these experiences, but also with loss of function such as colostomy, paralysis or infertility; and with loss of a part of the body, e.g. breast, limb, uterus.

grinder's asthma one of the many popular names for silicosis* arising from inhalation of metallic dust.

gripe *n* abdominal colic.

grocer's itch contact dermatitis, especially from flour or sugar.

groin *n* the junction of the thigh with the abdomen.

grommet *n* a type of ventilation tube inserted into the tympanic membrane. Frequently used in the treatment of glue* ear in children ⇒ myringotomy.

group psychotherapy ⇒ psychotherapy.

growing pains pain in the limbs during youth: the differential diagnosis is rheumatic fever.

growth hormone (GH, somatotropin*) secreted by the anterior pituitary gland in response to growth hormone releasing factor from the hypothalamus. Its main function is promotion of protein synthesis which is essential for healing including such pathology as infarct and inflammation. More than half the daily amount is released during early sleep. ⇒ dwarfism, gigantism.

growth hormone test (GHT) there is a reciprocal relationship between growth hormone (secreted by the pituitary* gland) and blood glucose. Blood is therefore estimated for GH during a standard 50 g oral glucose tolerance test. In acromegaly, not only is the resting level of GH higher, but it does not show normal suppression with glucose.

GTN *n* ⇒ glyceryl trinitrate.

guar *n* fibre derived from natural sources which disperses readily in fluid to produce a palatable drink.

guillotine *n* a surgical instrument for excision of the tonsils.

Guinea worm ⇒ *Dracunculus* medinensis.*

gullet *n* the oesophagus*.

GUM *abbr* genitourinary* medicine. ⇒ sexually transmitted disease.

gumboil *n* lay term for an abscess of gum tissue and periosteum (dentoalveolar abscess) which is usually very painful.

gumma *n* a localized area of vascular granulation tissue which develops in the later stages (tertiary) of syphilis. Obstruction to the blood supply results in necrosis, and gummata near a surface of the body tend to break down, forming chronic ulcers, which are probably not infectious—**gummata** *pl.*

gut *n* the intestines, large and small. *gut decontamination* the use of nonabsorbable antibiotics to suppress growth of microorganisms to prevent endogenous infection for patients undergoing bowel surgery or those who are neutropenic or immunocompromised.

Guthrie test assay of phenylalanine* to test for phenylketonuria* in the newborn. A drop of blood, usually taken from the heel, is dried on special filter paper. Carried out on the 6th day of life. It is necessary to confirm the diagnosis in those infants with a positive test.

gynaecologist *n* a surgeon who specializes in gynaecology*.

gynaecology *n* the science dealing with the diseases of the female reproductive system—**gynaecological** *adj.*

gynaecomastia *n* enlargement of the male mammary gland.

Gypsona *n* a proprietary readymade quick-setting plaster of

Paris bandage made by impregnating fine plaster of Paris into specially woven (interlock) cotton cloth. For immobilization in fracture treatment and orthopaedic conditions generally.

gypsum *n* plaster of Paris (calcium sulphate).

gyrectomy *n* surgical removal of a gyrus*.

gyrus *n* a convoluted portion of cerebral cortex.

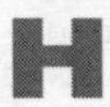

habilitation *n* the means by which a child gradually progresses towards the maximum degree of physical, psychological, and social independence of which he is capable. ⇒ rehabilitation.

habit *n* any learned behaviour that has a relatively high probability of occurrence in response to a particular situation or stimulus. Acquisition of habits may depend on both reinforcement and associative learning. *habit training* used in the care of people with a mental illness or a learning disability which requires them to relearn personal hygiene by constant repetition with encouragement.

habit retraining the patient voids at set times, according to the baseline frequency/volume chart, but may use the toilet at other times. ⇒ bladder retraining.

habitual abortion ⇒ abortion.

habituation *n* term to describe decreasing response to a stimulus when it becomes familiar through repeated presentation. It is often used in a negative sense in relation to drug use, where a psychological dependence develops through repeated use of a drug. ⇒ drug dependence.

haem *n* the pigment-carrying portion of haemoglobin*.

haemangioma *n* a malformation of blood vessels which may occur in any part of the body. When in the skin it is one form of birthmark, appearing as a red spot or a 'port wine stain'—**haemangiomata** *pl.*

haemarthrosis *n* the presence of blood in a joint cavity—**haemarthroses** *pl.*

haematemesis *n* the vomiting of blood, which may be bright red if recently swallowed. Otherwise it is of 'coffee ground' appearance due to the action of gastric juice.

haematin *n* an iron-containing constituent of haemoglobin. The hydroxide of haem, formed by oxidation from the ferrous to the ferric state. It may crystallize in the kidney tubules when there is excessive haemolysis.

haematinic *adj* any substance which is required for the production of the red blood cell and its constituents.

haematite *n* (*syn* miner's lung) a form of silicosis* occurring in the haematite (iron ore) industry.

haematocele *n* a swelling filled with blood.

haematocolpos *n* retained blood in the vagina. ⇒ cryptomenorrhoea.

haematocrit *n* the volume of red cells in the blood, expressed as a percentage of the total blood volume.

haematology *n* the science dealing with the formation, composition, functions and diseases of the blood—**haematological** *adj.*

haematoma *n* a swelling filled with blood—**haematomata** *pl.*

haematometra *n* an accumulation of blood (or menstrual fluid) in the uterus.

haematopoiesis *n* ⇒ haemopoiesis.

haematoporphyrin test 1–3 h after injection, haematoporphyrin localizes in rapidly multiplying cells and fluoresces under ultraviolet light. In many instances investigators can detect the exact extent of malignant or precancerous tissue.

haematosalpinx *n* (*syn* haemosalpinx) blood in the uterine tube. Often associated with tubal pregnancy.

haematozoa *npl* parasites living in the blood—**haematozoon** *sing.*

haematuria *n* blood in the urine; it may be from the kidneys, one or both ureters, the bladder or the urethra and may indicate trauma, infection or abnormal pathology—**haematuric** *adj.*

haemochromatosis *n* (*syn* bronzed diabetes) a congenital error in iron metabolism with increased iron deposition in tissues, resulting in brown pigmentation of the skin and cirrhosis of the liver—**haemochromatotic** *adj.*

haemoconcentration *n* relative increase of volume of red blood cells to volume of plasma.

haemocytometer *n* an instrument for measuring the number of blood corpuscles.

haemodialysis *n* removal of toxic solutes and excess fluid from the blood by dialysis* which is achieved by putting a semipermeable membrane between the blood and a rinsing solution called dialysate*. It is necessary when the patient is either in the end stage of renal failure (irreversible) or in acute renal failure (reversible).

haemodynamics *npl* the forces involved in circulating blood round the body.

haemofiltration *n* requires the same access to the blood circulation as haemodialysis*. The patient's cardiac output drives the blood through a small, highly permeable filter, permitting separation of fluid and solutes. This haemofiltrate is measured and discarded and is replaced with an isotonic solution. When large amounts of haemofiltrate are removed, haemodialysis is unnecessary. Particularly useful for patients in acute renal failure, in congestive heart failure with diuretic-resistant overhydration and in hypernatraemia resistant to drugs.

haemoglobin *n* the respiratory pigment in the red blood corpuscles. It is composed of an iron-containing substance called 'haem', combined with globin. It has the reversible function of combining with and releasing oxygen. At birth 45–90% of haemoglobin is of the fetal type which is replaced by adult haemoglobin at the end of the first year of life. ⇒ oxyhaemoglobin/deoxyhaemoglobin.

haemoglobinaemia *n* haemoglobin in the blood plasma*—**haemoglobinaemic** *adj.*

haemoglobinometer *n* an instrument for estimating the percentage of haemoglobin in the blood.

haemoglobinopathies *npl* includes various abnormalities of haemoglobin—**haemoglobinopathic** *adj.* ⇒ anaemia, haemolytic disease of the newborn, icterus.

haemoglobinuria *n* haemoglobin in the urine—**haemoglobinuric** *adj.*

haemolysin *n* an agent which causes disintegration of erythrocytes. ⇒ immunoglobulins.

haemolysis *n* disintegration of red blood cells, with liberation of contained haemoglobin—**haemolytic** *adj.* ⇒ anaemia, jaundice.

haemolytic disease of the newborn (*syn* erythroblastosis fetalis) a pathological condition in the newborn child due to Rhesus incompatibility between the child's blood and that of the mother. Red blood cell destruction occurs with anaemia, often jaundice and an excess of erythroblasts or primitive red blood cells in the circulating blood. Immunization of women at risk, using gammaglobulin containing a high titre of anti-D*, can prevent haemolytic disease of the newborn. Exchange transfusion of the infant may be essential.

haemolytic disorders febrile illnesses (including haemolytic uraemia syndrome) resembling gastroenteritis and followed by intravascular haemolysis which may also lead to hypertension and acute renal failure, manifested by oliguria. The longer this persists, the poorer the prognosis which can be chronic renal failure or death. A third do not develop oliguria and make a good recovery. It may be an autoimmune disease or an abnormal reaction to an uncommon virus.

haemopericardium *n* blood in the pericardial sac.

haemoperitoneum *n* blood in the peritoneal cavity.

haemophilias *npl* a group of conditions with congenital blood coagulation defects. In clinical practice the most commonly encountered are *haemophilia A,* factor VIII procoagulant deficiency: *haemophilia B* or Christmas disease, factor IX procoagulant deficiency. Both these conditions are X-linked recessive disorders exclusively affecting males and resulting in abnormalities in the clotting mechanism only. The bleeding usually occurs into deeply lying structures, muscles and joints. ⇒ blood clotting, haemophilic arthropathy, von Willebrand's disease.

haemophilic arthropathy joint damage seen in people suffering from haemophilia. The extent of the damage is staged as follows: (a) synovial thickening (b) epiphyseal overgrowth (c) minor joint changes and cyst formation (d) definite joint changes with loss of joint space (e) end-stage joint destruction and secondary changes leading to deformity.

Haemophilus *n* a genus of bacteria. Small Gram-negative rods which show much variation in shape (pleomorphism). Characteristically intracellular in polymorphonuclear leucocytes in exudate. They are strict parasites, and accessory substances present in blood are usually necessary for growth. *Haemophilus aegyptius* causes a form of acute infectious conjunctivitis. *Haemophilus ducreyi* causes chancroid. *Haemophilus influenzae* causes respiratory infections; a primary cause of bacterial meningitis and a common secondary cause of influenza infections. *Haemophilus pertussis* (now *Bordetella pertussis*) causes whooping cough.

haemopneumothorax *n* the presence of blood and air in the pleural cavity.

haemopoiesis *n* (*syn* haematopoiesis) the formation of blood. ⇒ erythropoiesis—**haemopoietic** *adj.*

haemoptysis *n* the coughing up of blood—**haemoptyses** *pl.*

haemorrhage *n* the escape of blood from a vessel. Arterial, capillary, venous designate the type of vessel from which it escapes—**haemorrhagic** *adj. primary haemorrhage* that which occurs at the time of injury or operation. *secondary haemorrhage* that which occurs some time after an injury or operation. *antepartum haemorrhage* ⇒ placental abruption. *intrapartum haemorrhage* that occurring during labour. *postpartum haemorrhage* excessive bleeding after delivery of child. In the UK it must be at least 500 ml to qualify as haemorrhage. *secondary postpartum haemorrhage* excessive uterine bleeding more than 24 h after delivery.

haemorrhagic disease of the newborn characterized by gastrointestinal, pulmonary or intracranial haemorrhage occurring from the 2nd to the 5th day of life. Caused by a physiological variation in clotting power due to change in prothrombin content, which falls on 2nd day and returns to normal at end of first week when colonization of gut with bacteria results in synthesis of vitamin K, thus permitting formation of prothrombin* by the liver. Responds to or prevented by administration of vitamin K.

haemorrhagic fever ⇒ mosquito-transmitted haemorrhagic fevers, viral haemorrhagic fevers.

haemorrhoidal *adj* **1** pertaining to haemorrhoids*. **2** applied to blood vessels and nerves in the anal region.

haemorrhoidectomy *n* surgical removal of haemorrhoids.

haemorrhoids *npl* (*syn* piles) varicosity of the veins around the anus. *external haemorrhoids* those outside the anal sphincter, covered with skin. *internal haemorrhoids* those inside the anal sphincter, covered with mucous membrane.

haemosalpinx *n* ⇒ haematosalpinx.

haemosiderosis *n* iron deposits in the tissues.

haemospermia *n* the discharge of blood-stained semen.

haemostasis *n* **1** arrest of bleeding. **2** stagnation of blood within its vessel.

haemostatic *adj* any agent which arrests bleeding. *haemostatic forceps* artery forceps.

haemothorax *n* blood in the pleural cavity.

HAI *abbr* hospital acquired infection. ⇒ infection.

hair *n* thread-like appendage present on all parts of human skin except palms, soles, lips, glans penis and that surrounding the terminal phalanges. The broken-off stump found at the periphery of spreading bald patches in alopecia areata is called an exclamation mark hair, from the characteristic shape caused by atrophic thinning of the hair shaft. *hair follicle* the sheath in which a hair grows. *hair root* the internal end of a hair; it is attached to the dimpled end of the hair follicle through which it receives its blood supply.

half life the time taken for a radioactive substance to decay by half. Can also be used to describe the time taken for half the dose of a drug to be excreted from the body.

halibut liver oil a very rich source of vitamins* A and D. The smaller dose required makes it more acceptable than cod liver oil.

halitosis *n* foul-smelling breath.

hallucination *n* a false perception occurring without any true sensory stimulus. A common symptom in severe psychoses including schizophrenia, paraphrenia and confusional states. Also common in delirium, during toxic states and following head injuries.

hallucinogens *npl* ⇒ psychotomimetics.

hallucinosis *n* a psychosis in which the patient is grossly hallucinated. Usually a subacute delirious state; the predominant symptoms are auditory illusions and hallucinations.

hallux *n* the big toe. *hallux valgus* ⇒ bunion. *hallux varus* the big toe is displaced towards the other foot. *hallux rigidus* ankylosis of the metatarsophalangeal articulation caused by osteoarthritis.

halo *n* a ring splint which encircles the head. ⇒ halopelvic traction.

halogen *n* any one of the non-metallic elements: bromine, chlorine, fluorine, iodine.

halopelvic traction a form of external fixation whereby traction can be applied to the spine between two fixed points. The device consists of three main parts (a) a halo (b) a pelvic loop and (c) four extension bars.

haloperidol *n* a psychotrophic agent used in the treatment of schizophrenia and other psychotic disorders for its tranquillizing properties. It can be taken orally, but if necessary, as in mania, it can be given by injection.

halothane *n* a clear colourless liquid used as an inhalation anaesthetic. Advantages: non-explosive and noninflammable in all circumstances. Odour is not unpleasant. It is non-irritant.

hammer toe a permanent hyperextension of the first phalanx and flexion of second and third phalanges.

hand *n* that part of the upper limb below the wrist.

hand-arm vibration syndrome (HAVS) an occupational hazard of certain machine or tool operators. The effects include vascular blanching of terminal digits known as Raynaud's phenomenon, and neurological numbness and tingling of terminal digits. It is a progressive disease and may lead to gangrene.

handicap *n* term formerly used to denote disadvantage arising from impairment or disability. It is no longer favoured by disability groups because this term carries negative connotations.

handicapped *adj* term, no longer considered acceptable, applied to a person with a defect that interferes with normal activity and achievement.

Hand-Schüller-Christian disease ⇒ histiocytosis.

handwashing *n* the most important activity in preventing infection*. It should include the wrists, the bulbar eminence of each thumb as well as between the fingers. Screw taps should not be touched with freshly-washed hands. The hands should be washed both before and after aseptic procedures. Handwashing is essential before and after emptying urine from a closed drainage system. The Infection* Control Committee usually advises about the circumstances to be followed by handwashing, in addition to those which have to be preceded, as well as followed by handwashing.

hangnail *n* a narrow strip of skin partly detached from the nailfold.

Hansen's bacillus ⇒ leprosy.

H_2 antagonist an agent which has a selective action against the H_2 histamine receptors and thereby decreases, e.g. the secretion of gastric juice. Cimetidine is an example.

haploid *adj* refers to the chromosome complement of the mature gametes (eggs and sperm) following meiosis (reduction division). This set represents the basic complement of 23 chromosomes in man. Its normal multiple is diploid, but abnormally three or more chromosome sets can be found (triploid, tetraploid, etc.).

hard drugs a term used in relation to drug misuse. There is not a standard classification but many people include amphetamine, barbiturates, cocaine, heroin, lysergic acid diethylamide (LSD) and morphine in the category. Current concern is about those who inject the drug and share dirty needles and syringes, not only exposing themselves but also others to the dangers of hepatitis B and HIV AIDS. ⇒ drug, over-the-counter drugs, soft drugs.

Harrington rod used in operations for scoliosis*: it provides internal fixation whereby the curve is held by the rod and is usually accompanied by a spinal fusion.

Hartmann's solution an electrolyte replacement solution. Contains sodium lactate and chloride, potassium chloride and calcium chloride.

Hartnup disease an inborn error of protein metabolism, associated with diffuse psychiatric symptoms or mild learning disability. It can be treated with nicotinamide and neomycin.

Hashimoto's disease an enlarged thyroid gland occurring in middle-aged females, and producing mild hypothyroidism. Result of sensitization of patient to her own thyroid protein, thyroglobulin.

hashish *n* ⇒ cannabis indica.

haustration *n* sacculation*, as of the colon—**haustrum** *sing*, **haustra** *pl*.

HAVS *abbr* hand-arm* vibration syndrome.

Hawthorne effect a positive result from introduction of change, of which people are less conscious with the passage of time. Nurses carrying out participant or non-participant observation in a research project allow for this reaction to their presence by not using the data collected in the first few days in the final analysis of the data. The term is derived from industrial management research at the Hawthorne factory in Illinois managed by the Western Electric Company.

Haygarth's nodes swelling of joints, sometimes seen in the finger joints of patients suffering from arthritis.

HBIG *abbr* hepatitis* B immunoglobulin.

HBV *abbr* hepatitis* B virus.

HCA *abbr* ⇒ health* care assistant.

HCG *abbr* human* chorionic gonadotrophin.

headache *n* pain most commonly experienced in the frontal or occipital region: it can accompany many illnesses which do not involve head structures. Causes of severe headache include conditions of the brain and meninges, such as inflammation; new growths which can be benign or malignant; increased intracranial pressure from trauma; and cardiovascular conditions, e.g. hypertension and stroke. Nursing intervention is based on nursing assessment and may be pharmacological, or use complementary therapies or health education. ⇒ migraine.

head injury usually the result of a blow to the head; there may or may not be fracture of the skull; concussion* can result. Damage to brain tissue can occur on the opposite side; if it is contusion, early return to consciousness can be expected. A severed blood vessel can cause subdural* haematoma. The varying level of consciousness/responsiveness can be measured by the Glasgow* coma scale.

head lice (Pediculus capitis) lay their eggs (nits) at the junction of the hair and skin. They hatch in 1 week and are fully grown in 3 and live for 5 weeks. They pierce the scalp to suck blood and cause intense itching; subsequent scratching can introduce infection. They spread quickly in schools and nurses are required to teach parents and children about head lice, how to be constantly vigilant for their presence, and how to treat an infestation.

Heaf test multiple puncture of the epidermis with a special 'gun' through a layer of filter paper soaked in tuberculin*, strength 1 in 1000 or 1 in 100. An inflammatory reaction is positive for tuberculosis.

healing *n* 1 the natural process of cure or repair of the tissues. 2 a term used in complementary medicine to imply the direct transmission of psychic energy for therapeutic purposes, either as faith healing or spiritual healing—**heal** *vt, vi. healing by first intention* when the edges of a clean wound are accurately held together, healing occurs with the minimum of scarring and deformity. *healing by second intention* when the edges of a wound are not held together, the gap is filled by granulation tissue before epithelium can grow over the wound.

health *n* a complex, abstract concept, which is difficult to define because people have different perceptions of what it means to be 'healthy'. In 1946, the World Health Organization (WHO) defined health as 'a state of complete physical, mental and social well-being, rather than solely as an absence of disease'. This definition has been criticized for being idealistic and unmeasurable. Health has several dimensions: physical, psychological, emotional, social and spiritual. The 1986 WHO first international conference on health promotion set out the action required to achieve 'health for all by the year 2000' (Ottawa charter) through building up public policy, and supporting and enabling people to improve their own health through developing personal skills and community action. *societal health* the impact of society, and the physical and socioeconomic factors of the environment, on the individual.

health care assistant (HCA) a health service employee who provides nursing support services under the direction of a qualified nurse. Formerly known as nursing auxiliaries, HCAs can now receive a nationally coordinated training, based on national vocational qualifications (NVQs).

health care system the means by which a government organizes administration of its health care policies.

health centre a building designated by a government to distribute its health care policies at local level. The personnel working in and from the centre are members of several professions, according to local needs and provisions.

health education the means by which people (individually or collectively) are informed of the pros and cons of particular personal behaviours which, according to current knowledge from research, either enhance or detract from the desirable state of health*. Coercion should not be part of this process: the objective is that people can make an informed choice.

heart *n* the hollow muscular organ which pumps the blood round the body; situated behind the sternum, lying obliquely between the two lungs It weighs about 225 g in the female and about 310 g in the male. *heart transplant* surgical transplantation of a heart from a suitable donor who has recently died. *heart block* partial or complete inhibition of the speed of conduction of the electrical impulse from the atrium to the ventricle of the heart (see Fig. 4). The cause may be an organic lesion or a functional disturbance. In its mildest form, it can only be detected electrocardiographically, whilst in its complete form the ventricles beat at their own slow intrinsic rate uninfluenced by the atria.

heartburn *n* ⇒ pyrosis, hot-fat heartburn syndrome.

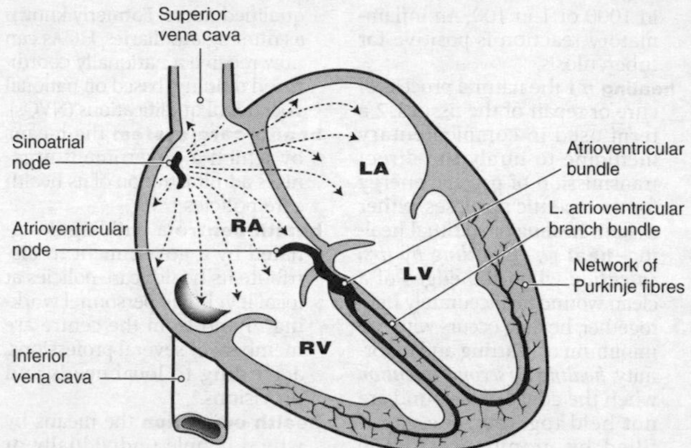

■ **Fig. 4** The electrical conduction system of the heart. Small groups of specialized neuromuscular cells in the myocardium initiate and conduct impulses of contraction over the heart muscle.

heart-lung machine a machine by means of which the blood can be removed from a vein for oxygenation, after which it is returned to the vein.

heat exhaustion (*syn* heat syncope) collapse, with or without loss of consciousness, suffered in conditions of heat and high humidity: largely resulting from loss of fluid and salt by sweating. If the surrounding air becomes saturated, heatstroke will ensue.

heatstroke *n* (*syn* sunstroke) final stage in heat exhaustion. When the body is unable to lose heat, hyperpyrexia occurs and death may ensue.

heat treatment the application of heat to a part of the body, either dry in the form of an electric pad or kaolin poultice; or moist in the form of a compress wrung out of hot water or an immersion bath.

hebephrenia *n* a common type of schizophrenia* characterized by a general disintegration of the personality. The onset is sudden and usually occurs in the teenage years. Symptoms include meaningless behaviour, inappropriate laughter, peculiar mannerisms, incoherent talk, and delusions—**hebephrenic** *adj.*

Heberden's disease angina* pectoris. *Heberden's nodes* small osseous swellings at terminal phalangeal joints occurring in many types of arthritis.

hedonism *n* excessive devotion to pleasure, so that a person's conduct is determined by an unconscious drive to seek pleasure and avoid unpleasant things.

Hegar's sign marked softening of the cervix in early pregnancy.

Heimlich manoeuvre an emergency technique to remove foreign body from upper part of lower respiratory tract. Wrap arms round victim's waist from behind; make a fist with one hand and place it against the victim's abdomen between the navel and the rib cage; clasp fist with free hand and press in with a quick forceful upward thrust. Repeat several times if necessary. The technique can be self-applied if the person is alone. Air is forced against the mass as pressure in a bottle can remove the cork.

Heinz body refractile, irregularly shaped body present in red blood cells in some haemoglobinopathies.

helium *n* an inert gas of low density. Sometimes mixed with oxygen for treatment of asthma, as it aids inspiration.

Heller's operation division of the muscle coat at the junction between the oesophagus and the stomach; used to relieve the difficulty in swallowing in cases of achalasia*.

helminthagogue *n* an anthelmintic*.

helminthiasis *n* the condition resulting from infestation with worms.

helminthology *n* the study of parasitic worms.

hemianopla *n* blindness in one half of the visual field of one or both eyes.

hemiatrophy *n* atrophy of one half or one side. *hemiatrophy facialis* a congenital condition, or a manifestation of scleroderma* in which the structures on one side of the face are shrunken.

hemichorea *n* choreiform movements limited to one side of the body. ⇒ chorea.

hemicolectomy *n* removal of approximately half the colon.

hemicrania *n* unilateral headache, as in migraine.

hemidiaphoresis *n* unilateral sweating of the body.

hemiglossectomy *n* removal of approximately half the tongue.

hemiparesis *n* a paralysis or weakness of one half of face or body.

hemiplegia *n* paralysis of one side of the body, usually resulting from a cerebrovascular accident on the opposite side—**hemiplegic** *adj*.

hemispherectomy *n* surgical removal of a cerebral hemisphere in the treatment of epilepsy. It may be either subtotal or total.

Henderson definition of nursing a much used definition of nursing, put forward by Virginia Henderson in 1969. The unique function of the nurse is to assist the individual, sick or well, in the performance of those activities contributing to health or recovery (or to a peaceful death) that the person would perform unaided if he or she had the necessary strength, will or knowledge, and to do this in such a way as to help him or her gain independence as rapidly as possible.

Henoch-Schönlein purpura (anaphylactoid purpura) *n* a syndrome of capillaritis mainly affecting children. It is characterized by purpuric bleeding into the skin, particularly shins and buttocks, and from the wall of the gut, resulting in abdominal colic and melaena; and bruising around joints. Nephritis can also occur. It may be idiopathic or follow a streptococcal infection.

hepar *n* the liver—**hepatic** *adj*.

heparin *n* an acid present in liver and lung tissue. When injected intravenously it inhibits coagulation of the blood, and it is widely used in the treatment of thrombosis, often in association with orally active anticoagulants such as warfarin*.

hepatectomy *n* excision of the liver, or more usually part of the liver.

hepatic *adj* pertaining to the liver.

hepatic coma there is impaired function of the central nervous system due to liver disease which prevents detoxication of many substances particularly ammonia. A 'mousy' odour of the breath is usually present. Nursing aims to keep the person as reality oriented as possible and prevent the potential problems of accident, infection, injury, malnutrition and pressure sores from becoming actual ones. Oral neomycin controls intestinal bacteria which favour ammonia production, and oral lactulose helps to decrease intestinal ammonia production.

hepaticocholedochostomy *n* end-to-end union of the severed hepatic and common bile ducts.

hepaticoenteric *adj* pertaining to the liver and intestine.

hepaticojejunostomy *n* anastomosis of the common hepatic duct to a loop of proximal jejunum*.

hepatitis *n* inflammation of the liver, commonly associated with viral infection but can be due to toxic agents. The onset is usually accompanied by vague symptoms, such as loss of appetite, nausea, vomiting and general fatigue. As the disease progresses, the patient becomes jaundiced and develops abdominal tenderness and pain in the right upper quadrant. Hepatitis is currently a serious public health problem. It is associated with a number of hepatitis viral types, most commonly hepatitis-A virus, hepatitis-B virus and hepatitis-C virus. *hepatitis-A* caused by an RNA enterovirus of the family *Picornaviridae*. Relatively common and may be epidemic, especially in institutions, e.g. schools. The incubation period is short (10–50 days) and the virus is transmitted by the faecooral route due to poor hygiene or contaminated food. Signs and symptoms range from mild to severe and occasionally can be fatal. *hepatitis-B* caused by a DNA virus of the family *Hepadnovirae*. Long incubation period (40–160 days) usually transmitted by injection of infected blood or blood products, or via contaminated equipment, e.g. needles. The virus is shed in saliva, semen and vaginal secretions. It is a common problem amongst drug users, and is an occupational hazard for health workers. Hepatitis-B virus may persist, causing chronic hepatitis, or a carrier state can develop. Virus particles carry the hepatitis-B surface antigen (HB_sAg) and at times when there is active viral replication hepatitis Be antigen (HB_eAg) can be detected free in the plasma, indicating a high degree of infectivity. An effective vaccine exists. *hepatitis-C* an example of a nonA nonB (NANB) virus type (incubation period is 30–90 days). It is an RNA virus and is transmitted mainly through blood transfusion and other blood products. Virus particles may remain in the blood for years and in 30–50% of infected people lead to chronic hepatitis, cirrhosis, liver failure and possibly cancer of the liver. The carrier state also exists. *hepatitis-D (Delta virus)* can only replicate in the presence of hepatitis-B and is therefore found infecting simultaneously with hepatitis-B, or as a superinfection in a person chronically carrying hepatitis-B. Delta virus may increase the severity of a hepatitis-B infection, increasing the risk of chronic liver disease.

hepatocellular *adj* pertaining to or affecting liver cells.

hepatocirrhosis *n* cirrhosis* of the liver.

hepatocyte *n* the main cell type in the liver, it carries out the functions performed by the liver, e.g. synthesis, bile production.

hepatoma *n* primary carcinoma of the liver—**hepatomata** *pl.*

hepatomegaly *n* enlargement of the liver, palpable below the costal margin.

hepatosplenic *adj* pertaining to the liver and spleen.

hepatosplenomegaly *n* enlargement of the liver and the spleen, so that each is palpable below the costal margin.

hepatotoxic *adj* having an injurious effect on liver cells—**hepatotoxicity** *n.*

herbalism *n* the therapeutic use of herbal and mineral remedies. There are restrictions on the availability of certain herbal remedies, such as ergot, scopalia and digitalis, which may only be prescribed by a doctor.

hereditary *adj* inherited; capable of being inherited.

heredity *n* transmission from parents to offspring of physical and mental attributes by means of the genetic material; the process by which this occurs, and the study of the biological laws that govern this transmission.

hermaphrodite *n* individual possessing both ovarian and testicular tissue. Although the individual may approximate either to male or female type, he or she is usually sterile from imperfect development of the gonads.

hermetic *adj* sealed by fusion to make airtight. Such a seal ensures that a wound is not exposed to air.

hernia *n* the abnormal protrusion of an organ, or part of an organ, through an aperture in the surrounding structures; commonly the protrusion of an abdominal organ through a gap in the abdominal wall. *diaphragmatic hernia* (*syn* hiatus hernia) protrusion through the diaphragm, the commonest one involving the stomach at the oesophageal opening. *femoral hernia* protrusion through the femoral canal, alongside the femoral blood vessels as they pass into the thigh. *incisional hernia* usually occurs as an emergency when there is an infected abdominal wound. *inguinal hernia* protrusion through the inguinal canal in the male. *irreducible hernia* when the contents of the sac cannot be returned to the appropriate cavity without surgical intervention. *strangulated hernia* hernia in which the blood supply to the organ involved is impaired, usually due to constriction by surrounding structures. *umbilical hernia* (*syn* omphalocele) protrusion of a portion of intestine through the area of the umbilical scar. *uterine hernia* protrusion of the uterus as part of a hernia. *vaginal hernia* protrusion of a loop of intestine into the vagina.

herniation *n* the formation of a hernia; rupture.

hernioplasty *n* an operation for hernia in which an attempt is made to prevent recurrence by refashioning the structures to give greater strength—**hernioplastic** *adj.*

herniorrhaphy *n* an operation for hernia in which the weak area is reinforced by some of the patient's own tissues or by some other material.

herniotome *n* a special knife with a blunt tip, used for hernia operations.

herniotomy *n* an operation to cure hernia by the return of its contents to their normal position and removal of the hernial sac.

heroin *n* ⇒ diamorphine.

herpangina *n* minute vesicles and ulcers at the back of the palate. Short, febrile form of pharyngitis in children caused by coxsackie virus Group A.

herpes *n* a vesicular eruption due to infection with the herpes* simplex virus. *genital herpes* infection with the herpes* simplex virus (HSV) Type I or II; it is a sexually transmitted disease. In the female, ulcers and vesicles can occur on the cervix, vagina, vulva and labia. In the male, these occur on the glans, prepuce and penal shaft and less commonly on the scrotum. In both sexes lesions may be seen on the pharynx, thighs, buttocks and perianal regions. *herpes gestationis* a rare skin disease peculiar to pregnancy. It clears in about 30 days after delivery.

herpes simplex virus (HSV) consists of two biologically and immunologically distinct types designated Type I, which generally causes oral disease and lesions above the waist, and Type II, most commonly associated with genital disease and lesions below the waist. Recurrent episodes are common as the virus remains latent in nerve ganglia after the initial infection. ⇒ herpes.

herpetiform *adj* resembling herpes*.

hesitancy *n* a delay in starting to pass urine, even when responding to a strong desire to void. A symptom of outflow obstruction.

Hess test a sphygmomanometer cuff is applied to the arm and is inflated. Petechial eruption in the surrounding area after 5 min denotes weakness of the capillary walls, characteristic of purpura.

heterogenous *adj* of unlike origin; not originating within the body; derived from a different species. ⇒ homogenous *opp.*

heterologous *adj* of different origin; from a different species. ⇒ homologous *opp.*

heterophile *n* a product of one species which acts against that of another, e.g. human antigen against sheep's red blood cells.

heterosexual *adj, n* literally, of different sexes; used to describe a person who is sexually attracted towards the opposite sex. ⇒ homosexual *opp.*

heterozygous *adj* having different genes or alleles at the same locus on both chromosomes of a pair (one of maternal and the other of paternal origin) ⇒ homozygous *opp.*

hexose *n* a class of simple sugars, monosaccharides containing six carbon atoms ($C_6H_{12}O_6$). Examples are glucose, mannose, galactose.

HGH *abbr* human growth* hormone.

HHNK *abbr* hyperglycaemic hyperosmolar nonketoacidotic coma. ⇒ diabetes.

hiatus *n* a space or opening. *hiatus hernia* ⇒ hernia—**hiatal** *adj.*

Hibb's operation operation for spinal fusion, following spinal tuberculosis. No bone graft is used, but the split vertebral spines are pressed outwards and laid in contact with the laminae. Bony union occurs and the spine is rigid.

hiccough *n* (*syn* hiccup). An involuntary inspiratory spasm of the respiratory organs, ending in a sudden closure of the glottis with the production of a characteristic sound.

hiccup ⇒ hiccough.

Hickman line proprietary name for a catheter which is used to provide a central* venous line.

hidrosis *n* sweat secretion.

Higginson's syringe a rubber bulb with tubes leading to and from it. One tube rests in a container of fluid, e.g. saline. Compression of the bulb forces fluid through the nozzle of the other tube for irrigation of a body cavity.

high density lipoprotein a plasma protein relatively high in protein, low in cholesterol. It is involved in transporting cholesterol and other lipids from plasma to the tissues.

hilum *n* a depression on the surface of an organ where vessels, ducts, etc. enter and leave–**hili** *pl,* **hilar** *adj. hilar adenitis* ⇒ adenitis.

hip bone (innominate bone) formed by the fusion of three separate bones: the ilium, ischium and pubis.

hip joint articulation of the head of femur within the acetabulum* to form a synovial, freely movable joint*.

hip replacement ⇒ arthroplasty.

hip spica enclosure of the lower trunk and one (single spica) or both (double spica) lower limb(s) in a plaster cast ⇒ spica.

Hippocrates *n* famous Greek physician and philosopher (460–367 BC) who established a school of medicine at Cos, his birthplace. He is often termed the 'Father of Medicine'.

Hirschsprung's disease congenital intestinal aganglionosis, leading to intractable constipation or even intestinal obstruction. There is marked hypertrophy and dilation of the colon (megacolon) above the aganglionic segment. There is an association with Down syndrome. Treatment involves surgical removal of the aganglionic segment.

hirsute *adj* hairy or shaggy.

hirsuties, hirsutism *n* excessive growth of hair in sites in which body hair is normally found. ⇒ hypertrichosis.

hirudin *n* a substance secreted by the medicinal leech*, which prevents the clotting of blood by acting as an antithrombin.

hirudo *n* ⇒ leech.

histamine *n* a naturally occurring chemical substance in body tissues which, in small doses, has profound and diverse actions on muscle, blood capillaries and gastric secretion. Sudden excessive release from the tissues, into the blood, is believed to be the cause of the main symptoms and signs in anaphylaxis*–**histaminic** *adj. histamine receptor cells* there are two types in the body, H_1 in the bronchial muscle and H_2 in the secreting cells in the stomach. *histamine test* designed to determine the maximal gastric secretion of hydrochloric acid. A Levin* tube is positioned in the most dependent part of the stomach of a fasting patient who has been weighed. Following the collection of a control specimen and the injection of an antihistamine and a histamine, gastric secretions are collected for a further hour. By titrating the collections against a standard alkaline solution, the acidity of the gastric secretions can be determined.

histidine *n* an essential amino acid which is widely distributed and is present in haemoglobin. It is a precursor of histamine*.

histiocytes *npl* macrophages derived from reticuloendothelial* cells; act as scavengers.

histiocytoma *n* benign tumour of histiocytes.

histiocytosis X *n* a rare disorder of the reticuloendothelial system (RES) in which there is an abnormal proliferation of histiocytes associated with local inflammatory reaction. Clinical features depend upon the organs or tissues involved. Three classical syndromes have been described: eosinophilic granuloma of bone, Hand-Schüller-Christian disease, and Letterer-Siwe disease. Treatment varies according to the type of disease. Local lesions may be excised or treated with radiotherapy; cytoxic therapy may be required for more severe forms of the disease.

histocompatibility antigens the antigens on nucleated cells which induce an allograft* response; important in organ transplantation.

histology *n* microscopic study of tissues—**histological** *adj,* **histologically** *adv.*

histolysis *n* disintegration of organic tissue—**histolytic** *adj.*

histones *npl* a special set of proteins closely associated with the chromosomal DNA of higher organisms, which coils and supercoils around histone molecules. These are therefore part of the way the DNA is organized to form the chromosomes.

histoplasmosis *n* an infection caused by inhaling spores of the fungus *Histoplasma capsulatum.* The primary lung lesion may go unnoticed or be accompanied by fever, malaise, cough and adenopathy. Progressive histoplasmosis can be fatal.

HIV *abbr* human immunodeficiency virus. ⇒ AIDS.

hives *n* nettlerash; urticaria*.

hoarseness *n* roughness of voice which can have many causes from laryngitis (acute or chronic) to cancer. Because of the possibility of cancer, nurses should advise patients who are not improving to consult a doctor. Nurses can offer steam inhalations and provide alternative means of communication to rest the larynx.

hobnail liver firm nodular liver which may be found in cirrhosis.

Hodgkin's disease a malignant disease of the lymphatic tissue, causing progressive enlargement of lymph nodes and eventually progressing to the spleen, liver and bone marrow. There are four stages of the disease, depending on its progression, and on which treatment is based.

Hoffman's exercises working the thumb and forefinger around the breast areola—an exercise for inverted and nonprotractile nipples in pregnant women. The benefit is unproven and some suggest that such antenatal interventions lead to a decrease in the number of women who breast feed.

Hogben test a female *Xenopus* toad is injected with a preparation obtained from the early morning urine of a woman suspected of pregnancy. In the case of pregnancy the toad lays eggs after 8–24 h. The test is over 99% accurate.

holistic *adj* in a nursing context, caring for the whole patient. ⇒ total patient care.

Homans' sign passive dorsiflexion of foot causes pain in calf muscles. Indicative of incipient or established venous thrombosis of leg.

home carers formerly termed home helps. Important members of social services community care teams who provide care for elderly and/or disabled people living in their own homes, in bathing, dressing, shopping and cooking meals. Less likely than formerly to do domestic work. A charge for home care services is usually made.

homeostasis *n* a physiological regulatory process whereby functions such as blood pressure, body temperature and electrolytes are maintained within a narrow range of normal.

homicide *n* killing of another person: manslaughter (Scots Law: culpable homicide) if accidental, murder if intentional.

homocystinuria *n* recessively inherited inborn error of metabolism. There is excretion of homocystine (a sulphur-containing amino acid, homologue of cystine) in the urine. Gives rise to slow development of varying degree; associated with lens dislocation, overgrowth of long bones, osteoporosis, pathological features, widespread vascular thrombosis, and other symptoms. May be diagnosed by a biochemical screening test—**homocystinuric** *adj.*

homogeneous *adj* of the same kind; of the same quality or consistency throughout.

homoeopathy *n* a method of treating disease by prescribing minute doses of drugs which, in maximum dose, would produce symptoms of the disease. First adopted by Hahnemann—**homoeopathic** *adj*.

homogenize *vt* to make into the same consistency throughout.

homogenous *adj* having a like nature, e.g. a tissue graft from another human being. ⇒ heterogenous *opp*.

homograft *n* a tissue or organ which is transplanted from one individual to another of the same species. ⇒ allograft.

homolateral *adj* on the same side.

homologous *adj* corresponding in origin and structure. ⇒ heterologous *opp*. *homologous chromosomes* those that pair during reduction cell division (meiosis) whereby mature gametes are formed. Their DNA has an identical arrangement and sequence of different genes. Of the two homologues, one is derived from the father, the other from the mother.

homonymous *adj* consisting of corresponding halves.

homosexual *adj, n* literally, of the same sex; used to describe a person who is sexually attracted to a member of the same sex. Homosexuals themselves prefer to be called 'gay' or 'lesbian'. Male homosexuals who have unprotected sex are at particular risk of contracting infection with hepatitis B_1 virus, cytomegalovirus, Epstein-Barr* virus, acquired immune* deficiency syndrome. ⇒ heterosexual *opp*.

homosexuality *n* attraction for, and desire to establish an emotional and sexual relationship with, a member of the same sex.

homozygous *adj* having identical genes or alleles in the same locus on both chromosomes of a pair (one of maternal and the other of paternal origin). ⇒ heterozygous *opp*.

hookworm *n* ⇒ Ancylostoma.

hordeolum *n* ⇒ stye.

hormone *n* specific chemical substance secreted by an endocrine gland and conveyed in the blood to regulate the functions of tissues and organs elsewhere in the body.

hormone replacement therapy (HRT) oestrogen treatment given to women for relief of menopausal symptoms and the prevention of osteoporosis. Administered orally, transdermally or by implant.

Horner syndrome clinical picture following paralysis of cervical sympathetic nerves on one side. There is myosis, slight ptosis with enophthalmos, and anhidrosis. Frequently associated with a diagnosis of lung cancer.

Horton syndrome severe headache due to the release of histamine in the body. To be differentiated from migraine*.

hospice *n* a place where terminally ill people are cared for by experienced staff in home-like surroundings which provide a friendly atmosphere. Patient and family participation is encouraged. Individualized pain control programmes are implemented so that patients and their families can learn to celebrate the life of the dying person, who being pain-free is relieved of the most common fear about dying.

hospital acquired infection (HAI) ⇒ infection.

hospital sterilization and disinfection unit (HSDU) central sterile supply units (CSSUs) which have extended their work to include disinfection of equipment.

host *n* the organic structure upon which parasites or bacteria thrive. *intermediate host* one in which the parasite passes its larval or cystic stage.

hot-fat heartburn syndrome due to reflux from stomach to oesophagus producing hypersensitivity in the oesophageal mucosa: tends to be worse after fatty or fried food or drinking coffee. May be associated with hiatus hernia*.

hour-glass contraction a circular constriction in the middle of a hollow organ (usually the stomach or uterus), dividing it into two portions following scar formation.

housemaid's knee ⇒ bursitis.

HPV *abbr* ⇒ human papilloma viruses.

HSDU *abbr* ⇒ hospital sterilization and disinfection unit.

HSSU *abbr* hospital sterile supply unit. ⇒ hospital sterilization and disinfection unit.

HSV *abbr* herpes* simplex virus.

HTLV. *abbr* human* T-cell lymphotropic viruses.

humanism *n* a philosophical movement which focusses on the nature and essence of the human individual. It explores and promotes the central importance of the human individual and has underpinned the reasonings behind human rights movements, patients' rights campaigns and patient-centred approaches to health care. It is one of the main philosophical movements underlying current theories of nursing practice.

human chorionic gonadotrophin (HCG) a hormone arising from the placenta. Used for cryptorchism, and sometimes for female infertility. The presence of HCG in urine is detectable in an early morning specimen of urine from the 4th week of pregnancy.

human immunodeficiency viruses (HIV) currently designates the AIDS* virus. It is the name recommended by the International Committee on the Taxonomy of Viruses, for the human T-cell lymphotropic virus type III which causes AIDS.

human needs the concept has been widely used in nursing; it is based on Maslow's analysis of human needs. The basic physiological needs for food, breathing and eliminating are at the bottom of the hierarchy and have to be at least minimally fulfilled before motivation is established to deal with safety and security needs; then love and belonging, and self-esteem needs are attended to; and at the top level achievement of self-actualisation brings satisfaction with living and a sense of fulfilment.

human papilloma viruses (HPV) belong to a group of wart viruses affecting human beings. HPV_{16} is implicated in genital warts and cervical cancer.

human T-cell lymphotropic viruses (HTLV) HTLV 1 associated with some forms of leukaemia; HTLV 2 with multiple sclerosis; HTLV 3 causes AIDS*. ⇒ lymphocyte.

humerus *n* the bone of the upper arm, between the elbow and shoulder joint—**humeri** *pl,* **humeral** *adj.*

humidity *n* the amount of moisture in the atmosphere, as measured by a hygrometer. *relative humidity* the ratio of the amount of moisture present in the air to the amount which would saturate it (at the same temperature).

humor *n* any fluid of the body. ⇒ aqueous, vitreous.

humoral immunity ⇒ immunity.

Hunter-Hurler syndrome ⇒ gargoylism.

Hunter syndrome one of the mucopolysaccharidoses*, designated Type II. A sex-linked recessive condition.

Huntington's chorea genetically determined heredofamilial disease with slow progresive degeneration of the nerve cells of the basal ganglia and cerebral cortex. Affects both sexes, and is due to a dominant gene of large effect. Develops in middle age, or later, and is associated with progressive dementia. ⇒ chorea.

Hurler syndrome one of the mucopolysaccharidoses*; designated Type II. Inherited as an autosomal recessive trait.

HUS *abbr* haemolytic* uraemic syndrome. ⇒ haemolytic disorders.

Hutchinson's teeth defect of the upper central incisors (second dentition) which is part of the facies of the congenital syphilitic person. The teeth are broader at the gum than at the cutting edge, with the latter showing an elliptical notch.

hyaline *adj* like glass; transparent. *hyaline degeneration* degeneration of connective tissue especially that of blood vessels in which tissue takes on a homogenous or formless appearance. *hyaline membrane disease* ⇒ respiratory distress syndrome.

hyaloid *adj* resembling hyaline* tissue. *hyaloid membrane* ⇒ membrane.

hydatid cyst *n* the cyst formed by larvae of a tapeworm, *Echinococcus,* which is found in dogs. The encysted stage normally occurs in sheep but can occur in man after he eats with soiled hands from petting a dog. The cysts are commonest in the liver and lungs: they grow slowly and only do damage by the space they occupy. If they leak, or become infected, urticaria and fever supervene and 'daughter' cysts can result. The treatment is surgical removal.

hydatidiform *adj* pertaining to or resembling a hydatid* cyst. *hydatidiform mole* a condition in which the chorionic villi of the placenta undergo cystic degeneration and the fetus is absorbed. The villi penetrate and destroy only the decidual layer of the uterus, but a hydatidiform mole may progress to become an invasive mole in which the villi penetrate the myometrium and can destroy the uterine wall and metastasize to the vagina or even the lungs and brain; these regress after evacuation of the mole. Invasive mole is benign but it may convert to choriocarcinoma.

hydraemia *n* a relative excess of plasma volume compared with cell volume of the blood; it is normally present in late pregnancy—**hydraemic** *adj.*

hydramnios *n* an excess of amniotic fluid.

hydrarthrosis *n* a collection of synovial fluid in a joint cavity. *intermittent hydrarthrosis* afflicts young women; probably due to allergy. Synovitis develops spontaneously, lasts a few days and disappears as mysteriously.

hydrate *vi* combine with water—**hydration** *n.*

hydroa *n* ⇒ dermatitis herpetiformis. *hydroa aestivale* **1** a vesicular or bullous disease occurring in atopic* children. It affects exposed parts and probably results from photosensitivity. **2** sun-induced dermatitis in some forms of porphyria. *hydroa vacciniforme* is a more severe form of this in which scarring ensues.

hydrocele *n* a swelling due to accumulation of serous fluid in the tunica vaginalis of the testis or in the spermatic cord.

hydrocephalus *n* (*syn* 'water on the brain') an excess of cerebrospinal fluid inside the skull due to an obstruction to normal CSF circulation—**hydrocephalic** *adj. external hydrocephalus* the excess of fluid is mainly in the subarachnoid space. *internal hydrocephalus* the excess of fluid is mainly in the ventricles of the brain. A Spitz*-Holter valve is used in drainage operations for this condition.

hydrochloric acid secreted by the gastric oxyntic cells and present in gastric juice (0.2%). The strong acid is caustic.

hydrocortisone *n* ⇒ cortisol.

hydrogen *n* a colourless, odourless, combustible gas. *hydrogen ion concentration* a measure of the acidity or alkalinity of a solution, ranging from pH 1 to pH 14, 7 being approximately neutral; the lower numbers denoting acidity; the higher ones denoting alkalinity. *hydrogen peroxide* H_2O_2, a powerful oxidizing and deodorizing agent, used for cleaning wounds; diluted with 4–8 parts of water as a mouthwash and with 50% alcohol as ear drops.

hydrolysis *n* the splitting into more simple substances by the addition of water—**hydrolytic** *adj,* **hydrolyse** *vt.*

hydrometer *n* an instrument for determining the specific gravity of fluids—**hydrometry** *n.*

hydronephrosis *n* distension of the kidney pelvis with urine, from obstructed outflow. If unrelieved, pressure eventually causes atrophy of kidney tissue. Surgical operations include nephroplasty and pyeloplasty.

hydropericarditis *n* pericarditis with effusion.

hydropericardium *n* fluid in the pericardial sac in the absence of inflammation. Can occur in heart and kidney failure.

hydroperitoneum *n* ⇒ ascites.

hydrophobia *n* ⇒ rabies.

hydrophylic *adj* having an affinity for water.

hydropneumopericardium *n* the presence of air and fluid in the membranous pericardial sac surrounding the heart. It may accompany pericardiocentesis*.

hydropneumoperitoneum *n* the presence of fluid and gas in the peritoneal cavity: it may accompany aspiration of that cavity; it may be due to perforation of the gut; or it may be due to gas-forming microorganisms in the peritoneal fluid.

hydropneumothorax *n* pneumothorax* further complicated by effusion of fluid into the pleural cavity.

hydrops *n* oedema*—**hydropic** *adj. hydrops fetalis* a severe form of erythroblastosis fetalis*.

hydrosalpinx *n* distension of a uterine tube with watery fluid.

hydrotherapy *n* the science of therapeutic bathing for diagnosed conditions.

hydrothorax *n* the presence of fluid in the pleural cavity.

hydroureter *n* abnormal distension of the ureter with urine.

hydroxybutyrate dehydrogenase a serum enzyme: high concentrations are indicative of myocardial infarction.

hydroxyl *n* a monovalent ion (OH), consisting of a hydrogen atom linked to an oxygen atom. Acts as a free radical so can cause tissue damage.

5-hydroxytryptamine (5-HT) *n* ⇒ serotonin.

hygiene *n* the science dealing with the maintenance and preservation of health, especially by the promotion of cleanliness—**hygienic** *adj.*

hygroma *n* malformation of the lymphatic trunks causing a cystic swelling containing watery fluid. *cystic hygroma* usually situated at the neck and present at birth, sometimes interfering with birth. Surgical excision is necessary before complications associated with infection develop—**hygromata** *pl,* **hygromatous** *adj.*

hygrometer *n* an instrument for measuring the amount of moisture in the air. ⇒ humidity.

hygroscopic *adj* readily absorbing water, e.g. glycerine.

hymen *n* a membranous perforated structure stretching across the vaginal entrance. *imperforate hymen* a congenital condition leading to haematocolpos. ⇒ cryptomenorrhoea.

hymenectomy *n* surgical excision of the hymen.

hymenotomy *n* surgical incision of the hymen. ⇒ haematocolpos.

hyoid *n* a U-shaped bone at the root of the tongue.

hyoscine *n* (*syn* scopolamine) a hypnotic alkaloid obtained from belladonna and hyoscyamus. Often used for preoperative sedation in association with morphine, papaveretum or pethidine. Also mydriatic and cycloplegic.

hyperacidity *n* excessive acidity. ⇒ hyperchlorhydria.

hyperactivity *n* excessive activity and distractability: modes of treatment incorporate techniques such as behaviour modification, dietary restrictions and drugs.

hyperaemia *n* excess of blood in an area. *active hyperaemia* caused by an increased flow of blood to a part. *passive hyperaemia* occurs when there is restricted flow of blood from a part—**hyperaemic** *adj.*

hyperaesthesia *n* excessive sensitiveness of a part—**hyperaesthetic** *adj.*

hyperaldosteronism *n* production of excessive aldosterone. *primary hyperaldosteronism* Conn* syndrome. *secondary hyperaldosteronism* the adrenal glands respond to an increased stimulus of extraadrenal origin.

hyperalgesia *n* excessive sensitivity to pain—**hyperalgesic** *adj.*

hyperalimentation *n* total* parenteral nutrition.

hyperbaric oxygen therapy a form of treatment in which a patient is entirely enclosed in a pressure chamber breathing 100% oxygen at greater than one atmosphere pressure. Used for patients with carbon monoxide poisoning, decompression sickness (caisson disease, the bends), clostridial infections such as gas gangrene, osteoradionecrosis, etc.

hyperbilirubinaemia *n* excessive bilirubin in the blood. When it rises above 1–1.5 mg per 100 ml, visible jaundice* occurs. Present in physiological jaundice of the newborn. ⇒ phototherapy—**hyperbilirubinaemic** *adj.*

hypercalcaemia *n* excessive calcium in the blood usually resulting from bone resorption as occurs in hyperparathyroidism, metastatic tumours of bone, Paget's disease and osteoporosis. It results in anorexia, abdominal pain, muscle pain and weakness. It is accompanied by hypercalciuria and can lead to nephrolithiasis*—**hypercalcaemic** *adj.*

hypercalciuria *n* greatly increased excretion of calcium in the urine. Occurs in diseases which result in bone resorption. *idiopathic hypercalciuria* is the term used when there is no known metabolic cause. Hypercalciuria is of importance in the pathogenesis of nephrolithiasis*.

hypercapnia *n* (*syn* hypercarbia) raised CO_2 tension in arterial blood—**hypercapnic** *adj.*

hypercarbia *n* ⇒ hypercapnia.

hypercatabolism *n* abnormal, excessive breakdown of complex substances into simpler ones within the body. Can occur in fevers and in acute renal failure—**hypercatabolic** *adj.*

hyperchloraemia *n* excessive chloride in the blood. One form of acidosis*—**hyperchloraemic** *adj.*

hyperchlorhydria *n* excessive hydrochloric acid in the gastric juice—**hyperchlorhydric** *adj.*

hypercholesterolaemia *n* excessive cholesterol in the blood.

Predisposes to atheroma and gallstones. Also found in myxoedema—**hypercholesterolaemic** *adj.*

hyperelectrolytaemia *n* dehydration (not manifested clinically), associated with high serum sodium and chloride levels.

hyperemesis *n* excessive vomiting. *hyperemesis gravidarum* excessive vomiting in pregnancy necessitating medical intervention.

hyperextension *n* overextension.

hyperflexion *n* excessive flexion.

hyperglycaemia *n* excessive glucose in the blood (normal range is from 3.0–5.0 mmol per litre), usually indicative of diabetes mellitus. The discovery of isolated high blood glucose readings in an otherwise symptomless diabetic is of little value, but during illness raised blood glucose readings may be a valuable guide to the need for extra insulin—**hyperglycaemic** *adj.*

hyperglycaemic coma ⇒ coma, diabetes.

hyperglycinaemia *n* excess glycine in the serum. Can cause acidosis and learning disability—**hyperglycinaemic** *adj.*

hyperhidrosis *n* excessive sweating—**hyperhidrotic** *adj.*

hyperinsulinism *n* intermittent or continuous loss of consciousness, with or without convulsions (a) due to excessive insulin from the pancreatic islets lowering the blood sugar (b) due to administration of excessive insulin.

hyperkalaemia (*syn* hyperpotassaemia) excessive potassium in the blood as occurs in renal failure; early signs are nausea, diarrhoea and muscular weakness—**hyperkalaemic** *adj.*

hyperkeratosis *n* hypertrophy of the stratum corneum, the horny layer of the skin—**hyperkeratotic** *adj.*

hyperkinesis *n* excessive movement—**hyperkinetic** *adj.*

hyperkinetic syndrome usually appears between the ages of 2 and 4 years. The child is slow to develop intellectually and displays a marked degree of distractability and a tireless unrelenting perambulation of the environment, together with aggressiveness (especially towards siblings) even if unprovoked. The child may appear to be fearless and undeterred by threats of punishment. The parents complain of his or her cold unaffectionate character and destructive behaviour. The child's history may suggest the possibility of minimal brain dysfunction. Careful management is required, with an individual programme arranged for each child. Amphetamine-related drugs may help some children; the exclusion of certain foods from the diet may relieve the hyperactivity.

hyperlipaemia *n* excessive total fat in the blood—**hyperlipaemic** *adj.*

hypermagnesaemia *n* excessive magnesium in the blood, found in kidney failure and in people who take excessive magnesium-containing antacids—**hypermagnesaemic** *adj.*

hypermetabolism *n* production of excessive body heat. Characteristic of thyrotoxicosis—**hypermetabolic** *adj.*

hypermetropia *n* longsightedness caused by faulty accommodation of the eye, with the result that the light rays are focused beyond, instead of on, the retina—**hypermetropic** *adj.*

hypermobility *n* excessive mobility.

hypermotility *n* increased movement, as peristalsis.

hypernatraemia *n* high levels of sodium in the blood caused by excessive loss of water and electrolytes through polyuria, diarrhoea, excessive sweating or inadequate fluid intake—**hypernatraemic** *adj.*

hypernephroma *n* (*syn* Grawitz tumour) a malignant neoplasm of the kidney whose structure resembles that of adrenocortical tissue—**hypernephromata** *pl*, **hypernephromatous** *adj*.

hyperonychia *n* excessive growth of the nails.

hyperosmolar diabetic coma coma characterized by a very high blood sugar without accompanying ketoacidosis.

hyperosmolarity *n* (*syn* hypertonicity) a solution exerting a higher osmotic pressure than another, is said to have a hyperosmolarity, with reference to it. In medicine, the comparison is usually made with normal plasma.

hyperostosis *n* ⇒ exostosis.

hyperoxaluria *n* excessive calcium oxalate in the urine—**hyperoxaluric** *adj*.

hyperparathyroidism *n* overaction of the parathyroid* glands with increase in serum calcium levels: may result in osteitis* fibrosa cystica with decalcification, leading to backache, joint and bone pain and possible spontaneous fracture of bones. ⇒ hypercalcaemia, hypercalciuria.

hyperperistalsis *n* excessive peristalsis—**hyperperistaltic** *adj*.

hyperphenylalaninaemia *n* excess of phenylalanine in the blood which results in phenylketonuria*.

hyperphosphataemia *n* excessive phosphates in the blood—**hyperphosphataemic** *adj*.

hyperpigmentation *n* increased or excessive pigmentation.

hyperpituitarism *n* overactivity of the anterior lobe of the pituitary* gland producing gigantism* or acromegaly*.

hyperplasia *n* excessive formation of cells—**hyperplastic** *adj*.

hyperpnoea *n* rapid, deep breathing; panting; gasping—**hyperpnoeic** *adj*.

hyperpotassaemia *n* ⇒ hyperkalaemia—**hyperpotassaemic** *adj*.

hyperprolactinaemia *n* excessive prolactin* in the blood. Can occur as an endocrine side-effect from certain antipsychotic drugs. In women, there may be breast enlargement, galactorrhoea* and secondary amenorrhoea. In men, there may be gynaecomastia*, loss of libido and impotence.

hyperpyrexia *n* body temperature above 40–41°C (105°F)—**hyperpyrexial** *adj*. *malignant hyperpyrexia* an inherited condition which presents during general anaesthesia; there is progressive rise in body temperature and if untreated may be fatal.

hypersecretion *n* excessive secretion.

hypersensitivity *n* a state of being unduly sensitive to a stimulus or an allergen*—**hypersensitive** *adj*.

hypersplenism *n* term used to describe depression of erythrocyte, granulocyte and platelet counts by enlarged spleen in presence of active bone marrow.

hypertelorism *n* genetically determined cranial anomaly (low forehead and pronounced vertex) associated with learning disability.

hypertension *n* abnormally high tension, by custom abnormally high blood pressure involving systolic and/or diastolic levels. There is no universal agreement of their upper limits of normal, especially in increasing age. Many cardiologists consider a resting systolic pressure of 160 mmHg, and/or a resting diastolic pressure of 100 mmHg, to be pathological. The cause may be renal, endocrine, mechanical or toxic (as in toxaemia of pregnancy) but in many cases it is unknown and this is then called 'essential hypertension'. ⇒ portal* hypertension, pulmonary* hypertension—**hypertensive** *adj.*

hyperthermia *n* very high body temperature. Can be therapeutically induced, e.g. for the treatment of cancer, and used in conjunction with radiotherapy or chemotherapy—**hyperthermic** *adj. local hyperthermia* localized heating of tumours to a temperature of 42.5°C. *whole body hyperthermia* treatment of cancer by heating the whole body to 40.2°C.

hyperthyroidism *n* thyrotoxicosis*.

hypertonia *n* increased tone in a muscular structure—**hypertonic** *adj,* **hypertonicity** *n.*

hypertonic *adj* **1** pertaining to hypertonia. **2** pertaining to saline. *hypertonic saline* has a greater osmotic pressure than normal physiological (body) fluid.

hypertonicity *n* ⇒ hyperosmolarity.

hypertrichosis *n* excessive hairiness in sites not usually bearing prominent hair, e.g. the forehead.

hypertrophy *n* increase in the size of tissues or structures, independent of natural growth. It may be congenital, compensatory, complementary or functional. ⇒ stenosis—**hypertrophic** *adj.*

hyperuricaemia *n* excessive uric acid in the blood. Characteristic of gout. Occurs in untreated reticulosis, but is increased by radiotherapy, cytotoxins and corticosteroids. ⇒ Lesch-Nyhan disease—**hyperuricaemic** *adj.*

hyperventilation *n* increased respiration rate above the body's metabolic requirements; may be active, as in salicylate poisoning or head injury, or passive as when it is imposed as part of a technique of general anaesthesia in intensive care.

hypervitaminosis *n* any condition arising from an excess of vitamins, especially vitamin D.

hypervolaemia *n* an increase in the volume of circulating blood.

hyphaema *n* blood in the anterior chamber of the eye.

hypnosis *n* a state resembling sleep, brought about by the hypnotist utilizing the mental mechanism of suggestion to produce relaxation of tense muscles. It can also be used during dental extractions, and, in suitable subjects, for smoking cessation—**hypnotic** *adj.*

hypnotherapy *n* treatment by a sleeplike state, hypnosis.

hypnotic *adj* **1** pertaining to hypnotism. ⇒ narcotic, sedative. **2** a drug which produces a sleep resembling natural sleep.

hypoaesthesia *n* diminished sensitiveness of a part—**hypoaesthetic** *adj.*

hypocalcaemia *n* decreased calcium in the blood—**hypocalcaemic** *adj.*

hypocapnia *n* reduced CO_2 tension in arterial blood; can be produced by hyperventilation—**hypocapnial** *adj.*

hypochloraemia *n* reduced chlorides in the circulating blood. A form of alkalosis*—**hypochloraemic** *adj.*

hypochlorhydria *n* decreased hydrochloric acid in the gastric juice—**hypochlorhydric** *adj.*

hypochlorite *n* salts of hypochlorous acid. They are easily decomposed to yield active chlorine, and have been widely used on that account in the treatment of wounds—Dakin's solution and eusol being examples. Milton is a proprietary product that contains a stabilizer and therefore retains its activity over a longer period.

hypochondria *n* excessive anxiety about one's health. Common in depressive and anxiety states—**hypochondriac, hypochondriacal** *adj,* **hypochondriasis** *n.*

hypochondrium *n* the upper lateral region (left and right) of the abdomen, below the lower ribs—**hypochondriac** *adj.*

hypochromic *adj* deficient in colouring or pigmentation. Of a red blood cell, having decreased haemoglobin or abnormally thin erythrocytes, as seen in thalassaemia.

hypodermic *adj* below the skin; subcutaneous—**hypodermically** *adv.*

hypofibrinogenaemia *n* low fibrin levels in blood—**hypofibrinogenaomic** *adj.*

hypofunction *n* diminished performance.

hypogammaglobulinaemia *n* decreased gammaglobulin in the blood, occurring either congenitally or, more commonly, as a sporadic disease in adults. Lessens resistance to infection. ⇒ dysgammaglobulinaemia—**hypogammaglobulinaemic** *adj.*

hypogastrium *n* that area of the anterior abdomen which lies immediately below the umbilical region. It is flanked on either side by the iliac fossae—**hypogastric** *adj.*

hypoglossal *adj* under the tongue. *hypoglossal nerve* the 12th pair of the 12 pairs of cranial nerves which arise directly from the brain.

hypoglycaemia *n* decreased blood glucose levels (normal range is from 3.0–5.0 mmol per litre), attended by anxiety, excitement, perspiration, delirium or coma. Hypoglycaemia occurs most commonly in diabetes* mellitus when it is due either to insulin overdosage or to inadequate intake of carbohydrate—**hypoglycaemic** *adj.*

hypoglycaemic coma ⇒ coma, diabetes.

hypokalaemia *n* (*syn* hypopotassaemia) abnormally low potassium level of the blood. ⇒ potassium deficiency—**hypokalaemic** *adj.*

hypomania *n* a less intense form of mania in which there is a mild elevation of mood with restlessness, distractability, increased energy and pressure of speech. The flight of ideas and grandiose delusions of frank mania* are usually absent—**hypomanic** *adj.*

hypometabolism *n* decreased production of body heat. Characteristic of myxoedema*.

hypomotility *n* decreased movement, as of the stomach or intestines.

hyponatraemia *n* decreased sodium in the blood—**hyponatraemic** *adj.*

hypoparathyroidism *n* underaction of the parathyroid* glands with decrease in serum calcium levels, producing tetany*.

hypopharynx *n* that portion of the pharynx* lying below and behind the larynx, more correctly called the laryngopharynx.

hypophoria *n* a state in which the visual axis in one eye is lower than the other.

hypophosphataemia *n* decreased phosphates in the blood—**hypophosphataemic** *adj.*

hypophysectomy *n* surgical removal of the pituitary gland.

hypophysis cerebri *n* ⇒ pituitary gland—**hypophyseal** *adj.*

hypopigmentation *n* decreased or poor pigmentation.

hypopituitarism *n* pituitary* gland insufficiency, especially of the anterior lobe. Absence of gonadotrophins* leads to failure of ovulation, uterine atrophy* and amenorrhoea in women, and loss of libido, pubic and axillary hair in both sexes. Lack of growth hormone in children results in short stature. Lack of corticotrophin (ACTH) and thyrotrophin (TSH) may result in lack of energy, pallor, fine dry skin, cold intolerance and sometimes hypoglycaemia. Usually due to tumour of or involving pituitary gland or hypothalamus but in other cases cause is unknown.

Occasionally due to postpartum infarction of the pituitary gland.

hypoplasia *n* defective development of any tissue—**hypoplastic** *adj*.

hypopotassaemia *n* ⇒ hypokalaemia.

hypoproteinaemia *n* deficient protein in blood plasma, from dietary deficiency or excessive excretion (albuminuria*)—**hypoproteinaemic** *adj*.

hypopyon *n* a collection of pus in the anterior chamber of the eye.

hyposecretion *n* deficient secretion.

hyposensitivity *n* lacking sensitivity to a stimulus.

hyposmia *n* decrease in the normal sensitivity to smell. Has been observed in patients following laryngectomy.

hypospadias *n* a congenital malformation of the male urethra. Subdivided into two types: (a) penile, when the terminal urethral orifice opens at any point along the posterior shaft of the penis (b) perineal, when the orifice opens on the perineum and may give rise to problems of sexual differentiation—**epispadias** *opp*.

hypostasis *n* 1 a sediment. 2 congestion of blood in a part due to impaired circulation—**hypostatic** *adj*.

hypotension *n* low blood pressure (systolic below 110 mmHg, diastolic below 70 mmHg); may be primary, secondary (e.g. caused by bleeding, shock, Addison's disease) or postural. It can be produced by the administration of drugs to reduce bleeding in surgery—**hypotensive** *adj*.

hypothalamus *n* literally, below the thalamus. Situated in the brain, just above the pituitary gland and combines functions of the nervous and endocrine systems. It is the main centre of the autonomic nervous system and controls various physiological functions such as emotion, hunger, thirst and circadian rhythms. Also has an important endocrine function as it produces releasing and some inhibiting hormones that act on the anterior pituitary* and regulate the release of its hormones. Also produces oxytocin* and vasopressin* that are stored and released by the posterior pituitary.

hypothermia *n* a severe fall in body temperature, ascertained by a low-reading thermometer. Can be fatal if untreated. Occurs particularly in the very young and in elderly people. An artificially induced hypothermia (30°C or 86°F) can be used in the treatment of head injuries and in cardiac surgery. It reduces the oxygen consumption of the tissues and thereby allows greater and more prolonged interference of normal blood circulation. *hypothermia of the newborn* failure of the newborn child to adjust to external cold; may be associated with infection. *local hypothermia* has been tried in the treatment of peptic ulcer.

hypothyroidism *n* defines those clinical conditions which result from low circulating levels of one or both thyroid hormones currently classified as: (a) overt, which if present at birth produces a cretin; if it occurs later, it is myxoedema* (b) mild (c) preclinical (d) autoimmune thyroid disease (Hashimoto's* disease).

hypotonic *adj* 1 ⇒ hypoosmolarity. 2 lacking in tone, tension, strength—**hypotonia, hypotonicity** *n*.

hypoventilation *n* diminished breathing or underventilation.

hypovolaemia (*syn* oligaemia) diminished quantity of total blood—**hypovolaemic** *adj*.

hypovolaemic shock shock* syndrome caused by hypovolaemia.

hypoxaemia *n* diminished amount of oxygen in the

arterial blood, shown by decreased arterial oxygen tension and reduced saturation—**hypoxaemic** *adj.*

hypoxia *n* diminished amount of oxygen in the tissues—**hypoxic** *adj. anaemic hypoxia* resulting from a deficiency of haemoglobin or a reduced number of erythrocytes. *histotoxic hypoxia* interference with the cells in their utilization of 0_2, e.g. in cyanide poisioning. *hypoxic hypoxia* interference with pulmonary oxygenation. *stagnant hypoxia* tissue blood volume is normal but blood flow is reduced due to impairment of venous outflow or in some cases reduced arterial flow.

hysterectomy *n* surgical removal of the uterus. *abdominal hysterectomy* effected via a lower abdominal incision. *subtotal hysterectomy* removal of the uterine body, leaving the cervix in the vaginal vault. Rarely performed because of the risk of a carcinoma developing in the cervical stump. *total hysterectomy* complete removal of the uterine body and cervix. *vaginal hysterectomy* carried out through the vagina. *Wertheim's hysterectomy* total removal of the uterus, adjacent lymphatic vessels and glands, with a cuff of the vagina.

hysteria *n* **1** the term previously used for conversion* disorder. **2** a state of tension or excitement in a person or group which results in a temporary loss of control over emotions—**hysterical** *adj.*

hysterosalpingectomy *n* surgical removal of the uterus and of one or both uterine tubes.

hysterosalpingography *n* ⇒ uterosalpingography.

hysterosalpingostomy *n* anastomosis between a uterine tube and the uterus.

hysterotomy *n* incision of the uterus to remove a pregnancy. The word is usually reserved for a method of abortion*.

hysterotrachelorrhaphy *n* repair of a lacerated cervix* uteri.

iatrogenic *adj* describes a secondary condition arising from treatment of a primary condition.

ibuprofen *n* nonnarcotic analgesic. Can be irritant to the gastrointestinal tract.

ICE *abbr* (Ice, Compress, Elevation) a mnemonic used in first aid for the treatment of bruises and swellings on the limbs. An ice compress is placed on the injured part which is then elevated to aid venous return.

ichthyoses *npl* a group of congenital conditions in which the skin is dry and scaly. Fish skin. Xeroderma. *ichthyosis hystrix* is a form of congenital naevus with patches of warty excrescences.

ICN *abbr* **1** International* Council of Nurses. **2** Infection* Control Nurse.

ICP *abbr* intracranial* pressure.

ICSH *abbr* interstitial*-cell stimulating hormone.

ICSI *abbr* intracytoplasmic* sperm injection.

icterus *n* ⇒ jaundice. *icterus gravis* acute diffuse necrosis of the liver. *icterus gravis neonatorum* one of the clinical forms of haemolytic* disease of the newborn. *icterus neonatorum* excess of the normal, or physiological, jaundice occurring in the first week of life as a result of excessive destruction of haemoglobin ⇒ phototherapy. *icterus index* measurement of concentration of bilirubin in the plasma. Used in diagnosis of jaundice.

id *n* that part of the unconscious mind which consists of a system of primitive urges (instincts) and, according to Freud, persists unrecognized into adult life.

IDDM *abbr* insulin dependent diabetes* mellitus.

ideation *n* the process concerned with the highest function of awareness, the formation of ideas. It includes thought, intellect and memory.

identical twins two offspring of the same sex, derived from a single fertilized ovum.

identification *n* recognition. In psychology, the way in which we form our personality by modelling it on a chosen person, e.g. identification with the parent of same sex helping to form one's sex role; identification with a person of own sex in the hero-worship of adolescence.

ideomotor *n* mental energy, in the form of ideas, producing automatic movement of muscles, e.g. mental agitation producing agitated movements of limbs.

idiopathic *adj* of a condition, of unknown or spontaneous origin, e.g. some forms of epilepsy. *idiopathic respiratory distress syndrome* ⇒ respiratory.

idiosyncrasy *n* **1** a peculiar variation of constitution or temperament. **2** unusual individual response to certain drugs, proteins, etc. whether by injection, ingestion, inhalation or contact.

idioventricular *adj* pertaining to the cardiac ventricles* and not affecting the atria.

Ig *abbr* ⇒ immunoglobulins.

IHD *abbr* ⇒ ischaemic heart disease.

ileal bladder ⇒ ileoureterostomy.

ileal conduit ⇒ ileoureterostomy.

ileitis *n* inflammation of the ileum*.

ileocaecal *adj* pertaining to the ileum and the caecum.

ileocolic *adj* pertaining to the ileum and the colon.

ileocolitis *n* inflammation of the ileum and the colon.

ileocolostomy *n* a surgically made fistula between the ileum and the colon, usually the transverse colon. Most often used to bypass an obstruction or inflammation in the caecum or ascending colon.

ileoproctostomy *n* an anastomosis between the ileum and rectum; used when disease extends to the sigmoid colon.

ileorectal *adj* pertaining to the ileum and the rectum.

ileosigmoidostomy *n* an anastomosis between the ileum and sigmoid colon; used where most of the colon has to be removed.

ileostomy *n* a surgically made fistula between the ileum and the anterior abdominal wall; usually a permanent form of artificial anus when the whole of the large bowel has to be removed, e.g. in severe ulcerative colitis. *ileostomy bags* rubber or plastic bags used to collect the liquid discharge from an ileostomy.

ileoureterostomy *n* (*syn* uretero-ileostomy) transplantation of the lower ends of the ureters from the bladder to an isolated loop of small bowel (ileal bladder) which, in turn, is made to open on the abdominal wall (ileal conduit).

ileum *n* the lower three-fifths of the small intestine, lying between the jejunum* and the caecum*—**ileal** *adj.*

ileus *n* intestinal obstruction. Usually restricted to paralytic as opposed to mechanical obstruction and characterized by abdominal distension, vomiting and the absence of pain⇒ meconium.

iliococcygeal *adj* pertaining to the ilium and coccyx.

iliofemoral *adj* pertaining to the ilium and the femur.

iliopectineal *adj* pertaining to the ilium and the pubis.

iliopsoas *adj* pertaining to the ilium and the loin*.

ilium *n* the upper part of the innominate (hip) bone; it is a separate bone in the fetus—**iliac** *adj.*

ill health, prevention of *primary prevention* involves taking measures which prevent disease or injury. *secondary prevention* refers to health care measures which are concerned with identifying and treating ill health; accomplished by screening programmes. *tertiary prevention* is concerned with mitigating the effects of illness and disease which have already occurred.

illusion *n* a misidentification of a sensation, e.g. of sight, a white sheet being mistaken for a ghost, the sheet being misrepresented in consciousness as a figure.

image *n* a revived experience of a percept recalled from memory (smell and taste).

imagery *n* imagination. The recall of mental images of various types depending upon the special sense organs involved when the images were formed, e.g. *auditory imagery* sound. *motor imagery* movement. *visual imagery* sight. *tactile imagery* touch. *olfactory imagery* smell. The technique of *guided imagery,* in which the patient is asked to imagine a particular situation or state, can induce a prehypnotic state and can be used by the nurse, e.g. to lessen the pain of a particular procedure.

imbalance *n* lack of balance. Term refers commonly to the upset of acid-base* relationship and the electrolytes* in body fluids. ⇒

drop attacks, Menière's disease, vertigo.

immersion foot ⇒ trench foot.

immune *adj* possessing the capacity to resist infection. *immune body* immunoglobulin*.

immune reaction, response that which causes a body to reject a transplanted organ, to respond to bacterial disease which develops slowly, and to act against malignant cells; cell mediated immunity*.

immunity *n* an intrinsic or acquired state of resistance to an infectious agent. *active immunity* is acquired, naturally during an infection or artificially by immunization*. *cell mediated immunity* T lymphocyte-dependent responses which cause graft rejection, immunity to some infectious agents and tumour rejection. *humoral immunity* from immunoglobulin produced by B-lymphocytes. Immunity can be innate (from inherited qualities), or it can be acquired, actively or passively, naturally or artificially. *passive immunity* is acquired, naturally when maternal antibody passes to the child via the placenta or in the milk, or artificially by administering sera containing antibodies from animals or human beings.

immunization *n* the administration of antigens to induce immunity*. Countries have different immunization programmes. In the UK, children are offered the triple vaccine against diphtheria, tetanus and pertussis at 2, 3 and 4 months, along with vaccination against poliomyelitis and Hib, one of the causative organisms of meningitis. Booster doses are offered usually preschool and in the early teens. A single, triple vaccine against measles, mumps and rubella is offered at around 12 months.

immunocompetent *adj* having the normal bodily capacity to develop an immune response following exposure to an antigen.

immunocompromized patients (*syn* immunosuppressed patients) patients with defective immune responses, often produced by treatment with drugs or irradiation or by AIDS. Also occurs in some patients with cancer and other diseases affecting the lymphoid system. Patients are liable to develop infections with opportunistic organisms such as *Candida, Pneumocystis carinii* and *Cryptococcus neoformans.*

immunodeficiency *n* the state of having defective immune responses, leading to increased susceptibility to infectious diseases.

immunodeficiency diseases inherited or acquired disorders of the immune system.

immunogenesis *n* the process of production of immunity*—**immunogenetic** *adj.*

immunogenetics *n* **1** the study of the interrelationship between immunity to disease and genetic makeup. **2** the branch of immunology that deals with the molecular and genetic bases of the immune response.

immunogenicity *n* the ability to produce immunity*—**immunogenic** *adj.*

immunoglobulins (Igs) *n* (*syn* antibodies) high molecular weight proteins produced by B lymphocytes which can combine with antigens such as bacteria and produce immunity or interfere with membrane signals to produce autoimmune disease, e.g. thyrotoxicosis. There are five classes of immunoglobulins—IgG, IgA, IgD, IgM and IgE—each with different characteristics and functions.

immunological response ⇒ immunity.

immunology *n* the study of the immune system of lymphocytes, inflammatory cells and associated cells and proteins, which affect an individual's response to antigens—**immunological** *adj,* **immunologically** *adv.*

immunopathology *n* the study of tissue injury involving the immune system.

immunosuppressed patients ⇒ immunocompromised patients.

immunosuppression *n* treatment which reduces immunological responsiveness.

immunosuppressive *n* that which reduces immunological responsiveness.

impacted *adj* firmly wedged, abnormal immobility, as of faeces in the rectum; fracture; a fetus in the pelvis; a tooth in its socket or a calculus in a duct. ⇒ faecal impaction, fracture.

impairment *n* loss or lack of part (e.g. a limb) or physiological function (e.g. hearing, walking).

impalpable *adj* not palpable; incapable of being felt by touch (palpation).

imperforate *adj* lacking a normal opening. *imperforate anus* a congenital absence of an opening into the rectum. *imperforate hymen* a fold of mucous membrane at the vaginal entrance which has no natural outlet for the menstrual fluid. ⇒ haematocolpos.

impetigo *n* an inflammatory, pustular skin disease usually caused by *Staphylococcus,* occasionally by *Streptococcus. impetigo contagiosa* a highly contagious form of impetigo, commonest on the face and scalp, characterized by vesicles which become pustules and then honey-coloured crusts. ⇒ ecthyma.

implantation *n* the insertion of living cells or solid materials into the tissues, e.g. accidental implantation of tumour cells in a wound; implantation of radium or solid drugs; implantation of the fertilized ovum into the endometrium.

implants *npl* tissues or drugs inserted surgically into the human body, e.g. implantation of pellets of testosterone under the skin in treatment of carcinoma of the breast, implants of deoxycortone acetate in Addison's disease, silastic implants in plastic surgery.

implementing *v* the third phase of the nursing process, when planned interventions to achieve the set goals are implemented and recorded on the patient's nursing notes, which provide cumulative information on the date set for evaluating*.

impotence *n* inability to participate in sexual intercourse, by custom referring to the male. It can be due to lack of erection or premature ejaculation.

impregnate *vt* fill; saturate; render pregnant.

impulse *n* **1** a sudden inclination, sometimes irresistible urge to act without deliberation. **2** the electrochemical process involved in neurotransmission of information and stimuli throughout the body.

impulsive action ⇒ action.

inaccessibility *n* in psychiatry, absence of patient response.

incarcerated *adj* describes the abnormal imprisonment of a part, as in a hernia which is irreducible or a pregnant uterus held beneath the sacral promontory.

incest *n* sexual intercourse between close blood relatives. The most common type of sexual abuse occurs between father and daughter; other types between mother and son and between siblings are known to occur. ⇒ child abuse.

incipient *adj* initial, beginning, in its early stages.

incision *n* the result of cutting into body tissue, using a sharp instrument—**incisional** *adj,* **incise** *vt.*

incisors *npl* the teeth first and second from the midline, four in each jaw used for cutting food.

inclusion bodies round, oval or irregularly shaped bodies found in the cytoplasm and nuclei of cells affected by viral infections such as smallpox or rabies.

incompatibility *n* usually refers to the bloods of donor and recipient in transfusion, when antigenic differences in the red cells result in reactions such as haemolysis or agglutination. When two or more medications are given concurrently or consecutively they can attenuate or counteract the desired effect of each.

incompetence *n* inadequacy to perform a natural function, e.g. mitral incompetence—**incompetent** *adj*.

incomplete abortion ⇒ abortion.

incomplete fracture ⇒ fracture.

incontinence *n* inability to control the evacuation of urine or faeces. Nursing aims include assessment of the pattern of incontinence so that appropriate nursing interventions can be planned. These may include treatment of urinary tract infections, habit training for continence, condom drainage for male patients, teaching and supervizing self-catheterization, preventing nosocomial infection, managing untreatable incontinence by using protective clothing and bedding, or using a self-retaining catheter and a closed urinary drainage system. *genuine stress incontinence* occurs when the intraabdominal pressure is raised as in coughing, giggling and sneezing; there is usually some weakness of the urethral sphincter muscle coupled with anatomical stretching and displacement of the bladder neck.*giggle incontinence* leakage of urine on laughing. Usually a problem with girls and is caused by a mixture of stress incontinence and detrusor* instability. *overflow incontinence* dribbling of urine from an overfull bladder. *urge incontinence* involuntary leakage of urine on the way to the toilet.

incoordination *n* inability to produce smooth, harmonious muscular movements.

incubation *n* **1** the period from entry of infection to the appearance of the first symptom. **2** the process of development, of an egg or of a bacterial culture, by means of artificial heat.

incubator *n* **1** apparatus used to provide a controlled environment. Facilitates observation and nursing of premature or sick babies. **2** a low-temperature oven in which bacteria are cultured.

incus *n* the anvil-shaped bone of the middle ear.

independent component of nursing assessing, planning, setting goals and evaluating in relation to problems which the patient is experiencing in everyday living activities which are amenable to nursing intervention: they may or may not be the product of the medical diagnosis.

indicanuria *n* excessive potassium salt in the urine. There are traces in normal urine; high levels are suggestive of intestinal obstruction ⇒ indole.

indicator *n* a substance which, when added in small quantities, is used to make visible the completion of a chemical reaction or the attainment of a certain pH.

indigenous *adj* of a disease etc., native to a certain locality or country, e.g. Derbyshire neck (simple colloidal goitre).

indigestion *n* (*syn* dyspepsia) a feeling of gastric discomfort, including fullness and gaseous distension, which is not necessarily a manifestation of disease.

indigocarmine *n* a dye used as an 0.4% solution for testing renal function. Given by intravenous or intramuscular injection. The urine is coloured blue in about 10 min if kidney function is normal.

individualized nursing nursing care that is planned and implemented according to an assessment of the patient's individual needs and agreed goals. Wherever possible, the patient is involved in care planning.

indole *n* a product of the decomposition of tryptophan* in the intestines: it is oxidized to indoxyl in the liver and excreted in urine as indican ⇒ indicanuria.

indolent *adj* a term applied to a sluggish ulcer which is generally painless and slow to heal.

indomethacin *n* a prostaglandin inhibitor with analgesic with antiinflammatory properties. Useful in the rheumatic disorders. Can be given orally but, to prevent nausea, capsules should be taken with a meal or a glass of milk. Also available as suppositories.

induction *n* the act of bringing on or causing to occur, as applied to anaesthesia and labour.

induration *n* the hardening of tissue, as in hyperaemia, infiltration by neoplasm, etc.—**indurated** *adj.*

industrial dermatitis ⇒ dermatitis.

industrial disease (*syn* occupational disease) a disease contracted by reason of occupational exposure to an industrial agent known to be hazardous, e.g. dust, fumes, chemicals, irradiation, etc., the notification of, safety precautions against and compensation for which are controlled by law.

industrial therapy current organization of simulated outside industrial working conditions within a unit in a psychiatric hospital. The main purpose is preparation of patients for their return to the working community.

inertia *n* inactivity. *uterine inertia* lack of contraction of parturient uterus. It may be primary due to constitutional weakness; secondary due to exhaustion from frequent and forcible contractions.

inevitable abortion ⇒ abortion.

in extremis at the point of death.

infant *n* a baby or a child of less than 1 year old.

infantile paralysis ⇒ poliomyelitis.

infantilism *n* general retardation of development with persistence of child-like characteristics into adolescence and adult life.

infarct *n* area of tissue affected when the end artery supplying it is occluded, e.g. in kidney or heart. Common complication of subacute endocarditis.

infarction *n* death of a section of tissue because the blood supply has been cut off. ⇒ myocardial infarction.

infection *n* the successful invasion, establishment and growth of microorganisms in the tissues of the host. It may be of an acute or chronic nature—**infectious** *adj. cross infection* occurs when pathogens are transferred from one person to another, or from animal to person. *endogenous infection* one caused by organisms originating from the patient's own body, resulting in disease at another site. *hospital-acquired (nosocomial) infection (HAI)* one which occurs in a patient who has been in hospital for more than 48 h and who did not have signs and symptoms of such infection on admission: approximately 10% of hospital patients develop a hospital-acquired infection. Urinary tract, respiratory, wound and skin infections are the most common types.

opportunistic infection an infection with a microorganism which normally has little or no pathogenic activity but which becomes pathogenic when the host's resistance is lowered, e.g. through disease, invasive treatments or drugs. ⇒ handwashing.

Infection Control Committee (ICC) a multidisciplinary committee which may consist of a medical microbiologist, an infection control nurse, a representative from each of the areas in which patients are nursed; a representative for domestic and portering staff, kitchen and meal serving staff. The committee formulates procedures to be carried out throughout the district to prevent hospital or community acquired infection.

Infection Control Nurse (ICN) a nurse who uses specialised knowledge and skills to encourage nurses in the clinical areas to carry out efficiently the policy of the Infection Control Committee. The pattern of incidents of nosocomial* infection is studied, and if it clusters in a particular ward, or in a particular group of patients, e.g. those whose operation was performed in a particular theatre, further investigation is carried out to identify the source of infection. Many countries have a special association to which ICNs belong and they have an international association.

infection, prevention of an essential element of nursing. It includes all activities which achieve social* cleanliness of articles which come into contact with patients; personal* hygiene of patients and staff; as well as aseptic* techniques. ⇒ closed urinary drainage, disinfection, handwashing, infection, infection control committee, infection control nurse, perineal toilet.

infectious disease a disease caused by a specific, pathogenic organism and capable of being transmitted to another individual by direct or indirect contact.

infectious mononucleosis (*syn* glandular fever) a contagious self-limiting disease caused by the Epstein-Barr virus. Characterized by fever, sore throat, enlargement of superficial lymph nodes and appearance of atypical lymphocytes resembling monocytes. Specific antibodies to Epstein-Barr virus are present in the blood as well as an abnormal antibody which has 'heterophile' activity directed against sheep's red blood cells–the basis of the Paul*-Bunnell test which is positive in infectious mononucleosis. One attack confers complete immunity and also lifelong harbouring of virus particles in the lymphocytes and in the saliva, hence the synonym 'kissing disease'.

infective *adj* infectious. Disease transmissible from one host to another. *infective hepatitis* ⇒ hepatitis.

inferior *adj* lower; beneath.

infertility *n* lack of ability to reproduce. Psychological and physical causes play their part. The abnormality can be in either or both parties. Special clinics exist to investigate this condition.

infestation *n* the presence of animal parasites in or on the human body–**infest** *vt*.

infibulation *n* ⇒ circumcision.

infiltration *n* penetration of the surrounding tissues; the oozing or leaking of fluid into the tissues. *infiltration anaesthesia* analgesia produced by infiltrating the tissues with a local anaesthetic.

inflammation *n* the reaction of living tissues to injury, infection, or irritation; characterized by pain, swelling, redness and heat. The degree of redness can be measured by a tintometer*—**inflammatory** *adj*.

influenza *n* an acute viral infection of the nasopharynx and respiratory tract which occurs in epidemic or pandemic form—**influenzal** *adj*.

informed choice the means by which patients/clients can make decisions about their own care and management. Nurses and other health care professionals provide accurate, appropriate information about the person's condition, and about the treatment options available, and on this the client decides how to proceed. Professionals may not always agree with the client's decisions, but the latter should take precedence.

informed consent in the UK the Medical Defence Union recommends consent forms which include a signed declaration by the doctor that he has explained the nature and purpose of the operation to the patient in non-technical terms. Some forms contain a clause 'and any other procedures which may become necessary during the operation'. A patient can be distressed to find that a mastectomy or colostomy has been 'considered necessary'. Should a patient, after signing the form, ask the nurse about the operation, the question should be referred back to the doctor.

infra-red rays long wavelength, invisible rays of the electromagnetic spectrum.

infundibulum *n* any funnel-shaped passage—**infundibula** *pl*, **infundibular** *adj*.

infusion *n* **1** fluid flowing by gravity into the body. **2** an aqueous solution containing the active principle of a drug, made by pouring boiling water on the crude drug. **3** amniotic* fluid infusion.

ingestion *n* **1** the act of taking food or medicine into the stomach. **2** the means by which a phagocytic cell takes in surrounding solid material such as microorganisms.

Ingram regime a treatment for psoriasis using dithranol paste, tar baths and ultraviolet light.

ingrowing toenail spreading of the nail into the lateral tissue, causing inflammation.

inguinal *adj* pertaining to the groin. *inguinal canal* a tubular opening through the lower part of the anterior abdominal wall, parallel to and a little above the inguinal (Poupart's) ligament. In the male it contains spermatic cord; in the female the uterine round ligaments. *inguinal hernia* ⇒ hernia.

inhalation *n* a medicinal substance which is inhaled.

inherent *adj* innate; inborn.

inhibition *n* the process of restraining one's impulses or behaviour as a result of conscious or unconscious influences.

injection *n* **1** the act of introducing a fluid (under pressure) into the tissues, a vessel, cavity or hollow organ. **2** the substance injected.

innate *adj* inborn, dependent on genetic constitution.

innervation *n* the nerve supply to a part.

innocent *adj* benign; not malignant.

innocuous *adj* harmless.

innominate *adj* unnamed ⇒ hip bone.

inoculation *n* **1** the injection of substances, especially vaccine, into the body. **2** introduction of microorganisms into culture medium for propagation. *accidental inoculation* a term pertaining to staff, it includes contamination of an abrasion or burn, heavy soiling of skin with blood or body fluid, or spillage into the eyes or mouth, as well as needlestick* injury.

inorganic *adj* neither animal nor vegetable in origin.

inotropic *adj* affecting the force of muscle contraction, applied particularly to cardiac muscle. An inotrope is a drug which increases the contractile force of the heart.

inquest *n* in England and Wales, a legal enquiry, held by a coroner into the cause of sudden or unexpected death.

insecticide *n* an agent which kills insects—**insecticidal** *adj*.

insemination *n* introduction of semen into the vagina, normally by sexual intercourse. *artificial insemination* instrumental injection of semen into the vagina ⇒ AID, AIH, DI.

insensible *adj* without sensation or consciousness. Too small or gradual to be perceived, as insensible perspiration.

insertion *n* **1** the act of setting or placing in. **2** the attachment of a muscle to the bone it moves.

insidious *adj* having an imperceptible commencement, as of a disease with a late manifestation of definite symptoms.

insight *n* ability to accept one's limitations but at the same time to develop one's potentialities. Also: (a) knowing that one is ill (b) a developing knowledge of one's present attitudes and past experiences and the connection between them.

in situ in the correct position, undisturbed. Also describes a cancer which has not invaded adjoining tissue.

insomnia *n* sleeplessness.

inspiration *n* the drawing of air into the lungs; inhalation—**inspiratory** *adj*, **inspire** *vt*.

inspissated *adj* thickened, as by evaporation or withdrawal of water, applied to sputum and culture media used in the laboratory.

instep *n* the arch of the foot on the dorsal surface.

instillation *n* insertion of drops into a cavity, e.g. conjunctival sac, external auditory meatus.

instinct *n* an inborn tendency to act in a certain way in a given situation, e.g. *paternal, maternal instinct* to protect children—**instinctive** *adj*, **instinctively** *adv*.

institutionalization *n* a condition of apathy resulting from lack of motivation characterizing people living (or working) in institutions who have been subjected to a rigid routine with deprivation of decision-making.

insufflation *n* the blowing of air along a tube (eustachian, uterine) to establish patency. The blowing of powder into a body cavity.

insulin *n* a pancreatic hormone produced by the beta cells in the islets of Langerhans. Its secretion is regulated by the level of glucose in the bloodstream, i.e. a negative feedback mechanism. Its action is opposite to that of glucagon* produced in the alpha cells and it has an effect on the metabolism of carbohydrate, protein and fat by stimulating the transport of glucose into cells. An absolute or relative lack of insulin results in hyperglycaemia, a high blood glucose with decreased utilization of carbohydrate and increased breakdown of fat and protein. This condition is known as diabetes mellitus. Three types of insulin are produced: from the pancreas of cows (bovine), from pigs (porcine), and human insulin, produced using genetic engineering techniques. Clear insulins have a shorter span of action (8–10 hours) than the cloudy insulins, which have an intermediate or longer activity span (12–24 hours). Mixtures of clear and cloudy insulins in varying proportions are also available. Insulin is produced in U100 strength, i.e. 100 units per ml, a standardization replacing the previous 20, 40 and 80 unit strengths. The most common method of administration is by subcutaneous injection using disposable plastic syringes. Preloaded pen devices are also popular, containing cartridges of insulin and allowing the dose to be dialled in 1 or 2 unit increments. Click count and preset syringes are also available for those having difficulty in drawing up the correct dosage, e.g. due to poor eyesight. Common injection sites are abdomen, buttocks, thigh, arm and sometimes calves. Rotation of sites is advised to prevent lipoatrophy or lipohypertrophy, i.e. hollows or swelling of fatty tissue. Subcutaneous injection of insulin using a syringe drive or infusion pump may have a limited use in some patients. Insulin may also be administered intravenously, e.g. prior to surgery or during an acute ketoacidotic episode. Diluted soluble insulin is given via an infusion pump, the amount being dictated by blood glucose levels. An excess of insulin administration may lead to hypoglycaemia, i.e. a low blood glucose. ⇒ insulin dependent diabetes mellitus (IDDM).

insulinoma *n* adenoma of the islets of Langerhans in the pancreas.

intake and output a crude measure of a person's fluid balance. The amount of fluid taken orally, intravenously, by nasogastric tube or gastrostomy is recorded on a special chart. All urine excreted is measured and recorded: most charts advise how much has to be added for estimated loss by perspiration, respiration and defaecation. The amount of intake and output is usually totalled each 24 h.

integument *n* a covering, especially the skin.

intellect *n* reasoning power, thinking faculty.

intelligence *n* inborn mental ability. *intelligence tests* designed to determine the level of intelligence. *intelligence quotient (IQ)* the ratio of mental age to chronological (actual) age.

intensive therapy unit (ITU) a unit in which highly specialized monitoring, resuscitation and therapeutic techniques are used.

intention tremor ⇒ tremor.

interaction *n* when two or more things or people have a reciprocal influence on each other ⇒ care, drug interaction.

interarticular *adj* between joints.

interatrial *adj* between the two atria of the heart.

intercellular *adj* between cells.

intercostal *adj* between the ribs.

intercourse *n* 1 human communication. 2 coitus*.

intercurrent *adj* describes a second disease arising in a person already suffering from one disease.

interferon *n* a protein effective against some viruses. When a virus infects a cell, it triggers off the cell's production of interferon. This then interacts with surrounding cells and renders them resistant to virus attack. Interferon has caused regression of tumour in some cases of multiple myelomatosis. Two human types are available, one prepared from cultured leucocytes and the other prepared from cultured fibroblasts.

interlobar *adj* between the lobes, e.g. interlobar pleurisy.

interlobular *adj* between the lobules.

intermenstrual *adj* between the menstrual periods.

intermittent *adj* occurring at intervals. *intermittent claudication* ⇒ claudication. *intermittent peritoneal dialysis* ⇒ dialysis.

intermittent pneumatic compression (IPC) a stocking worn to prevent deep vein thrombosis of upper and lower limb.⇒ phlebothrombosis. *intermittent positive pressure* ⇒ positive pressure ventilation. *intermittent self-catheterization* ⇒ self-catheterization.

intermittent positive pressure ventilation (IPPV) mechanically applied ventilation of the lungs for controlled ventilation as part of general anaesthesia or intensive care. Respiratory rate and tidal volume are preset, with no patient effort required, though modern ventilators may allow patient-initiated breaths.

internal *adj* inside. *internal ear* that part of the ear which comprises the vestibule, semicircular canals and the cochlea. *internal respiration* ⇒ respiration. *internal secretions* those produced by the ductless or endocrine glands and passed directly into the blood stream; hormones. *internal version* ⇒ version.

International Council of Nurses (ICN) at international level the ICN, founded in 1899, represents worldwide national nurses' associations. The headquarters are in Geneva and among its many duties it organizes a quadrennial congress (each in a different country) which is open to nurses throughout the world.

interosseous *adj* between bones.

interphalangeal *adj* between the phalanges*.

interserosal *adj* between serous membrane, as in the pleural peritoneal and pericardial cavities—**interserosally** *adv.*

intersexuality *n* the possession of both male and female characteristics ⇒ Turner syndrome, Klinefelter syndrome.

interspinous *adj* between spinous processes, especially those of the vertebrae.

interstices *npl* spaces.

interstitial *adj* situated in the interstices of a part; distributed through the connective structures. *interstitial-cell stimulating hormone (ICSH)* a hormone released from the anterior lobe of the pituitary gland; causes production of testosterone* in the male.

intertrigo *n* superficial inflammation occurring in moist skin folds—**intertrigenous** *adj.*

intertrochanteric *adj* between trochanters*, usually referring to those on the proximal femur.

interventricular *adj* between ventricles, as those of the brain or heart.

intervertebral *adj* between the vertebrae, as discs and foramina. ⇒ nucleus, prolapse.

interviewing *v* one of the methods used to collect data at the initial assessment. Prompting and reflecting techniques may be required to help the patient give the necessary information.

intestine *n* a part of the alimentary canal extending from the stomach to the anus. It comprises the small intestine and the large intestine.—**intestinal** *adj.*

intima *n* the internal coat of a blood vessel—**intimal** *adj.*

intolerance *n* the manifestation of various unusual reactions to particular substances such as nutrients or medications.

intraamniotic *adj* within, or into the amniotic fluid.

intraarticular *adj* within a joint.

intrabronchial *adj* within a bronchus.

intracanalicular *adj* within a canaliculus*.

intracapillary *adj* within a capillary.

intracapsular *adj* within a capsule, e.g. that of the lens or a joint ⇒ extracapsular *opp.*

intracardiac *adj* within the heart.

intracaval *adj* within the vena cava, by custom referring to the inferior vena cava—**intracavally** *adv.*

intracellular *adj* within cells ⇒ extracellular *opp.*

intracerebral *adj* within the cerebrum.

intracranial *adj* within the skull.

intracranial pressure (ICP) maintained at a normal level by brain tissue, intracellular and extracellular fluid, cerebrospinal* fluid and blood. A change in any of these compartments can increase the pressure.

intracutaneous *adj* within the skin tissues—**intracutanoously** *adv.*

intracytoplasmic sperm injection (ICSI) the direct insertion in vitro of a chosen sperm into the female gamete. Fertilized ova are then placed in the uterus as preembryos.

intradermal *adj* within the skin—**intradermally** *adv.*

intradural *adj* inside the dura mater.

intragastric *adj* within the stomach.

intragluteal *adj* within the gluteal muscle comprising the buttock—**intragluteally** *adv.*

intrahepatic *adj* within the liver.

intralobular *adj* within the lobule, as the vein draining a hepatic lobule.

intraluminal *adj* within the hollow of a tube-like structure—**intraluminally** *adv.*

intralymphatic *adj* within a lymphatic gland or vessel.

intramedullary *adj* within the bone marrow.

intramural *adj* within the layers of the wall of a hollow tube or organ—**intramurally** *adv.*

intramuscular *adj* within a muscle—**intramuscularly** *adv.*

intranasal *adj* within the nasal cavity.

intranatal *adj* ⇒ intrapartum—**intranatally** *adv.*

intraocular *adj* within the globe of the eye. *intraocular lens (IOL)* artificial lens placed inside the eye to provide correction of vision following cataract surgery.

intraoral *adj* within the mouth, as an intraoral appliance.

intraorbital *adj* within the orbit.

intraosseous *adj* inside a bone.

intrapartum *adj* (*syn* intranatal) at the time of birth; during labour, as asphyxia, haemorrhage or infection.

intraperitoneal *adj* within the peritoneal cavity.

intrapharyngeal *adj* within the pharynx.

intrapleural *adj* within the pleural cavity.

intrapulmonary *adj* within the lungs, as intrapulmonary pressure.

intrapunitive *adj* a tendency to blame oneself.

intraretinal *adj* within the retina.

intraspinal *adj* within the spinal canal.

intrasplenic *adj* within the spleen.

intrasynovial *adj* within a synovial membrane or cavity.

intrathecal *adj* within the meninges; into the subarachnoid space.

intrathoracic *adj* within the cavity of the thorax.

intratracheal *adj* within the trachea.

intrauterine *adj* within the uterus. *intrauterine contraceptive device (IUCD, IUD)* a device which is implanted in the cavity of the uterus to prevent conception. Its exact mode of action is not known. *intrauterine growth retardation (IUGR)* associated with a poor delivery of maternal blood to the placental bed, diminished placental exchange or a poor fetal transfer from the placental area. Serial ultrasonography has been shown to be beneficial in high-risk pregnancies to measure fetal growth and wellbeing. *intrauterine insemination (IUI)* prepared, fresh semen sample is inserted into the uterus via the cervix, ovulation having usually already been induced using hormone injections and under ultrasound supervision. Fertilization should take place naturally in the uterine tubes.

intravaginal *adj* within the vagina—**intravaginally** *adv.*

intravascular *adj* within the blood vessels—**intravascularly** *adv.*

intravenous *adj* within or into a vein. *intravenous feeding* ⇒ parenteral. *intravenous infusion* commonly referred to as a 'drip': the closed administration of fluids from a containing vessel into a vein for such purposes as hydrating the body, correcting electrolyte imbalance or introducing nutrients. *intravenous injection* the introduction of drugs, including anaesthetics, into a vein. It is not a continuous procedure. ⇒ eutetic mixture of local anaesthetics (EMLA), venepuncture. *intravenous pyelogram* ⇒ urography.

intraventricular *adj* within a ventricle, especially a cerebral ventricle.

intrinsic *adj* inherent or inside; from within; real; natural. *intrinsic factor* a protein released by gastric glands, essential for the satisfactory absorption of the extrinsic factor vitamin B_{12}.

introitus *n* any opening in the body; an entrance to a cavity, particularly the vagina.

introjection *n* a mental process whereby a person incorporates another person's or group's standards and values into his own personality.

introspection *n* study by a person of his own mental processes. Seen in an exaggerated form in schizophrenia*.

introversion *n* the direction of thoughts and interest inwards to the world of ideas, instead of outwards to the external world.

introvert *n* an individual whose characteristic interests and modes of behaviour are directed inwards towards the self. ⇒ extrovert *opp.*

intubation *n* insertion of a tube into a hollow organ. Tracheal intubation is used during anaesthesia to maintain an airway and to permit suction of the respiratory tract. *duodenal intubation* a double tube is passed as far as the pyloric antrum under fluoroscopy. The inner tube is then passed along to the duodenojejunal flexure. Barium sulphate suspension can then be passed to outline the small bowel. ⇒ extubation *opp.*

intussusception *n* a condition in which one part of the bowel telescopes into the adjoining distal bowel, causing severe colic and intestinal obstruction. It occurs most commonly in infants around the time of weaning, presenting as an acute emergency requiring surgical treatment.

intussusceptum *n* the invaginated portion of an intussusception.

inunction *n* the act of rubbing an oily or fatty substance into the skin.

invagination *n* the act or condition of being ensheathed; a pushing inward, forming a pouch—**invaginate** *vt.*

invasion *n* the entry of bacteria into the body.

inversion turning inside out, as inversion of the uterus. ⇒ procidentia.

invertase *n* (*syn* β-fructofuranosidase) a sugar-splitting enzyme in intestinal juice.

investigations *npl* procedures which are done either to establish diagnosis or to monitor the course of a disease or its treatment. They are classified as invasive, e.g. a barium enema, or noninvasive, for instance taking the blood pressure. They all have potential for increasing patient anxiety and research has shown that well-informed patients are less anxious.

in vitro in glass, as in a test tube. *in vitro fertilization (IVF)* a method of fertilizing human ova and spermatozoa under specialized laboratory conditions, outside the body. The resulting embryo(s) are implanted in the uterus for a potentially normal gestation.

in vivo in living tissue.

involucrum *n* a sheath of new bone, which forms around necrosed bone, in such conditions as osteomyelitis. ⇒ cloaca.

involuntary *adj* independent of the will, as muscle of the thoracic and abdominal organs.

involution *n* **1** the normal shrinkage of an organ after fulfilling its functional purpose, e.g. uterus after labour. **2** in psychiatry, the period of decline after middle life. ⇒ subinvolution—**involutional** *adj*.

iodides *npl* compounds of iodine and a base. Potassium* iodide and sodium* iodide are the most common medicinal iodides.

iodine *n* powerful bactericide used as a tincture for skin preparation and emergency treatment of small wounds. Orally it is antithyroid, i.e. it decreases release of the hormones from the thyroid gland. *povidone iodine* ⇒ povidone. *radioactive iodine* ⇒ radioactive.

iodism *n* poisoning by iodine* or iodides*; the symptoms are those of a common cold and the appearance of a rash.

iodopsin *n* a protein substance which, within vitamin A, is a constituent of visual purple present in the rods in the retina of the eye.

ion *n* a charged atom or radical. In electrolysis, ions in solution pass to one or the other pole, or electrode—**ionic** *adj*.

ionization *n* **1** the dissociation of a substance in solution into ions. **2** iontophoresis*.

ionizing radiation a form of radiation which destabilizes an atom, forming an ion. X-rays, gamma rays and particle radiation are all examples of ionizing radiation.

iontophoresis *n* (*syn* iontherapy) treatment whereby ions of various soluble salts (e.g. zinc, chlorine, iodine, histamine) are introduced into the tissues by means of a constant electrical current; a form of electroosmosis.

IPD *abbr* intermittent peritoneal dialysis*.

ipecacuanha *n* dried root from Brazil and other South American countries. Has expectorant properties and is widely used in acute bronchitis and relief of dry cough. A safe emetic in larger doses.

IPP *abbr* intermittent positive pressure. ⇒ positive pressure ventilation.

IPPV *abbr* ⇒ intermittent positive pressure ventilation.

ipsilateral *adj* on the same side—**ipsilaterally** *adv*.

IQ *abbr* intelligence* quotient.

iridectomy *n* excision of a part of the iris, thus forming an artificial pupil to improve drainage of aqueous* humor.

iridencleisis *n* an older type of filtering operation. Scleral incision made at angle of anterior chamber; meridian cut in iris; either one or both pillars are left in scleral wound to contract as scar tissue. Decreases intraocular tension in glaucoma*.

iridium *n* (Iridium 192) a radioactive metal used in brachytherapy* to treat tumours in anus, tongue, breast as implanted wires or hair pins.

iridocele *n* (*syn* iridoptosis) protrusion of part of the iris through a corneal wound (prolapsed iris).

iridocyclitis *n* inflammation of the iris* and ciliary* body.

iridodialysis *n* a separation of the iris from its ciliary attachment.

iridoplegia *n* paralysis of the iris.

iridotomy *n* an incision into the iris.

iris *n* the circular coloured membrane forming the anterior one-sixth of the middle coat of the eyeball. It is perforated in the centre by an opening, the pupil. Contraction of its muscle fibres regulates the amount of light entering the eye. *iris bombe* bulging forward of the iris due to pressure of the aqueous* behind, when posterior synechiae are present around the pupil.

iritis *n* inflammation of the iris.

irradiation *n* exposure to any form of radiant energy, e.g. heat, light or X-ray.

irreducible *adj* unable to be brought to desired condition. *irreducible hernia* ⇒ hernia.

irritable *adj* capable of being excited to activity; responding easily to stimuli—**irritability** *n. irritable bowel syndrome* unusual motility of both small and large bowel which produces discomfort and intermittent pain, for which no organic cause can be found.

irritant *adj, n* describes any agent which causes irritation.

ISC *abbr* intermittent self-catheterization*.

ischaemia *n* deficient blood supply to any part of the body. ⇒ angina, Volkmann—**ischaemic** *adj.*

ischaemic heart disease (IHD) deficient blood supply to cardiac muscle causing central chest pain of varying intensity which may radiate to arms and jaws. The lumen of the blood vessels is usually narrowed by atheromatous plaques. If treatment with vasodilator drugs is unsuccessful, bypass surgery may be considered. ⇒ angina pectoris, myocardial infarction.

ischiorectal *adj* pertaining to the ischium and the rectum, as in ischiorectal abscess which occurs between these two structures.

ischium *n* the lower part of the innominate bone of the pelvis; the bone on which the body rests when sitting—**ischial** *adj.*

islets of Langerhans collections of special cells scattered throughout the pancreas. They secrete insulin which is absorbed directly into the blood stream.

isoantibody *n* an antibody produced by one individual that reacts with the isoantigen* of another individual of the same species.

isoantigen *n* an antigen existing in an alternative form in a species, thus inducing an immune response when one form is transferred to a member of the species that lacks it; typical antigens are the blood group antigens; also called *alloantigens.*

isoimmunization *n* development of anti-Rh agglutinins in the blood of an Rh-negative person who has been given an Rh-positive transfusion, or who is carrying an Rh-positive fetus.

isolation *n* separation of a patient from others for a variety of reasons. ⇒ containment isolation, exclusion isolation, protective isolation, source isolation.

isoleucine *n* one of the essential amino* acids.

isometric *adj* of equal proportions. *isometric exercises* carried out without movement; maintain muscle tone.

isotonic *adj* equal tension; applied to any solution which has the same osmotic pressure as blood. Also refers to muscle contraction at constant tension. *isotonic saline* (*syn* normal saline, physiological saline), 0.9% solution of salt in water.

isotopes *npl* two or more forms of the same element having identical chemical properties and the same atomic number but different mass numbers. Those isotopes with radioactive properties are used in medicine for research, diagnosis and treatment of disease.

isotope scanning injection of an isotope before a scan*. ⇒ isotopes.

isoxazole penicillins can be taken orally. After absorption give high blood levels of penicillin in a freely available form to act against staphylococci. Particularly effective for boils and carbuncles.

isthmus *n* a narrowed part of an organ or tissue such as that connecting the two lobes of the thyroid gland.

itch *n* a sensation on the skin which makes one want to scratch. ⇒ scabies. itch mite Sarcoptes* scabiei.

ITU *abbr* intensive* therapy unit.

IUCD *abbr* intrauterine* contraceptive device.

IUD *abbr* intrauterine* (contraceptive) device.

IUGR *abbr* ⇒ intrauterine growth retardation.

IUI *abbr* intrauterine* insemination.

IVC *abbr* inferior* vena çava ⇒ vena cava.

IVF *abbr* in* vitro fertilization.

IVU, IVP *abbr* intravenous urogram/pyelogram ⇒ urography. Pyelogram indicates examination of kidneys–ureters and bladder.

J

Jacksonian epilepsy ⇒ epilepsy.

Jacquemier's sign blueness of the vaginal mucosa seen in early pregnancy.

jargon *n* specialized or technical language which is only understood by a particular group. The word is often used to describe the use of obscure and pretentious language, together with a roundabout way of expression.

jaundice *n* (*syn* icterus) a condition characterized by a raised bilirubin level in the blood (hyperbilirubinaemia). Minor degrees are only detectable chemically *latent jaundice*. Major degrees are visible in the yellow skin, sclerae and mucosae *overt* or *clinical jaundice*. Jaundice may be due to (a) obstruction anywhere in the biliary tract *(obstructive jaundice)* (b) excessive haemolysis of red blood cells *(haemolytic jaundice)* (c) toxic or infective damage of liver cells *(hepatocellular jaundice)* (d) bile stasis *(cholestatic jaundice)*. *acholuric jaundice* (*syn* spherocytosis*) jaundice without bile in the urine. *infective jaundice* most commonly due to a virus; infective hepatitis*. *leptospiral jaundice* ⇒ Weil's disease. *malignant jaundice* acute diffuse necrosis of the liver. *jaundice of the newborn* icterus* gravis neonatorum.

jaw-bone *n* either the maxilla (upper jaw) or mandible (lower jaw).

jejunal biopsy a test used in the diagnosis of coeliac disease. A tube is passed through the mouth and into the jejunum. A small piece of jejunal mucosa is removed and sent for histological and enzyme examinations.

jejunostomy *n* a surgically made fistula between the jejunum and the anterior abdominal wall; used temporarily for feeding where passage of food through the stomach is impossible or undesirable.

jejunum *n* that part of the small intestine between the duodenum* and the ileum*—**jejunal** *adj*.

jigger *n* a flea, *Tunga penetrans,* prevalent in the tropics. It burrows under the skin to lay its eggs, causing intense irritation. Secondary infection is usual.

joint *n* the articulation of two or more bones (arthrosis). There are three main classes: (a) fibrous (synarthrosis), e.g. the sutures of the skull (b) cartilaginous (synchondrosis), e.g. between the manubrium and the body of the sternum and (c) synovial, e.g. elbow or hip. ⇒ Charcot's joint.

joule *n* the SI unit for energy, work and quantity of heat. The unit (J) is the energy expended when 1 kg (kilogram) is moved 1 m (metre) by a force of gravity. The kilojoule (kJ = 10^3J) and the megajoule (MJ = 10^6J) are used by physiologists and nutritionists for measuring large amounts of energy.

jugular *adj* pertaining to the throat. *jugular veins* two veins passing down either side of the neck.

junket *n* milk predigested by the

addition of rennet; curds and whey.

junk food a term used to describe convenience or 'fast' foods with added chemicals, e.g. monosodium* glutamate.

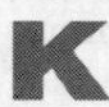

Kahn test a serological test for the diagnosis of syphilis*. The patient's serum reacts with a heterologous antigen prepared from mammalian tissue: flocculation occurs if syphilitic antibodies are present.

kala-azar *n* a generalized form of leishmaniasis* occurring in the tropics. There is anaemia, fever, splenomegaly and wasting. It is caused by the parasite *Leishmania donovani* and is spread by sandflies.

Kanner's syndrome autism*.

kaolin *n* natural aluminium silicate. When given orally it absorbs toxic substances, hence useful in diarrhoea, colitis and food poisoning. Also used in dusting powders and poultices.

Kaposi's disease ⇒ xeroderma.

Kaposi's sarcoma a malignant, multifocal neoplasm of reticuloendothelial cells. It first appears as brown or purple patches on the feet and spreads on the skin, metastasizing on the lymph nodes and viscera. Originally common in Africa but currently of interest because it can complicate acquired* immune deficiency syndrome.

Kaposi's varicelliform eruption occurs in eczematous children. Generalized bullous eczema.

Kardex *n* a proprietary piece of stationery which permits the storing of a given number of patients' nursing or medication records.

karyotype *n* creation of an orderly array of chromosomes, usually derived from the study of cultured cells. This is usually done for diagnostic purposes on abnormal persons, or persons prone to produce chromosomally abnormal children, or for the prenatal detection of fetal abnormality in women at risk of producing chromosomally abnormal fetuses, for example, because of advancing age.

Keller's operation for hallux* valgus or rigidus. Excision of the proximal half of the proximal phalanx, plus any osteophytes and exostoses on the metatarsal head. The toe is fixed in the corrected position; after healing a pseudarthrosis results.

Kell factor a blood group factor found in about 10% of Caucasians: inherited according to Mendelian laws of inheritance. Anti-Kell antibodies can cross the placenta.

Kelly-Paterson syndrome ⇒ Plummer-Vinson syndrome.

keloid *n* an overgrowth of scar tissue, which may produce a contraction deformity or large bulbous scar. Keloid scarring occurs in some pigmented skins; it tends to get progressively worse. ⇒ disfigurement, pressure garment.

keratectomy *n* surgical excision of a portion of the cornea. ⇒ photorefractive keratectomy, radial keratectomy.

keratin *n* a protein found in all horny tissue. Once used to coat pills given for their intestinal effect, since keratin can withstand gastric juice.

keratinization *n* conversion into horny tissue. Occurs as a pathological process in vitamin A deficiency.

keratitic precipitates (KP) large cells adherent to the posterior surface of the cornea*; present in inflammation of iris, ciliary body and choroid.

keratitis *n* inflammation of the cornea*.

keratoconjunctivitis *n* inflammation of the cornea and conjunctiva. *epidemic keratoconjunctivitis* due to an adenovirus. Present as an acute follicular conjunctivitis with preauricular and submaxillary adenitis. *keratoconjunctivitis sicca* ⇒ Sjögren syndrome.

keratoconus *n* a cone-like protrusion of the cornea, usually due to a noninflammatory thinning.

keratoiritis *n* inflammation of the cornea and iris.

keratolytic *adj* having the property of breaking down keratinized epidermis.

keratoma *n* ⇒ callosity*—**keratomata** *pl.*

keratomalacia *n* softening of the cornea; ulceration may occur; frequently caused by lack of vitamin A.

keratome *n* a special knife with a trowel-like blade for incising the cornea.

keratopathy *n* any disease of the cornea—**keratopathic** *adj.*

keratophakia *n* surgical introduction of a biological 'lens' into the cornea to correct hypermetropia*.

keratoplasty *n* ⇒ corneal graft—**keratoplastic** *adj.*

keratosis *n* thickening of the horny layer of the skin. Also referred to as hyperkeratosis. Has the appearance of warty excrescences. *keratosis palmaris et plantaris* (*syn* tylosis) a congenital thickening of the horny layer of the palms and soles.

kerion *n* a boggy suppurative mass of the scalp associated with ringworm* of the hair.

kernicterus *n* bile staining of the basal ganglia in the brain which may result in mental deficiency; it occurs in icterus* gravis neonatorum.

Kernig's sign inability to straighten the leg at the knee joint when the thigh is flexed at right angles to the trunk. Occurs in meningitis.

ketoacidosis *n* (*syn* ketosis) acidosis* due to accumulation of ketone bodies β-hydroxybutyric acid, acetoacetic acid and acetone, products of the metabolism of fat. Primarily a complication of insulin dependent diabetes. Symptoms include drowsiness, headache and deep respiration—**ketoacidotic** *adj.*

ketogenic diet a high fat content producing ketosis (acidosis).

ketonaemia *n* ketone bodies in the blood—**ketonaemic** *adj.*

ketones *npl* organic compounds (e.g. ketosteroids) containing the carbonyl group, C = 0, whose carbon atom occurs within a carbon chain. By-product of the breakdown of fats, e.g. as a result of raised blood glucose levels; become apparent in the urine and blood. *ketone bodies* (*syn* acetone bodies) a term which includes acetone, acetoacetic acid and β-hydroxybutyric acid. ⇒ diabetes mellitus.

ketonuria *n* ketone bodies in the urine—**ketonuric** *adj.*

ketosis *n* ketoacidosis*—**ketotic** *adj.*

ketosteroids *npl* steroid hormones which contain a ketone group, formed by the addition of an oxygen molecule to the basic ring structure. The 17-ketosteroids (which have this oxygen at carbon-17) are excreted in normal urine and are present in excess in overactivity of the adrenal glands and the gonads.

khat *n* the leaves contain two psychostimulants structurally similar to amphetamine. Chewing the leaves is a widespread habit in countries such as East Africa and Arabia. It is becoming increasingly available in the UK.

kidney *n* a pair of organs situated one on either side of the vertebral column in the upper posterior abdominal cavity. Their main function is secretion of urine* which flows into the ureters*. They secrete renin* and renal* erythropoietic factor. *horseshoe kidney* an anatomical variation in which the inner lower border of each kidney is joined to give a horseshoe shape. Usually symptomless and only rarely interferes with drainage of urine into ureters. *kidney failure* ⇒ renal failure. *kidney machine* ⇒ dialyser. *kidney transplant* surgical transplantation of a kidney from a previously tested suitable live donor or one who has recently died. Kidneys may also be transplanted from the renal bed to other sites in the same individual in cases of ureteric disease or trauma. *kidney function tests* various tests are available for measuring renal function. All require careful collection of urine specimens. Those in common use are: para-aminohippuric acid clearance test for measuring renal blood flow; creatinine clearance test for measuring glomerular filtration rate; ammonium chloride test for measuring tubular ability to excrete hydrogen ions; urinary concentration and dilution tests for measuring tubular function. ⇒ indigocarmine.

kilojoule (kJ) *n* replaces the calorie*; the large calorie which was in diatetic use is equal to 4.2 kJ. 1 g of fat yields 38 kJ, 1 g of protein 17 kJ, and 1 g of carbohydrate yields 16 kJ.

Kimmelstiel-Wilson syndrome intercapillary glomerulosclerosis* develops in diabetics, who have hypertension, albuminuria and oedema.

kinaesthesis *n* muscle sense; perception of movement—**kinaesthetic** *adj.*

kinase *n* enzymes which catalyse the transfer of a high-energy group of a donor, usually adenosine triphosphate, to some acceptor, usually named after the acceptor (e.g. fructokinase).

kineplastic surgery operative measures, whereby certain muscle groups are isolated and utilized to work certain modified prostheses.

kinetic *adj* pertaining to or producing motion.

Kirschner wire a wire drilled into a bone to apply skeletal traction. A hand or electric drill is used, a stirrup is attached and the wire is rendered taut by means of a special wire-tightener.

Klebsiella *n* a Gram-negative bacillus (rod-shaped). *Klebsiella pneumoniae* is the cause of a rare form of severe pneumonia resulting in tissue necrosis and abscess formation.

Klebs-Loeffler bacillus *Corynebacterium* diphtheriae.*

kleptomania *n* compulsive stealing due to mental disturbance, usually of the obsessional type—**kleptomaniac** *n, adj.*

Klinefelter syndrome a chromosomal abnormality affecting boys, usually with 47 chromosomes including XXY sex chromosomes. Puberty is frequently delayed, with small firm testes, often with gynaecomastia. Associated with sterility, which may be the only symptom.

Klumpke's paralysis paralysis and atrophy of muscles of the forearm and hand, with sensory and pupillary disturbances due to injury to lower roots of brachial plexus and cervical sympathetic nerves. Claw-hand results.

knee *n* the hinge joint formed by

the lower end of the femur and the head of the tibia. *kneecap* the patella*. *knee jerk* a reflex contraction of the relaxed quadriceps muscle elicited by a tap on the patellar tendon: usually performed with the lower femur supported behind, the knee bent and the leg limp. Persistent variation from normal usually signifies organic nervous disorder.

knuckles *npl* the dorsal aspect of any of the joints between the phalanges and the metacarpal bones, or between the phalanges.

Koch's bacillus *Mycobacterium* tuberculosis*, the organism that causes tuberculosis.

Koch-Weeks bacillus *Haemophilus* aegyptius.*

Köhler disease osteochondritis* of the tarsal navicular bone. Confined to children of 3–5 years. Tenderness, redness, swelling and sometimes pain occur over the tarsal navicular bone on the medial side of the foot.

koilonychia *n* spoon-shaped nails, characteristic of iron deficiency anaemia.

Koplik's spots small white spots inside the mouth, during the first few days of the invasion (prodromal) stage of measles*.

Korsakoff psychosis, syndrome alcoholic dementia; polyneuritic psychosis. A condition which follows delirium and toxic states. Often due to alcoholism. The consciousness is clear and alert, but the patient is disorientated for time and place, with grossly impaired memory, especially for recent events (patient often confabulates to fill in the gaps). Afflicts more men than women in the 45–55 age group.

KP *abbr* keratitic* precipitates.

Krabbe disease genetically determined degenerative disease of the central nervous system associated with mental subnormality.

kraurosis vulvae a degenerative condition of the vaginal introitus associated with postmenopausal lack of oestrogen.

Krukenberg tumour a secondary malignant tumour of the ovary. The primary growth is usually in the stomach or gastrointestinal tract.

Küntscher nail used for intramedullary fixation of fractured long bones, especially the femur. The nail has a 'clover-leaf' cross-section.

Kusman's sign venous pulsus* paradoxus.

Kveim test an intracutaneous test for sarcoidosis* using tissue prepared from a person known to be suffering from the condition.

kwashiorkor *n* a nutritional disorder of infants and young children when the diet is persistently deficient in essential protein; commonest where maize is the staple diet. Characteristic features are anaemia, wasting, dependent oedema and a fatty liver. Untreated, it progresses to death. Aflatoxin* has been found at postmortem in people who died from kwashiorkor.

KY jelly a proprietary mucilaginous lubricating jelly.

kymograph *n* an apparatus for recording movements, e.g. of muscles, columns of blood. Used in physiological experiments—**kymographic** *adj*, **kymographically** *adv*.

kypholordosis *n* coexistence of kyphosis* and lordosis*.

kyphoscoliosis *n* coexistence of kyphosis* and scoliosis*.

kyphosis *n* an excessive curvature of the dorsal spine, seen as round shoulder deformity, humpback—**kyphotic** adj.

L

labia *npl* lips. *labia majora* two large lip-like folds of skin extending from the mons veneris to encircle the vagina. *labia minora* two smaller folds lying within the labia majora—**labium** *sing,* **labial** *adj.*

labile *adj* unstable; readily changed, as many drugs when in solution; and blood pressure.

lability *n* instability. *emotional lability* rapid change in mood. Occurs especially in the mental disorders of old age.

labioglossolaryngeal *adj* relating to the lips, tongue and larynx. *labioglossolaryngeal paralysis* a nervous disease characterized by progressive paralysis of the lips, tongue and larynx.

labioglossopharyngeal *adj* relating to the lips, tongue and pharynx.

labour *n* (*syn* parturition) the act of giving birth to a child. The first stage lasts from onset until there is full dilation of the cervical os; the second stage lasts until the baby is delivered; the third stage until the placenta is expelled.

labyrinth *n* part of the inner ear which includes the semicircular canals and the cochlea. *bony labyrinth* that part which is directly hollowed out of the temporal bone. *membranous labyrinth* the membrane which lines the bony labyrinth—**labyrinthine** *adj.*

labyrinthectomy *n* surgical removal of part or the whole of the membranous labyrinth of the internal ear. Sometimes carried out for Menière's disease.

labyrinthitis *n* inflammation of the internal ear.

lacerated wound one in which the tissues are torn, usually by a blunt instrument, biting or pressure: likely to become infected and to heal by second intention. ⇒ healing.

lachrymal *adj*

lacrimal, lachrymal, lacrymal *adj* pertaining to tears. *lacrimal bone* a tiny bone at the inner side of the orbital cavity. *lacrimal duct* connects lacrimal gland to upper conjunctival sac. *lacrimal gland* situated above the upper, outer canthus of the eye. ⇒ dacryocyst.

lacrimation *n* an outflow of tears; weeping.

lacrimonasal *adj* pertaining to the lacrimal and nasal bones and ducts.

lacrymal *adj* ⇒ lacrimal.

lactagogue *n* any substance given to stimulate lactation. ⇒ galactagogue.

lactalbumin *n* the more easily digested of the two milk proteins. ⇒ caseinogen.

lactase *n* (*syn* β-galactosidase) a saccharolytic enzyme of intestinal juice; it splits lactose* into glucose* (dextrose) and galactose*. *lactase deficiency* the clinical syndrome of milk sugar intolerance. In severe congenital intolerance the infant may pass a litre or more of fluid stool per day. Temporary intolerance can follow neonatal alimentary tract obstructions, but rarely gives long-term problems.

lactate dehydrogenase (LDH) an enzyme, of which there are five isozymes, that catalyses the interconversion of lactate and pyruvate. LDH-1 is the one found in the heart; its blood level rises rapidly when heart tissues die, e.g. after a myocardial infarction. After heart transplant, rejection is imminent when the LDH-1 activity is greater than that of its isozyme LDH-2 during the first 4 postoperative weeks. After 6 months this diagnostic indicator disappears. *lactate dehydrogenase test* when tissue of high metabolic activity dies the ensuing tissue necrosis is quickly reflected by an increase of the serum enzyme lactate dehydrogenase.

lactation *n* 1 secretion of milk. 2 the period during which the child is nourished from the breast.

lacteals *npl* blind ending lymphatic ducts in the intestinal villi; they absorb microchylors* (digested fat particles) and convey them to the receptaculum* chyli.

lactic acid the acid that causes the souring of milk. It is obtained by the fermentation of lactose*. Produced naturally in the body through the metabolism of glucose. A build up of the acid in the muscles can cause cramp.

lactiferous *adj* conveying or secreting milk.

Lactobacillus *n* a genus of bacteria. A large Gram-positive rod which is active in fermenting carbohydrates, producing acid. No members are pathogenic.

lactogenic *adj* stimulating milk production.

lactometer *n* an instrument for measuring the specific gravity of milk.

lactose *n* milk sugar, a disaccharide of glucose* and galactose*. Less soluble and less sweet than ordinary sugar. Used in infant feeding to increase the carbohydrate content of diluted cow's milk. In some infants the gut is intolerant to lactose. ⇒ lactase.

lactulose *n* a sugar which is not metabolized so that it reaches the colon unchanged. Sugar-splitting bacteria then act on it, promoting a softer stool.

lacuna *n* a space between cells; usually used in the description of bone—**lacunae** *pl*, **lacunar** *adj*.

laevulose *n* ⇒ fructose.

lambliasis *n* ⇒ giardiasis.

lamella *n* a thin plate-like scale or partition—**lamellae** *pl*.

lamina *n* a thin plate or layer, usually of bone—**laminae** *pl*.

laminectomy *n* removal of vertebral laminae to expose the spinal cord nerve roots and meninges. Most often performed in the lumbar region, for removal of degenerated invertebral disc.

Lancefield's groups subdivision of the genus *Streptococcus* on the basis of antigenic structure. The members of each group have a characteristic capsular polysaccharide. The most dangerous streptococci of epidemiological importance to man belong to Group A.

Landry's paralysis an acute ascending condition accompanied by fever; it may terminate in respiratory stasis and death. ⇒ paralysis.

lanae hydrosus ⇒ lanolin.

language *n* the usual interpretation involves verbal language (spoken and written), which uses a set of letters, 26 in English, from which many thousands of words can be computed. Also using these letters, particular groups of people may construct a verbal language (jargon*) to explain their work. Body* or non-verbal language conveys accurately the person's current mood. Dysphasic and deaf people can learn to use sign* language. Profoundly deaf people benefit from the use of sign language, both personally and by their family, friends and colleagues.

lanolin *n* (*syn* adeps lanae hydrosus) wool fat containing 30% water. *Anhydrous lanolin* is the fat obtained from sheep's wool. Used in ointment bases, as such bases can form water-in-oil emulsions with aqueous constituents, and are readily absorbed by the skin. Contact sensitivity to lanolin products may occur.

lanugo *n* the soft, downy hair sometimes present on newborn infants, especially when they are premature. Usually replaced before birth by vellus hair.

laparoscope *n* a type of endoscope* inserted through the abdominal wall to facilitate examination of or surgery on the peritoneal cavity.

laparoscopy *n* endoscopic examination of or surgery to internal organs by the transperitoneal route. Specially designed instruments are introduced through the abdominal wall via small incisions into a preformed pneumoperitoneum*, under video control. A variety of surgical procedures can now be performed in this way, including biopsy, aspiration of cysts, division of adhesions, tubal ligation, appendicectomy and cholecystectomy. The procedure minimizes trauma of access and shortens the length of hospital stay—**laparoscopic** *adj,* **laparoscopically** *adv.*

laparotomy *n* incision of the abdominal wall. Usually reserved for exploratory operation.

Larsen syndrome multiple joint dislocations and deformities.

larva *n* an embryo which is independent before it has assumed the characteristic features of its parents. *larva migrans* itching tracks in the skin with formation of blisters; caused by the burrowing of larvae of some species of fly, and the normally animal-infesting *Ancylostoma*—**larvae** *pl,* **larval** *adj.*

larvicide *n* any agent which destroys larvae—**larvicidal** *adj.*

laryngeal *adj* pertaining to the larynx.

laryngectomy *n* surgical removal of the larynx.

laryngismus stridulus momentary sudden attack of laryngeal spasm with a crowing sound on inspiration. It occurs in inflammation of the larynx, in connection with rickets, and as an independent disease.

laryngitis *n* inflammation of the larynx; can be acute or chronic. ⇒ hoarseness.

laryngologist *n* a specialist in diseases of the larynx.

laryngology *n* the study of diseases affecting the larynx.

laryngoparalysis *n* paralysis of the larynx.

laryngopharyngectomy *n* excision of the larynx and lower part of pharynx.

laryngopharynx *n* the lower portion of the pharynx—**laryngopharyngeal** *adj* ⇒ hypopharynx.

laryngoscope *n* instrument for exposure and visualization of larynx, for diagnostic or therapeutic purposes or during the procedure of tracheal intubation*—**laryngoscopy** *n,* **laryngoscopic** *adj.*

laryngospasm *n* convulsive involuntary muscular contraction of the larynx, usually accompanied by spasmodic closure of the glottis.

laryngostenosis *n* narrowing of the glottic aperture.

laryngotomy *n* the operation of opening the larynx.

laryngotracheal *adj* pertaining to the larynx* and trachea*.

laryngotracheitis *n* inflammation of the larynx* and trachea*.

laryngotracheobronchitis *n* inflammation of the larynx*, trachea* and bronchi*.

laryngotracheoplasty *n* an operation to widen a stenosed airway—**laryngotracheoplastic** *adj.*

larynx *n* the organ of voice situated below and in front of the pharynx* and at the upper end of the trachea*—**laryngeal** *adj.*

laser *n* acronym for Light Amplification by Stimulated Emission of Radiation. Energy is transmitted as heat which can coagulate tissue. Has been used for detached retina and cancer. Precautions must be taken by those using lasers as blindness can be an occupational hazard if precautions are neglected.

Lassa fever one of the viral* haemorrhagic fevers. The incubation period is 3–16 days; early symptoms resemble typhoid* and septicaemia*. By the sixth day ulcers develop in the mouth and throat; fever is variable, sometimes being very high. Fatality rate in some areas is as high as 67%. Infected people must be nursed in strict isolation.

latent heat that heat which is used to bring about a change in state, not in temperature.

lateral *adj* at or belonging to the side; away from the median line—**laterally** *adv. lateral position* lying on one or other side. *modified lateral position* lying on the right side with both legs drawn up so that the knees are as near the bowed head as possible. Used to facilitate entry to the rectum and in lumbar* puncture. ⇒ colonic washout, enema, suppository.

lavage *n* irrigation of or washing out a body cavity.

laxatives *npl* (*syn* aperients) drugs which produce peristalsis and promote evacuation of the bowel, usually to relieve constipation. The more powerful laxatives are known as purgatives, and drastic purgatives are termed cathartics. Laxatives are further classified, either relating to the constituents or to the function, as saline, vegetable, synthetic, bulk-increasers (bulking), or lubricators (lubricants).

LE *abbr* lupus* erythematosus. *LE cells* characteristic cells found in patients with lupus* erythematosus.

lead *n* a soft metal with toxic salts. *lead poisoning* (*syn* plumbism) acute poisoning is unusual, but chronic poisoning due to absorption of small amounts over a period is less uncommon. This can occur in young children by sucking articles made of lead alloys, or painted with lead paint. Where the water supply is soft, lead poisoning may occur because drinking water picks up lead from water pipes. In spite of legislation and safety precautions, industrial poisoning is still the commonest cause. Anaemia, loss of appetite, and the formation of a blue line round the gums are characteristic. Nervous symptoms, including convulsions*, are seen in severe cases.

learning disability the preferred term to describe people who are slow learners of the skills needed for everyday living. Individualized programmes, that offer a range of educational and/or therapeutic techniques, enable many people with a learning disability to achieve independence in these skills. ⇒ disability, impairment, mental.

lecithinase *n* (*syn* phospholipase D) an enzyme which catalyses the decomposition of lecithin (phosphatidylcholine) and occurs in the toxin of *Clostridium perfringens.*

lecithins *npl* a group of phosphoglycerides esterified with the alcohol group of choline*. Found in animal tissues, mainly in cell membranes. They are present in surfactant*.

leech *n Hirudo medicinalis.* An aquatic worm which can be applied to the human body to suck blood. Its saliva contains hirudin*, an anticoagulant.

Legionella haemophila a small Gram-negative nonacid-fast bacillus which causes Legionnaire's* disease and Pontiac* fever.

Legionnaire's disease a severe and often fatal pneumonia caused by *Legionella* pneumophila:* the outbreak first affected an American Legion convention. There is pneumonia, dry cough, and often nonpulmonary involvement such as gastrointestinal symptoms, renal impairment and confusion. A cause of both community and hospital-acquired pneumonia. ⇒ Pontiac fever.

legumes *npl* pulse vegetables, e.g. peas, beans, lentils.

Leishman-Donovan bodies the rounded forms of the protozoa *Leishmania* found in the endothelial cells and macrophages of patients suffering from leishmaniasis*.

Leishmania *n* genus of flagellated protozoon. *Leishmania donovani* responsible for disease of kala-azar* or leishmaniasis*.

leishmaniasis *n* infestation by *Leishmania,* spread by sandflies. Generalized manifestation is kala-azar*. Cutaneous manifestation is such as oriental* sore; nasopharyngeal manifestation is espundia.

lens *n* the small biconvex crystalline body which is supported in the suspensory ligament immediately behind the iris of the eye. On account of its elasticity, the lens can alter in shape, enabling light rays to focus exactly on the retina.

lenticular *adj* pertaining to or resembling a lens*.

lentigo *n* a freckle with an increased number of pigment cells. ⇒ ephelides—**lentigines** *pl.*

lentil *n* a nutritious legume containing a large amount of protein.

leontiasis *n* enlargement of the face and head giving a lion-like appearance; most often caused by fibrous dysplasia of bone.

leprologist *n* one who specializes in the study and treatment of leprosy*.

leprology *n* the study of leprosy* and its treatment.

lepromata *npl* the granulomatous cutaneous eruption of leprosy—**leproma** *sing,* **lepromatous** *adj.*

leprosy *n* a progressive and contagious disease, endemic in warmer climates and characterized by granulomatous formation in the nerves or on the skin. Caused by *Mycobacterium leprae* (Hansen's bacillus). BCG* vaccination conferred variable protection in different trials. Leprosy can be controlled but not cured by long-term treatment with sulphone drugs—**leprous** *adj.*

leptocytosis *n* thin, flattened, circulating red blood cells (leptocytes). Characteristic of thalassaemia*. Also seen in jaundice, hepatic disease and sometimes after splenectomy. Sometimes known as 'target cells' (resemble a target).

leptomeningitis *n* inflammation of the inner covering membranes (arachnoid* and pia* mater) of brain or spinal cord.

Leptospira *n* a genus of bacteria. Very thin, finely coiled bacteria which require dark ground microscopy for visualization. Common in water as saprophytes; pathogenic species are numerous in many animals and may infect man. *Leptospira interrogans* serotype *icterohaemorrhagiae* causes Weil's* disease in man; *Leptospira interrogans* serotype *canicola* causes 'yellows' in dogs and pigs; transmissible to man. ⇒ leptospirosis.

leptospiral agglutination tests serological tests used in the diagnosis of specific leptospiral infections e.g. Weil's* disease.

leptospirosis *n* infection of man by *Leptospira* from rats, dogs, pigs, foxes, mice, voles and possibly cats. There is high fever, headache, conjunctival congestion, jaundice, severe muscular pains, rigors and vomiting. As the fever abates in about a week, the jaundice disappears. ⇒ Weil's disease.

lesbianism *n* sexual attraction of one woman to another.

Lesch-Nyhan disease X-linked recessive genetic disorder. Overproduction of uric acid, associated with brain damage, resulting in cerebral palsy and learning disability. Victims are compelled, by a self-destructive urge, to bite away the sides of their mouth, lips and fingers.

lesion *n* pathological change in a bodily tissue.

lethargy *n* apathy, indifference and sluggishness in an environment to which the person usually responds positively.

leucine *n* one of the essential amino* acids. Leucine-induced hypoglycaemia is a genetic metabolic disorder due to a person's sensitivity to leucine.

leucocidin *n* a bacterial exotoxin* which selectively destroys white blood cells.

leucocytes *npl* the white corpuscles of the blood, some of which are granular and some nongranular. In the bloodstream they are colourless, nucleated masses, and some are motile and phagocytic. The different types are: basophil*, eosinophil*, lymphocyte*, monocyte*, neutrophil*—**leucocytic** *adj.*

leucocytolysis *n* destruction and disintegration of white blood cells—**leucocytolytic** *adj.*

leucocytosis *n* increased number of leucocytes* in the blood. Often a response to infection and haematological disorders—**leucocytotic** *adj.*

leucoderma *n* defective skin pigmentation, especially when it occurs in patches or bands.

leuconychia *n* white spots on the nails.

leucopenia *n* decreased number of white blood cells in the blood—**leucopenic** *adj.*

leucopoiesis *n* the formation of white blood cells—**leucopoietic** *adj.*

leucorrhoea *n* a sticky, whitish vaginal discharge. Normal unless it becomes copious, malodorous or abnormal in colour—**leucorrhoeal** *adj.*

leukaemia *n* a malignant disease producing abnormal proliferation of white blood cells. Can be acute or chronic and may involve different cell lines, e.g. myeloid*, causing myeloblastic or granulocytic leukaemia, and lymphoid*, causing lymphatic, lymphoblastic or lymphocytic leukaemia. Leukaemia is complicated by anaemia, vulnerability to infection and haemorrhage. Other symptoms include fever, joint pain and lymphadenopathy. Untreated leukaemia is progressive and fatal—**leukaemic** *adj.*

leukoma *n* white opaque spot on the cornea—**leukomata** *pl,* **leukomatous** *adj.*

leukoplakia *n* white, thickened patch occurring on mucous membranes. Occurs on lips, inside mouth or on genitalia. Sometimes denotes precancerous change. Sometimes due to syphilis. ⇒ kraurosis vulvae.

levator *adj* **1** a muscle which acts by raising a part. **2** an instrument for lifting a depressed part (bone).

Levin tube a French plastic catheter used for gastric intubation; it has a closed weighted tip and an opening on the side.

levodopa (L-dopa) *n* a synthetic anti-Parkinson drug. In Parkinson's disease there is inadequate dopamine* (a transmitter substance) in the basal ganglia. In these ganglia levodopa is converted into dopamine and replenishes the stores. Unlike dopamine, levodopa can cross the blood-brain barrier.

levonorgestrel *n* a hormone widely used in oral contraceptives. Also contained in a contraceptive implant, consisting of six small rubber capsules containing levonorgestrel. They are inserted under the skin of a woman's forearm; the implants release small amounts of the drug; the effect is achieved in 24 h and lasts for 5 years.

LGVCFT *abbr* lymphogranuloma* venereum complement fixation test.

LHBI *abbr* lower hemibody irradiation.

liaison nurse usually refers to a nurse who is appointed to organize the necessary resources in the community so that when a person is discharged from hospital these resources will be available.

libido *n* Freud's name for the urge to obtain sensual satisfaction which he believed to be the mainspring of human behaviour. Sometimes more loosely used to mean sexual urge. Freud's meaning was satisfaction through all the senses.

lice *n* ⇒ Pediculus.

lichen *n* aggregations of papular skin lesions—**lichenoid** *adj*. *lichen nitidus* characterized by minute, shiny, flat-topped, pink papules of pinhead size. *lichen planus* an eruption of unknown cause showing purple, angulated, shiny, flat-topped papules. *lichen scrofulosorum* a form of tuberculide. *lichen simplex* ⇒ neurodermatitis. *lichen spinulosus* a disease of children characterized by very small spines protruding from the follicular openings of the skin and resulting from vitamin A deficiency. *lichen urticarus* papular urticaria*.

lichenification *n* thickening of the skin, usually secondary to scratching. Skin markings become more prominent and the area affected appears to be composed of small, shiny rhomboids. ⇒ neurodermatitis.

lienitis *n* inflammation of the spleen*.

life crisis a term which describes an unexpected unpleasant happening such as an accident, sudden illness or life event (such as divorce).

life event a sociological term which describes the major happenings in a lifetime such as starting or changing school, getting married or divorced, changing house or work or suffering a bereavement, etc.

life expectancy the average age at which death occurs. It is not only affected by health/illness but also by social factors such as education and industry; and environmental factors such as housing, sanitation and a piped water supply.

lifespan *n* the span of human life from birth to death, however long or short it might be. From collected data, different countries can predict the expected lifespan which is increasing in the West and is lower in the developing countries. Some nursing specialities are predicated on patients' stage on the lifespan, e.g. neonatal nursing, paediatric nursing, midwifery and the nursing of elderly people.

lifestyle *n* the pattern which each individual has developed in relation to the everyday activities of living. These are investigated at the initial assessment of a person entering the health care service, so that the nursing contribution can be individualized.

lifting *v* in a nursing context the word is usually taken to mean lifting a patient up or down the bed, from bed to chair and vice versa, from bed to trolley and vice versa, on and off a bedpan. Since much more than the actual lifting is involved in these and the majority of nursing activities, many professionals now prefer the term 'patient* handling'. ⇒ log roll.

ligament *n* a strong band of fibrous tissue serving to bind bones or other parts together, or to support an organ—**ligamentous** *adj*.

ligate *vt* to tie off blood vessels etc. at operation—**ligation** *n*.

ligation tying off; usually reserved for *ligation of the uterine tubes,* a method of sterilization.

ligature *n* the material used for tying vessels. Silk, catgut, nylon and man-made absorbable and nonabsorbable materials, e.g. Vicryl, can be used.

lightening *n* a word used to denote the relief of pressure on the diaphragm by the abdominal viscera, when the presenting part of the fetus descends into the pelvis in the last 3 weeks of a first pregnancy.

lightning pains symptomatic of tabes* dorsalis. Occur as paroxysms of swift-cutting (lightning) stabs in the lower limbs.

lignocaine *n* a local anaesthetic with a more powerful and prolonged action than procaine. The strength of solution varies from 0.5% for infiltration anaesthesia to 2% for nerve block. Adrenaline* is usually added to delay absorption. Also effective for surface anaesthesia as ointment (2%) and for urethral anaesthesia as a 2% gel. Now widely accepted as an antiarrhythmic agent, especially in the management of ventricular tachycardia and ventricular ectopic beats occurring as complications of acute myocardial infarction.

liminal *adj* of a stimulus, of the lowest intensity which can be perceived by the human senses. ⇒ subliminal.

linctus *n* a sweet, syrupy liquid, used to soothe coughing.

linea *n* a line. *linea alba* the white line visible after removal of the skin in the centre of the abdomen, stretching from the ensiform cartilage to the pubis, its position on the surface being indicated by a slight depression. *linea nigra* pigmented line from umbilicus to pubis which appears in pregnancy. *lineae albicantes* white lines which appear on the abdomen after reduction of tension as after childbirth, tapping of the abdomen, etc.

linear accelerator a mega-voltage machine which accelerates electrons and produces high energy X-rays which are used in the treatment of malignant disease.

lingua *n* the tongue—**lingual** *adj*.

liniment *n* a liquid to be applied to the skin by gentle friction.

linolenic acid an unsaturated, essential fatty acid found in vegetable fats.

lipaemia *n* increased lipoids (especially cholesterol) in the blood—**lipaemic** *adj*.

lipase *n* any fat-splitting enzyme. *pancreatic lipase* steapsin.

lipid *n* any water-insoluble fat or fat-like substance extractable by nonpolar solvents such as alcohol. Lipids serve as a source of fuel and are an important constituent of cell membranes.

lipoid *adj, n* (a substance) resembling fats or oil. Serum lipoids are raised in thyroid deficiency.

lipoidosis *n* disease due to disorder of fat metabolism—**lipoidoses** *pl*.

lipolysis *n* the chemical breakdown of fat by lipolytic enzymes—**lipolytic** *adj*.

lipoma *n* a benign tumour containing adipose tissue—**lipomata** *pl,* **lipomatous** *adj.*

lipoprotein *n* a fatty protein present in blood plasma. Mainly synthesized in the liver and classified according to composition and density as chylomicrons, high-density lipoproteins (HDLs)*, low-density lipoproteins (LDLs) or very-low-density lipoproteins (VLDLs). ⇒ lipid.

lipotrophic substances factors which cause the removal of fat from the liver by transmethylation.

liquor *n* a solution. *liquor amnii* the fluid surrounding the fetus. *liquor epispasticus* a blistering fluid. *liquor folliculi* the fluid surrounding a developing ovum in a graafian follicle. *liquor picis carb* an alcoholic extract of coal tar. Used in eczema and other conditions requiring mild tar treatment. *liquor sanguinis* the fluid part of blood (plasma*).

listening *v* a cluster of skills used in communicating: the nurse gives her whole attention to what is being said as well as how it is being said, and whether or not it is congruent with nonverbal signals.

lithiasis *n* any condition in which there are calculi*.

lithopaedion *n* a dead fetus retained in the abdominal cavity, the result of an abdominal pregnancy. The fetus becomes mummified and sometimes impregnated with lime salts. Rare.

lithotomy *n* surgical incision of the bladder for the removal of calculi: achieved by the abdominal or the perineal route. *lithotomy position* patient lying on her back, feet brought up towards her buttocks, soles of her feet facing each other and knees dropped apart, for gynaecological examination.

lithotripsy *n* the treatment of choice for a person who has a renal calculus. ⇒ lithotriptor.

lithotriptor(er) *n* a machine which sends shock waves through renal calculi causing them to crumble and leave the body naturally via the urine.

lithotrite *n* an instrument for crushing a stone in the urinary bladder.

litmus *n* a vegetable pigment used as an indicator of acidity (red) or alkalinity (blue). Often stored as paper strips impregnated with blue or red litmus: blue litmus paper turns red when in contact with an acid; red litmus paper turns blue when in contact with an alkali.

Little's area anterior part of nasal septum, most common site for epistaxis.

Little's disease diplegia* of spastic type causing 'scissor leg' deformity. A congenital disease in which there is cerebral atrophy or agenesis.

liver *n* the largest organ in the body, varying in weight in the adult from 13.6–18.1 kg or about one-thirtieth of body weight. It is relatively much larger in the fetus. It is situated in the right section of the abdominal cavity. It secretes bile*, forms and stores glycogen* and plays an important part in the metabolism of proteins and fats. *liver transplant* surgical transplantation of a liver from a suitable donor who has recently died.

livid *adj* showing blue discolouration due to bruising, congestion or insufficient oxygenation.

living will ⇒ Ethics box, p. 134.

LMP *abbr* last menstrual period.

LOA *abbr* left occipitoanterior; used to describe the position of the fetus in the uterus.

lobe *n* a rounded section of an organ, separated from neighbouring sections by a fissure or septum etc.—**lobar** *adj.*

lobectomy removal of a lobe, e.g. of the lung for lung abscess or localized bronchiectasis.

lobule *n* a small lobe or a subdivision of a lobe—**lobular, lobulated** *adj.*

local anaesthesia ⇒ anaesthesia.

localize *vt* 1 to limit the spread. 2 to determine the site of a lesion—**localization** *n.*

lochia *n* the vaginal discharge which occurs during the puerperium*. At first pure blood, it later becomes paler, diminishes in quantity and finally ceases—**lochial** *adj.*

lockjaw *n* ⇒ tetanus.

locomotor *adj* can be applied to any tissue or system used in human movement. Usually refers to nerves and muscles. Sometimes includes the bones and joints. *locomotor ataxia* the disordered gait and loss of sense of position in the lower limbs, which occurs in tabes* dorsalis. Tabes dorsalis is still sometimes called 'locomotor ataxia'.

loculated *adj* divided into numerous cavities.

Logan bow a thin metal device, shaped like a bow; it is used after cleft lip surgery to reduce tension on the suture line.

log roll the patient lies on his back with legs extended and arms folded across chest and is rolled by the nurse on to one or other side.

loiasis *n* special form of filariasis (caused by the worm *Filaria Loa loa*) which occurs in West Africa, Nigeria and the Cameroons. The vector, a large horse-fly, *Chrysops,* bites in the daytime. Larvae take 3 years to develop and may live in man for 17 years. They creep about and cause intense itching. Accompanied by eosinophilia*.

loin *n* that part of the back between the lower ribs and the iliac crest; the area immediately above the buttocks.

loneliness *n* a feeling which some people describe as devastating; it is sometimes accompanied by one of hopelessness. It can be experienced by people who are physically in the presence of others whom they find incompatible, as well as by those in the community who have few social contacts. Others can be alone for long periods yet do not experience loneliness. When the assessment data reveal that a person lives alone and has few social contacts, nurses should explore with him the significance of these facts. Special arrangements may need to be made to overcome their negative effects after discharge from hospital. ⇒ liaison nurse, suicide.

longsighted *adj* hypermetropic. ⇒ hypermetropia.

lordoscoliosis *n* lordosis* complicated by the presence of scoliosis*.

lordosis *n* an exaggerated forward, convex curve of the lumbar spine—**lordotic** *adj.*

loupe *n* a magnifying lens used in ophthalmology.

louse *n* ⇒ Pediculus—**lice** *pl.*

low birthweight term used to indicate a weight of 2.5kg or less at birth, indicating the baby is premature* and/or 'small-for-dates'.

lower respiratory tract infection (LRTI) ⇒ pneumonia, bronchitis.

low reading thermometer ⇒ thermometer.

LP *abbr* lumbar* puncture.

LRTI *abbr* lower respiratory tract infection. ⇒ pneumonia, bronchitis.

lubb-dupp *n* words descriptive of the heart sounds as appreciated in auscultation.

lubricants *npl* drugs which are emollient in nature and facilitate the easy and painless evacuation of faeces. ⇒ laxatives.

lucid *adj* clear; describing mental clarity. *lucid interval* a period of mental clarity which can be of variable length, occurring in people with organic mental disorder such as dementia.

Ludwig's angina ⇒ cellulitis.

lues *n* syphilis*–**luetic** *adj.*

lumbar *adj* pertaining to the loin or lower region of spine. *lumbar puncture (LP)* the withdrawal of cerebrospinal fluid through a hollow needle inserted into the subarachnoid space in the lumbar region. The fluid can be examined for its chemical, cellular and bacterial content; its pressure can be measured by the attachment of a manometer. The procedure is hazardous if the pressure is high, but the pressure for an adult has a wide range ó50–200 mm water, so a better guide is examination of the optic fundi for papilloedema. *lumbar sympathectomy* surgical removal of the sympathetic chain in the lumbar region; used to improve the blood supply to the lower limbs by allowing the blood vessels to dilate.

lumbocostal *adj* pertaining to the loin and ribs.

lumbosacral *adj* pertaining to the loin or lumbar vertebrae and the sacrum.

Lumbricus *n* a genus of earthworms. ⇒ ascarides, ascariasis.

lumen *n* the space inside a tubular structure–**lumina** *pl,* **luminal** *adj.*

lumpectomy *n* the surgical excision of a tumour with removal of minimal surrounding tissue. Increasingly being carried out for breast cancer.

lungs *npl* the two main organs of respiration which occupy the greater part of the thoracic cavity; they are separated from each other by the heart and other contents of the mediastinum. They are concerned with the oxygenation of blood.

lunula *n* the semilunar pale area at the root of the nail.

lupus *n* several destructive skin conditions, with different causes. ⇒ collagen. *lupus erythematosus (LE)* an autoimmune process. The discoid variety is characterized by patulous follicles, adherent scales, telangiectasis and atrophy; commonest on nose, malar regions, scalp and fingers. The disseminated or systemic variety is characterized by large areas of erythema on the skin, pyrexia, toxaemia, involvement of serous membranes (pleurisy, pericarditis) and renal damage. Occurs most commonly in younger women. *lupus pernio* a form of sarcoidosis. *lupus vulgaris* the commonest variety of skin tuberculosis; ulceration occurs over cartilage (nose or ear) with necrosis and facial disfigurement.

luteotrophin *n* secreted by the anterior pituitary gland; it assists the formation of the corpus luteum* in the ovary. In the male it acts on Leydig cells in the testis which produce androgens*.

luteum *adj* yellow. *corpus luteum* a yellow mass which forms in the ovary after rupture of a Graafian follicle. It secretes progesterone* and persists and enlarges if pregnancy supervenes.

luxation *n* dislocation of bone at a joint site. ⇒ subluxation.

lymph *n* the fluid contained in the lymphatic vessels. It is transparent, colourless or slightly yellow. Unlike blood, lymph contains only one type of cell, the lymphocyte*. *lymph circulation* that of lymph collected from the tissue spaces; it then passes via capillaries, vessels, glands and ducts to be poured back into the bloodstream. *lymph nodes* accumulations of lymphatic tissue at intervals along lymphatic vessels. They mainly act as filters.

lymphadenectomy *n* excision of one or more lymph nodes.

lymphadenitis *n* inflammation of a lymph node.

lymphadenopathy *n* any disease of the lymph nodes—**lymphadenopathic** *adj.*

lymphangiectasis *n* dilation of the lymph vessels—**lymphangiectatic** *adj.*

lymphangiography *n* ⇒ lymphography.

lymphangioma *n* a simple tumour of lymph vessels—**lymphangiomata** *pl,* **lymphangiomatous** *adj.*

lymphangioplasty *n* replacement of lymphatics by artificial channels (buried silk threads) to drain the tissues. Relieves lymphoedema after radical mastectomy—**lymphangioplastic** *adj.*

lymphangitis *n* inflammation of a lymph vessel.

lymphatic *adj* pertaining to, conveying or containing lymph*.

lymphaticovenous *adj* implies the presence of both lymphatic vessels and veins to increase drainage from an area.

lymphoblast *n* immature lymphocyte found in acute lymphoblastic leukaemia*.

lymphoblastoma *n* malignant lymphoma in which single or multiple tumours arise from lymphoblasts* in lymph nodes. Sometimes associated with acute lymphatic leukaemia.

lymphocyte *n* one variety of white blood cell. The lymphocytic stem cells undergo transformation to T lymphocytes (in the thymus) which provide cellular immunity involved in graft or organ acceptance/rejection: and B lymphocytes which form antibodies and provide humoral immunity. The transformation is usually complete a few months after birth. ⇒human T-cell lymphotropic viruses—**lymphocytic** *adj.*

lymphocytosis *n* an increase in lymphocytes in the blood.

lymphoedema *n* excess of fluid in the tissues from obstruction of lymph vessels. ⇒ elephantiasis, filariasis.

lymphoepithelioma *n* rapidly growing malignant pharyngeal tumour. May involve the tonsil. Often has metastases in cervical lymph nodes—**lymphoepitheliomata** *pl.*

lymphogranuloma inguinale a tropical venereal disease caused by a virus. Primary lesion on the genitalia may be an ulcer or herpetiform eruption. Soon buboes appear in regional lymph nodes. They form a painful mass called poradenitis* and commonly produce sinuses. Further spread by lymphatics may cause severe periproctitis or rectal stricture in women. Patch skin test (lygranum) and a complement-fixation test of patient's serum are used in diagnosis.

lymphography *n* X-ray examination of the lymphatic system after it has been rendered radiopaque—**lymphographical** *adj,* **lymphograph** *n,* **lymphographically** *adv.*

lymphoid *adj* pertaining to lymph*.

lymphokines *npl* chemical substances derived from stimulated T lymphocytes.

lymphology *n* study of the lymphatic system.

lymphoma *n* a benign tumour of lymphatic tissue. *malignant lymphoma* malignant tumours arising in lymph nodes—**lymphomata** *pl,* **lymphomatous** *adj.*

lymphorrhagia *n* an outpouring of lymph from a severed lymphatic vessel.

lymphosarcoma *n* a malignant tumour arising from lymphatic tissue ⇒ nonHodgkin's lymphoma—**lymphosarcomata** *pl,* **lymphosarcomatous** *adj.*

Lyofoam C *n* a proprietary wound dressing: it is a polyethylene foam with a hydrophilic membrane on its surface. It provides a moist wound environment with a degree of absorption which encourages healing. ⇒ moist wound healing.

lyophilization *n* a special method of preserving such biological substances as plasma, sera, bacteria and tissue.

lyophilized skin skin which has been subjected to lyophilization. It is reconstituted and used for temporary skin replacement.

lysin *n* a cell dissolving substance in blood. ⇒ bacteriolysin, haemolysin.

lysine *n* an essential amino* acid necessary for growth.

lysis *n* **1** destruction or decomposition of a cell, or other substances, under the influence of a specific agent. **2** gradual abatement of the symptoms of an infectious disease. **3** surgery to loosen from restraining adhesions—**lytic** *adj*.

lysozyme *n* a basic enzyme which acts as an antibacterial agent and is present in various body fluids such as tears and saliva.

M

maceration *n* softening of the horny layer of the skin by moisture, e.g. in and below the toes (in tinea pedis), or in perianal area (in pruritus ani). Maceration reduces the protective quality of the integument and so predisposes to penetration by bacteria or fungi.

Mackenrodt's ligaments the transverse cervical or cardinal ligaments which are the chief uterine supports.

Macmillan nurses specialist nurses who provide palliative care, emotional support and advice on symptom control to cancer patients and their families either in hospices*, hospitals or in the community. ⇒ Cancer Relief Macmillan Fund.

McMurray's osteotomy division of femur between lesser and greater trochanter. Shaft displaced inwards beneath the head and abducted. This position maintained by a nail plate. Restores painless weight bearing. In congenital dislocation of hip, deliberate pelvic osteotomy renders the outer part of the socket (acetabulum) more horizontal.

macrocephaly *n* excessive size of the head, not caused by hydrocephalus*—**macrocephalic** *adj.*

macrocheilia *n* enlargement of the lips.

macrocytosis *n* an increased number of macrocytes.

macrodactyly *n* excessive development of the fingers or toes.

macroglossia *n* an abnormally large tongue.

macromastia *n* an abnormally large breast.

macronutrients *npl* a group of nutrients which includes carbohydrates, fat, protein, water, calcium, phosphorus, potassium, sodium, chloride and magnesium.

macrophages *npl* mononuclear cells, which scavenge foreign bodies and cell debris. Monocytes are precursors of macrophages. Macrophages play a major role in the immune response. Part of the reticuloendothelial* system. ⇒ histiocytes.

macroscopic *adj* visible to the naked eye; gross. ⇒ microscopic *opp.*

macula *n* a spot. *macula lutea* the yellow spot on the retina, the area of clearest central vision—**maculae** *pl,* **macular** *adj.*

macule *n* a nonpalpable localized area of change in skin colour—**macular** *adj.*

maculopapular *adj* the presence of macules and raised palpable spots (papules) on the skin.

madura foot (*syn* mycetoma) fungus disease of the foot found in India and tropical Africa. Characterized by swelling and the development of nodules and sinuses. May terminate in death from sepsis.

magnesium carbonate a powder widely used as an antacid in peptic ulcer and as a laxative.

magnesium hydroxide a valuable antacid and laxative. It is sometimes preferred to magnesium and other carbonates, as it does not liberate carbon dioxide in the stomach. Also used as an antidote in poisoning by mineral acids.

magnesium sulphate (*syn* Epsom salts) an effective rapid-acting laxative, especially when given in dilute solution on an empty stomach. It is used as a 25% solution as a wet dressing for inflamed conditions of the skin, and as a paste with glycerin for the treatment of boils and carbuncles. It has been given by injection for magnesium deficiency.

magnesium trisilicate tasteless white powder with a mild but prolonged antacid action. It is therefore used extensively in peptic ulcer, often combined with more rapidly acting antacids. It does not cause alkalosis, and large doses can be given without side-effects.

magnetic resonance imaging (MRI) (*syn* nuclear magnetic resonance (NMR)) a technique of imaging by computer using a strong magnetic field and radiofrequency signals to examine thin slices through the body. Has the advantage over computed* tomography in that no X-rays are used, thus no biological harm is thought to be caused to the subject.

magnum *adj* large or great, as foramen magnum in occipital bone.

Makaton *n* one of the sign languages.

mal *n* disease. *mal de mer* seasickness. *grand mal, petit mal* ⇒ epilepsy.

malabsorption *n* poor or disordered absorption of nutrients from the digestive tract. *malabsorption syndrome* loss of weight and steatorrhoea*, varying from mild to severe. Caused by: (a) lesions of the small intestine (b) lack of digestive enzymes or bile salts (c) surgical operations.

malacia *n* softening of a part. ⇒ keratomalacia, osteomalacia.

maladjustment *n* poor adaptation to environment, socially, mentally or physically.

malaise *n* a feeling of illness and discomfort.

malalignment *n* faulty alignment as of the teeth, or bones after a fracture.

malar *adj* relating to the cheek.

malaria *n* a tropical disease caused by one of the genus *Plasmodium* and carried by infected mosquitoes of the genus Anopheles. *Plasmodium falciparum* causes *malignant tertian malaria*. *Plasmodium vivax* causes *benign tertian malaria* and *Plasmodium malariae* causes *quartan malaria*. Signs and symptoms are caused by the presence in the blood cells of the erythrocytic (E) stages of the parasite. In the falciparum malaria *only* the blood-forms of the parasite exist. There is an additional persistent infection in the liver (the extraerythrocytic or EE form) in vivax malaria, it is the factor responsible for relapses. Clinical picture is one of recurring rigors, anaemia, toxaemia and splenomegaly—**malarial** *adj.*

malassimilation *n* poor or disordered assimilation*.

malathion *n* organophosphorus compound, used as an insecticide in agriculture. Powerful and irreversible anticholinesterase action follows excessive inhalation; potentially dangerous to man for this reason. Used to treat head lice and scabies.

malformation *n* abnormal shape or structure; deformity.

malignant *adj* virulent and dangerous; that which is likely to have a fatal termination—**malignancy** *n*. *malignant growth or tumour* ⇒ cancer, sarcoma. *malignant pustule* ⇒ anthrax.

malingering *n* deliberate (volitional) production of symptoms to evade an unpleasant situation.

malleolus *n* a part or process of a bone shaped like a hammer. *external malleolus* at the lower end of the fibula*. *internal malleolus* situated at the lower end of the tibia*—**malleoli** *pl,* **malleolar** *adj.*

malleus (hammer) *n* the hammer-shaped lateral bone of the middle ear which is in contact with the tympanic membrane.

malnutrition *n* the state of being poorly nourished. May be caused by inadequate intake of one or more of the essential nutrients or by malassimilation

malocclusion *n* failure of the upper and lower teeth to meet properly when the jaws are closed.

malodour *n* an unpleasant odour* usually due to decomposing discharge from an infected wound, faeces or urine ⇒ deodorants.

malposition *n* any abnormal position of a part.

malpractice *n* unethical professional behaviour; improper or injurious medical or nursing treatment.

malpresentation *n* any unusual presentation of the fetus in the pelvis.

Malta fever ⇒ brucellosis.

maltase *n* (*syn* α-glucosidase) a sugar splitting (saccharolytic) enzyme found especially in intestinal juice.

maltose *n* malt sugar. A disaccharide produced by the hydrolysis of starch by amylase during digestion. Used as a nutrient and sweetener.

malunion *n* the union of a fracture in a bad position.

mamma *n* the breast—**mammae** *pl,* **mammary** *adj.*

mammaplasty *n* plastic surgery reconstruction of the breast as may be done to augment or reduce its size—**mammaplastic** *adj.*

mammilla *n* 1 the nipple. 2 a small papilla—**mammillae** *pl.*

mammogram *n* the product of mammography.

mammography *n* radiographic demonstration of the breast by use of specially low-penetration (long wavelength) X-rays. Used in the diagnosis of or screening for breast cancer—**mammographic** *adj,* **mammographically** *adv.*

mammotrophic *adj* having an effect upon the breast.

Manchester Repair ⇒ Fothergill's operation.

mandatory minute volume (MMV) a mode of mechanical ventilation. Allows the patient to breathe spontaneously but ensures a mandatory volume of air is delivered by the machine.

mania *n* one phase of manic depressive psychosis in which the prevailing mood is one of undue elation and there is pronounced psychomotor overactivity and often pathological excitement. Flight of ideas and grandiose delusions are common—**manic** *adj.*

manic depressive psychosis/manic depression a type of mental disorder in which the patient's mood alternates between phases of excitement and phases of depression. Often between these phases there are periods of complete normality. Also known as bipolar depression or bipolar affective disorder. ⇒ depression.

manipulation *n* using the hands skilfully as in reducing a fracture or hernia, or changing the fetal position.

mannitol *n* a natural sugar that is not metabolized in the body and acts as an osmotic diuretic. Especially useful in some cases of drug overdose and in cerebral oedema.

manometer *n* an instrument for measuring the pressure exerted by liquids or gases.

Mantoux reaction intradermal

injection of old tuberculin or PPD (purified protein derivative, a purified type of tuberculin) into the anterior aspect of forearm. Inspection after 48–72 h. If positive, there will be an area of induration and inflammation greater than 5 mm in diameter.

manual evacuation of bowel a nursing intervention only rarely carried out. After oral medication to lubricate/soften hardened faeces, the nurse introduces a gloved finger into the rectum and tries to dislodge pieces of faeces. It is an unpleasant experience for both nurse and patient and each needs psychological support. It is important that training is received before attempting this technique.

manubrium *n* a handle-shaped structure; the upper part of the breast bone or sternum.

many-tailed bandage composed of five narrow strips joined in their middle third: it is used to cover the abdomen or chest.

MAOI *abbr* monoamine* oxidase inhibitor.

maple syrup urine disease recessively inherited disorder of amino acid metabolism. Leucine*, isoleucine* and valine* are excreted in excess in urine giving the smell of maple syrup. Symptoms include spasticity, poor feeding and respiratory difficulties; convulsions and severe damage to the CNS may occur. A diet low in the three amino acids may be effective if started sufficiently early, otherwise the disorder is rapidly fatal. Genetic counselling may be indicated. Diagnosis can be made by a biochemical screening test on the blood of newborn babies.

marasmus *n* severe form of protein-energy deficiency as a result of malnutrition. Rarely seen in western societies but still common in areas of famine. Affected infants usually have a good appetite and respond to feeding. ⇒ failure* to thrive–**marasmic** *adj.*

marble bones ⇒ osteopetrosis.

Marburg disease a severe and highly infectious haemorrhogic fever caused by the Marburg/Ebola virus (first cases were amongst laboratory workers in Marburg, Germany, who had handled monkey tissue from Uganda). Incubation period is 3–7 days and there is a wide range of symptoms, including fever, severe headache, vomiting, diarrhoea and bleeding from mucous membranes. No specific treatment is available and the mortality rate is high, from 75–95%.

Marfan's syndrome a hereditary genetic disorder of unknown cause which affects connective tissue. There is dislocation of the lens, congenital heart disease and arachnodactyly with hypotonic musculature and lax ligaments, occasionally excessive height and abnormalities of the iris.

marihuana *n* ⇒ cannabis indica.

marker *n* ⇒ tumour* marker.

Marshall-Marchetti-Krantz operation for stress incontinence. A form of abdominal cystourethropexy usually undertaken in patients who have not been controlled by a colporrhaphy*.

marsupialization *n* an operation for cystic abdominal swellings, which entails stitching the margins of an opening made into the cyst to the edges of the abdominal wound, thus forming a pouch.

Maslow's hierarchy of human needs ⇒ human needs.

masochism *n* the deriving of pleasure from pain inflicted on self by others or occasionally by oneself. It may be a conscious or unconscious process and is frequently of a sexual nature. ⇒ sadism *opp.*

massage *n* the soft tissues are kneaded, rubbed, stroked or tapped for the purpose of improving circulation, metabolism and muscle tone, breaking down of adhesions and generally relaxing the patient. *cardiac* massage* done for cardiac arrest. With the patient on his back on a firm surface, the lower portion of sternum is depressed 37–50 mm each second to massage the heart.⇒ resuscitation.

mastalgia *n* pain in the breast.

mast cells connective tissue cells which contain heparin and histamine in their granules. These substances are released as a cellular defence mechanism in response to infection* injury.

mastectomy *n* surgical removal of the breast. ⇒ breast–self-examination of, lumpectomy. *simple mastectomy* removal of the breast with the overlying skin. May be combined with radiotherapy and possibly chemotherapy as treatment for carcinoma of the breast. *radical mastectomy* removal of the breast with the skin and underlying pectoral muscle together with all the lymphatic tissue of the axilla: carried out for carcinoma when there has been spread to the glands.

mastication *n* the act of chewing.

mastitis *n* inflammation of the breast. May occur during breast-feeding. *chronic mastitis* the name formerly applied to the nodular changes in the breasts now usually called fibrocystic* disease.

mastoid *adj* nipple-shaped. *mastoid air cells* extend in a backward and downward direction from the antrum. *mastoid antrum* the air space within the mastoid process, lined by mucous membrane continuous with that of the tympanum and mastoid cells. *mastoid process* the prominence of the mastoid portion of the temporal bone just behind the ear.

mastoidectomy *n* drainage of the mastoid air-cells and excision of diseased tissue. *cortical mastoidectomy* all the mastoid cells are removed making one cavity which drains through an opening (aditus) into the middle ear. The external meatus and middle ear are untouched. *radical mastoidectomy* the mastoid antrum and middle ear are made into one continuous cavity for drainage of infection. Loss of hearing is inevitable. *modified radical mastoidectomy* tympanic membrane preserved.

mastoiditis *n* inflammation of the mastoid air-cells.

masturbation *n* the production of sexual excitement by friction of the genitals.

materia medica the science dealing with the origin, action and dosage of drugs.

maternal deprivation failure to thrive, child abuse.

matrix *n* the foundation substance in which the tissue cells are embedded.

maturation *n* the process of attaining full development.

Maurice Lee tube a double-bore tube which combines nasogastric aspiration and jejunal feeding.

maxilla *n* the jawbone; in particular the upper jaw—**maxillary** *adj*.

maxillofacial *adj* pertaining to the maxilla and face.

MBC *abbr* maximal breathing capacity. ⇒ respiratory function tests.

McBurney's point a point one-third of the way between the anterior superior iliac spine and the umbilicus, the site of maximum tenderness in cases of acute appendicitis.

ME *abbr* myalgic* encephalomyelitis. Also known as benign myalgic encephalomyelitis (BME). A flu-like illness with symptoms including dizziness, muscle fatigue and spasm, headaches and other neurological pain. A high percentage of ME sufferers have a higher level of Coxsackie B antibodies in their blood than the rest of the population.

meals-on-wheels element of community care provided by social services for disabled and/or elderly clients in their own homes. Provides either a ready-cooked meal, or packs of frozen meals (to be cooked by the client), throughout the week. Usually delivered by WRVS volunteers, thus also providing brief form of company for housebound. A charge is usually made.

measles *n* (*syn* morbilli) an acute infectious disease caused by a virus. Characterized by fever, a blotchy rash and catarrh of mucous membranes. Endemic and worldwide in distribution. In the UK, children are usually immunized against measles during infancy.

meatotomy *n* surgery to the urinary meatus for meatal ulcer and stricture in men.

meatus *n* an opening or channel—**meatal** *adj.*

Meckel's diverticulum a blind, pouch-like sac sometimes arising from the free border of the lower ileum. Occurs in 2% of population: usually symptomless. May cause gastrointestinal bleeding; may intussuscept or obstruct.

meconium *n* the infant's first stool, normally passed shortly after birth. It is a greenish-black, viscid substance. *meconium ileus* obstruction of the bowel by thick intestinal secretions; one way in which cystic* fibrosis can present.

media 1 *n* the middle coat of a vessel. 2 *npl* nutritive jellies used for culturing bacteria. ⇒ medium.

medial *adj* pertaining to or near the middle—**medially** *adv.*

median *adj* the middle. *median line* an imaginary line passing through the centre of the body from a point between the eyes to between the apposed feet.

mediastinoscopy *n* a minor surgical procedure for visual inspection of the mediastinum. May be combined with biopsy of lymph nodes for histological examination.

mediastinum *n* the space between the lungs containing the heart and great vessels—**mediastinal** *adj.*

medical diagnosis attribution of the disease exhibited by a patient into a specific category, using an international classification of same. Some people have multiple medical diagnoses and occasionally a patient's characteristics cannot be allocated to a specific disease category, an example being pyrexia of unknown origin.

medical history the main objective of a history taken by a doctor is to enable the making of a medical diagnosis, according to an international classification.

medical jurisprudence ⇒ forensic medicine.

medical model in a nursing context, the term signifies that the focus of nursing is the medical diagnosis allocated by the doctor. ⇒ diagnosis.

medicament *n* a remedy or medicine. ⇒ drug.

medicated *adj* impregnated with a drug or medicine.

medication *n* therapeutic substance taken orally or administered by injection subcutaneously, intramuscularly, intravenously; also by inhalation, suppository and topical application. ⇒ drug, noncompliance, skin patch.

medicinal *adj* pertaining to a medicine.

medicine *n* **1** science or art of healing, especially as distinguished from surgery* and obstetrics*. **2** a therapeutic substance. ⇒ drug.

medicochirurgical *adj* pertaining to both medicine and surgery.

medicosocial *adj* pertaining to medicine and sociology.

mediolateral *adj* pertaining to the middle and one side.

Mediterranean anaemia thalassaemia*.

Mediterranean fever a genetically inherited disease characterized by polyserositis*.

medium *n* a substance used in bacteriology for the growth of organisms—**media** *pl.*

medulla *n* **1** the marrow in the centre of a long bone. **2** the soft internal portion of glands, e.g. kidneys, adrenals, lymph nodes, etc. *medulla oblongata* the upper part of the spinal cord between the foramen magnum of the occipital bone and the pons cerebri—**medullary** *adj.*

medullated *adj* containing or surrounded by a medulla* or marrow, particularly referring to nerve fibres.

medulloblastoma *n* malignant, rapidly growing tumour occurring in children; appears in the midline of the cerebellum.

megacephalic *adj* (*syn* macrocephalic, megalocephalic) large headed.

megacolon *n* dilatation and hypertrophy of the colon. *aganglionic megacolon* due to congenital absence of ganglionic cells in a distant segment of the large bowel with loss of motor function resulting in hypertrophic dilatation of the normal proximal colon. *acquired megacolon* associated with chronic constipation in the presence of normal ganglion cell innervation: it can accompany amoebic or ulcerative colitis.

megakaryocyte *n* large cell with lobulated nucleus which produces the blood platelets.

megaloblast *n* a large, nucleated, primitive red blood cell formed where there is a deficiency of vitamin B_{12} or folic acid—**megaloblastic** *adj.*

megalocephalic *adj* ⇒ megacephalic.

megalomania *n* delusion of grandeur, characteristic of GPI*.

Meibomian cyst a cyst* on the edge of the eyelid from retained secretion of the Meibomian glands.

Meibomian glands sebaceous glands lying in grooves on the inner surface of the eyelids, their ducts opening on the free margins of the lids.

Meigs syndrome a benign fibroma of the ovary associated with ascites* and hydrothorax*.

meiosis *n* the process which, through two successive cell divisions, leads to the formation of mature gametes, ova* and sperm*. The process starts by the pairing of the partner chromosomes, which then separate from each other at the meiotic divisions, so that the diploid* chromosome number (i.e. 23 pairs in man) is halved to 23 chromosomes, only one member of each original pair: this set constitutes the haploid complement. ⇒ mitosis.

melaena *n* black, tar-like stools. Evidence of gastrointestinal bleeding.

melancholia *n* term reserved in psychiatry to mean severe forms of depression—**melancholic** *adj.*

melanin *n* a black pigment found in hair, skin and the choroid of the eye.

melanoma *n* a tumour arising from the pigment-producing cells of the deeper layers in the skin, or of the eye. *malignant* *melanoma* the most serious form of skin cancer. The incidence is rising worldwide, especially in countries populated with fair-skinned races. Thought to be caused mainly by intense exposure to sunlight—**melanomata** *pl,* **melanomatous** *adj.*

melanosarcoma *n* one form of malignant melanoma—**melanosarcomata** *pl,* **melanosarcomatous** *adj.*

melanosis *n* dark pigmentation of surfaces as in sunburn, Addison's disease, etc.—**melanotic** *adj.*

melatonin *n* a catecholamine* hormone produced by the pineal gland. It appears to inhibit numerous endocrine functions.and to decrease pigmentation of the skin.

melitensis *n* ⇒ brucellosis.

membrane *n* a thin lining or covering substance—**membranous** *adj. basement membrane* a thin layer beneath the epithelium of mucous surfaces. *cell membrane* thin, semipermeable membrane surrounding the cytoplasm of cells. *hyaloid membrane* the transparent capsule surrounding the vitreous humor of the eye. *mucous membrane* contains glands which secrete mucus. It lines the cavities and passages that communicate with the exterior of the body. *serous membrane* a lubricating membrane lining the closed cavities, and reflected over their enclosed organs. *synovial membrane* the membrane lining the intraarticular parts of bones and ligaments. It does not cover the articular surfaces. *tympanic membrane* the eardrum.

memory lapses many adults experience a memory loss and some time later retrieve the appropriate information. Many people experience increasing incidents as they become older. ⇒ Alzheimer's disease, dementia.

menarche *n* when the menstrual periods commence.

Mendel's law the fundamental theory of heredity and its laws, evolved by an Austrian monk, Gregor Mendel. The laws determine the inheritance of different characters, particularly the interaction of dominant and recessive traits in cross-breeding, the maintenance of the purity of such characters during hereditary transmission and the independent segregation of genetically different characteristics (see Fig. 5). ⇒ gene.

Mendelson syndrome inhalation of regurgitated stomach contents, which can cause rapid death from anoxia, or it may produce extensive lung damage or pulmonary oedema with severe bronchospasm.

Menière's disease distension of membranous labyrinth of inner ear from excess fluid. Pressure causes failure of function of nerve of hearing and balance, thus there is fluctuating deafness, tinnitus and repeated attacks of vertigo, which may be accompanied by vomiting.

meninges *npl* the surrounding membranes of the brain and spinal cord. They are three in number: (a) the dura mater (outer) (b) arachnoid membrane (middle) (c) pia mater (inner)—**meninx** *sing,* **meningeal** *adj.*

meningioma *n* a slowly growing fibrous tumour arising in the meninges—**meningiomata** *pl,* **meningiomatous** *adj.*

meningism *n* (*syn* meningismus) a condition presenting with signs and symptoms of meningitis (e.g. neck stiffness); meningitis does not develop.

meningitis *n* inflammation of the meninges. The main causative organisms are *Haemophilus influenzae* Type B (Hib), *Neisseria meningitidis* (meningococcus) and *Streptococcus pneumoniae*

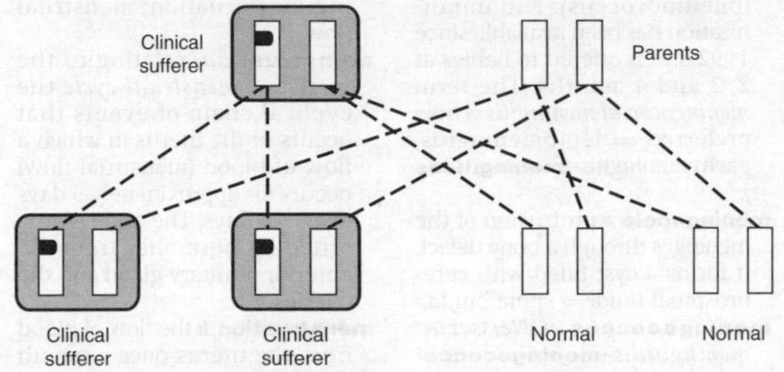

Autosomal dominant inheritance

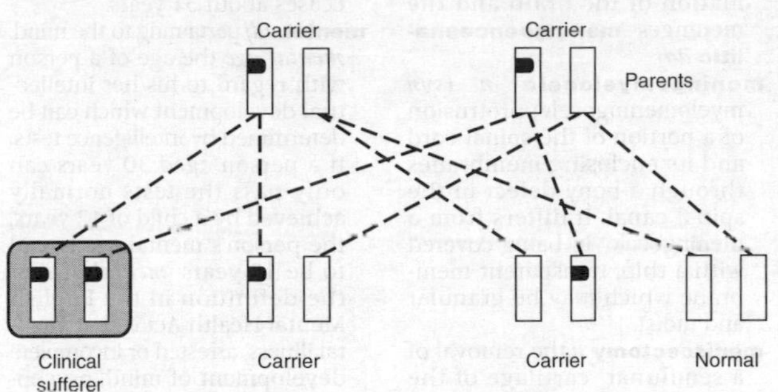

Autosomal recessive inheritance

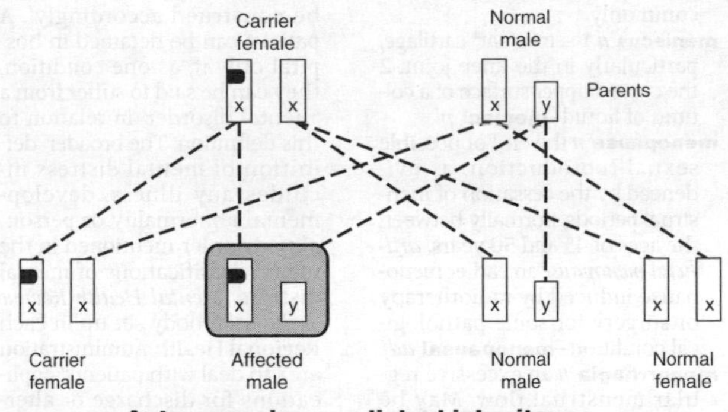

Autorecessive sex-linked inheritance

■ **Fig. 5** Mendelian laws of inheritance: how characteristics are inherited via dominant and recessive genes.

(pneumococcus). Hib immunization has been available since 1992 and is offered to babies at 2, 3 and 4 months. The term *meningococcal meningitis* is now preferred. ⇒ leptomeningitis, pachymeningitis—**meningitides** *pl.*

meningocele *n* protrusion of the meninges through a bony defect. It forms a cyst filled with cerebrospinal fluid. ⇒ spina bifida.

meningococcus *n Neisseria* meningitidis*—**meningococcal** *adj.*

meningoencephalitis *n* inflammation of the brain and the meninges—**meningoencephalitic** *adj.*

meningomyelocele *n* (*syn* myelomeningocele) protrusion of a portion of the spinal cord and its enclosing membranes through a bony defect in the spinal canal. It differs from a meningocele* in being covered with a thin, transparent membrane which may be granular and moist.

meniscectomy *n* the removal of a semilunar* cartilage of the knee joint, following injury and displacement. The medial cartilage is damaged most commonly.

meniscus *n* **1** semilunar* cartilage, particularly in the knee joint. **2** the curved upper surface of a column of liquid—**menisci** *pl.*

menopause *n* the end of possible sexual reproduction, as evidenced by the cessation of menstrual periods, normally between the ages of 45 and 50 years. *artificial menopause* an earlier menopause induced by radiotherapy or surgery for some pathological condition—**menopausal** *adj.*

menorrhagia *n* an excessive regular menstrual flow. May be associated with IUD*, fibroids or systemic disease.

menses *n* the sanguineous fluid discharged from the uterus during menstruation; menstrual flow.

menstrual *adj* relating to the menses*. *menstrual cycle* the cyclical chain of events that occurs in the uterus in which a flow of blood (menstrual flow) occurs for approximately 5 days every 28 days. The cycle is governed by hormones from the anterior pituitary gland and the ovaries.

menstruation *n* the flow of blood from the uterus once a month in the female. It commences about the age of 13 years and ceases about 51 years.

mental *adj* pertaining to the mind. *mental age* the age of a person with regard to his/her intellectual development which can be determined by intelligence tests. If a person aged 30 years can only pass the tests normally achieved by a child of 12 years, the person's mental age is said to be 12 years. *mental distress* the definition in the English Mental Health Act is that 'mental illness, arrested or incomplete development of mind, psychopathic disorder and any other disorder or disability of mind, and "mentally disordered" shall be construed accordingly'. A patient can be detained in hospital only if, as one condition, they can be said to suffer from a 'mental disorder' in relation to this definition. The broader definition of mental distress includes any illness, developmental abnormality or personality disorder mentioned in the major classifications of mental distress. *Mental Health Review Tribunal* a body set up in each Regional Health Administration area to deal with patients' applications for discharge or alteration of their conditions of detention in hospital (in England and Wales, with a separate, similar system in Northern Ireland).

In Scotland, the same function is performed by requests for review of detention to the Mental Welfare Commission, or appeal to the sheriff. *Approved Social Worker (ASW)* appointed by the Local Health Authority to deal with: (a) applications for compulsory or emergency admission to hospital, or for conveyance of patients there (b) applications concerning guardianship, the functions of the nearest relative, or acting as nearest relative if so appointed (c) returning patients absent without leave, or apprehending patients escaped from legal custody. In addition the ASW may have a wide range of functions in the care and aftercare of the mentally disordered in the community. This includes home visiting, training centres, clubs and general supervision of the discharged patient. The Scottish equivalent is the Mental Health Officer (MHO). The MHO is also a social worker with special experience in mental disorder (mental distress is the preferred term). MHOs can make application for admission of a patient under the Mental Health (Scotland) Act 1984, or for guardianship under the same Act. They have a duty to provide reports on the social circumstances of patients who are detained in hospital and of certain other functions under the Act.

mental defence/coping mechanisms processes which the mind uses, sometimes consciously and sometimes unconsciously, in response to particular life experiences. ⇒ compensation, conversion, denial, displacement, fantasy, identification, projection, rationalization, regression, repression, sublimation, suppression, withdrawal.

mental handicap ⇒ learning disability.

mental health a sense of well-being in the emotional, personal, spiritual and social domains of people's lives. ⇒ Mental health nursing box.

menthol *n* mild analgesic obtained from oil of peppermint. Used in liniments and ointments for rheumatism, and as an inhalation or drops for nasal catarrh.

mentoanterior *adj* forward position of the fetal chin in the maternal pelvis in a face presentation.

mentoposterior *adj* backward position of the fetal chin in the maternal pelvis in a face presentation.

mentorship *n* a system which provides support to students during their training. A mentor–a qualified and experienced nurse–works with the student on clinical placements, ensuring he or she receives the appropriate experience. ⇒ preceptorship.

mercurialism *n* toxic effects on human body of mercury, the ancient cure for syphilis. May result from use of calomel-containing teething powders or calomel (as an abortifacient). Symptomatology includes stomatitis, loosening of teeth, gastroenteritis and skin eruptions.

mercurochrome *n* a red dye containing mercury in combination. Has antiseptic properties.

mercury *n* the only common metal that is liquid at room temperature. Used in measuring instruments such as thermometers and sphygmomanometers. Forms two series of salts: mercurous ones are univalent, and mercuric ones are bivalent. ⇒ mercurialism.

mesarteritis *n* inflammation of the middle coat of an artery.

mesencephalon *n* the midbrain.

mesentery *n* a large sling-like fold of peritoneum passing between a portion of the intestine and the

MENTAL HEALTH NURSING

Mental health nursing is the branch of nursing which is concerned with helping people to enhance, maintain or improve their emotional, personal, spiritual and social lives. It is an area of care that was first called 'mental nursing' and then 'psychiatric nursing'. Psychiatric nurses, increasingly, care for people in the community as the UK government's policy of community care develops. Modern mental health nursing concentrates, particularly, on the enhancement or maintenance of mental health and one of the aims of mental health nursing is to help prevent the onset of breakdown or illness where this is possible. The skills of a mental health nurse include a range of interpersonal and therapeutic skills, such as listening, responding, problem-solving and enabling the release of emotion.

The Butterworth Report (Department of Health 1994) highlighted the need for a flexible response to future mental health needs. Its recommendations included:

- An improvement in the understanding of racial and cultural needs.
- The establishment of research.
- Representation and participation of service users.
- Links with the criminal justice system.
- A focus on work with severe mental illness.
- Availability of mental health nursing skills to the primary health care team.
- Establishment of clinical supervision.
- Development of a framework for good practice.

Mental health nursing is a branch of the nursing diploma course and of many bachelor's degree courses in nursing. Increasingly, it can also be studied at a postgraduate level.

posterior abdominal wall, containing blood vessels, nerves and lymphatics (see Fig. 9, p. 281)—**mesenteric** *adj.*

mesothelioma *n* a rapidly fatal tumour that spreads over the mesothelium of the pleura, pericardium or peritoneum. Of current interest because of its association with the asbestos industry.

mestoderm *n* the middle of the three primitive germ layers of the embryo, lying between the ectoderm* and the endoderm*. From it are derived the connective tissue, bone, cartilage, muscle, blood and blood vessels, lymphatics, lymphoid glands, pleura, pericardium, peritoneum, kidneys and gonads.

metabolic *adj* pertaining to metabolism. *basal metabolic rate (BMR)* the expression of basal metabolism in terms of kJ per m^2 of body surface per hour—**metabolically** *adv.*

metabolism *n* the continuous series of chemical changes in the living body by which life is maintained. Food and tissues are broken down (catabolism), new substances are created for growth and rebuilding (anabolism) and energy is released in anabolism and utilized in catabolism and heat production ⇒ adenosine diphosphate, adenosine triphosphate—**metabolic** *adj. basal metabolism* the minimum energy expended in the maintenance of respiration, circulation, peristalsis, muscle tonus, body temperature and other vegetative functions of the body.

metabolite *n* by-product of metabolism. An *essential metabolite* is a substance which is necessary for normal metabolism, e.g. vitamins.

metacarpophalangeal *adj* pertaining to the metacarpus* and the phalanges*.

metacarpus *n* the five bones which form that part of the hand between the wrist and fingers—**metacarpal** *adj*.

metastasis *n* the spread of tumour cells from one part of the body to another, usually by blood or lymph. A secondary growth—**metastases** *pl*, **metastasize** *vi*.

metatarsalgia *n* pain under the metatarsal heads. *Morton's metatarsalgia* neuralgia caused by a neuroma on the digital nerve, most commonly that supplying the third toe cleft.

metatarsophalangeal *adj* pertaining to the metatarsus and the phalanges.

metatarsus *n* the five bones of the foot between the ankle and the toes—**metatarsal** *adj*.

meteorism *n* ⇒ tympanites.

methadone *n* a synthetic morphine*-like analgesic, but with a reduced sedative action. Can be given orally or by injection. Particularly valuable in visceral pain and useful in the treatment of useless cough. May cause addiction if treatment is prolonged. Can be used in withdrawal programmes for heroin addicts.

methaemalbumin *n* abnormal compound in blood from combination of haem with plasma albumin.

methaemoglobin *n* a form of haemoglobin consisting of a combination of globin with an oxidized haem, containing ferric iron. This pigment is unable to transport oxygen. It may be formed following the administration of a wide variety of drugs, including the sulphonamides*. It may be present in the blood as a result of a congenital abnormality.

methaemoglobinaemia *n* methaemoglobin in the blood. If large quantities are present, individuals may show cyanosis, but otherwise no abnormality except, in severe cases, breathlessness on exertion, because the methaemoglobin cannot transport oxygen—**methaemoglobinaemic** *adj*.

methaemoglobinuria *n* methaemoglobin* in the urine—**methaemoglobinuric** *adj*.

methane *n* CH_4 a colourless, odourless, inflammable gas produced as a result of putrefaction and fermentation of organic matter.

methicillin *n* a semisynthetic penicillin given by injection and active against penicillin-resistant staphylococci. The emergence of resistant strains of staphylococci has led to the decline of methicillin and more potent derivatives such as cloxacillin are now preferred.

methionine *n* one of the essential sulphur-containing amino* acids. Occasionally used in hepatitis, paracetamol overdose and other conditions associated with liver damage.

methylated spirit alcohol containing 5% of wood naphtha to make it nonpotable. The methylated spirit used for spirit stoves etc. is less pure, and is coloured to distinguish it from the above.

methylcellulose *n* a compound which absorbs water and gives bulk to intestinal contents thus encouraging peristalsis.

metritis *n* inflammation of the uterus.

metropathia haemorrhagica irregular episodes of anovular uterine bleeding due to excessive and unopposed oestrogens* in the blood stream. Usually associated with a follicular cyst in the ovary.

metrorrhagia *n* uterine bleeding between the menstrual periods.

Michel's clips small metal clips used instead of sutures for the closure of a wound.

microangiopathy *n* thickening and reduplication of the basement membrane in blood vessels. It occurs in diabetes mellitus, the collagen diseases, infections and cancer. Common manifestations are kidney failure and purpura.

microbe *n* ⇒ microorganism—**microbial, microbic** *adj.*

microbiology *n* the science that studies microorganisms and their effects on humans and animals. A medical microbiologist is a member of the Infection Control Committee—**microbiological** *adj,* **microbiologically** *adv.*

microcephalic *adj* pertaining to an abnormally small head.

microchylors *npl* emulsified fat droplets that have been acted upon by the enzyme lipase, and which are capable of being absorbed into the lymphatic circulation in the villi of the small intestine.

microcirculation *n* blood flow throughout the system of smaller vessels of the body, i.e.arterioles, blood capillaries and venules.

Micrococcus *n* a genus of bacteria. Gram-positive spherical bacteria occurring in irregular masses. They comprise saprophytes, parasites and pathogens.

microcyte *n* an undersized red blood cell found especially in iron deficiency anaemia. *microcytosis* an increased number of microcytes—**microcytic** *adj.*

microenvironment *n* the environment at the microscopic or cellular level immediately surrounding the body.

microfilaria *n* a genus of tiny worms which cause filariasis*.

micrognathia *n* small jaw, especially the lower one; associated with Pierre Robin syndrome.

micron *n* a millionth part of a metre, represented by the Greek letter mu (μ).

micronutrients *npl* trace* elements. Includes the vitamins and those minerals required in very small amounts, only a few mg daily. ⇒ macronutrients.

microorganism *n* (*syn* microbe) a microscopic cell. Often synonymous with bacterium but includes virus, protozoon, rickettsia, fungus, alga and lichen.

microscopic *adj* extremely small; visible only with the aid of a microscope. ⇒ macroscopic *opp.*

Microsporum *n* a genus of fungi. Parasitic, living in keratin-containing tissues of man and animals. *Microsporum audouini* is the commonest cause of scalp ringworm*.

microsurgery *n* use of the binocular operating microscope during the performance of operations—**microsurgical** *adj.*

microvascular *adj* capillary* vessels which are too small to be seen by the naked eye.

microvascular surgery surgery carried out on blood vessels using a binocular operating microscope.

microvilli *npl* microscopic projections from the free surface of cell membranes whose purpose is to increase the exposed surface of the cell, e.g. cells of proximal convoluted tubules, intestinal epithelium.

micturating cystogram after intravenous injection of a contrast medium (or, more commonly, after contrast is introduced via a urinary catheter until micturating begins), sequential X-rays are taken during the act of passing urine. Can be part of an investigation into urinary incontinence.

micturition *n* (*syn* urination) the act of passing urine.

middle ear (tympanum) an air-containing cavity bounded by the tympanic membrane on the outer side and the internal ear (cochlea*) on the inner side. ⇒ ear, glue ear, grommet.

midriff *n* the diaphragm*.

midwife *n* (mid=with; wife= woman) a person, usually a woman, who has undergone specific role preparation and who attends an expectant mother in childbirth; she also teaches and supports women during pregnancy and after the birth.

migraine *n* recurrent localized headaches which are often associated with vomiting and visual and sensory disturbances (the aura); caused, it is thought, by intracranial vasoconstriction—**migrainous** *adj.*

milestone *n* a 'norm' against which the physical, social and psychological development of a child is assessed. Used especially by health visitors, paediatric and school nurses.

miliaria *n* (*syn* strophulus) prickly heat common in the tropics, and affects waistline, cubital fossae and chest. Vesicular and erythematous eruption, caused by blocking of sweat ducts and their subsequent rupture, or their infection by fungi or bacteria.

miliary *adj* resembling a millet seed. *miliary tuberculosis* ⇒ tuberculosis.

milium *n* condition in which tiny, white, cystic excrescences appear on the face, especially about the eyelids; associated with seborrhoea*.

milk *n* secretion of the mammary glands. Provided that the mother is taking an adequate diet, human milk contains all the essential nutrients required by the newborn in the correct proportions. It contains IgA and lactoferrin which increases the newborn infant's resistance to infection. Cow's milk is not recommended as a main drink for infants under one year of age. *milk sugar* lactose*.

Miller-Abbot tube a double lumen rubber tube used for intestinal suction. The second channel leads to a balloon near the tip of the tube. This balloon is inflated when the tube reaches the duodenum and it is then carried down the intestine by peristaltic activity.

Milton *n* a stabilized solution of sodium hypochlorite. Used as 2.5–5% solution for wounds and other antiseptic purposes, as 1% solution for sterilizing babies' feeding bottles. In wounds it has a chemical debriding action which is not specific to necrotic tissue.

Milwaukee brace a body splint which is worn at all times during the treatment period for correction of spinal curvature (scoliosis). It applies fixed traction between the occiput and the pelvis.

mineralocorticoid *n* ⇒ aldosterone.

minerals *npl* inorganic substances which play a vital role in some of the body's functions.

miner's anaemia hookworm disease. ⇒ ancylostomiasis.

miner's lung ⇒ haematite.

miosis (myosis) *n* constriction of the pupil of the eye.

miotic (myotic) *adj* pertaining to or producing miosis*, usually refers to a drug.

miscarriage *n* spontaneous loss of pregnancy during the first or second trimester. ⇒ abortion.

missed abortion ⇒ abortion.

Misuse of Drugs Act (1971) designed to control the manufacture, sale, prescribing and dispensing of certain habit-forming drugs to which an addiction may arise; these are called 'controlled' drugs and are available to the public by medical prescription only; heavy penalties may follow any illegal sale or supply. The principal drugs concerned are opium*, morphine*, cocaine*, diamorphine*, cannabis* indica and the many synthetic morphine substitutes such as pethidine*.

mitochondrion *n* membrane-bound cytoplasmic organelles that are the principal sites of ATP synthesis. They contain DNA, RNA and ribosomes, replicate independently, and synthesize some of their own proteins—**mitrochondria** *pl.*

mitosis *n* the ordinary type of nuclear (cell) division, preceded by the faithful replication of chromosomes. Through this process, daughter cells, derived from division of a mother cell, retain the diploid chromosome number, 46 in man. ⇒ meiosis—**mitotic** *adj.*

mitral *adj* mitre-shaped, as the valve between the left atrium and ventricle of the heart (bicuspid valve). *mitral incompetence* a defect in the closure of the mitral valve whereby blood tends to flow backwards into the left atrium from the left ventricle. *mitral stenosis* narrowing of the mitral orifice, usually due to rheumatic fever. *mitral valvulotomy (valvotomy)* an operation for splitting the cusps of a stenosed mitral valve.

mittelschmerz abdominal pain midway between menstrual periods, at time of ovulation.

MLNS *abbr* mucocutaneous* lymph node syndrome.

MMV *abbr* mandatory minute volume.

mobility *n* in a nursing context, refers to a person's ability to walk, rise from and return to a bed, chair, lavatory and so on, as well as movements of the upper limbs. It is included in an assessment of a patient's activities of living in order to plan individualized nursing care.

moist wound healing achieved by application of an occlusive, semipermeable dressing which permits the exudate to collect under the film to carry out its bactericidal functions. ⇒ LyofoamC, OpSite.

molar teeth the teeth 4th and 5th in the deciduous dentition and 6th, 7th and 8th in the permanent dentition, used for grinding food.

mole *n* a pigmented area on the skin, usually brown. Some moles are flat, some are raised and occasionally have hairs growing from them. Malignant changes can occur in them, characterized by changes in colour, size and shape. ⇒ naevus.

molecule *n* a combination of two or more atoms to form a specific chemical substance—**molecular** *adj.*

mollities *n* softness. *mollities ossium* osteomalacia*.

molluscum *n* a soft tumour. *molluscum contagiosum* an infectious condition common in infants caused by a virus. Tiny translucent papules with a central depression are formed. *molluscum fibrosum* the superficial tumours of von Recklinghausen's* disease.

monarticular *adj* relating to one joint.

Mönckeberg's sclerosis senile degenerative change resulting in calcification of the median muscular layer in arteries, especially of the limbs; leads to intermittent claudication and possibly to gangrene, if atherosclerosis coexists.

mongol *n* a person afflicted with Down* syndrome.

mongolism *n* ⇒ Down syndrome.

Monilia *n* ⇒ Candida.

moniliasis *n* ⇒ candidiasis.

Monitor *n* an anglicized version of the Rush Medicus quality assurance programme for use in hospitals. ⇒ quality assurance.

monitoring *n* sequential recording. Term usually reserved for automatic visual display of such measurements as temperature, pulse, respiration and blood pressure.

monoamine oxidase an enzyme which causes the breakdown of serotonin* and catecholamines* in the brain. *monoamine oxidase inhibitors (MAOIs)* drugs which inhibit this action, used in the treatment of exogenous or reactive depression. In patients receiving MAOIs, certain drugs (e.g. adrenaline, noradrenaline and amphetamine), alcohol and certain foods (cheese, broad beans, Marmite and Bovril) should be avoided as the build-up of substances normally broken down by monoamine oxidase can cause serious episodic hypertension.

monoclonal *adj* refers to antibodies produced by fusion of an immunoglobulin-producing cell with a lymphocyte making a specific antibody. The cell and its progeny continue to make a single antibody. Widely used for production of highly specific antibodies for diagnostic and therapeutic uses.

monocular *adj* pertaining to one eye.

monocyte *n* a mononuclear* white blood cell—**monocytic** *adj.*

monomania *n* obsession with a single idea.

mononuclear *adj* with a single nucleus. Usually refers to a type of blood cell (monocyte), the largest of the cells in the normal blood with a round, oval or indented nucleus.

mononucleosis *n* an increase in the number of circulating monocytes (mononuclear* cells) in the blood. *infectious mononucleosis* ⇒ infectious*.

monoplegia *n* paralysis of only one limb—**monoplegic** *adj.*

monosaccharide *n* a simple sugar carbohydrate with the general formula CH_2O. Examples are glucose*, fructose* and galactose*.

monosodium glutamate a chemical which can be added to food as a flavour enhancer. Often found in Chinese cooking and in many preprepared meals.

monosomy *n* state resulting from the absence of a chromosome from an otherwise diploid* chromosome complement (e.g. monosomy for chromosome 21).

monovular *adj* ⇒ uniovular.

mons veneris the eminence formed by the pad of fat which lies over the pubic bone in the female and covered by pubic hair after puberty.

mood *n* an involuntary state of mind or feeling. Variations in mood are normal but frequent swings from depression* to over-excitement may be considered abnormal. ⇒ mania.

Mooren's ulcer a gutter-like excoriation of the peripheral cornea with a tendency to spread.

morbidity *n* the state of being diseased.

morbilli *n* ⇒ measles.

morbilliform *adj* describes a rash resembling that of measles*.

moribund *adj* in a dying state.

Moro reflex (startle reflex) a reflex normally present in the newborn. On being startled the baby throws out its arms, then brings them together in an embracing movement. An asymmetrical response may indicate nerve damage or a fracture of the arm or clavicle.

morphine *n* one of the narcotics*. Derived from opium. Widely used as a powerful analgesic, particularly in advanced pain, e.g. due to terminal cancer. May cause some respiratory depression, especially in full doses. Vomiting and constipation are other associated side-effects.

morphology *n* the science which deals with the form and structure of living things—**morphological** *adj*, **morphologically** *adv*.

mortality *n* number or frequency of deaths. *mortality rate* the death rate; the ratio of the total number of deaths to the total population.

mortification *n* death of tissue. ⇒ gangrene.

Morton's metatarsalgia ⇒ metatarsalgia.

morula *n* cleavage of the fertilised ovum gives rise to the morula which is a solid ball of cells.

mosquito-transmitted haemorrhagic fevers infections which occur mainly in a tropical climate: they result in bleeding particularly into joints, muscles and the skin. The important ones are chikungunya, dengue, Rift valley fever and yellow fever.

motile *adj* capable of spontaneous movement—**motility** *n*.

motion *n* an evacuation of the bowel.

motivate *v* provision of an incentive or purpose for ensuing action.

motive *n* that which induces a person to act, examples being circumstance, desire, fear.

motor *adj* pertaining to action. ⇒ neurone.

motor neurone disease a progressive degenerative disease of the motor part of the nervous system. It occurs in middle age and results in increasing muscle weakness and wasting.

mould *n* a multicellular fungus. Often used synonymously with fungus (excluding the yeasts). A member of the plant kingdom with no differentation into root, stem or leaf, and without chlorophyll. Structurally it consists of filaments or hyphae, which aggregate into a mycelium. Propagation is by means of spores. Occurs in infinite variety, as common saprophytes contaminating foodstuffs, and more rarely as pathogens.

moulding *n* the compression of the fetal head during its passage through the genital tract in labour.

mountain sickness symptoms of sickness, tachycardia and dyspnoea caused by low oxygen content of rarefied air at high altitude.

mouth *n* a cavity bounded by the closed lips and facial muscles, the hard and soft palate, and lower jaw. It contains the upper and lower teeth and the tongue. Glands pour saliva into it. Some drugs cause a dry mouth and patients should be warned of this side-effect and advised to drink more frequently to keep the mouth comfortably moist. *mouth care* (oral hygiene) adequate use of a small baby toothbrush is the most effective way of removing plaque from another person's teeth. Sordes are softened with glycerine 20%, then removed by a swab dipped in mouthwash solution wrapped round a finger. Vaseline on lips lubricates for longer than glycerine. Adequate hydration is essential in preventing and treating a dirty mouth.

MRI *abbr* magnetic* resonance imaging.

MRSA *abbr* methicillin-resistant *Staphylococcus aureus*.

MS *abbr* ⇒ multiple sclerosis.

mucilage *n* the solution of a gum in water—**mucilaginous** *adj*.

mucin *n* a mixture of glycoproteins found in and secreted by many cells and glands. Can be used as a diagnostic indicator for gastric metaplasia—**mucinous** *adj*.

mucinase *n* a specific mucin-dissolving substance contained in some aerosols. Useful in cystic fibrosis.

mucinolysis *n* dissolution of mucin*—**mucinolytic** *adj*.

mucocele *n* distension of a cavity with mucus*.

mucocutaneous *adj* pertaining to mucous membrane* and skin. *mucocutaneous lymph node syndrome (MLNS)* a disease affecting mainly babies and children first noticed in Japan in the late 1960s. Characterized by fever, dry lips, red mouth and strawberry-like tongue. A rash in a glove-and-stocking distribution (i.e. on hands and legs) is followed by desquamation. There is cervical adenitis, polymorphonuclear leucocytosis and a raised ESR.

mucoid *adj* resembling mucus*.

mucolytics *npl* drugs which reduce viscosity of secretion from the respiratory tract.

mucopolysaccharidoses *npl* a group of inherited neurometabolic conditions in which genetically determined specific enzyme defects lead to accumulation of abnormal amounts of mucopolysaccharides. ⇒ gargoylism, Hunter syndrome.

mucopurulent *adj* containing mucus and pus.

mucopus *n* mucus containing pus.

mucosa *n* a mucous membrane*—**mucosae** *pl*, **mucosal** *adj*.

mucositis *n* inflammation of a mucous membrane*.

mucous *adj* pertaining to or containing mucus*. *mucous colitis* also called mucomembranous colitis. Possibly a functional disorder, manifested by passage of mucus in the stool, obstinate constipation and occasional colic. *mucous polypus* a growth (adenoma) of mucous membrane which becomes pedunculated. *mucous membrane* ⇒ membrane.

mucoviscidosis *n* cystic* fibrosis.

mucus *n* the viscid fluid secreted by mucous glands—**mucous, mucoid** *adj*.

multicellular *adj* constructed of many cells.

multidisciplinary team within the health care system, a varying number of professionals are working towards the same objective—optimal independence of the patient/client according to his or her circumstances and available resources.

multigravida *n* (*syn* multipara) a woman who has had more than one pregnancy—**multigravidae** *pl*.

multilobular *adj* possessing many lobes.

multilocular *adj* possessing many small cysts, loculi or pockets.

multinuclear *adj* possessing many nuclei, e.g. hepatocytes—**multinucleate** *adj*.

multipara a woman who has had more than one birth—**multiparae** *pl*.

multiple sclerosis (MS) (*syn* disseminated sclerosis) now considered as one of the muscular dystrophies. It is a variably progressive disease of the nervous system, most commonly first affecting young adults in which patchy, degenerative changes occur in nerve sheaths in the brain, spinal cord and optic nerves, followed by sclerosis*. The presenting symptoms can be diverse, ranging from diplopia to weakness or unsteadiness of a limb; disturbances of micturition are common. Characterized by periods of remission followed by a worsening of the disease.

mumps *n* (*syn* infectious parotitis) an acute, specific inflammation of the parotid* glands, caused by a virus.

Munchausen syndrome patients consistently produce false stories so they receive needless medical investigations, operations and treatments. *Munchausen syndrome by proxy* is the term used when the mother produces false stories for her child.

mural *adj* pertaining to the wall of a cavity, organ or vessel.

murmur *n* (*syn* bruit) abnormal sound heard on auscultation of heart or great vessels. *presystolic murmur* characteristic of mitral stenosis in regular rhythm.

Musca *n* genus of the common house-fly, capable of transmitting many enteric infections.

muscle *n* strong, contractile tissue which produces movement in the body—**muscular** *adj. cardiac muscle* makes up the middle wall of the heart; it is involuntary, striated and innervated by autonomic nerves. *skeletal muscle* surrounds the skeleton; it is voluntary, striated and innervated by the peripheral nerves of the central nervous system. *visceral (internal) muscle* is non-striated and involuntary and is innervated by the autonomic nerves. *muscle relaxants* a group of drugs which reduce tension in muscles. Widely used in surgery, in tetanus to prevent spasm and in mechanically aided respiration. Muscle relaxants paralyse all skeletal muscles, including those of breathing. They have no sedative action.

muscular dystrophies a group of genetically transmitted diseases; they are all characterized by progressive atrophy of different groups of muscles with loss of strength and increasing disability and deformity. Pseudohypertrophic or Duchenne type is the most severe. Presents in early childhood. ⇒ Duchenne muscular dystrophy.

muscular rheumatism ⇒ fibrositis.

musculature *n* the muscular system, or any part of it.

musculocutaneous *adj* pertaining to muscle and skin.

musculoskeletal *adj* pertaining to the muscular and skeletal systems.

music therapy may be used as an aid to socialisation and expression or to help people with physical or learning disabilities to keep moving, listening and thinking.

mustine *n* a nitrogen* mustard.

mutagen *n* an agent which induces gene or chromosome mutation.

mutagenesis *n* the production of mutations—**mutagenic, mutagenetic** *adj*, **mutagenetically** *adv*.

mutagenicity *n* the capacity to produce gene mutations or chromosome aberrations.

mutant *n* a cell (or individual) which carries a genetic change or mutation.

mutation *n* an alteration in genes or chromosomes of a living cell gives rise to genetic change, as a result of which the characters of the cell alter. The change is heritable. *induced mutation* a gene mutation or change produced by known agents outside the cell that interact with and affect the chromosomal DNA and may alter chromosome structure or number, e.g. ionizing radiation and mutagenic chemicals, ultraviolet radiation, etc. *spontaneous mutation* a genetic mutation taking place without apparent influence from outside the cell.

mute *adj* unable to speak.

mutilation *n* the removal of a limb or other part of the body. It results in a change of body image, to which there has to be considerable physical, psychological and social adjustment for a successful outcome.

mutism *n* (*syn* dumbness) inability or refusal to speak. It may be due to congenital causes, the most common being deafness; it may be the result of physical disease, the most common being a stroke, and it can be a manifestation of mental disease.

myalgia *n* pain in the muscles—**myalgic** *adj. epidemic myalgia* ⇒ Bornholm disease.

myalgic encephalomyelitis debilitating illness which is difficult to diagnose and which can last for years. Its many symptoms include malaise and exhaustion, inability to concentrate, digestive problems, memory loss and depression.

myasthenia *n* muscular weakness—**myasthenic** *adj. myasthenia gravis* a disorder characterized by marked fatiguability of voluntary muscles, especially those of the face and neck. Due to a deficiency of acetylcholine, a functional abnormality of acetylcholine or an excess of cholinesterase at neuromuscular junctions. There is considerable evidence for an autoimmune process.

myasthenic crisis a sudden deterioration with weakness of respiratory muscles due to an increase in severity of myasthenia. It is distinguished from cholinergic* crisis by giving edrophonium chloride 10 mg intravenously. Marked improvement confirms myasthenic crisis. ⇒ edrophonium test.

mycelium *n* a mass of branching filaments (hyphae) of moulds or fungi—**mycelial** *adj.*

mycetoma *n* ⇒ madura foot.

Mycobacterium *n* a genus of rod-shaped acid-fast bacteria. *Mycobacterium avium* ⇒ avian. *Mycobacterium leprae* causes leprosy and *Mycobacterium tuberculosis* causes tuberculosis.

mycologist *n* a person who has expert knowledge of mycology* and the methods used to study it.

mycology *n* the study of fungi—**mycological** *adj,* **mycologically** *adv.*

Mycoplasma *n* a genus of microscopic organisms considered the smallest free-living organisms. Some are parasites, some are saprophytes and others are pathogens. *Mycoplasma pneumoniae* causes primary atypical pneumonia, previously called viral pneumonia. *Mycoplasma hominis* is associated with inflammatory disease of the female upper genital tract and *Ureaplasma* with nongonococcal urethritis.

mycosis *n* disease caused by any fungus—**mycotic** *adj. mycosis fungoides* is a chronic and usually fatal lymphomatous disease, not fungal in origin. It is manifested by generalized pruritus, followed by skin eruptions of diverse character which become infiltrated and finally develop into granulomatous ulcerating tumours.

mycotoxins *npl* the secondary metabolites of moulds or microfungi. About 100 chemical substances have been identified as mycotoxins, many capable of causing cancer as well as other diseases—**mycotoxic** *adj.*

mydriasis *n* dilation of the pupil of the eye.

mydriatics *npl* drugs which cause mydriasis*.

mydricaine *n* a mixture of atropine*, cocaine* and adrenaline*; usually used for subconjunctival injections to dilate the pupil.

myelin *n* the white, fatty substance constituting the medullary sheath of various nerve fibres.

myelitis *n* inflammation of the spinal cord.

myeloblasts *npl* the earliest identifiable cells which after several stages develop into granulocytic white blood cells—**myeloblastic** *adj.*

myelocele *n* a spina* bifida defect, commonly in the lumbar region, wherein development of the spinal cord itself has been arrested, and the central canal of the cord opens on the skin surface exposing the meninges and discharging cerebrospinal fluid.

myelocytes *npl* precursor cells of granulocytic white blood cells normally present only in bone marrow–**myelocytic** *adj*.

myelofibrosis *n* formation of fibrous tissue within the bone marrow cavity. Interferes with the formation of blood cells.

myelogenous *adj* produced in or by the bone marrow.

myelography *n* radiographic examination of the spinal canal by injection of a contrast medium into the subarachnoid space–**myelographic** *adj*, **myelograph** *n*, **myelographically** *adv*.

myeloid *adj* pertaining to the granulocyte precursor cells, myeloblasts* and myelocytes* in the bone marrow.

myeloma *n* a malignant condition arising from plasma cells, usually in the bone marrow–**myelomata** *pl*, **myelomatous** *adj*. *multiple myeloma* the formation of a number of myelomata in bones.

myelomatosis *n* plasma cell neoplasia. Crowding of the bone marrow by abnormal plasma cells; suppression of normal blood cells leads to anaemia, thrombocytopenia and neutropenia. Consequently the patient is immunosuppressed and is therefore susceptible to infection. May produce changes in serum globulins and Bence-Jones proteinuria.

myelomeningocele *n* ⇒ meningomyelocele.

myelopathy *n* disease of the spinal cord. Can be a serious complication of cervical spondylosis–**myelopathic** *adj*.

myocardial infarction death of a part of the myocardium* from deprivation of blood. The deprived tissue becomes necrotic and requires time for healing. The patient experiences a 'heart attack' with sudden intense chest pain which may radiate to arms and jaws. Because of the danger of ventricular fibrillation many patients are nursed in a coronary care or intensive care unit. ⇒ angina (pectoris), ischaemic heart disease.

myocarditis *n* inflammation of the myocardium*.

myocardium *n* the middle layer of the heart wall. ⇒ muscle–**myocardial** *adj*.

myocele *n* protrusion of a muscle through its ruptured sheath.

myoclonus *n* clonic contractions of individual or groups of muscles.

myoelectric *adj* pertaining to the electrical properties of muscle.

myofibrosis *n* excessive connective tissue in muscle. Leads to inadequate functioning of part–**myofibroses** *pl*.

myogenic *adj* originating in or starting from muscle.

myoglobin ⇒ myohaemoglobin.

myoglobinuria *n* ⇒ myohaemoglobinuria.

myohaemoglobin *n* (*syn* myoglobin) a muscle protein resembling a single subunit of haemoglobin and thus of much lower molecular weight than blood haemoglobin. It combines with the oxygen released by the erythrocytes, stores it and transports it to the muscle cell mitochondria where energy is generated for synthesis and heat production.

myohaemoglobinuria *n* (*syn* myoglobinuria) excretion of myohaemoglobin in the urine as in crush syndrome.

myokymia *n* muscle twitching. In the lower eyelid it is benign. *facial* *myokymia* may result from long use of phenothiazine* drugs; has also been observed in patients with multiple sclerosis.

myoma *n* a benign fibroid tumour of the uterine muscle tissue—**myomata** *pl,* **myomatous** *adj.*

myomalacia *n* softening of muscle, as occurs in the myocardium after infarction.

myomectomy *n* removal of uterine fibroid(s)*.

myometrium *n* the thick muscular wall of the uterus.

myoneural *adj* pertaining to muscle and nerve.

myopathy *n* any disease of the muscles. ⇒ glycogenosis—**myopathic** *adj.*

myope *n* a shortsighted person—**myopic** *adj.*

myopia *n* shortsightedness. The light rays come to a focus in front of, instead of on, the retina—**myopic** *adj.*

myoplasty *n* plastic surgery on muscle, in which portions of partly detached muscle are utilized to repair defects or deformities—**myoplastic** *adj.*

myosarcoma *n* a malignant tumour derived from muscle—**myosarcomata** *pl,* **myosarcomatous** *adj.*

myosin *n* one of the main proteins of muscle; reacts with actin in the muscle cell to cause contraction.

myosis *n* ⇒ miosis—**myotic** *adj.*

myositis *n* inflammation of a muscle. *myositis ossificans* deposition of active bone cells in muscle, resulting in hard swellings.

myotomy *n* cutting or dissection of muscle tissue.

myotonia *n* a condition in which there is prolonged contraction of muscle fibres (tonic spasm of muscle)—**myotonic** *adj.* *myotonia congenita* a genetically-determined form of congenital muscular spasticity, usually presenting in infancy and due to degeneration of anterior horn cells in the spinal cord. Fibrillation of affected muscles is characteristic.

myringitis *n* inflammation of the eardrum* (tympanic membrane).

myringoplasty *n* operation designed to close a defect in the tympanic membrane—**myringoplastic** *adj.*

myringotomy *n* incision into the eardrum* (tympanic membrane). Performed for the drainage of pus or fluid from the middle ear. Middle ear ventilation maintained by insertion of a grommet or Teflon tube.

myxoedema *n* clinical syndrome of hypothyroidism*. Patient becomes slow in movement and dull mentally; there is bradycardia, low temperature, dry skin and swelling of limbs and face. Associated with low serum thyroxine (T4) and raised thyroid stimulating hormone (TSH) levels—**myxoedematous** *adj.* *pretibial myxoedema* violaceous indurated areas of skin, usually on foreleg, in some cases of thyrotoxicosis*. May be associated with exophthalmos and clubbing of fingers.

myxoma *n* a connective tissue tumour composed largely of mucoid material—**myxomata** *pl,* **myxomatous** *adj.*

myxosarcoma *n* a malignant tumour of connective tissue with a soft, mucoid consistency—**myxosarcomata** *pl,* **myxosarcomatous** *adj.*

myxoviruses *npl* name for the influenza group of viruses.

N

nabothian follicles cystic distension of chronically inflamed cervical glands of uterus, where the duct of the gland has become obliterated by a healing epithelial covering and the normal mucus cannot escape.

Naegele's obliquity tilting of the fetal head to one or other side to decrease the transverse diameter presented to the pelvic brim.

naevoid amentia ⇒ Sturge-Weber syndrome.

naevus *n* a mole; a circumscribed lesion of the skin arising from pigment-producing cells (melanoma) or due to a developmental abnormality of blood vessels (angioma)—**naevi** *pl,* **naevoid** *adj.*

NAI *abbr* nonaccidental injury.

nails *npl* an epidermal horny cell structure forming flat plates on the dorsal surface of the terminal phalanges, differentially called toe and finger nails. *nail bed* the epidermis underlying a nail. *hang nail* a break in the continuity of cuticle surrounding a nail. *ingrowing toe nail* penetration of the nail edge into soft tissue and can be the site of painful inflammatory reaction and superimposed infection. ⇒ onychocryptosis.

named nurse ⇒ The named nurse box.

nape *n* the back of the neck; the nucha.

napkin (nappy) rash an erythema of the napkin area. It can vary from a simple erythema on the buttocks and labia/scrotum, to excoriation and maceration of the total napkin area. Usual causes are ammoniacal decomposition of urine, thrush, infantile psoriasis, allergy to detergents, excoriation from diarrhoea.

THE NAMED NURSE

The concept of the named nurse was introduced in the *Patient's Charter* of 1991, which promised that:

'Each patient will be told the name of the qualified nurse or midwife who will be responsible for his or her nursing/midwifery care when admitted to hospital; or midwife, community nurse or health visitor when in need of care in the community.'

One qualified nurse, midwife or health visitor is accountable for the care of each patient or client and, wherever possible, the same nurse should care for, or supervize care for, the same patient during the time that person needs nursing, midwifery or health visiting care.

The named nurse concept can be operated within a primary nursing, team nursing, or patient allocation model.

See also: primary nursing, team nursing.

narcissism *n* self-love. In psychiatry the narcissistic type of personality is one where the sexual love-object is the self.

narcoanalysis *n* analysis of mental content under light anaesthesia, usually an intravenous barbiturate—**narcoanalytic** *adj*, **narcoanalytically** *adv*.

narcolepsy *n* an irresistible tendency to go to sleep. It is more usual to speak of the narcolepsies rather than of narcolepsy, for sudden, repetitive attacks of sleep occurring in the daytime arise in diverse clinical conditions—**narcoleptic** *adj*.

narcosis *n* unconsciousness produced by a drug. *carbon dioxide narcosis* full bounding pulse, muscular twitchings, mental confusion and eventual coma due to increased CO_2 in the blood. *continuous narcosis* treatment by prolonged sleep by spaced administration of narcotics. Used occasionally in mental illness to cut short attacks of excitement or for severe emotional upset.

narcosynthesis *n* the building up of a clearer mental picture of an incident involving the patient by reviving memories of it, under light anaesthesia, so that both he and the therapist can examine the incident in clearer perspective.

narcotic *n, adj* describes a drug which produces abnormally deep sleep. Strong analgesic narcotics, morphine and opiates, cause profound respiratory depression which is reversible by the use of narcotic antagonists*. ⇒ hypnotics, sedative.

nares *npl* (*syn* choanae) the nostrils—**naris** *sing*. *anterior nares* the pair of openings from the exterior into the nasal cavities. *posterior nares* the pair of openings from the nasal cavities into the nasopharynx*.

nasal *adj* pertaining to the nose.

nasendoscope *n* an endoscope for viewing the nasal passages and postnasal space and larynx.

nasogastric *adj* pertaining to the nose and stomach, as passing a *nasogastric tube* via this route, usually for suction, lavage or feeding. ⇒ enteral.

nasojejunal *adj* pertaining to the nose and jejunum, usually referring to a tube passed via the nose into the jejunum.

nasolacrimal *adj* pertaining to the nose and lacrimal apparatus.

nasooesophageal *adj* pertaining to the nose and the oesophagus, as passing a tube via this route.

nasopharynx *n* the portion of the pharynx above the soft palate—**nasopharyngeal** *adj*.

natural flora ⇒ flora.

natural killer cells cells capable of mediating cytotoxic reactions without themselves being specifically sensitized against the target.

naturopathy *n* a system of therapeutics based on natural foods grown without chemical fertilizers, and medicines which are prepared from herbs, spices and plants. Advocates believe that these procedures enable the natural body processes an optimal environment for healing—**naturopathic** *adj*.

nausea *n* a feeling of impending vomiting—**nauseate** *vt*, **nauseous** *adj*.

navel *n* ⇒ umbilicus.

navicular *adj* shaped like a canoe (as in bone of the foot).

nebula *n* a greyish, corneal opacity.

nebulizer *n* an apparatus for converting a liquid into a fine spray. It can contain medicaments for application to the skin, or nose, or throat. Widely used in the treatment of asthma.

NEC *abbr* necrotizing* enterocolitis.

Necator *n* a genus of hookworms*.

necropsy *n* the examination of a dead body.

necrosis *n* localized death of tissue–**necrotic** *adj.*

necrotizing enterocolitis (NEC) a condition occurring primarily in preterm or low birthweight neonates. Probably caused by hypoxia leading to ischaemia of the bowel. Parts of the bowel wall become necrotic with the development of obstruction and peritonitis.

needlestick injury a term used to describe accidental injury with blood contaminated injection needle. Of current interest as a transmitter of hepatitis* B and AIDS. ⇒ accident form, accidental inoculation*, acquired immune deficiency syndrome.

needs *n* ⇒ human needs.

negative anxiety ⇒ anxiety.

negativism *n* active refusal to cooperate, usually shown by the patient consistently doing the exact opposite of what he is asked. Common in schizophrenia*.

negligence *n* in law, want of proper care or attention resulting in damage to another person. Medical negligence is failure by a doctor or nurse to treat a patient with that standard of care and skill commensurate with his/her training, qualifications and experience. It is a professional duty to avoid patient injury or suffering caused in this way. It can become the basis of litigation for damages.

Neisseria *n* a genus of bacteria. Gram-negative cocci, usually arranged in pairs, which are found as commensals of man and animals, e.g. *Neisseria catarrhalis,* or pathogens to man. *Neisseria gonorrhoeae* causes gonorrhoea and *Neisseria meningitidis* causes meningitis.

Nelaton's line an imaginary line joining the anterior superior iliac spine to the ischial tuberosity. The great trochanter of the femur normally lies on or below this line.

Nelson syndrome associated with a pituitary tumour. The skin changes colour, that is white becomes black and black becomes white. Almost all patients find there is an associated racial stigma.

nematodes *npl* wormlike creatures that have two sexes and an intestinal canal. Various species are parasitic to man and can be divided into two groups: (a) those that mainly live in the intestine, e.g. hookworms and whipworms (b) those that are mainly tissue parasites, e.g. guinea worms, filarial worms.

neoadjuvant therapy treatment, usually involving drugs, to reduce the size of a tumour before surgery or radiation therapy.

neologism *n* a specially coined word, often nonsensical; may express a thought disorder.

neomycin *n* an antibiotic frequently used with corticosteroids in the treatment of inflamed and infected skin conditions. Sometimes given orally for intestinal infections.

neonatal period the first 28 days after birth, during which an infant adjusts to an extrauterine environment. It is the most hazardous time for any infant. *neonatal mortality* the death rate of babies in the first month of life. *neonatal herpes* a comparatively rare disease acquired during vaginal delivery from a mother actively shedding herpes simplex virus. It is a devastating illness with a 75% mortality rate and a high incidence of severe neurological sequelae among survivors. *neonatal respiratory distress syndrome* occurs most frequently in premature infants–the more immature the greater the risk of this condition, which may be fatal. Deficiency in pulmonary surfactant leading to atelectasis and hypoxia necessitates assisted ventilation in more seriously ill infants.

neonate *n* a newborn baby up to 4 weeks old.

neonatology *n* the scientific study of the newborn.

neonatorum *adj* pertaining to the newborn.

neoplasia *n* literally, the formation of new tissue. By custom refers to the pathological process in tumour formation—**neoplastic** *adj.*

neoplasm *n* a new growth; a tumour which is either cancerous or noncancerous—**neoplastic** *adj.*

nephralgia *n* pain in the kidney. ⇒ Dietl's crisis*.

nephrectomy *n* surgical removal of a kidney.

nephritis *n* a term embracing a group of conditions in which there is either an inflammatory or an inflammatory-like reaction, focal or diffuse, in the kidneys. ⇒ glomerulonephritis, glomerulosclerosis, nephrotic syndrome, renal failure—**nephritic** *adj.*

nephrocalcinosis *n* multiple areas of calcification within the kidney.

nephrocapsulectomy *n* surgical removal of the kidney capsule. Occasionally done for polycystic* renal disease.

nephrogenic *adj* arising in or produced by the kidney.

nephrography *n* the technique of imaging renal shadow following injection of contrast medium—**nephrographical** *adj,* **nephrograph** *n,* **nephrographically** *adv.*

nephrolithiasis *n* the presence of stones in the kidney.

nephrolithotomy *n* surgical removal of a stone from the kidney. Now also accomplished by extracorporeal shock-wave lithotripsy (ESWL). ⇒ Dornier lithotriptor. *percutaneous nephrolithotomy* currently the treatment of choice: the kidney pelvis is punctured under X-ray control, and a guide wire inserted through which, using an endoscope, the stone is removed. The patient's stay in hospital has been reduced to between 2–4 days.

nephrology *n* special study of the kidneys and the diseases which afflict them.

nephron *n* the basic unit of the kidney, comprising a glomerulus*, Bowman's capsule, proximal and distal convoluted tubules, with the loop of Henle connecting them; a straight collecting tubule follows via which urine is conveyed to the renal pelvis (see Fig. 6, p. 250).

nephropathy *n* kidney disease. May be of vasomotor origin, when it is often reversible—**nephropathic** *adj.*

nephroplasty *n* any plastic operation on the kidney, especially for large aberrant renal vessels that are dissected off the urinary tract and the kidney folded laterally upon itself. ⇒ hydronephrosis.

nephropyosis *n* pus formation in the kidney.

nephrosclerosis *n* renal insufficiency from hypertensive vascular disease, developing into a clinical picture identical with that of chronic nephritis. ⇒ renal failure—**nephrosclerotic** *adj.*

nephroscope *n* an endoscope* for viewing kidney tissue. It can be designed to create a continuous flow of irrigating fluid and provide an exit for the fluid and accompanying debris—**nephroscopic** *adj.*

nephrosis *n* any degenerative, noninflammatory change in the kidney—**nephrotic** *adj.*

nephrostomy *n* a surgically established fistula from the pelvis of the kidney to the body surface.

nephrotic syndrome characterized by reduction in blood

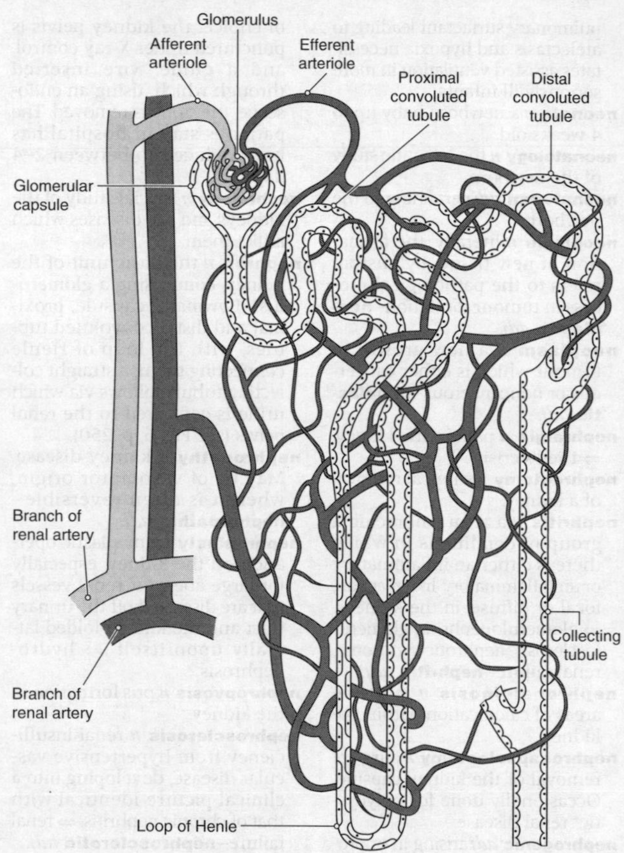

■ **Fig. 6** Diagram of a nephron, including the arrangement of blood vessels.

plasma albumen, albuminuria and oedema, usually with hyperlipaemia. There are minimal histological changes in the kidneys. It may occur in other conditions such as amyloid disease and glomerulosclerosis* complicating diabetes.

nephrotomogram *n* a tomograph* of the kidney.

nephrotomy *n* an incision into the kidney substance.

nephrotoxic *adj* any substance which inhibits or prevents the functions of kidney cells, or causes their destruction—**nephrotoxin** *n*.

nephroureterectomy *n* removal of the kidney along with a part or the whole of the ureter.

nerve *n* an elongated bundle of fibres which serves for the transmission of impulses between the periphery and the nerve centres. *afferent nerve* one conveying impulses from the tissues to the nerve centres; also known as 'receptor' and 'sensory' nerves. *efferent nerve* one which conveys impulses outwards from the nerve centres; also known as 'effector', 'motor', 'secretory', 'trophic', 'vasoconstrictor', 'vasodilator', etc. according to function and location.

nerve entrapment syndrome ⇒ prolapse.

nervous *adj* **1** relating to nerves or nerve tissue. **2** referring to a state of restlessness or timidity. *nervous breakdown* a euphemistic term for mental illness. There is some controversy about an exact meaning for 'mental illness' but it is generally conceded that the psychoses and neuroses are included. *nervous system* the structures controlling the actions and functions of the body; it comprises the brain and spinal cord and their nerves (central nervous system), and the ganglia and fibres forming the autonomic* system (peripheral, sympathetic).

nettlerash *n* ⇒ urticaria.

neural *adj* pertaining to nerves. *neural canal* ⇒ vertebral column. *neural tube* formed from fusion of the neural folds from which the brain and spinal cord arise. *neural tube defect* any of a group of congenital malformations involving the neural tube including anencephaly*, hydrocephalus* and spina* bifida.

neuralgia *n* pain in the distribution of a nerve—**neuralgic** *adj*.

neurapraxia *n* temporary loss of function in peripheral nerve fibres. Most commonly due to crushing or prolonged pressure. ⇒ axonotmesis.

neurasthenia *n* a frequently misused term, the precise meaning of which is an uncommon nervous condition consisting of lassitude, inertia, fatigue and loss of initiative. Restless fidgeting, over-sensitivity, undue irritability and often an asthenic physique are also present—**neurasthenic** *adj*.

neurectomy *n* excision of part of a nerve.

neurilemma *n* the thin membranous outer covering of a nerve fibre surrounding the myelin sheath.

neuritis *n* inflammation of a nerve—**neuritic** *adj*.

neuroblast *n* a primitive nerve cell.

neuroblastoma *n* malignant tumour arising in adrenal medulla from tissue of sympathetic origin. Most cases show a raised urinary catecholamine excretion—**neuroblastomata** *pl*, **neuroblastomatous** *adj*.

neurodermatitis *n* (*syn* lichen simplex) leathery, thickened patches of skin secondary to pruritus and scratching. As the skin thickens, irritation increases, scratching causes further thickening and so a vicious circle is set up. The appearance of the patch develops characteristically as a thickened sheet dissected into small, shiny, flat-topped papules. Common manifestation of atopic* dermatitis.

neurofibroma *n* a tumour arising from the connective tissue of nerves—**neurofibromata** *pl*.—**neurofibromatous** *adj*.

neurofibromatosis *n* a genetically determined condition in which there are many fibromata.⇒ Recklinghausen's disease.

neurogenic *adj* originating within or forming nervous tissue. *neurogenic bladder* interference with the nerve control of the urinary bladder causing either retention of urine, which presents as incontinence, or continuous dribbling without retention. When

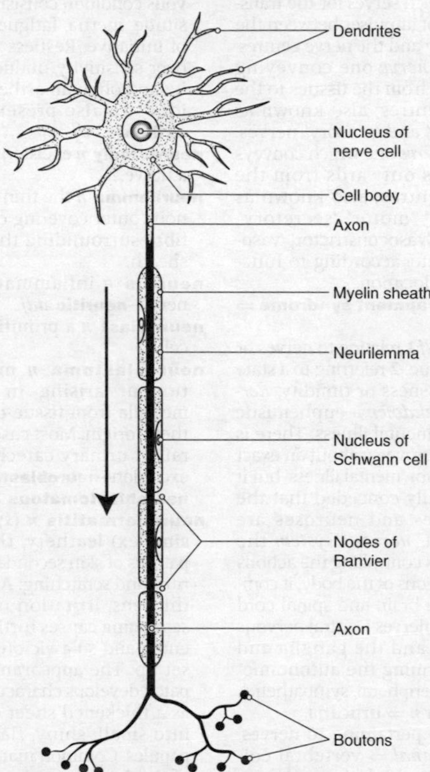

■ **Fig. 7** Electrical conduction along a neuron (the arrow shows the direction of impulse conduction).

necessary the bladder is emptied by exerting manual pressure on the anterior abdominal wall.

neuroglia *n* (*syn* glia) the supporting tissue of the brain and cord—**neuroglial** *adj.*

neuroglycopenia *n* shortage of glucose in nerve cells, which is the immediate cause of brain dysfunction when it occurs in hypoglycaemia—**neuroglycopenic** *adj.*

neuroleptics *npl* drugs acting on the nervous system. Includes the major antipsychotic tranquillizers. *depot neuroleptic* an antipsychotic drug given as a depot* injection to a client who is failing to take medication regularly.

neurologist *n* a specialist in neurology*.

neurology *n* the science and study of nerves their structure, function and pathology—**neurological** *adj.*

neuromuscular *adj* pertaining to nerves and muscles.

neuron(e) *n* the basic structural unit of the nervous system comprising fibres (dendrites) which convey impulses to the nerve cell; the nerve cell itself, and the fibres (axons) which convey impulses from the cell (see Fig. 7). ⇒ motor neurone disease—**neuronal, neural** *adj. lower motor neurone* the cell is in the spinal cord and the axon passes to skeletal muscle. *upper motor neurone* the cell is in the cerebral cortex and the axon passes down the spinal cord to arborize with a lower motor neurone.

neuronotmesis *n* ⇒ axonotmesis.

neuropathic *adj* relating to disease of the nervous system—**neuropathy** *n.*

neuropathology *n* a branch of medicine dealing with diseases of the nervous system—**neuropathological** *adj.*

neuropeptides *npl* chemical substances secreted continually in the brain, and currently associated with moods and states. They include the endorphins*.

neuropharmacology *n* the branch of pharmacology dealing with drugs which affect the nervous system—**neuropharmacological** *adj.*

neuroplasticity *n* the capacity of nerve cells to regenerate.

neuroplasty *n* surgical repair of nerves—**neuroplastic** *adj.*

neuropsychiatry *n* the combination of neurology and psychiatry. Speciality dealing with organic and functional disease—**neuropsychiatric** *adj.*

neurorrhaphy *n* suturing the ends of a divided nerve.

neurosis *n* (*syn* psychoneurosis) the symptoms of a neurosis differ from normal experience only in degree, e.g. someone suffering from an anxiety neurosis has symptoms indistinguishable from normal anxiety but out of context, or more severely than the situation warrants. People usually know that their experiences are abnormal, even though they might not be able to do anything about them. Other neuroses include obsessional* compulsive disorders (OCD) and phobias*. ⇒ psychosis, for comparison—**neuroses** *pl,* **neurotic** *adj.*

neurosurgery *n* surgery of the nervous system—**neurosurgical** *adj.*

neurosyphilis *n* infection of brain or spinal cord, or both, by *Treponema pallidum.* The variety of clinical pictures produced is large, but the two common syndromes encountered are tabes* dorsalis and GPI*. The basic pathology is disease of the blood vessels, with later development of pathological changes in the meninges and the underlying nervous tissue. Very often symptoms of the disease do not arise until 20 years or more after the date of primary infection. ⇒ Argyll Robertson pupil—**neurosyphilitic** *adj.*

neurotmesis *n* ⇒ axonotmesis.

neurotomy *n* surgical cutting of a nerve.

neurotoxic *adj* poisonous or destructive to nervous tissue—**neurotoxin** *n.*

neurotropic *adj* with predilection for the nervous system. *Treponema pallidum* often produces neurosyphilitic complications. Neurotropic viruses (rabies, poliomyelitis, etc.) make their major attack on the cells of the nervous system.

neutropenia *n* shortage of neutrophils, i.e. less than 500 circulating neutrophils per μl blood, but not sufficient to warrant the description 'agranulocytosis*'—**neutropenic** *adj.*

neutrophil *n* the most common

form of granulocyte and white blood cell in the blood, in which the granules are neither strongly basophilic nor strongly acidophilic.

next of kin an item frequently requested on the document used for recording data collected at the initial assessment of a patient. Great tact is required when acquiring information as a spouse may be the legal next of kin, but may be estranged from the patient. ⇒ significant other.

NGU *abbr* nongonococcal* urethritis.

NHS *abbr* National Health Service.

nicotinic acid one of the essential food factors of the vitamin B complex. The vasodilator action of the compound is useful in chilblains, migraine, etc.

NICU *abbr* neonatal intensive care unit.

nidation *n* implantation of the early embryo in the uterine mucosa.

NIDDM *abbr* noninsulin dependent diabetes* mellitus.

nidus *n* the focus of an infection. A septic focus.

Niemann-Pick disease a lipoid metabolic disturbance, chiefly in female Jewish infants. Now thought to be due to absence or inadequacy of enzyme sphingomyelinase. There is enlargement of the liver, spleen and lymph nodes with mental subnormality. Now classified as a lipid reticulosis.

night blindness (*syn* nyctalopia) sometimes occurs in vitamin A deficiency and is a maladaptation of vision to darkness.

night cry a shrill noise, uttered during sleep. May be of significance in hip disease when pain occurs in the relaxed joint.

Nightingale ward a rectangular ward housing as many as 36 patients whose beds are arranged along the walls between the windows.

night sweat profuse sweating, usually during sleep; typical of tuberculosis*.

nihilistic *adj* involving delusions and ideas of unreality; of not existing.

Nikolsky's sign slight pressure on the skin causes 'slipping' of apparently normal epidermis, in the way that a rubber glove can be moved on a wet hand. Characteristic of pemphigus*.

nipple *n* the conical eminence in the centre of each breast, containing the outlets of the milk ducts. Stimulation can cause erection of the nipple in both men and women. *inverted nipple* concavity of the nipple which may be a factor in unsuccessful breastfeeding. *nonprotractile nipple* a nipple which does not become erect on stimulation; may contribute to unsuccessful breastfeeding. *nipple shield* ⇒ breast shell.

NIPPV *abbr* noninvasive positive pressure ventilation.

nit *n* the egg of the head louse (*Pediculus* capitis).* It is firmly cemented to the hair.

nitrogen *n* **1** an almost inert gaseous element; the chief constituent of the atmosphere, but it cannot be utilized directly by man. However, certain bacteria in the soil and roots of legumes are capable of nitrogen fixation. It is an important constituent of many complements of living cells, e.g. proteins. **2** the essential constituent of protein foods **3** nitrogenous *adj*. nitrogen balance is when a person's daily intake of nitrogen from proteins equals the daily excretion of nitrogen: a negative balance occurs when excretion of nitrogen exceeds the daily intake. Nitrogen is excreted mainly as urea in the urine: ammonia, creatinine and uric acid account for a further small amount. Less than 10% total nitrogen excreted in faeces. *nitrogen mustards* a group of cytotoxic drugs, derivatives of mustard gas.

nitrogenous foods those containing proteins*.

nitrous oxide (*syn* laughing gas) gas used in combination with other agents for induction and maintenance of anaesthesia.

NMR *abbr*

nocturia *n* the arousal from sleep to pass urine.

nocturnal *adj* nightly; during the night.

node *n* a protuberance or swelling. A constriction. *atrioventricular node* the commencement of the bundle* of His in the right atrium of the heart. *node of Ranvier* the constriction in the neurilemma of a myelinated nerve fibre. *sinoatrial node* situated at the opening of the superior vena cava into the right atrium; the wave of contraction begins here, then spreads over the heart.

nodule *n* a small node—**nodular** *adj*.

noise induced hearing loss (*syn* occupational deafness) substantial sensorineural hearing loss caused by occupational noise. The average of pure tone losses measured by audiometry over the 1, 2 and 3 kHz frequencies.

nonaccidental injury (NAI) injuries, usually to children, that cannot be explained by natural disease or simple accident. The term is now preferred to 'battered baby syndrome'. The lesions are frequently multiple and typically involve the head, soft tissues, long bones and the thoracic cage. Usually there is accompanying psychological damage. ⇒ abuse.

noncompliance *n* a term used when patients who understand their drug or general treatment regime do not comply with it.

nongonococcal urethritis (NGU) (*syn* nonspecific urethritis, NSU) a common sexually transmitted disease. About half the cases are caused by *Chlamydia;* other causatory organisms are *Ureaplasma* and *Mycoplasma genitalium.*

nonHodgkin's lymphoma a malignant disease of lymphoid tissue, as distinct from Hodgkin's disease.

noninsulin dependent diabetes mellitus (NIDDM) ⇒ diabetes.

noninvasive *adj* describes any diagnostic or therapeutic technique which does not require penetration of the skin or of any cavity or organ.

noninvasive positive pressure ventilation (NIPPV) a mode of mechanical ventilation which uses a nasal or full-face mask rather than an endotracheal or tracheostomy tube.

nonnursing duties duties such as serving meals or doing clerical, administrative and domestic work which it may be argued detract from direct clinical care and could equally well be done by others.

nonprotein nitrogen (NPN) nitrogen derived from all nitrogenous substances other than protein, i.e. urea, uric acid, creatinine, creatine and ammonia.

nonsense syndrome Ganser* syndrome.

nonspecific urethritis nongonococcal* urethritis.

nonstarch polysacchrides (NSP) NSP has replaced the term 'dietary fibre'. There are many different types of NSP, found in differing amounts in all plant structures—in cell walls and within the cells of roots, leaves, stems, seeds and fruits. NSP has many functions (not all of which are completely understood) but it is an essential component of a well-balanced diet, e.g. it prevents constipation by reducing colonic transit time and increasing the frequency of defaecation; the incidence of diabetes mellitus increases if the diet is rich in refined, sugary foods (NSP is removed from a carbohydrate * food when it is refined). ⇒ bran.

nonsteroidal antiinflammatory drugs (NSAID) large group of drugs, used to treat minor pains, e.g. headache, but also useful in the rheumatological diseases. They can produce gastric ulceration and bleeding from the alimentary mucous membrane.

nonverbal communication ⇒ body language.

Noonan syndrome (*syn* Bonnevie-Ullrich syndrome) in either males or females, with eyes set apart (hypertelorism) and other ocular and facial abnormalities; short stature, sometimes with neck webbing (and other Turner*-like features). The commonest and most characteristic cardiac abnormality is congenital pulmonary stenosis. Generally not chromosomal; most cases sporadic; a few either dominantly or recessively inherited.

noradrenaline *n* endogenous noradrenaline is a neurohumoral transmitter which is released from adrenergic nerve endings. Although small amounts are associated with adrenaline in the adrenal medulla, its role as a hormone is a secondary one. It has an intense peripheral vasoconstrictor action, and is given by slow intravenous injection in shock and peripheral failure.

norm *n* a measure of a phenomenon, against which other measures of the phenomenon can be measured.

normalisation *n* a word which is currently used in relation to people with a learning disability. Programmes of behaviour modification and individualized goal setting can help in acquiring the skills of daily living.

normoblast *n* a normal sized nucleated red blood cell, the precursor of the erythrocyte—**normoblastic** *adj.*

normocyte *n* a red blood cell of normal size—**normocytic** *adj.*

normoglycaemic *adj* a normal amount of glucose in the blood—**normoglycaemia** *n.*

normotension *n* normal tension, by current custom alluding to blood pressure—**normotensive** *adj.*

normothermia *n* normal body temperature, as opposed to hyperthermia* and hypothermia*—**normothermic** *adj.*

normotonic *adj* normal strength, tension, tone, by current custom referring to muscle tissue. Spasmolytic drugs induce normotonicity in muscle, and can be used before radiography—**normotonicity** *n.*

Norton scale a numerical scale for assessing people who are at risk of developing pressure sores. Norton in 1987 advised that a person with a score of 15 or below denotes need for intensive preventive nursing interventions.

nosocomial *adj* pertaining to a hospital. ⇒ infection.

nostalgia *n* homesickness; a longing to return to a 'place' to which, and where, one may be emotionally bound—**nostalgic** *adj.*

nostrils *npl* the anterior openings in the nose; the anterior nares; choanae.

NRDS *abbr* neonatal* respiratory distress syndrome.

NSAIDs *abbr* nonsteroidal antiinflammatory drugs. An abbreviation used to differentiate them from corticosteroids*.

NSP *abbr* nonstarch polysaccharides.

NSU *abbr* ⇒ nonspecific urethritis.

nucha *n* the nape* of the neck—**nuchal** *adj.*

nuclear family the simplest of all family groups, consisting of one or two parents and their offspring.

nuclear magnetic resonance (NMR) ⇒ magnetic resonance imaging.

nucleated *adj* possessing one or more nuclei.

nucleoproteins *npl* proteins found in the nuclei of cells, consisting of a protein conjugated with nucleic acid. They are broken down during digestion to produce purine and pyramidine bases. An end product of nucleoprotein metabolism is uric acid which is excreted in the urine.

nucleotoxic *adj* poisonous to cell nuclei. The term may be applied to chemicals and viruses—**nucleotoxin** *n.*

nucleus *n* **1** the combination of atoms forming the central element or basic framework of the molecules of a specific compound or class of compounds. **2** the dense core of an atom, called the atomic nucleus. **3** a circumscribed accumulation of nerve cells in the central nervous system associated with a particular function—**nuclei** *pl,* **nuclear** *adj. nucleus pulposus* the soft core of an intervertebral disc which can prolapse into the spinal cord and cause sciatica.

null cells lymphocytes that lack the surface antigens characteristic of B and T lymphocytes; such cells are seen in active systemic lupus* erythematosus.

nullipara *n* a woman who has not borne a child—**nulliparous** *adj,* **nulliparity** *n.*

nummular *adj* coin shaped; resembling rolls of coins, as the sputum in phthisis.

nurse *n* a word protected by law in many countries. Only those whose name appears on the central register after having successfully undergone the prescribed educational programme can legally be called a nurse. ⇒ The named nurse box.

nurse practitioner a nurse who has undergone specific role preparation to enable him or her to function at an advanced level within a particular working environment. This may be within primary health care, in an accident and emergency setting or working with certain client groups—such as homeless people. Nurse practitioners can offer a nurse-led service and invariably have highly developed skills in client assessment.

nursing auxiliary ⇒ health* care assistant

nursing models frameworks that identify, describe and explain a range of nursing concepts; traditionally named after the writers who first propound them, e.g. Roy's model, Rogers' model, Roper, Logan, Tierney model. Nursing models may or may not be developed out of research

nursing process a systematic approach to nursing care. It comprises four phases; assessing, planning, implementing and evaluating. Only for purposes of description can they be sequential: in reality they overlap and occur and recur throughout the period a person is receiving nursing care.

nursing theory theory that explains, illuminates, or offers practical guidance about the field of nursing; generated by nursing research or, rationally, through the development of nursing ideas.

nutation *n* nodding; applied to uncontrollable head shaking.

nutrient *n, adj* a substance serving as or providing nourishment. ⇒ macronutrients, micronutrients. *nutrient artery* one which enters a long bone. *nutrient foramen* hole in a long bone which admits the nutrient artery.

nutrition *n* the total process by which the living organism receives and utilizes the materials necessary for survival, growth and repair of worn-out tissues.

nux vomica the nuts from which strychnine* is obtained. Occasionally used with other bitters as a gastric stimulant.

nyctalgia *n* pain occurring during the night.

nyctalopia *n* ⇒ night blindness.

nyctophobia *n* irrational fear of the night and darkness.

nymphomania *n* excessive sexual desire in a female—**nymphomaniac** *adj*.

nystagmus *n* involuntary and jerky repetitive movement of the eyeballs.

nystatin *n* an antifungal antibiotic effective in the treatment of candidiasis. Prevents intestinal fungal overgrowth during broad spectrum antibiotic treatment.

O

oat cell carcinoma a small cell carcinoma of the lung. Accounts for one third of lung cancer diagnoses, usually related to tobacco use. Sensitive to radiotherapy and chemotherapy but recurrence is common.

obesity *n* the deposition of excessive fat around the body, particularly in the subcutaneous tissue. The intake of food is in excess of the body's energy requirements. Obesity can be measured by weighing and measuring height and calculating the Body Mass Index (BMI), and by measuring the thickness of skin folds.

objective *adj* pertaining to things external to one's self. ⇒ subjective *opp. objective signs* those which the observer notes, as distinct from the symptoms of which the patient complains.

obligate *adj* characterized by the ability to survive only in a particular set of environmental conditions, e.g. an obligate parasite cannot exist other than as a parasite.

OBS *abbr* organic brain syndrome. ⇒ dementia.

observations *npl* in a nursing context, the regular measurement of the patient's physiological status–blood pressure, temperature, pulse and respiration.

observing *v* one of the many complex skills required by nurses.

obsessional neurosis two types are recognized: (a) obsessive compulsive thoughts: constant preoccupation with a constantly recurring morbid thought which cannot be kept out of the mind, and enters against the wishes of the patient who tries to eliminate it. The thought is almost always painful and out of keeping with the person's normal personality (b) obsessive compulsive actions: a feeling of compulsion to perform repeatedly a simple act, e.g. handwashing, touching door knobs. Ideas of guilt frequently form the basis of an obsessional state. ⇒ neurosis.

obstetrician *n* a qualified doctor who practises the science and art of obstetrics.

obstetrics *n* the science dealing with the care of the pregnant woman during the antenatal, parturient and puerperal stages; midwifery.

obstruction *n* any of the body's organs which are hollow tubes can be obstructed by something in the lumen, abnormality in the wall, or pressure from outside. Obstruction can occur as an 'emergency' requiring immediate treatment or operation. ⇒ Heimlich manoeuvre.

obturator *n* that which closes an aperture. *obturator foramen* the opening in the innominate bone which is closed by muscles and fascia. *obturator internus* obturator nerve.

occipital *adj* pertaining to the back of the head. *occipital bone* characterized by a large hole through which the spinal cord passes.

occipitoanterior *adj* describes a presentation when the fetal occiput lies in the anterior half of the maternal pelvis.

occipitofrontal *adj* pertaining to the occiput* and forehead.

occipitoposterior *adj* describes a presentation when the fetal occiput is in the posterior half of the maternal pelvis.

occiput *n* the posterior region of the skull.

occlusion *n* the closure of an opening, especially of ducts or blood vessels. In dentistry, the fit of the teeth as the two jaws meet–**occlusal** *adj*.

occult blood ⇒ blood.

occupational disease ⇒ industrial disease.

occupational health assessment a one-to-one interaction between a client (the employee or prospective employee) and an occupational health professional, usually a doctor or a nurse, for the puposes of assessing the physical and/or mental health status of the client.

occupational health nursing client care offered by nurses specially educated to deliver care in the workplace. It includes examination of the workplace for accident/illness risk, preventive teaching, assessment of new workers, maintaining records as well as running health promotion sessions or surgeries.

occupational therapy the treatment of physical and psychiatric conditions through specific activities in order to help people reach their maximum level of function and independence in all aspects of daily life.

ocular *adj* pertaining to the eye. *ocular motility* eye movements.

oculist *n* a medically qualified person who treats eye disease.

oculogenital *adj* pertaining to the eye and genital region, as the virus TRIC*, which is found in the male and female genital canals and in the conjunctival sacs of the newborn.

oculomotor *n* the third cranial nerve which moves the eye and supplies the upper eyelid.

odontalgia *n* toothache.

odontic *adj* pertaining to the teeth.

odontoid *adj* resembling a tooth.

odontology *n* dentistry.

odontoma *n* a tumour developing from or containing tooth structures–**odontomata** *pl*, **odontomatous** *adj*.

odontotherapy *n* the treatment of diseases of the teeth.

odour *n* the property of a substance which is individually perceived by a person's sense of smell as pleasant, unpleasant or odourless. ⇒ malodour.

oedema *n* abnormal infiltration of tissues with fluid. There are many causes–it can be in the blood, or disease of the cardiopulmonary system, the urinary system and the liver. ⇒ anasarca, angioneurotic oedema, ascites–**oedematous** *adj*.

Oedipus complex an unconscious attachment of a son to his mother resulting in a feeling of jealousy towards the father and then guilt, producing emotional conflict. This process was described by Freud as part of his theory of infantile sexuality and he considered it to be normal in male infants.

oesophageal *adj* pertaining to the oesophagus*. *oesophageal speech* a patient who has undergone a laryngectomy may learn to use this method of speech production, producing a pseudovoice using the top of the oesophagus. *oesophageal ulcer* ulceration of the oesophagus due to gastrooesophageal reflux caused by hiatus hernia*. *oesophageal varices* varicosity of the veins in the lower oesophagus due to portal hypertension; they often extend below the cardia into the stomach. These varices can bleed and cause a massive haematemesis, but this occurs only in a minority of patients.

Others present with iron deficiency anaemia or melaena ⇒ Sengstaken tube.

oesophagectasis *n* a dilated oesophagus*.

oesophagectomy *n* excision of part or the whole of the oesophagus*.

oesophagitis *n* inflammation of the oesophagus*.

oesophagogastroduodenoscopy (OGD) *n* endoscopic* examination of the upper alimentary tract.

oesophagoscope *n* an endoscope* for passage into the oesophagus*—**oesophagoscopy** *n,* **oesophagoscopic** *adj.*

oesophagostomy *n* a surgically established fistula between the oesophagus and the skin in the root of the neck. Used temporarily for feeding after excision of the pharynx for malignant disease.

oesophagotomy *n* an incision into the oesophagus.

oesophagus *n* the musculomembranous canal, 23 cm in length, extending from the pharynx* to the stomach*—**oesophageal** *adj.*

oestriol *n* an oestrogen metabolite present in the urine of pregnant woman. The fetus and placenta are concerned in its production. Oestriol excretion has been used as an indicator of fetal wellbeing.

oestrogen *n* a generic term referring to ovarian hormones. Three 'classical' ones: oestriol, oestrone and oestradiol. Urinary excretion of these substances increases throughout normal pregnancy—**oestrogenic** *adj.*

olecranon process the large process at the upper end of the ulna; it forms the tip of the elbow when the arm is flexed. *olecranon bursitis* ⇒ bursitis.

OGD *abbr* oesophagogastroduodenoscopy*.

oleum ricini castor* oil.

olfactory *adj* pertaining to the sense of smell—**olfaction** *n.* *olfactory nerve* the nerve supplying the olfactory region of the nose; the first cranial nerve. *olfactory organ* the nose.

oligaemia *n* ⇒ hypovolaemia—**oligaemic** *adj.*

oligohydramnios *n* deficient amniotic fluid.

oligomenorrhoea *n* infrequent menstruation; normal cycle is prolonged beyond 35 days.

ombudsman *n* a person officially appointed to investigate complaints about the health service, for which the complainer has not received a satisfactory explanation at local level. Also called Health Services Commission.

omentum *n* a sling-like fold of peritoneum—**omental** *adj. gastrosplenic omentum* connects the stomach and spleen. The functions of the omentum are protection, repair and fat storage. *greater omentum* the fold which hangs from the lower border of the stomach and covers the front of the intestines. *lesser omentum* a smaller fold, passing between the transverse fissure of the liver and the lesser curvature of the stomach.

omphalitis *n* inflammation of the umbilicus*.

omphalocele *n* ⇒ hernia.

Onchocerca *n* a genus of filarial worms.

onchocerciasis *n* infestation of man with *Onchocerca*. Adult worms encapsulated in subcutaneous connective tissue. Can cause 'river blindness' if the larvae migrate to the eyes.

oncogene *n* an abnormal gene thought to be made active by a chemical when it becomes capable of making 'forged' chemical keys and locks that can trick cells into uncontrollable cancerous growth.

oncogenic *adj* capable of tumour production.

oncology *n* the scientific and medical study of tumours—

oncological *adj,* **oncologically** *adv.*

oncolysis *n* destruction of a neoplasm. Sometimes used to describe reduction in size of tumour—**oncolytic** *adj.*

onychia *n* acute inflammation of the nail matrix; suppuration may spread beneath the nail, causing it to become detached and fall off.

onychocryptosis *n* ingrowing of the nail.

onychogryphosis, oncogryposis *n* a ridged, thickened deformity of the nails, common in the elderly.

onycholysis *n* loosening of toe or finger nail from the nail bed—**onycholytic** *adj.*

onychomycosis *n* a fungal infection of the nails.

o'nyong-nyong fever (*syn* jointbreaker fever) caused by a virus transmitted by mosquitoes in East Africa. First noted in 1952.

oocyte *n* an immature ovum.

oogenesis *n* the production and formation of ova* in the ovary—**oogenetic** *adj.*

oophorectomy *n* (*syn* ovariectomy, ovariotomy) removal of an ovary*.

oophoritis *n* (*syn* ovaritis) inflammation of an ovary*.

opacity *n* nontransparency; cloudiness; an opaque spot, as on the cornea or lens.

operant conditioning ⇒ conditioning.

operating microscope an illuminated binocular microscope enabling surgery to be carried out on delicate tissues such as nerves and blood vessels. Some models incorporate a beam splitter and a second set of eyepieces to enable a second person to view the operation site.

operation *n* surgical procedure upon a part of the body.

ophthalmia *n* (*syn* ophthalmitis) inflammation of the eye. *ophthalmia neonatorum* defined by law in 1914 as a 'purulent discharge from the eyes of an infant commencing within 21 days of birth'. Only 6% of total cases are gonorrhoeal, but all are notifiable including chlamydial. *sympathetic ophthalmia* iridocyclitis of one eye secondary to injury or disease of the other.

ophthalmic *adj* pertaining to the eye.

ophthalmitis *n* ⇒ ophthalmia.

ophthalmologist *n* a person who studies ophthalmology*.

ophthalmology *n* the science which deals with the structure, function and diseases of the eye—**ophthalmological** *adj,* **ophthalmologically** *adv.*

ophthalmoplegia *n* paralysis of one or more muscles which move the eye—**ophthalmoplegic** *adj.*

ophthalmoscope *n* an instrument fitted with a lens and illumination for examining the interior of the eye—**ophthalmoscopic** *adj.*

opisthotonos *n* extreme extension of the body occurring in tetanic spasm. Patient may be supported on his heels and his head alone—**opisthotonic** *adj.*

opium *n* the dried juice of opium poppy capsules. Contains morphine*, codeine* and other alkaloids. Valuable analgesic, but more constipating than morphine. Also used as tincture of opium and as paregoric (camphorated tincture of opium).

opportunistic infection ⇒ infection.

OpSite *n* a proprietary brand of permeable, adhesive polyurethane membrane designed to retain wound exudate, thereby creating a moist wound environment. It permits the exchange of oxygen and carbon dioxide and the passage of water as a vapour, but it is impermeable to bacteria, viruses and water. It therefore fulfils the requirements for moist* wound healing with its many advantages. It can be used in the prevention of pressure sores when it is placed over intact skin.

opsonic index a figure obtained by experiment which indicates the ability of phagocytes to ingest foreign bodies such as bacteria.

opsonin *n* an antibody which unites with an antigen, usually part of intact cells, and renders the cells more susceptible to phagocytosis*. ⇒ immunoglobulins—**opsonic** *adj.*

optic *adj* pertaining to sight. *optic chiasma* ⇒ chiasma. *optic disc* the point where the optic nerve enters the eyeball.

optical aberration imperfect focus of light rays by a lens.

optician *n* one who prescribes spectacles to correct refractive errors.

optics *n* the branch of physics which deals with light rays and their relation to vision.

optimum *adj* most favourable. *optimum position* that which will be least awkward and most useful should a limb remain permanently paralysed.

optometry *n* measurement of visual acuity.

oral *adj* pertaining to the mouth—**orally** *adv. oral hygiene* ⇒ mouth care. *oral rehydration solution (ORS)* a particular liquid for the treatment of diarrhoeal dehydration containing glucose, sodium chloride, sodium bicarbonate and potassium chloride dissolved in one litre of water. *oral rehydration therapy (ORT)* administration of oral rehydration solution by mouth to correct dehydration*.

orbicular *adj* resembling a globe; spherical or circular.

orbit *n* the bony socket containing the eyeball and its appendages—**orbital** *adj.*

orchidectomy *n* excision of a testis*.

orchidopexy *n* the operation of bringing an undescended testis* into the scrotum*, and fixing it in this position.

orchis *n* the testis.

orchitis *n* inflammation of a testis.

orf *n* skin lesions caused by a virus normally affecting sheep.

organic *adj* pertaining to an organ. Associated with life. *organic brain syndrome* ⇒ dementia. *organic disease* one in which there is structural change.

organism *n* a living cell or group of cells differentiated into functionally distinct parts which are interdependent.

organogenesis *n* the formation and development of body organs from embryonic tissue. The concept of 'preconceptual care' enables a woman to be experiencing maximum health when she conceives, so that organogenesis can proceed normally.

organ transplantation ⇒ transplant.

orgasm *n* the climax of sexual excitement.

oriental sore (*syn* Delhi boil) a form of cutaneous leishmaniasis* producing papular, crusted, granulomatous eruptions of the skin. A disease of the tropics and subtropics.

orientation *n* clear awareness of one's position relative to the environment. In mental conditions, orientation 'in space and time' means that the patient knows where he is and recognizes the passage of time, i.e. can give the correct date. Disorientation means the reverse.

orifice *n* a mouth or opening.

origin *n* the commencement or source of anything. *origin of a muscle* the end that remains relatively fixed during contraction of the muscle.

ornithosis *n* human illness resulting from disease of birds. ⇒ Chlamydia.

orogenital *adj* pertaining to the

mouth and the external genital area.

oropharyngeal *adj* pertaining to the mouth and pharynx.

oropharynx *n* that portion of the pharynx which is below the level of the soft palate and above the level of the hyoid bone.

orphenadrine *n* an anticholinergic agent used in Parkinson's disease. May reduce drug-induced parkinsonism caused by tranquillizers.

ORS *abbr* oral* rehydration solution.

ORT *abbr* oral* rehydration therapy.

orthodontics *n* a branch of dentistry dealing with prevention and correction of irregularities of the teeth.

orthodox sleep *n* lasts approximately one hour in each sleep* cycle. The metabolic rate and therefore oxygen consumption is lowered.

orthopaedics *n* formerly a specialty devoted to the correction of deformities in children. It is now a branch of surgery dealing with all conditions affecting the locomotor system.

orthopnoea *n* breathlessness necessitating an upright, sitting position for its relief—**orthopnoeic** *adj.*

orthoptics *n* the study and treatment of ocular motility.

orthosis *n* a device which can be applied to or around the body in the care of physical impairment or disability. ⇒ prosthesis—**orthoses** *pl*—**orthotic** *adj.*

orthostatic *adj* caused by the upright stance. *orthostatic albuminuria* occurs in some healthy subjects only when they take the upright position. When lying in bed the urine is normal.

orthotics *n* the scientific study and manufacture of devices which can be applied to or around the body in the care of physical impairment or disability.

orthotist *n* a person who practises orthotics*.

Ortolani's sign a test performed shortly after birth to discern dislocation of the hip.

os *n* a mouth or opening. *external os* the opening of the cervix into the vagina. *internal os* the opening of the cervix into the uterine cavity—**ora** *pl.*

oscillation *n* a swinging or moving to and fro; a vibration.

oscillometry *n* measurement of vibration, using a special apparatus (oscillometer). Measures the magnitude of the pulse wave more precisely than palpation.

Osgood-Schlatter's disease ⇒ Schlatter's disease.

Osler's nodes small painful areas in pulp of fingers or toes, or palms and soles caused by emboli and occurring in subacute bacterial endocarditis.

osmolality *n* the number of osmoles* per kilogram of solution.

osmolarity *n* the osmotic* pressure exerted by a given concentration of osmotically active solute in aqueous solution, defined in terms of the number of active particles per unit volume.

osmole *n* the standard unit of osmotic pressure which is equal to the gram molecular weight of a solute divided by the number of particles or ions into which it dissociates in solution.

osmosis *n* the passage of pure solvent across a semipermeable membrane under the influence of osmotic* pressure (see Fig. 8).

osmotic pressure the pressure with which solvent molecules are drawn across a semipermeable membrane separating two concentrations of solute (such as sodium chloride, sugars, urea) dissolved in the same solvent, when the membrane is impermeable to the solute but permeable to the solvent.

osseous *adj* pertaining to or resembling bone.

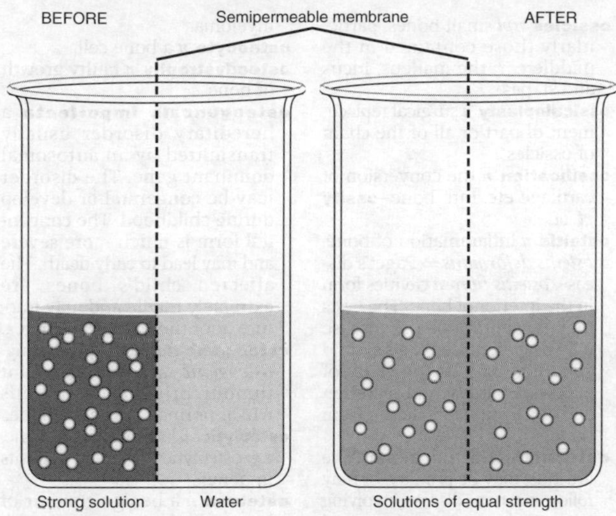

DIFFUSION

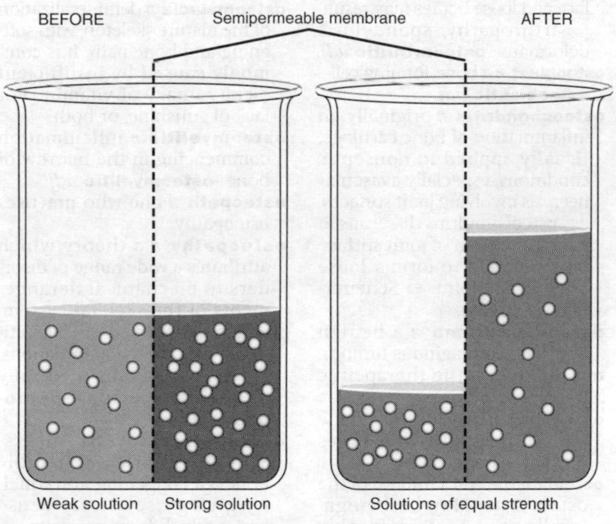

OSMOSIS

■ **Fig. 8** Osmosis and diffusion across a membrane.

ossicles *npl* small bones, particularly those contained in the middle ear; the malleus, incus and stapes.

ossiculoplasty *n* surgical replacement of part or all of the chain of ossicles*.

ossification *n* the conversion of cartilage etc. into bone—**ossify** *vt, vi.*

osteitis *n* inflammation of bone. *osteitis deformans* ⇒ Paget's disease. *osteitis fibrosa* cavities form in the interior of bone. The cysts may be solitary or the disease may be generalized. This second condition may be the result of excessive parathyroid secretion and absorption of calcium from bone.

osteoarthritis *n* degenerative arthritis; may be primary, or may follow injury or disease involving the articular surfaces of synovial joints. The articular cartilage becomes worn, osteophytes form at the periphery of the joint surface and loose bodies may result. ⇒ arthropathy, spondylosis deformans—**osteoarthritic** *adj.*

osteoblast *n* a bone-forming cell—**osteoblastic** *adj.*

osteochondritis *n* originally an inflammation of bone cartilage. Usually applied to nonseptic conditions, especially avascular necrosis involving joint surfaces, e.g. osteochondritis dissecans in which a portion of joint surface may separate to form a loose body in the joint. ⇒ Scheuermann's disease.

osteochondroma *n* a benign bony and cartilaginous tumour.

osteoclasis *n* the therapeutic fracture of a bone.

osteoclast *n* bone destroyer; the cell which dissolves or removes unwanted bone.

osteoclastoma *n* a tumour of the osteoclasts. May be benign, locally recurrent, or frankly malignant. The usual site is near the end of a long bone. ⇒ myeloma.

osteocyte *n* a bone cell.

osteodystrophy *n* faulty growth of bone.

osteogenesis imperfecta a hereditary disorder usually transmitted by an autosomal dominant gene. The disorder may be congenital or develop during childhood. The congenital form is much more severe and may lead to early death. The affected child's bones are extremely fragile and may fracture after the mildest trauma.

osteogenic *adj* bone-producing. *osteogenic sarcoma* malignant tumour originating in cells which normally produce bone.

osteolytic *adj* destructive of bone, e.g. osteolytic malignant deposits in bone.

osteoma *n* a benign tumour of bone which may arise in the compact tissue *(ivory osteoma)* or in the cancellous tissue. May be single or multiple.

osteomalacia *n* demineralization of the mature skeleton, with softening and bone pain. It is commonly caused by insufficient dietary intake of vitamin D or lack of sunshine, or both.

osteomyelitis *n* inflammation commencing in the marrow of bone—**osteomyelitic** *adj.*

osteopath *n* one who practises osteopathy.

osteopathy *n* a theory which attributes a wide range of disorders to mechanical derangements of the skeletal system, which it is claimed can be rectified by suitable manipulations. Often practised by medically unqualified persons—**osteopathic** *adj.*

osteopetrosis (*syn* Albers-Schönberg disease, marble bones) a congenital abnormality giving rise to very dense bones which fracture easily.

osteophyte *n* a bony outgrowth or spur, usually at the margins of joint surfaces, e.g. in osteoarthritis–**osteophytic** *adj.*

osteoplasty *n* reconstructive operation on bone–**osteoplastic** *adj.*

osteoporosis *n* reduction in bone density which can affect the skeleton so that a fracture can occur with minimal trauma. Caused by excessive absorption of calcium and phosphorus from the bone, due to progressive loss of the protein matrix of bone which normally carries the calcium deposits. Most common in women following the menopause. Treatment includes oestrogen hormone replacement therapy and calcium supplements–**osteoporotic** *adj.*

osteosarcoma *n* a sarcomatous tumour growing from bone–**osteosarcomata** *pl,* **osteosarcomatous** *adj.*

osteosclerosis *n* increased density or hardness of bone–**osteosclerotic** *adj.*

osteotome *n* an instrument for cutting bone; it is similar to a chisel, but it is bevelled on both sides of its cutting edge.

osteotomy *n* division of bone followed by realignment of the ends to encourage union by healing. *McMurray's osteotomy* ⇒ McMurray's.

ostium *n* the opening or mouth of any tubular passage–**ostia** *pl.*–**ostial** *adj.*

OT *abbr* 1 occupational* therapy. 2 operating theatre.

otalgia *n* earache.

OTC *abbr* over-the-counter drugs/medicines.

otitis *n* inflammation of the ear. ⇒ grommet. *otitis externa* inflammation of the skin of the external auditory canal. *malignant otitis externa* caused by *Pseudomonas aeruginosa,* can erode bone and be fatal. *otitis media* inflammation of the middle ear cavity. The effusion tends to be serous, mucoid or purulent. Nonpurulent effusions in children are often called glue* ear.

otologist *n* a person who specializes in otology.

otology *n* the science which deals with the structure, function and diseases of the ear.

otorhinolaryngology *n* the science which deals with the structure, function and diseases of the ear, nose and throat; each of these three may be considered a specialty. ⇒ laryngology, otology, rhinology.

otorrhoea *n* a discharge from the external auditory meatus.

otosclerosis *n* new bone formation affecting primarily the footplate of the stapes* and a common cause of progressive conductive deafness–**otosclerotic** *adj.*

ototoxic *adj* having a toxic action on the ear.

outcome *n* a word which can be used synonymously with patient goal* or objective. It implies the outcome which is expected from implementing the planned nursing intervention.

outflow obstruction usually refers to the passage of urine and may be caused by prostatic enlargement, urethral stenosis or stricture or chronic constipation.

ova *npl* the female reproductive cells–**ovum** *sing. ovum donation* ova are retrieved from a donor following superovulation* and used to help another achieve a pregnancy, combined with IVF* techniques. HIV screening is now expected of the donor.

ovarian *adj* pertaining to the ovaries. *ovarian cyst* a tumour of the ovary, usually containing fluid: may be benign or malignant. It may reach a large size and can twist on its stalk creating an acute emergency surgical condition.

ovariectomy *n* ⇒ oopherectomy.

ovariotomy *n* literally means incision of an ovary, but usually applied to the removal of an ovary (oophorectomy).

ovaritis *n* ⇒ oophoritis.

ovary *n* one of two small oval bodies situated on either side of the uterus on the posterior surface of the broad ligament. The structures in which the ova* are developed—**ovarian** *adj. cystic ovary* retention cysts in ovarian follicles. Cysts contain oestrogen-rich fluid which causes menorrhagia.

overcompensation *n* name given to any type of behaviour which a person adopts in order to cover up a deficiency. Thus a person who is afraid may react by becoming arrogant or boastful or quarrelsome.

over-the-counter drugs/medicines (OTC) medicines which can be sold over-the-counter as opposed to prescription*-only. Countries vary as to which drugs are included in this category At the initial assessment, the person should be asked whether or not any of these are, or have been taken. ⇒ drug.

ovulation *n* the maturation and rupture of a Graafian* follicle with the discharge of an ovum.

oxaluria *n* excretion of urine containing calcium oxalate crystals; associated often with dyspepsia.

Oxford grading system used for assessing pelvic floor strength for patients with genuine stress incontinence* prior to designing an individual pelvic floor exercise plan.

oxidase *n* any enzyme which promotes oxidation.

oxidation *n* the act of oxidizing or state of being oxidized. It involves an increase of positive charges on an atom or the loss of a pair of hydrogen atoms or the addition of oxygen. Oxidation must be accompanied by reduction of an acceptor molecule. Part of the process of metabolism, resulting in the release of energy.

oximeter *n* an instrument attached to the ear to 'sense' the oxygen saturation of arterial blood. An accurate noninvasive transcutaneous technique.

Oxycel a proprietary preparation of oxidized cellulose; used to achieve haemostasis when conventional methods of ligature, sutures or diathermy have failed. The material is subsequently absorbed by the tissues.

oxygen *n* a colourless, odourless, gaseous element; necessary for life and combustion. Constitutes 20% by weight of atmospheric air. Used medicinally as an inhalation, when precautions must be taken against fire. Supplied in cylinders (black with a white top) in which the gas is at a high pressure. ⇒ hyperbaric oxygen therapy. *oxygen concentrator* a device for removing nitrogen from the air to provide a high concentration of oxygen.

oxygenation *n* the saturation of a substance (particularly blood) with oxygen. Arterial oxygen tension indicates degree of oxygenation; reference range 13.1 kPa—**oxygenated** *adj.*

oxygenator *n* artificial 'lung' as used in heart surgery.

oxyhaemoglobin *n* oxygenated haemoglobin, an unstable compound formed from haemoglobin on exposure to alveolar gas in the lungs.

oxyntic *adj* producing acid. *oxyntic cells* the cells in the gastric mucosa which produce hydrochloric acid.

oxytocic *adj, n* hastening parturition; an agent promoting uterine contractions.

oxytocin *n* one of the posterior pituitary hormones. Causes contraction of uterine muscle. Synthetic preparation Syntocinon is used for the induction and augmentation of labour, often combined with ergometrine and used in the active management of the third stage of labour and for the prevention and treatment of postpartum* haemorrhage. Also causes contraction of the milk ducts and is part of the milk ejection reflex. Has been used as a nasal spray to enhance lactation.

Oxyuris *n* a genus of nematodes, commonly called threadworms.

ozone *n* an allotropic form of oxygen, O_3. Has powerful oxidizing properties and is therefore antiseptic and disinfectant. It is both irritating and toxic in the pulmonary system.

P

^{32}P *abbr* radioactive phosphorus.

pacemaker *n* the region of the heart which initiates atrial contraction and thus controls heart rate. The natural pacemaker is the sinoatrial node which is situated at the opening of the superior vena cava into the right atrium; the wave of contraction begins here, then spreads over the heart. *artificial pacemaker* ⇒ cardiac.

pachyblepharon *n*

pachycephalia *n* a thick skull.

pachychilia *n* thick lip(s).

pachydermia *n* thick skin. ⇒ elephantiasis.

pachymeningitis *n* inflammation of the dura mater (pachymeninx).

paediatrician *n* a specialist in children's diseases.

paediatrics *n* the branch of medicine dealing with children and their diseases—**paediatric** *adj.*

paedophilia *n* sexual attraction to children—**paedophiliac** *adj.* ⇒ child abuse, incest.

Paget-Schroetter syndrome axillary or subclavian vein thrombosis, often associated with effort in fit young persons.

Paget's disease 1 (*syn* osteitis deformans) excess of the enzyme alkaline phosphatase causes too rapid bone formation; consequently bone is thin. There is loss of stature, crippling deformity, enlarged head, collapse of vertebrae and neurological complications can result. Sufferers are particularly susceptible to sarcoma of bone. **2** erosion of the nipple caused by invasion of the dermis by intraduct carcinoma of the breast.

pain *n* because pain is a subjective experience, one person's pain cannot be compared with another's. Acute pain is usually of sudden onset and acts as a warning whereas chronic pain is 'useless' pain and is seldom life-threatening. ⇒ backache, colic, pain assessment, phantom pain, referred pain.

pain assessment an important function of the nurse's role, especially with children and infants who are unable to articulate their pain experience. There are several pain assessment tools. Most of them include a longitudinal scale, at one end of which is 0 for 'no pain', and at the other 10 for 'the pain is as bad as it could possibly be'. The patient points to the number which equates with the current experience of pain. Several pain assessment tools have been developed for use with children of varying ages, e.g. the Whaley and Wong 'faces scale', in which the child points to the facial expression corresponding to his pain experience.

painful arc syndrome pain in the shoulder and upper arm as it is actively abducted.

painter's colic ⇒ colic.

palate *n* the roof of the mouth—**palatal, palatine** *adj. cleft palate* ⇒ cleft palate. *hard palate* the front part of the roof of the mouth formed by the two palatal bones. *soft palate* situated at the posterior end of the palate and consisting of muscle covered by mucous membrane.

palatine *adj* pertaining to the palate. *palatine arches* the bilateral double pillars or arch-like folds formed by the descent of the soft palate as it meets the pharynx.

palatoplegia *n* paralysis of the soft palate—**palatoplegic** *adj.*

palliative *adj, n* (describes) anything which serves to alleviate but cannot cure a disease—**palliation** *n.*

pallidectomy *n* destruction of a predetermined section of globus* pallidus. ⇒ chemopallidectomy, stereotactic surgery.

palm *n* the anterior or flexor surface of the hand.

palmar *adj* pertaining to the palm* of the hand. *palmar arches* superficial and deep, are formed by the anastomosis of the radial and ulnar arteries.

palpable *adj* capable of being palpated or felt by manual examination.

palpation *n* the act of manual examination—**palpate** *vt.*

palpebra *n* an eyelid—**palpebrae** *pl,* **palpebral** *adj.*

palpitation *n* rapid forceful beating of the heart of which the patient is aware.

palsy *n* paralysis*. A word which is only retained in compound forms—Bell's* palsy, cerebral* palsy and Erb's* palsy.

panarthritis *n* inflammation of all the structures of a joint.

pancarditis *n* inflammation of all the structures of the heart.

pancreas *n* a tongue-shaped glandular organ lying below and behind the stomach. Its head is encircled by the duodenum and its tail touches the spleen. It is about 18 cm long and weighs about 100 g. It secretes the hormones insulin* and glucagon, and also pancreatic juice which contains enzymes involved in the digestion of fats, proteins and carbohydrates in the small intestine.

pancreatectomy *n* excision of part or the whole of the pancreas.

pancreatic function test Levin's tubes are positioned in the stomach and second part of duodenum. The response of the pancreatic gland to various hormonal stimuli can be measured by analysing the duodenal aspirate.

pancreatitis *n* inflammation of the pancreas*. The lipase level of blood and urine is used as an indicator of pancreatitis. *acute pancreatitis* usually the result of damage to the biliary tract; characterized by severe abdominal and back pain, nausea and vomiting. *chronic pancreatitis* chronic inflammation following acute attacks. Pancreatic failure can lead to diabetes mellitus.

pancreatrophic *adj* having an affinity for or an influence on the pancreas. Some of the anterior pituitary hormones have a pancreatrophic action.

pancreozymin *n* a hormone secreted by the duodenal mucosa; it stimulates the flow of pancreatic enzymes, especially amylase.

pancytopenia *n* describes peripheral blood picture when red cells, granular white cells and platelets are reduced as occurs in suppression of bone marrow function.

pandemic *n* an infection spreading over a whole country or the world.

pannus *n* corneal vascularization, often associated with conjunctival irritation.

panophthalmitis *n* inflammation of all the tissues of the eyeball.

panosteitis *n* inflammation of all constituents of a bone—medulla, bony tissue and periosteum.

pantothenic acid a constituent of the vitamin B complex.

PAO *abbr* peak acid output.

PaO_2 *abbr* pulmonary arterial oxygen saturation and tension.

papilla *n* a minute nipple-shaped eminence—**papillae** *pl,* **papillary** *adj.*

papillitis *n* **1** inflammation of the optic disc. **2** inflammation of a papilla. Can arise in the kidney after excessive intake of phenacetin, an old analgesic now replaced by paracetamol.

papilloedema *n* (*syn* choked disc) oedema of the optic disc; suggestive of increased intracranial pressure.

papilloma *n* a simple tumour arising from a nonglandular epithelial surface—**papillomata** *pl,* **papillomatous** *adj.*

papillomatosis *n* the growth of benign papillomata on the skin or a mucous membrane. Removal by laser means fewer recurrences.

Pap test (Papanicolaou) a smear of epithelial cells taken from the cervix is stained and cytologically examined to detect abnormal cervical cells.

papule *n* (*syn* pimple) a small circumscribed elevation of the skin—**papular** *adj.*

papulopustular *adj* pertaining to both papules* and pustules*.

paraaminobenzoic acid filters the ultraviolet rays from the sun and in a cream or lotion protects the skin from sunburn or harmful exposure to sunlight.

paraaortic *adj* near the aorta*.

paracentesis *n* ⇒ aspiration—**paracenteses** *pl.*

paracetamol *n* a mild analgesic; has virtually no antiinflammatory properties and is of no value in rheumatic conditions. Also an antipyretic and is used in children's preparations for this purpose. Does not cause indigestion or gastric bleeding. Overdose may cause severe liver damage.

paradoxical respiration ⇒ respiration.

paradoxical sleep (*syn* REM sleep) constitutes about a quarter of sleeping time. Characterized by rapid eye movements during which dreaming occurs.

paraesthesia *n* any abnormality of sensation.

paraffin *n* medicinal paraffins are: *liquid paraffin,* used as a laxative; *soft paraffin,* the familiar ointment base; and *hard paraffin,* used in wax baths for rheumatic conditions.

paraganglioma *n* ⇒ phaeochromocytoma.

parainfluenzavirus *n* causes acute upper respiratory infection. One of the myxoviruses.

paralysis *n* complete or incomplete loss of nervous function to a part of the body. This may be sensory or motor or both. *paralysis agitans* ⇒ paraplegia, parkinsonism, tetraplegia.

paralytic *adj* pertaining to paralysis. *paralytic ileus* paralysis of the intestinal muscle so that the bowel content cannot pass onwards even though there is no mechanical obstruction. ⇒ aperistalsis.

paramedian *adj* near the middle.

paramedical *adj* associated with the medical profession. The paramedical services include occupational, physical and speech therapy and medical social work.

paramenstruum *n* the four days before the start of menstruation and the first four days of the period itself.

parameter *n* boundary, constraint or limitation; for instance, one of the parameters of nursing is that it has to provide a 24 h service.

parametritis *n* inflammation of the cellular tissue adjacent to the uterus.

parametrium *n* the connective tissues immediately surrounding the uterus—**parametrial** *adj.*

paranoia *n* a mental disorder characterized by the insidious onset of delusions of persecution—**paranoid** *adj.*

paranoid behaviour acts denoting suspicion of others.

paranoid schizophrenia a form of schizophrenia* dominated by delusions and, to a lesser extent, hallucinations.

paraoesophageal *adj* near the oesophagus.

paraphimosis *n* retraction of the prepuce* behind the glans* penis so that the tight ring of skin interferes with the blood flow in the glans.

paraphrenia *n* a psychiatric illness in the elderly, characterized by well-circumscribed delusions, usually of a persecutory nature—**paraphrenic** *adj.*

paraplegia *n* paralysis of the lower limbs, usually including the bladder and rectum—**paraplegic** *adj.*

parapsychology *n* the study of extrasensory perception, telepathy and other psychic phenomena.

paraquat *n* widely used as a weed killer. If ingested it causes delayed toxic effects in the lungs, liver and kidneys. Poisoning may cause death from progressive pneumonia.

pararectal *adj* near the rectum.

parasitaemia *n* parasites in the blood—**parasitaemic** *adj.*

parasite *n* an organism which obtains food or shelter from another organism, the 'host'—**parasitic** *adj.* ⇒ commensals.

parasiticide *n* an agent which will kill parasites.

parasomnias *npl* a broad class of disturbances around sleep; it includes behaviours such as sleepwalking, nightmares and bruxism*.

parasuicide *n* also known as deliberate self-harm (DSH). A suicidal gesture: an act such as self-mutilation or drug overdose which may or may not be motivated by a genuine desire to die. It is common in young people who are distressed but not mentally ill.

parasympathetic *adj* describes a portion of the autonomic nervous system derived from some of the cranial and sacral nerves belonging to the central nervous system.

parasympatholytic *adj* capable of antagonizing the effect of parasympathetic stimulation, usually an anticholinergic.

parathion *n* an organic phosphate used as insecticide in agriculture. Has a powerful and irreversible anticholinesterase action. Potentially dangerous to man for this reason.

parathormone *n* a hormone secreted by the parathyroid* glands, which controls the level of calcium in the blood, partly by its effect on calcium content of bone. Excess hormone causes mobilization of calcium from the bones, which become rarefied.

parathyroidectomy *n* excision of one or more parathyroid* glands.

parathyroid glands *npl* four small endocrine glands lying close to or embedded in the posterior surface of the thyroid* gland. They secrete a hormone, parathormone (PTH), which helps to maintain a normal serum calcium level in association with calcitonin and vitamin D.

paratracheal *adj* near the trachea.

paratyphoid fever a variety of enteric fever, less severe and prolonged than typhoid* fever. Caused by *Salmonella paratyphi A* and *B,* and more rarely *C.* ⇒ TAB.

paraurethral *adj* near the urethra.

paravaginal *adj* near the vagina.

paravertebral *adj* near the spinal column. *paravertebral block anaesthesia* (more correctly, 'analgesia') is induced by infiltration of local anaesthetic around the spinal nerve roots as they emerge from the intervertebral foramina. *paravertebral injection* of local anaesthetic into sympathetic chain, can be used as a test in ischaemic limbs to see if sympathectomy will be of value.

parenchyma *n* the parts of an organ concerned with its function, as distinct from its interstitial tissue—**parenchymal, parenchymatous** *adj*.

parenteral *adj* not via the alimentary tract. *parenteral feeding* is necessary when it is impossible to provide adequate nutrition via the gastrointestinal tract. A sterile solution of nutrients is infused into a silicone catheter inserted into a large peripheral or, more usually, a large central vein (e.g. the vena cava). An infusion pump regulates the number of drops per minute. Patients and their families can learn to manage parenteral feeding at home. Mouth hygiene needs special attention—**parenterally** *adv*.

paresis *n* partial or slight paralysis; weakness of a limb—**paretic** *adj*.

pareunia *n* coitus*.

parietal *adj* pertaining to a wall. *parietal bones* the two bones which form the sides and vault of the skull.

parity *n* status of a woman with regard to the number of children she has borne.

parkinsonism *n* a syndrome of mask-like expression, shuffling gait, tremor of the limbs and pill-rolling movements of the fingers. Can be induced by antipsychotic drugs. The postencephalitic type comes on in the 30–40 age group and there may or may not be a clear history of encephalitis (sporadic type). Degenerative type of parkinsonism (paralysis agitans) comes on during middle life; arteriosclerotic type comes on in the elderly. Characterized by a distinctive clinical pattern of tremor and rigidity. There is a distinction between Parkinson's disease, which is a degenerative process associated with ageing, and parkinsonism, the causes of which are multiple and include such factors as injury, stroke, atherosclerosis, various toxic agents and the viral infection encephalitis lethargica. ⇒ dyskinesia, tardive.

paronychia *n* (*syn* whitlow) inflammation around a fingernail which may be bacterial or fungal. The virus of herpes simplex may also cause multiple vesicles over inflamed skin *herpetic paronychia*.

parosmia *n* perverted sense of smell, usually of hallucinatory nature.

parotid gland the salivary gland situated in front of and below the ear on either side.

parotitis *n* inflammation of a parotid* gland. *infectious parotitis* mumps*. *septic parotitis* refers to ascending infection from the mouth via the parotid duct, when a parotid abscess may result.

parous *adj* having borne a child or children.

paroxysm *n* a sudden, temporary attack.

paroxysmal *adj* coming on in attacks or paroxysms. *paroxysmal dyspnoea* occurs mostly at night in patients with cardiac disease. *paroxysmal fibrillation* occurs in the atrium of the heart and is associated with a ventricular tachycardia and total irregularity of the pulse rhythm. *paroxysmal tachycardia* may result from ectopic impulses arising in the atrium or in the ventricle itself.

parrot disease ⇒ psittacosis*.

Parrot's nodes bossing of frontal bones in the congenital syphilitic. ⇒ pseudoparalysis.

partial pressure pressure exerted by gas in a mixture of gases in proportion to concentration.

parturient *adj* pertaining to childbirth.

parturition *n* labour* and giving birth.

passive *adj* inactive. ⇒ active *opp. passive hyperaemia* ⇒ hyperaemia. *passive immunity* ⇒ immunity. *passive movement* performed by the therapist, the patient being relaxed.

Pasteurella *n* a genus of bacteria. Short Gram-negative rods, staining more deeply at the poles (bipolar staining). Pathogenic in man and animals.

pasteurization *n* a process whereby pathogenic organisms in fluid (especially milk) are killed by heat. *flash method of pasteurization* (HT, ST–high temperature, short time), the fluid is heated to 72°C, maintained at this temperature for 15 s, then rapidly cooled. *holder method of pasteurization* the fluid is heated to 63–65.5°C, maintained at this temperature for 30 min, then rapidly cooled.

Patau's syndrome trisomy of chromosome 13. Closely associated with learning disability. There are accompanying physical defects.

patch test a skin test for identifying reaction to allergens which are incorporated in an adhesive patch applied to the skin. Allergy is apparent by redness and swelling.

patella *n* a triangular, sesamoid bone; the kneecap—**patellae** *pl,* **patellar** *adj.*

patellectomy *n* excision of the patella*.

patent *adj* open; not closed or occluded—**patency** *n. patent ductus arteriosus* failure of ductus arteriosus to close soon after birth, so that the abnormal shunt between the pulmonary artery and the aorta is preserved. *patent interventricular septum* a congenital defect in the dividing wall between the right and left ventricles of the heart.

pathogen *n* a disease-producing agent, usually restricted to a living agent—**pathogenic** *adj,* **pathogenicity** *n.*

pathogenesis *n* the origin and development of disease—**pathogenetic** *adj.*

pathogenicity *n* the capacity to produce disease.

pathognomonic *adj* characteristic of or peculiar to a disease.

pathology *n* the science which deals with the cause and nature of disease—**pathological** *adj,* **pathologically** *adv.*

pathophobia *n* a morbid dread of disease—**pathophobic** *adj.*

pathophysiology *n* the science which deals with abnormal functioning of the human being—**pathophysiological** *adj,* **pathophysiologically** *adv.*

patient *n* **1** designates a person whose name is on the list of a general practitioner, whether or not he or she is attending the doctor's surgery or health clinic. **2** designates a person who is attending a hospital outpatient clinic at intervals; or is being visited in his home by a district nurse; or is an inpatient in hospital. ⇒ client, sickness certificate, sick role. *patient advocate* this includes the notion that a nurse argues on behalf of a patient, e.g. when the patient does not want to take a drug or undergo treatment prescribed by a doctor. ⇒ ombudsman. *patient compliance* a term used for the situation when a patient follows correctly the prescribed treatment regimen. ⇒ patient noncompliance *opp. patient handling* a term preferred by many professionals to lifting*. It includes lifting, but it also encompasses many of the transfers with which nurses help patients move from one surface to another; and techniques to help patients get into and out of a bath, and equipment to help them with walking. ⇒ backache. *patient* *participation* nurses are encouraged to interact with patients, especially in the initial assessment interview to support, prompt, reflect and help them to give their perception of their current health problem. Identification of problems with everyday living, actual and anticipated; goal setting; interventions to achieve the goal, all require patient participation which is a criterion of good nursing practice. *patient problems* in a nursing context those related to everyday living activities which are amenable to nurse-initiated intervention. Some other interventions to relieve a problem will be doctor prescribed and are therefore collaborative nursing interventions.

Paul-Bunnell test a serological test used in the diagnosis of infectious mononucleosis.

Paul-Mikulicz operation a method for excision of a portion of the colon whereby the two cut ends of the bowel are kept out on the surface of the abdomen, and are joined at a later date without entering the peritoneal cavity. The method was designed to lessen the risk of peritonitis from leakage at the suture line.

Pawlik's grip a method of determining the engagement or otherwise of the fetal head in the maternal pelvic brim.

PCM *abbr* protein* calorie malnutrition.

peak expiratory flow rate the measured amount of air in a forced exhalation over one second. Used to indicate presence or severity of respiratory disease, especially asthma.

peau d'orange term applied to the appearance of the skin over the breast in acute inflammation or in advanced carcinoma, when lymphoedema causes the orifices of the hair follicles to appear as dimples, resembling the pits in the skin of an orange.

pectoral *adj* pertaining to the breast.

pectus *n* the chest. *pectus carinatum* ⇒ pigeon chest. *pectus excavatum* ⇒ funnel chest.

pedal *adj* pertaining to the foot.

pedicle *n* a stalk, e.g. the narrow part by which a tumour is attached to the surrounding structures.

pediculosis *n* infestation with lice (pediculi).

Pediculus *n* a genus of parasitic insects (lice) important as vectors of disease. *Pediculus capitis* the head louse. *Pediculus corporis* the body louse. *Pediculis* (more correctly, *Phthirius) pubis* the pubic or crab louse. In some parts of the world body lice are involved in transmitting relapsing fever and typhus.

pedopompholyx *n* ⇒ cheiropompholyx.

peduncle *n* a stalk-like structure, often acting as a support—**peduncular, pedunculated** *adj.*

peeling *n* desquamation*.

peer support support from other members of a group to which one belongs, either temporarily or permanently. It is known for instance that new patients perceive established patients as providing support. Likewise nurses use their peer groups to gain and provide support, particularly in stressful circumstances.

PEG *abbr* percutaneous* endoscopic gastrostomy.

pellagra *n* a deficiency disease caused by lack of vitamin B complex and protein. Syndrome includes glossitis, dermatitis, peripheral neuritis and spinal cord changes (even producing ataxia), anaemia and mental confusion.

pellet *n* a little pill. ⇒ implant.

pelvic floor a mainly muscular partition with the pelvic cavity above and the perineum below.

In the female, weakening of these muscles, e.g. after childbirth, can contribute to urinary incontinence and uterine prolapse; they can be toned with pelvic floor exercises.

pelvic floor repair ⇒ Fothergill's operation.

pelvic girdle the bony pelvis comprising two innominate bones, the sacrum and coccyx.

pelvic inflammatory disease (PID) a sexually transmitted condition caused by bacteria, commonly Chlamydia* or gonorrhoea*. It causes inflammation of the uterine tubes and uterus, and can lead to reduced fertility and chronic pain if not treated at an early stage.

pelvic pain syndrome pelvic pain which occurs in women but for which no pathological cause is evident. Investigation can reveal congested pelvic blood vessels which may be treated with progestogens. Counselling is also beneficial.

pelvimetry *n* the measurement of the dimensions of the pelvis—**pelvimetric** *adj.*

pelvis *n* **1** a basin-shaped cavity, e.g. pelvis of the kidney. **2** the large bony basin-shaped cavity formed by the innominate bones and sacrum, containing and protecting the bladder, rectum and, in the female, the reproductive organs.—**pelvic** *adj. contracted pelvis* one in which one or more diameters are smaller than normal; this may result in difficulties in childbirth. *false pelvis* the wide expanded part of the pelvis above the brim. *true pelvis* that part of the pelvis below the brim.

pemphigoid *n* allied to pemphigus*. A bullous eruption in the latter half of life which is of autoimmune cause. Histological examination of the base of a blister differentiates it from pemphigus.

pemphigus *n* skin conditions with bullous (blister) eruptions, but more correctly used of a group of dangerous diseases called pemphigus vulgaris, pemphigus vegetans and pemphigus erythematosus. The latter two are rare. *pemphigus neonatorum* (a) a dangerous form of impetigo* occurring as an epidemic in the hospital nursery (b) bullous eruption in congenital syphilis of the newborn. *pemphigus vulgaris* a bullous disease of middle-age and later, of autoimmune aetiology. Oedema of the skin results in blister formation in the epidermis, with resulting secondary infection and rupture, so that large raw areas develop. Bullae develop also on mucous membranes. Death is from malnutrition or intercurrent disease.

pendulous *adj* hanging down. *pendulous abdomen* a relaxed condition of the anterior wall, allowing it to hang down over the pubis.

penetrating ulcer an ulcer* which is locally invasive and may erode a blood vessel causing haematemesis or melaena in the case of gastric or duodenal ulcer respectively.

penetrating wound (*syn* puncture wound) caused by a sharp, usually slim object, or a missile, which passes through the skin into the tissues beneath.

penicillin *n* the first antibiotic, also known as 'penicillin G' or 'benzyl penicillin'. Widely used by injection in many infections due to Gram-positive bacteria, some cocci and spirochaetes. High blood levels are obtained rapidly, and can be supplemented by injections of the slower acting procaine-penicillin (Depocillin) or the longer acting benethamine penicillin. The dose of penicillin varies widely according to the severity of infection, the largest being given in bacterial endocarditis (2 000 000 units).

penicillinase *n* an enzyme which destroys penicillin*.

Penicillium *n* a genus of moulds. The hyphae bear spores characteristically arranged like a brush. A common contaminant of food. *Penicillium chrysogenum* is now used for the commercial production of the antibiotic. *Penicillium notatum* is a species shown by Fleming (1928) to produce penicillin.

penis *n* the male organ of copulation—**penile** *adj*.

pentosuria *n* pentose in the urine. Can be due to a metabolic disorder—**pentosuric** *adj*.

pepsin *n* a proteolytic enzyme secreted by the stomach in the gastric juice. Breaks down proteins to polypeptides. It is stimulated by food and has an optimum pH of 1.5–2.0.

pepsinogen *n* a proenzyme secreted mainly by the chief cells in the gastric mucosa and converted into pepsin by contact with hydrochloric acid (gastric acid) or pepsin itself.

peptic *adj* pertaining to pepsin or to digestion generally. *peptic ulcer* a nonmalignant ulcer* in those parts of the digestive tract which are exposed to the gastric secretions; hence usually in the stomach or duodenum but sometimes in the lower oesophagus or with a Meckel's diverticulum.

peptides *npl* low molecular weight compounds which yield two or more amino acids on hydrolysis, e.g. dipeptides, tripeptides and polypeptides.

peptones *npl* substances produced when a proteolytic enzyme (e.g. pepsin) or an acid acts upon a native protein during the first stage of protein digestion.

percept *n* the mental product of a sensation; a sensation plus memories of similar sensations and their relationships.

perception *n* the reception of a conscious impression through the senses by which we distinguish objects one from another and recognize their qualities according to the different sensations they produce.

percolation *n* the process by which fluid slowly passes through a hard but porous substance.

percussion *n* tapping to determine the resonance or dullness of the area examined. Normally a finger of the left hand is laid on the patient's skin and the middle finger of the right hand (plexor) is used to strike the left finger.

percutaneous *adj* through the skin. *percutaneous endoscopic gastrostomy* a gastroscope* is used to aid the insertion of a feeding tube into the stomach which exits via the abdominal wall. ⇒ cholangiography.

perforation *n* a hole in an intact sheet of tissue. Used in reference to perforation of the tympanic membrane, or the wall of the stomach or gut (perforating ulcer*), constituting a surgical emergency.

Performance Indicators (PIs) quantitative measures of the activities and resources used in delivering health care.

periadenitis *n* inflammation in soft tissues surrounding glands. Responsible for the 'bull' neck in rubella.

perianal *adj* surrounding the anus.

periarterial *adj* surrounding an artery.

periarteritis *n* inflammation of the outer sheath of an artery and the periarterial tissue. *periarteritis nodosa* ⇒ polyarteritis.

periarthritis *n* inflammation of the structures surrounding a joint. Sometimes applied to frozen* shoulder.

periarticular *adj* surrounding a joint.

pericardectomy *n* surgical removal of the pericardium*.

pericardiocentesis *n* aspiration of the pericardial sac.

pericarditis *n* inflammation of the outer, serous covering of the heart. It may or may not be accompanied by an effusion and formation of adhesions between the two layers. ⇒ Broadbent's sign, pericardectomy.

pericardium *n* the double membranous sac which envelops the heart. The layer in contact with the heart is called 'visceral'; the outer is called 'parietal'. Between the two is the pericardial cavity, which normally contains a small amount of serous fluid—**pericardial** *adj*.

perichondritis *n* condition affecting the pinna; can result in gross deformity of the ear. Caused by a pyogenic infection of the perichondrium or a progressive systemic condition in which elastic cartilage elsewhere in the body is affected (relapsing polychondritis).

perichondrium *n* the membranous covering of cartilage—**perichondrial** *adj*.

pericolic *adj* around the colon.

pericranium *n* the periosteal covering of the cranium—**pericranial** *adj*.

perifollicular *adj* around a follicle.

perilymph *n* the fluid contained in the internal ear, between the bony and membranous labyrinth.

perimetrium *n* the peritoneal covering of the uterus—**perimetrial** *adj*.

perinatal *adj* currently used to describe the weeks before a birth, the birth and the succeeding few weeks. ⇒ death, stillbirth.

perineometer *n* a pressure gauge inserted into the vagina to register the strength of contraction in the pelvic floor muscles.

perineorrhaphy *n* an operation for the repair of a torn perineum.

perineotomy *n* episiotomy*.

perineal toilet the term usually applies to the female perineum. Girls from an early age should learn to cleanse the area from front to back so that bacteria from faeces do not reach the short urethra and travel to the bladder where they can be pathogenic and cause cystitis.

perinephric *adj* surrounding the kidney.

perineum *n* the portion of the body included in the outlet of the pelvis—**perineal** *adj*.

periodic breathing a period of apnoea in a newborn baby of 5–10 seconds followed by a period of hyperventilation at a rate of 50–60 breaths a minute, for a period of 10–15 seconds. The overall respiratory rate remains between 30 and 40 breaths per minute. Apnoea occurs quite frequently in very low birthweight babies, often without definite cause. Attacks are only a problem if they are prolonged and do not respond to simple stimulation.

perionychia *n* red and painful swelling around nail fold. Common in hands that are much in water or have poor circulation. Due to infection from the fungus *Candida*. More common now because of the use of antibiotics which subdue organisms that previously curtailed the activity of *Candida*. Secondary infection can occur.

periodontal disease commonly an inflammatory disease of the periodontal tissues resulting in the gradual loss of the supporting membrane and bone around the root of the tooth and a deepened gingival sulcus* or periodontal pocket. ⇒ pyorrhoea.

perioperative *adj* refers to the period during which a surgical operation is carried out, as well as to the pre and postoperative periods.

perioral *adj* around the mouth. *perioral dematitis* a red scaly or papular eruption around the mouth. Common in young adult females. Thought to be due to the use of corticosteroids* on the face.

periosteum *n* the membrane which covers a bone. In long bones only the shaft as far as the epiphyses is covered. It is protective and essential for regeneration—**periosteal** *adj.*

periostitis *n* inflammation of the periosteum*. *diffuse periostitis* that involving the periosteum of long bones. *haemorrhagic periostitis* that accompanied by bleeding between the periosteum and the bone.

peripheral *adj* pertaining to the outer parts of an organ or of the body. *peripheral nervous system* a term usually reserved for those nerves which supply the musculoskeletal system and surrounding tissues to differentiate from the autonomic nervous* system. *peripheral resistance* the force exerted by the arteriolar walls which is an important factor in the control of normal blood pressure. *peripheral vascular disease (PVD)* any abnormal condition arising in the blood vessels outside the heart, the main one being atherosclerosis*, which can lead to thrombosis and occlusion of the vessel resulting in gangrene. *peripheral vision* that surrounding the central field of vision.

periportal *adj* surrounding the portal vein.

periproctitis *n* inflammation around the rectum and anus.

perirenal *adj* around the kidney.

perisplenitis *n* inflammation of the peritoneal coat of the spleen and of the adjacent structures.

peristalsis *n* the characteristic movement of the intestines by which the contents are moved along the lumen. It consists of a wave of contraction preceded by a wave of relaxation—**peristaltic** *adj.*

peritoneal dialysis ⇒ dialysis.

peritoneoscopy ⇒ laparoscopy.

peritoneum *n* the delicate serous membrane which lines the abdominal and pelvic cavities and also covers the organs contained in them (see Fig. 9)—**peritoneal** *adj.*

peritonitis *n* inflammation of the peritoneum, usually secondary to disease of one of the abdominal organs.

peritonsillar abscess (quinsy) acute inflammation of the tonsil and surrounding loose tissue, with abscess formation.

peritrichous *adj* applied to bacteria which possess flagella on all sides of the cell. ⇒ Bacillus.

periumbilical *adj* surrounding the umbilicus.

periurethral *adj* surrounding the urethra, as a periurethral abscess.

perivascular *adj* around a blood vessel.

perleche *n* dryness and cracking at the angles of the mouth with maceration, fissuring, or crust formation. May result from persistent lip licking or use of poorly fitting dentures, bacterial infection, thrush infestation, vitamin deficiency, drooling or thumbsucking.

permeability *n* in physiology, the extent to which substances dissolved in the body fluids are able to pass through the membranes of cells or layers of cells (e.g. the walls of capillary blood vessels, or secretory or absorptive tissues).

permeable *adj* pervious; permitting passage of a substance.

pernicious *adj* deadly, noxious.

pernicious anaemia ⇒ anaemia.

perniosis *n* chronic chilblains. The smaller arterioles go into spasm readily from exposure to cold.

peromelia *n* a teratogenic malformation of a limb.

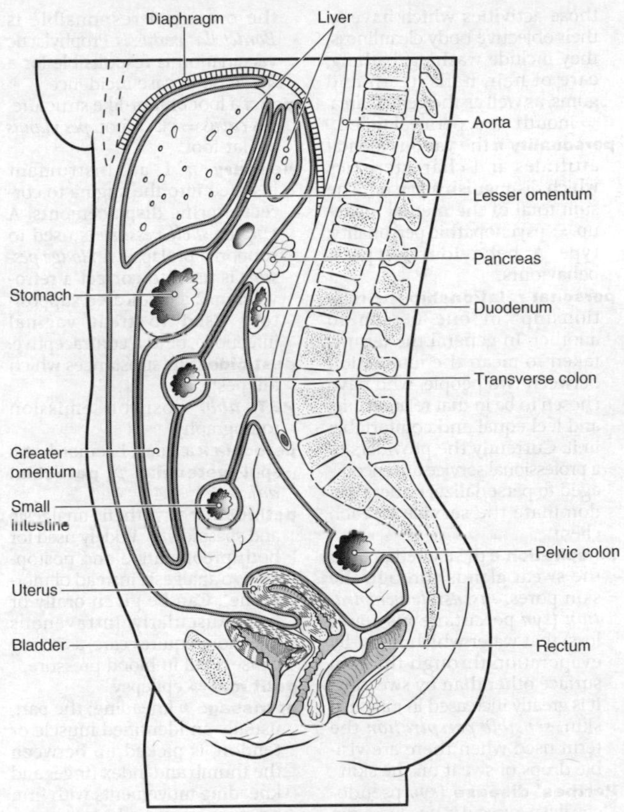

■ **Fig. 9** The mesentery and the peritoneum, showing how the peritoneum attaches the stomach and intestines to the abdominal wall.

peroral *adj* through the mouth.

peroxide *n* hydrogen* peroxide.

perseveration *n* constant repetition of a meaningless word or phrase.

persistent generalized lymphadenopathy (PGL) palpable lymph node enlargement at several sites which persists for more than 3 months in the absence of an identifiable cause other than HIV* infection. May be seen in the second and otherwise symptom-free stage of AIDS*.

persistent vegetative state (PVS) a condition resulting from brain damage, in which the person is without consciousness or the ability to initiate voluntary action.

persona *n* what one presents of one's 'self' to be perceived by others.—**personae** *pl.*

personal hygiene includes all

those activities which have as their objective body cleanliness; they include washing, bathing, care of hair, nails, teeth and gums, as well as the genital area. ⇒ mouth care, perineal toilet.

personality *n* the various mental attitudes and characteristics which distinguish a person. The sum total of the mental make-up. ⇒ psychopathic personality, type A behaviours, type B behaviours.

personal relationship the relationship* of one person to another. In general the term is taken to mean the interaction between two people, who have chosen to be in that relationship, and feel equal and comfortable in it. Currently the providers of a professional service are encouraged to personalize, rather than dominate the service to each client.

perspiration *n* the excretion from the sweat glands through the skin pores. *insensible perspiration* (*syn* percutaneous water loss) that water which is lost by evaporation through the skin surface other than by sweating. It is greatly increased in inflamed skin. *sensible perspiration* the term used when there are visible drops of sweat on the skin.

Perthes' disease (*syn* pseudocoxalgia) avascular degeneration of the upper femoral epiphysis in children; revascularization occurs, but residual deformity of the femoral head may subsequently lead to arthritic changes.

pertussis *n* (*syn* whooping cough) an infectious disease of children with attacks of paroxysmal coughing which in older children may end in an inspiratory whoop. In infants the cough is often associated with vomiting, and they can become cyanosed or apnoeic during coughing spasms. The basis of the condition is respiratory catarrh and the organism responsible is *Bordetella* pertussis.* Prophylactic vaccination is responsible for a decrease in case incidence.

pes *n* a foot or foot-like structure. *pes cavus* ⇒ claw-foot. *pes planus* ⇒ flat-foot.

pessary *n* **1** an instrument inserted into the vagina to correct uterine displacements. A *ring* or *shelf pessary* is used to support a prolapse. A *Hodge pessary* is used to correct a retroversion. **2** a medicated suppository used to treat vaginal infections, or as a contraceptive.

pesticides *npl* substances which kill pests.

PET *abbr* positron emission tomography*.

petechia *n* a small, haemorrhagic spot—**petechiae** *pl*, **petechial** *adj*.

pethidine *n* a synthetic analgesic and spasmolytic. Widely used for both preoperative and postoperative analgesia instead of morphine*. Can be given orally or intramuscularly. Intravenous injection requires care, as it may cause a fall in blood pressure.

petit mal ⇒ epilepsy.

pétrissage *n* kneading; the part, usually an identified muscle or tendon, is picked up between the thumb and index finger and kneading movements with firm pressure are carried out in a centripetal direction.

Peyer's patches flat patches of lymphatic tissue situated in the small intestine but mainly in the ileum; they are the seat of infection in typhoid fever; also known as 'aggregated lymph nodules'.

Peyronie's disease deformity and painful erection of penis due to fibrous tissue formation from unknown cause. Often associated with Dupuytren's* contracture.

pH *abbr* the concentration of hydrogen ions expressed as a negative logarithm. A neutral solution has a pH 7.0. With increasing acidity the pH falls and with increasing alkalinity it rises.

phacoemulsification *n* ⇒ phakoemulsification.

phaeochromocytoma *n* (*syn* paraganglioma) a condition in which there is a tumour of the adrenal medulla, or of the structurally similar tissues associated with the sympathetic chain. It secretes adrenaline and allied hormones and the symptoms are due to the excess of these substances. Aetiology unknown.

phagocyte *n* a cell capable of engulfing bacteria and other particulate material—**phagocytic** *adj.*

phagocytosis *n* the engulfment by phagocytes of bacteria or other particles.

phakoemulsification, phacoemulsification *n* ultrasonic vibration is used to liquefy mature lens fibres. The liquid lens matter is then sucked out.

phalanges *npl* the small bones of the fingers and toes—**phalanx** *sing,* **phalangeal** *adj.*

phallus *n* the penis*—**phallic** *adj.*

phantasy *n* ⇒ fantasy.

phantom limb the sensation that a limb is still attached to the body after it has been amputated. Phantom pain is experienced as coming from the amputated limb.

phantom pregnancy (*syn* pseudocyesis) signs and symptoms simulating those of early pregnancy; it occurs in a childless person who has an overwhelming desire to have a child.

pharmacogenetic *adj* produced by drugs, usually referring to side-effects.

pharmacokinetics *n* the study of the way in which drugs are absorbed, distributed and excreted from the body. It increases knowledge of drug concentrations in different parts of the body at different times throughout each 24 hours.

pharmacology *n* the science dealing with drugs—**pharmacological** *adj,* **pharmacologically** *adv.*

pharyngeal pouch pathological dilatation of the lower part of the pharynx*.

pharyngectomy *n* surgical removal of part of the pharynx.

pharyngismus *n* spasm of the pharynx*.

pharyngitis *n* inflammation of the pharynx*.

pharyngolaryngeal *adj* pertaining to the pharynx* and larynx*.

pharyngolaryngectomy *n* surgical removal of the pharynx and larynx.

pharyngoplasty *n* any plastic operation to the pharynx.

pharyngotomy *n* the operation of opening into the pharnynx.

pharyngotympanic tube ⇒ eustachian tube.

pharynx *n* the cavity at the back of the mouth. It is cone shaped, varies in length (average 75 mm), and is lined with mucous membrane; at the lower end it opens into the oesophagus*. The eustachian tubes pierce its lateral walls and the posterior nares pierce its anterior wall. The larynx lies immediately below it and in front of the oesophagus—**pharyngeal** *adj.*

PHC *abbr* primary* health care.

phenobarbitone *n* long-acting barbiturate and anticonvulsant. Used as a general sedative, and in epilepsy.

phenol *n* (*syn* carbolic acid) the first disinfectant which paved the way to the current era of aseptic surgery. It has been replaced for most purposes by more active and less toxic compounds. It is still used in calamine lotion for its local anaesthetic effect in relieving itching.

phenothiazines *npl* powerful tranquillizing drugs used to produce a sense of calm, without making the client feel sleepy. Includes chlorpromazine and promazine.

phenylalanine *n* an essential amino* acid. Those unable to metabolize it develop phenylketonuria*.

phenylketonuria (PKU) *n* metabolites of phenylalanine* (the best known being the phenylketones) in urine. Occurs in hyperphenylalaninaemia, owing to the lack of inactivity of the phenylalanine hydroxylase enzyme in the liver which converts dietary phenylalanine into tyrosine*. Autosomal recessive disease, resulting in mental subnormality unless discovered by screening and treated with an appropriate diet from birth. ⇒ Guthrie test—**phenylketonuric** *adj.*

phimosis *n* tightness of the prepuce so that it cannot be retracted over the glans penis.

phlebectomy *n* excision of a vein. *multiple cosmetic phlebectomy (MCP)* removal of varicose veins through little stab incisions which heal with minimal scarring.

phlebitis *n* inflammation of a vein—**phlebitic** *adj.*

phlebography ⇒ venography.

phlebolith *n* a concretion which forms in a vein.

phlebothrombosis *n* thrombosis in a vein due to sluggish flow of blood rather than to inflammation in the vein wall, occurring chiefly in bedfast patients and affecting the deep veins of the lower limbs or pelvis. The loosely attached thrombus is liable to break off and lodge in the lungs as an embolus. ⇒ intermittent pneumatic compression, pulmonary.

phlebotomist *n* a technician who is trained to carry out phlebotomy.

phlebotomy *n* venotomy* ⇒ venesection.

phlegm *n* the secretion of mucus expectorated from the bronchi.

phlegmatic *adj* describes an emotionally stable person.

phlyctenule *n* a minute blister (vesicle) usually occurring on the conjunctiva or cornea—**phlyctenular** *adj.*

phobia *n* irrational fear, either of a disease, e.g. pathophobia*, cardiac phobia, cancer phobia, or of an object or state, e.g. agoraphobia*—**phobic** *adj.*

phocomelia (seal limbs) *n* an intercalary deficiency of long bones, with relatively good development of hands and feet attached at or near the shoulders or hips. Most reduction deformities are associated with primary defects of development. Prosthetic* devices are fitted whenever possible and at the earliest possible stage of development. (A series of severe limb abnormalities in the 1960s was associated with women who had taken the drug thalidomide during pregnancy.)

phonation *n* the production of voice by vibration of the vocal cords.

phospholipase D *n* ⇒ lecithinase.

phosphonecrosis *n* 'fossy-jaw' occurring in workers engaged in the manufacture of matches made with white phosphorus; necrosis of the jaw with loosening of the teeth.

phosphorus *n* a nonmetallic element forming an important constituent of bone and nerve tissue.

photalgia *n* pain in the eyes from exposure to intense light.

photochemotherapy *n* the effect of the administered drug is enhanced by exposing the patient to ultraviolet light.

photocoagulation *n* burning of the tissues with a powerful, focused light source.

photoendoscope *n* an endoscope to which a camera is attached for the purpose of making a permanent record—**photoendoscopic** *adj*, **photoendoscopically** *adv*.

photophobia *n* inability to expose the eyes to light—**photophobic** *adj*.

photorefractive keratectomy (PRK) surgical reshaping of the cornea, using a laser, in order to correct refractive error, usually myopia* and/or astigmatism.

photosensitive *adj* sensitive to light, as the pigments in the eye.

phototherapy *n* exposure to artificial blue light. In hyperbilirubinaemia* it appears to dehydrogenate the bilirubin to biliverdin. Used for neonatal jaundice and to prevent jaundice in premature infants.

phren *n* pertaining to the diaphragm—**phrenic** *adj*.

phrenicotomy *n* division of the phrenic nerve to paralyse one half of the diaphragm.

phrenoplegia *n* paralysis of the diaphragm—**phrenoplegic** *adj*.

physical abuse ⇒ abuse, nonaccidental injury.

physician *n* customarily used to differentiate a medical doctor who uses the title Dr, from a surgeon who is entitled Mr.

physicochemical *adj* pertaining to physics and chemistry.

physiological *adj* in accordance with natural processes of the body. Adjective often used to describe a normal process or structure, to distinguish it from an abnormal or pathological feature (e.g. the physiological level of glucose in the blood is from 3.0–5.0 mmol per litre; higher and lower levels are pathological and indicative of disease). *physiological age* ⇒ biological age. *physiological saline* ⇒ isotonic. *physiological solution* a fluid isotonic* with the body fluids and containing similar salts.

physiology *n* the science which deals with the normal functions of the body—**physiological** *adj*, **physiologically** *adv*.

physiotherapy *n* treatment and rehabilitation by using physical agents such as cold, electricity, water and light, as well as massage, manipulation, therapeutic exercises and teaching patients to use equipment to help with walking.

pia, pia mater *n* the innermost of the meninges; the vascular membrane which lies in close contact with the substance of the brain and spinal cord.

pica *n* a desire for extraordinary articles of food, a feature of some pregnancies.

Pick's disease 1 syndrome of ascites, hepatic enlargement, oedema and pleural effusion occurring in constrictive pericarditis. **2** a type of cerebral atrophy which produces mental changes similar to presenile dementia*.

picornavirus *n* from pico (very small) and RNA (ribonucleic acid). Small RNA viruses. The group includes polio, coxsackie, echo and rhinoviruses.⇒ virus.

PID *abbr* **1** prolapse of an intervertebral disc. ⇒ prolapse. **2** pelvic* inflammatory disease.

pigeon chest (*syn* pectus carinatum) a narrow chest, bulging anteriorly in the breast bone region.

pigeon-toed *adj* walking with the toes of one or both feet turned inwards.

pigment *n* any colouring matter of the body.

pigmentation *n* the deposit of pigment, especially when abnormal or excessive.

piles *n* ⇒ haemorrhoids.

pilomotor nerves tiny nerves attached to the hair follicle; innervation causes the hair to stand upright and give the appearance of 'goose flesh'.

pilonidal *adj* hair-containing. *pilonidal sinus* a sinus containing hairs which is usually found in hirsute people in the cleft between the buttocks. In this situation it is liable to infection.

pilosebaceous *adj* pertaining to the hair follicle and the sebaceous gland opening into it.

pimple *n* ⇒ papule.

Pinard's stethoscope trumpet-shaped instrument enabling direct auscultation of the fetal heart through the abdominal wall.

pineal body a small reddish-grey conical structure on the dorsal surface of the midbrain. Its functions are not fully understood but there is some evidence that, encouraged by direct sunlight, it secretes melatonin*, the levels of which rise at night and drop at dawn. ⇒ depression.

pinguecula *n* a yellowish, slightly elevated thickening of the bulbar conjunctiva near the lid aperture. Associated with the ageing eye.

pink-eye *n* a popular name for acute contagious conjunctivitis, which spreads rapidly in closed communities or institutions where children mix the face-cloths.

pinna *n* that part of the ear which is external to the head; the auricle.

pinnaplasty *n* corrective surgery for bat ears.

pinta *n* colour changes in patches of skin due to *Treponema pinta,* identical with the spirochaete of syphilis* and yaws*.

pitting *n* **1** making an indentation in oedematous tissues. **2** depressed scar left on the skin at the sites of former pustules*.

pituitary gland (*syn* hypophysis cerebri) a small oval endocrine gland lying in the pituitary fossa of the sphenoid bone. The anterior lobe secretes several hormones; growth hormone, corticotrophin, thyrotrophin, luteotrophin, follicle stimulating hormone and prolactin. The posterior lobe secretes oxytocin* and ADH*. It is under the control of the hypothalamus*. The overall function of pituitary hormones is to regulate growth and metabolism.

pityriasis *n* scaly (branny) eruption of the skin. *pityriasis alba* a common eruption in children characterized by scaly hypopigmented macules on the cheeks and upper arms. *pityriasis capitis* dandruff. *pityriasis rosea* a slightly scaly eruption of ovoid erythematous lesions which are widespread over the trunk and proximal parts of the limbs. There may be mild itching. It is a self-limiting condition. *pityriasis rubra pilaris* a chronic skin disease characterized by tiny red papules of perifollicular distribution. *pityriasis versicolor* called also 'tinea versicolor', is a yeast infection which causes the appearance of buff-coloured patches on the chest.

Pityrosporum *n* genus of yeasts. *P. orbiculare (Malassezia furfur)* is associated with pityriasis versicolor.

PKU *abbr* phenylketonuria*.

placebo *n* a harmless substance given as medicine. In experimental research an inert substance, identical in appearance with the material being tested. Neither the physician nor the patient knows which is which.

placement *n* a period of time a student spends in a specific clinical area for explicit learning purposes.

placenta *n* the afterbirth, a vascular structure developed about the third month of pregnancy and attached to the inner wall of the uterus. Through it the fetus is supplied with nourishment and oxygen and through it the fetus gets rid of its waste products. In normal labour it is expelled within an hour of the birth of the child. When this does not occur it is termed a *retained placenta* and may be an *adherent placenta.* The placenta is usually attached to the upper segment of the uterus; when it lies in the lower uterine segment it is called a *placenta praevia* and usually causes painless antepartum haemorrhage.

placental abruption (*syn* antepartum haemorrhage*) bleeding after the 28th week of pregnancy and before labour, caused by partial or complete separation of the placenta, usually associated with abdominal pain and tenderness and shock. Bleeding may be concealed or revealed via the vagina.

placental insufficiency inefficiency of the placenta. Can occur due to maternal disease giving rise to a 'small-for-dates' baby, or to postmaturity of fetus.

placentography *n* X-ray examination of the placenta after injection of opaque substance.

plague *n* very contagious epidemic disease caused by *Yersinia pestis,* and spread by infected rats. Transfer of infection from rat to man is through the agency of fleas. The main clinical types are bubonic, septicaemic or pneumonic.

planning *v* regarded as the second phase of the nursing process. After identification of the patient's actual and potential problems with everyday living activities, the patient participates in setting appropriate goals to be achieved by the selected nursing interventions. A date is set for evaluation of whether or not the goals have been achieved. ⇒ assessing, implementing, evaluating.

plantar *adj* pertaining to the sole of the foot. *plantar arch* the union of the plantar and dorsalis pedis arteries in the sole of the foot. *plantar flexion* downward movement of the big toe.

plaque *n* ⇒ dental plaque.

plasma *n* the fluid fraction of blood. *blood plasma* is used for infusion in cases of haemoconcentration* of the patient's blood, as in severe burns. *dried plasma* is in the form of a yellow powder which must be 'reconstituted' before being used for infusion. Various plasma substitutes are available, e.g. Dextran, Plasmosan. *plasma cell* a normal cell with an eccentric nucleus derived from the B lymphocyte and reticuloendothelial system and concerned with the production of antibodies; abnormally produced in myelomatosis.

plasmin *n* a protease which digests fibrin.

plasminogen *n* precursor of plasmin*. Release of activators from damaged tissue promotes the conversion of plasminogen into plasmin.

Plasmodium *n* a genus of protozoa. Parasites in the blood of warm-blooded animals which complete their sexual cycle in blood-sucking arthropods. Four species cause malaria* in man—**plasmodial** *adj.*

Plastazote *n* proprietary lightweight thermoplastic material used for splints, supports and appliances.

plaster of Paris ⇒ gypsum.

plastic *adj* capable of taking a form or mould. *plastic surgery* reconstruction and refashioning of soft tissue to repair defects and deformities, and to restore and create form.

platelet *n* ⇒ thrombocyte. Disc-shaped particles playing an important role in blood coagulation.

platyhelminth *n* flat worm; fluke. ⇒ schistosomiasis.

play therapist a qualified person who uses play constructively to help children to come to terms with their illness or to prepare for various aspects of treatment. Other staff may be employed to play with children in hospital under the direction of the play therapist.

pleomorphism *n* denotes a wide range in shape and size of individuals in a bacterial population—**pleomorphic** *adj.*

plethysmograph *n* an instrument which measures accurately the blood flow in a limb—**plethysmographic** *adj.*

pleura *n* the serous membrane covering the surface of the lung (visceral pleura), the diaphragm, the mediastinum and the chest wall (parietal pleura) enclosing a potential space, the pleural cavity, to allow frictionless movement in respiration—**pleural** *adj.*

pleural effusion ⇒ hydrothorax.

pleurectomy *n* stripping off parietal pleura to obliterate pleural space and prevent recurrence of pneumothoraces.

pleurisy, pleuritis *n* inflammation of the pleura*. May be fibrinous (dry), be associated with an effusion (wet), or be complicated by empyema*—**pleuritic** *adj.*

pleurodesis *n* adherence of the visceral to the parietal pleura. Can be achieved therapeutically to treat recurrent pleueral effusion by instilling a sclerosing substance, such as iodized talc.

pleurodynia *n* intercostal myalgia or muscular rheumatism (fibrositis). It is a feature of Bornholm disease.

pleuropulmonary *adj* pertaining to the pleura and lung.

plexus *n* a network of vessels or nerves.

plication *n* a surgical procedure of making tucks or folds to decrease the size of an organ—**plica** *sing,* **plicate** *adj, vt.*

plombage *n* extrapleural compression of a tuberculous lung cavity.

plumbism *n* ⇒ lead poisoning.

Plummer-Vinson syndrome (*syn* Kelly-Paterson syndrome) a combination of severe glossitis with dysphagia and nutritional iron deficiency anaemia. Iron taken orally usually leads to complete recovery.

pluriglandular *adj* pertaining to several glands, as mucoviscidosis.

PMS *abbr* premenstrual* syndrome.

pneumaturia *n* the passage of flatus with urine, usually as a result of a vesicocolic (bladder-bowel) fistula.

pneumococcus *n Streptococcus pneumoniae,* a coccal bacterium arranged characteristically in pairs. A common cause of lobar pneumonia and other infections—**pneumococcal** *adj.*

pneumoconiosis *n* (*syn* dust disease) fibrosis of the lung caused by long continued inhalation of dust in industrial occupations. The most important complication is the occasional superinfection with tuberculosis—**pneumoconioses** *pl. rheumatoid pneumoconiosis* fibrosing alveolitis occurring in patients suffering from rheumatoid arthritis. ⇒ anthracosis, asbestosis, byssinosis, siderosis, silicosis.

Pneumocystis carinii a microorganism which causes pneumonia. The most usual victims are immunosuppressed or debilitated patients or infants: mortality is high.

pneumocytes *npl* special cells which line the alveolar walls in the lungs. Type I are flat, Type II are cuboidal and secrete surfactant.

pneumoencephalography *n* radiographic examination of cerebral ventricles after injection of air by means of a lumbar or cisternal puncture—**pneumoencephalogram** *n.*

pneumogastric *adj* pertaining to the lungs and stomach. ⇒ vagus.

pneumomycosis *n* fungus infection of the lung such as

aspergillosis, actinomycosis, candidiasis—**pneumomycotic** *adj*.

pneumonectomy *n* excision of a lung.

pneumonia *n* traditionally used for inflammation of the lung; when resulting from allergic reaction it is often referred to as alveolitis; that which is due to physical agents is pneumonitis, the word 'pneumonia' being reserved for invasion by microorganisms.

pneumonitis *n* inflammation of lung tissue.

pneumoperitoneum *n* air or gas in the peritoneal cavity. Can be introduced for diagnostic or therapeutic purposes.

pneumothorax *n* air or gas in the pleural cavity separating the visceral from the parietal pleura so that lung tissue is compressed. A pneumothorax can be secondary to asthma, carcinoma of bronchus, chronic bronchitis, congenital cysts, emphysema, intermittent positive pressure ventilation, pneumonia, trauma or tuberculosis—**pneumothoraces** *pl. artificial pneumothorax* deliberate introduction of air/gas into the pleural space to collapse the lung. *spontaneous pneumothorax* occurs when an overdilated pulmonary air sac ruptures, permitting communication of respiratory passages and pleural cavity. *tension pneumothorax* occurs when a valve-like wound allows air to enter the pleural cavity at each inspiration but not to escape on expiration, thus progressively increasing intrathoracic pressure and constituting an acute medical emergency.

PNI *abbr* psychoneuroimmunology*.

podalic version ⇒ version.

podiatrist *n* (*syn* chiropodist) one who specializes in the care and treatment of feet—**podiatry** *n*.

podopompholyx *n* pompholyx* on the feet.

polioencephalitis *n* inflammation of the cerebral grey matter—**polioencephalitic** *adj*.

poliomyelitis *n* (*syn* infantile paralysis) an epidemic viral infection which attacks the motor neurones of the anterior horns in the brain stem (*bulbar poliomyelitis)* and spinal cord. An attack may or may not lead to paralysis of the lower motor neurone type with loss of muscular power and flaccidity. Vaccination against the disease is desirable—in the UK, all children are offered the vaccine in infancy as part of the regular immunization schedule. When it occurs within two days of vaccination with any alum-containing prophylactic, the term *provocative paralytic poliomyelitis* is used. ⇒ Sabin vaccine, Salk vaccine.

polioviruses cause poliomyelitis*. ⇒ virus.

Politzer's bag a rubber bag for inflation of the eustachian tube.

pollenosis *n* an allergic condition arising from sensitization to pollen.

pollicization *n* a surgical procedure whereby the index finger is rotated and shortened to produce apposition as a thumb.

pollution *n* diminished purity or quality. *air pollution* the government's declaration of smoke-free zones in which it is an offence to burn ordinary coal in a domestic fire, together with regulations about emission of smoke from tall industrial chimneys has done much to rid the air of smog—fog made worse by smoke. Currently attention is being paid to lead in petrol, the fumes from which can be inhaled; and also to pollution of the atmosphere by tobacco smoke. *noise pollution* a term introduced in the last few decades. Excessive environmental noise can cause such conditions as deafness, lessened concentration and insufficient sleep. *water pollution* natural lakes, rivers and seas can become polluted from land seepage and untreated sewage rendering them unfit for swimming and poisoning fish which are rendered unsafe for human consumption.

Polya operation partial gastrectomy*.

polyarteritis *n* inflammation of many arteries. In *polyarteritis nodosa* (*syn* periarteritis nodosa) aneurysmal swellings and thrombosis occur in the affected vessels. Further damage may lead to haemorrhage and the clinical picture presented depends upon the site affected. ⇒ collagen.

polyarthralgia *n* pain in several joints.

polyarthritis *n* inflammation of several joints at the same time. ⇒ Still's disease.

polycystic *adj* composed of many cysts. Polycystic renal disease is a genetically inherited condition which results in enlarged, spongy kidneys; it is also associated with cysts in the liver and other organs. There are several varieties of the disease (the infantile form can be fatal).

polycythaemia *n* increase in the number of circulating red blood cells. This may result from dehydration or be a compensatory phenomenon to increase the oxygen carrying capacity, as in congenital heart disease. *polycythaemia vera* (*syn* erythraemia) is an idiopathic condition in which the red cell count is very high. The patient complains of headache and lassitude, and there is danger of thrombosis and haemorrhage.

polydactyly, polydactylism *n* having more than the normal number of fingers or toes.

polydipsia *n* excessive thirst.

polygraph *n* instrument which records several variables simultaneously.

polyhydramnios *n* an excessive amount of amniotic fluid.

polymorphonuclear *adj* having a many-shaped or lobulated nucleus, usually applied to the phagocytic neutrophil leucocytes (granulocytes) which constitute 70% of the total white blood cells.

polymyalgia rheumatica a syndrome occurring in elderly people comprising of a sometimes crippling ache in the shoulders, pelvic girdle muscles and spine, with pronounced morning stiffness and a raised ESR*. There is an association with temporal arteritis. Clinically different from rheumatoid arthritis. ⇒ arthritis.

polymyositis *n* manifests as muscle weakness, most commonly in middle age. Microscopic examination of muscle reveals inflammatory changes: they respond to corticosteroid drugs. ⇒ dermatomyositis.

polyneuritis *n* multiple neuritis—**polyneuritic** *adj.*

polyoma *n* one of the tumour-producing viruses.

polyp, polypus a pedunculated tumour arising from any mucous surface, e.g. cervical, uterine, nasal, etc. Usually benign but may become malignant—**polypi** *pl,* **polypous** *adj.*

polypectomy *n* surgical removal of a polyp.

polypeptides *npl* proteins which on hydrolysis yield more than two amino acids.

polypharmacy *n* a word used when several oral drugs are prescribed for the same patient. It increases the risk of patient noncompliance* and noncomprehension*.

polypoid *adj* resembling a polyp(us).

polyposis *n* a condition in which

there are numerous polypi in an organ. *polyposis coli* a dominantly-inheritable condition in which polypi occur throughout the large bowel and which can often lead to carcinoma of the colon. Prevention is by removal of polyps.

polysaccharide *n* carbohydrates ($C_6H_{10}O_5$) containing a large number of monosaccharide groups. Starch, inulin, glycogen, dextrin and cellulose are examples.

polyserositis *n* inflammation of several serous membranes. A genetic type is called familial Mediterranean fever. ⇒ amyloidosis.

polyuria *n* excretion of an excessive amount of urine—**polyuric** *adj.*

pompholyx *n* vesicular skin eruption associated with itching or burning. ⇒ cheiropompholyx.

pons *n* a bridge; a process of tissue joining two sections of an organ. *pons varolii* the white convex mass of nerve tissue at the base of the brain which serves to connect the various lobes of the brain—**pontine** *adj.*

Pontiac fever a flu-like illness with little or no pulmonary involvement and no mortality—caused by *Legionella* pneumophila.*

popliteal *adj* pertaining to the popliteus. *popliteal space* the diamond-shaped depression at the back of the knee joint, bounded by the muscles and containing the popliteal nerve and vessels.

popliteus *n* a muscle in the popliteal space which flexes the leg and aids it in rotating.

poradenitis *n* painful mass of iliac glands, characterized by abscess formation. Occurs in lymphogranuloma* inguinale.

pore *n* a minute surface opening. One of the mouths of the ducts (leading from the sweat glands) on the skin surface; they are controlled by fine papillary muscles, contracting and closing in the cold and dilating in the presence of heat.

porphyria *n* an inborn error in porphyrin metabolism, usually hereditary, causing pathological changes in nervous and muscular tissue in some varieties and photosensitivity in others, depending on the level of the metabolic block involved. Excess porphyrins or precursors are found in the urine (porphyrinuria) or stools or both. In some cases attacks are precipitated by certain drugs. Prognosis is good if diagnosed early, if attention is given to management of fluids and diet, and avoidance of contraindicated drugs.

porphyrins *npl* light-sensitive organic compounds which form the basis of respiratory pigments, including haemoglobin. Naturally occurring porphyrins are uroporphyrin and coproporphyrin* ⇒ porphyria.

porta *n* the depression (hilum) of an organ at which the vessels enter and leave—**portal** *adj. porta hepatis* the transverse fissure through which the portal vein, hepatic artery and bile ducts pass on the under surface of the liver.

Portacath *n* proprietary device which has an injectionable port underneath the skin with a catheter leading from it to provide a central* venous line. Allows repeated venous access without the need for venepuncture.

portacaval, portocaval *adj* pertaining to the portal vein and inferior vena cava. *portacaval anastomosis* a fistula made between the portal vein and the inferior vena cava with the object of reducing the pressure within the portal vein in cases of cirrhosis of the liver.

Portage system based on behaviour modification techniques

PORTFOLIO

A portfolio is a personal and private collection of evidence, which demonstrates the owner's continuing professional and personal development. It documents the acquisition of knowledge, skills, attitudes, understanding and achievements; in recording these events, it deals with the past. It contains reflections on current practice and progress, and in doing this it deals with the present. However, it also contains an action plan for future career and personal development, and in this it looks to the future. It does not simply record outcomes, but rather it documents the journey taken *en route* to the outcomes. As such it is a valuable tool in your continuing professional development. Note that from your portfolio you should be able to select profiles for a number of different purposes.

See also: profile.

which are used by family members and a home visitor who work together to help children with a physical or learning disability to develop and acquire skills required for everyday living. The kit includes a checklist, box of teaching cards, an activity chart and a system for monitoring progress.

portahepatitis *n* inflammation around the transverse fissure of the liver.

portal circulation that of venous blood (collected from the intestines, pancreas, spleen and stomach) to the liver before return to the heart.

portal hypertension increased pressure in the portal vein. Usually caused by cirrhosis of the liver; results in splenomegaly, with hypersplenism and alimentary bleeding. ⇒ oesophageal varices.

portal vein that conveying blood into the liver; it is about 75 mm long and is formed by the union of the superior mesenteric and splenic veins.

portfolio *n* ⇒ Portfolio box.

position *n* posture.

positive pressure ventilation (PPV) positive pressure inflation of lungs to produce inspiration. Exhaled air, a manual respirator or more sophisticated apparatus can be used. Expiration results from elastic recoil of the lung. ⇒ continuous positive airways pressure, intermittent positive pressure ventilation, mandatory minute volume, noninvasive positive pressure ventilation, pressure support ventilation, synchronized intermittent mandatory ventilation.

posseting *n* regurgitation of small amounts of milk in infants, usually after feeding; associated with swallowing air during the feed.

possum *n* Patient-Operated Selector Mechanism. An apparatus which can be operated by a slight touch, or by suction using the mouth if no other muscle movement is possible. It may transmit messages or be adapted for typing, telephoning and other activities.

postanal *adj* behind the anus.

postcoital *adj* after sexual intercourse. The word describes the 'morning after' contraceptive.

postconcussional syndrome the association of headaches, giddiness and a feeling of faintness, which may persist for a considerable time after a head injury.

postdiphtheritic *adj* following an attack of diphtheria. Refers especially to the paralysis of limbs and palate.

postencephalitic *adj* following encephalitis lethargica. The adjective is commonly used to describe the syndrome of parkinsonism, which often results from an attack of this type of encephalitis.

postepileptic *adj* following on an epileptic seizure. *postepileptic automatism* is a fugue state, following on a fit, when the patient may undertake a course of action, even involving violence, without having any memory of this (amnesia).

posterior *adj* situated at the back. ⇒ anterior *opp.* posterior chamber of the eye the space between the anterior surface of the lens and the posterior surface of the iris. ⇒ aqueous

postganglionic *adj* situated after a collection of nerve cells (ganglion) as in postganglionic nerve fibre.

postgastrectomy syndrome covers two sets of symptoms, those of hypoglycaemia when the patient is hungry, and those of a vasovagal attack immediately after a meal.

posthepatic *adj* behind the liver.

postherpetic *adj* after shingles*.

posthitis *adj* inflammation of the prepuce*.

posthumous *adj* occurring after death. *posthumous birth* delivery of a baby by caesarian section after the mother's death, or birth occurring after the death of the father.

postmature *adj* past the expected date of delivery. A baby is postmature when labour is delayed beyond the usual 40 weeks. Intervention is now often delayed to 42 or 43 weeks provided the maternal and fetal wellbeing is monitored and gives no cause for concern—**postmaturity** *n.*

postmenopausal *adj* occurring after the menopause* has been established.

postmortem *adj* after death, usually implying dissection of the body. ⇒ antemortem *opp,* autopsy. *postmortem wart* ⇒ verruca.

postmyocardial infarction syndrome pyrexia and chest pain associated with inflammation of the pleura, lung or pericardium. Due to sensitivity to released products from dead muscle.

postnasal *adj* situated behind the nose and in the nasopharynx—**postnasally** *adv.*

postnatal *adj* after delivery. ⇒ antenatal *opp. postnatal blues* describes a low mood experienced by some mothers for a few days following the birth of a baby; sometimes called 'fourth-day blues'. Less severe than *postnatal depression* ⇒ puerperal* psychosis. *postnatal examination* routine examination 6 weeks after delivery

postoperative *adj* after operation—**postoperatively** *adv.*

postpartum *adj* after a birth (parturition).

postprandial *adj* following a meal.

postural *adj* pertaining to posture. *postural albuminuria* orthostatic* albuminuria. *postural drainage* usually infers drainage from the respiratory tract, by elevation of the foot of the bed or by using a special frame. The chest is percussed and sputum coughed into a disposable carton. Children with cystic fibrosis need to have this treatment at home and family members learn to do it.

posture *n* active or passive arrangement of the whole body, or a part, in a definite position.

postvagotomy diarrhoea three types: (a) transient diarrhoea shortly after operation, lasting from a few hours to a day or two. These episodes disappear in 3–6 months. (b) if they recur later than this and the attacks last longer, the term 'recurrent episodic diarrhoea' is used. (c) an increased daily bowel frequency; may be of disabling severity, but often acceptable in contrast to preoperative constipation.

potassium chlorate a mild antiseptic used in mouthwashes and gargles. Distinguish from potassium chloride.

potassium chloride used in potassium replacement solutions, and as a supplement in thiazide diuretic therapy.

potassium deficiency disturbed electrolyte balance; can occur after excessive vomiting, and/or diarrhoea; after prolonged use of diuretics, steroids, etc. The signs and symptoms are variable, but nausea and muscle weakness are often present. Heart failure can quickly supervene.

potassium permanganate purple crystals with powerful disinfectant and deodorizing properties. Used as lotion 1 in 1000; 1 in 5000 to 10 000 for baths.

potter's rot one of the many popular names for silicosis* arising in workers in the pottery industry.

Pott's disease spondylitis; spinal caries; spinal tuberculosis. The resultant necrosis of the vertebrae causes kyphosis.

Pott's fracture a fracture-dislocation of the ankle joint. A fracture of the lower end of the tibia and fibula, 75 mm above the ankle joint, and a fracture of the medial malleolus of the tibia.

pouch *n* a pocket or recess. *pouch of Douglas* the rectouterine pouch.

povidone iodine a liquid from which iodine is slowly liberated when in contact with the skin and mucous membranes. It is therefore useful for preoperative skin preparation and as a douche.

powerlessness *n* a feeling that one is trapped and unable to deal with inadvertent circumstances. ⇒ depression, institutionalization.

PPD *abbr* purified protein derivative. ⇒ Mantoux reaction.

PPLO *abbr* pleuropneumonia-like organism, similar to the agent that causes contagious pleuropneumonia in cattle. ⇒ Mycoplasma.

PPV *abbr* ⇒ positive pressure ventilation.

PR *abbr* per rectum: describes the route used for examination of the rectum, or introduction of substances into the body.

practice nurses registered nurses who are employed by general practitioners to carry out minor procedures, advise on health problems and offer health promotion. As members of the primary health care team they are also responsible for the clinical nursing care of the practice population together with the community nursing team.

practitioner *n* in a nursing context a clinician*. In a wider health context, any professional who works with patients/clients. ⇒ general practitioner, nurse practitioner.

Prader-Willi syndrome a metabolic condition characterized by congenital hypotonia, hyperphagia, obesity and mental retardation. Diabetes mellitus develops in later life.

praecordial *adj* ⇒ precordial.

precancerous *adj* occurring before cancer, with special reference to nonmalignant pathological changes which are believed to lead on to, or to be followed by, cancer unless treated.

preceptorship *n* a system to help the newly qualified nurse achieve confidence in the early months of registered practice, under the guidance of a preceptor.

precipitin *n* an antibody which is

capable of forming an immune complex with an antigen and becoming insoluble—a precipitate. This reaction forms the basis of many delicate diagnostic serological tests for the identification of antigens in serum and other fluids ⇒ immunoglobulins.

preconceptual *adj* before conception. Health education stresses that attention to an adequate diet, avoidance of alcohol and smoking in the months before a couple decide to have a baby reduces the risk of complications.

precordial, praecordial *adj* pertaining to the area of the chest immediately over the heart. *precordial thump* direct blow with closed fist over precordium. Sometimes used in the initial stages of resuscitation to shock the heart into sinus rhythm.

precursor *adj* forerunner.

prediabetes *n* potential predisposition to diabetes* mellitus. Preventive mass urine testing can detect the condition. Early treatment prevents ketoacidosis and may help to prevent the more serious complications such as retinopathy and neuropathy—**prediabetic** *adj, n.*

predisposition *n* a natural tendency to develop or contract certain diseases.

prednisolone *n* a synthetic hormone with properties similar to those of cortisone* but side-effects, such as salt and water retention, are markedly reduced. Widely prescribed for connective tissue diseases, conditions involving immune reaction including autoimmune disorders.

prednisone converted into prednisolone* in the liver, therefore prescribed for the same conditions as prednisolone.

preeclampsia *n* a condition of pregnancy characterized by albuminuria, hypertension and oedema, arising usually in the latter part of pregnancy and endangering the health of both mother and fetus ⇒ eclampsia—**preeclamptic** *adj.*

prefrontal *adj* situated in the anterior portion of the frontal lobe of the cerebrum.

preganglionic *adj* preceding or in front of a collection of nerve cells (ganglia), as a preganglionic nerve fibre.

pregnancy *n* being with child, i.e. gestation from last menstrual period to parturition, normally 40 weeks or 280 days. ⇒ ectopic pregnancy, phantom pregnancy. *pregnancy-induced hypertension* solely a disease of pregnancy, most commonly of the primigravida. Blood pressure returns to normal and protein and urea, if present in the blood, resolve quickly after delivery in nearly all instances.

pregnanediol *n* a urinary excretion product from progesterone*.

prehensile *adj* equipped for grasping.

prejudice *n* a preconceived opinion or bias which can be negative or positive; it can be for or against members of minority groups, or people practising a particular religion.

premature *adj* occurring before the proper time. *premature (preterm) baby/birth* in English law, the birth of a baby after 24 but before 37 weeks' gestation. The baby is likely to be of low birthweight* and possibly small-for-dates* or dysmature* through placental* insufficiency.

premedication *n* drugs given before the administration of another drug, e.g. those given before an anaesthetic. The latter are of several types: (a) sedative or anxiolytic, e.g. morphine, papaveretum, pethidine, which also have sedative properties (b) drugs which inhibit the secretion of saliva and of mucus from the upper respiratory tract and cause tachycardia, e.g. atropine glycopyrrolonium.

premenstrual *adj* preceding menstruation. *premenstrual (cyclical) syndrome (PMS)*, also known as premenstrual tension (PMT), a group of physical and mental changes which begin any time between 2 and 14 days before menstruation and which are relieved almost immediately the flow starts. Research has revealed a deficiency of essential fatty acids. Some women are treated successfully with pyridoxine*, evening primrose oil, progestogens or oestrogens.

premolars *npl* the teeth, also called bicuspids, situated fourth and fifth from the midline of the jaws, used with the molars for gripping and grinding food.

prenatal *adj* pertaining to the period between the last menstrual period and birth of the child, normally 40 weeks or 280 days—**prenatally** *adv.*

preoperative *adj* before operation—**preoperatively** *adv.*

PREP ⇒ PREP box.

preparalytic *adj* before the onset of paralysis, usually referring to the early stage of poliomyelitis.

prepatellar *adj* in front of the kneecap, as applied to a large bursa. ⇒ bursitis.

prepubertal *adj* before puberty.

prepuce *n* the foreskin of the penis.

prerenal *adj* literally, before or in front of the kidney, but used to denote states in which, for instance, renal failure has arisen not within the nephrons but in the vascular fluid compartment, as in severe dehydration.

presbycusis *n* sensorineural deafness seen in the elderly.

presbyopia *n* longsightedness, due to failure of accommodation, typically in those of 45 years and over—**presbyopic** *adj,* **presbyope** *n.*

prescribed diseases a list of occupational diseases prescribed under the UK industrial injuries scheme. It is the responsibility of the Industrial Injuries Advisory Council. The council advises the Secretary of State whether to accept or reject the arguments for prescription. There are currently approximately 65 prescribed diseases.

prescription *n* a written formula, signed by a physician, directing the pharmacist to supply the required drugs.

prescription only medicines (POM) medicines which require a written prescription signed by a qualified doctor as opposed to over-the-counter* drugs. ⇒ drug.

presenile dementia ⇒ dementia, Alzheimer's disease.

presentation *n* the part of the fetus which first enters the pelvic brim and will be felt by the examining finger through the cervix in labour. May be vertex, face, brow, shoulder, breech or footling.

pressor *n* a substance which raises the blood pressure.

pressure areas the bony prominences of the body, over which the flesh of bedfast and chairfast patients is denuded of its blood supply as it is compressed between the bone and an external source of pressure; the latter is usually the bed, but may be a splint, plaster, upper bedclothes, chair, etc.

pressure garment a garment for a particular part of the body. It is made of a strong, flesh-coloured Lycra material which produces firm, even pressure to the part. Often used in the treatment of varicose veins; and burns and scalds to prevent keloid. ⇒ disfigurement.

pressure point a place at which an artery passes over a bone, against which it can be compressed, to stop bleeding.

PREP

PREP stands for Postregistration Education and Practice. In 1990, the United Kingdom Central Council for Nursing, Midwifery and Health Visiting (UKCC) published a discussion document on educational needs following registration that became known as the PREP project. After 4 years of discussion and debate, the proposals were finalized in 1994 in a report from the UKCC entitled *The Council's Standards for Education and Practice following Registration.* The report focused on the following areas:

- Standards for Professional Practice.
- Standards in Specialist Nursing Practice, Specialist Community Nursing Practice and Midwifery Practice (all pitched at degree level).
- Standards for Education and Teaching in all these areas.
- Advanced Nursing and Midwifery Practice (pitched at Masters level).

Much of the discussion relating to PREP has been concerned with the standards for professional practice, particularly the UKCC's requirements. Professional practice is seen as building on the foundation of preregistration education. It is concerned with safeguarding the interests of patients and clients by:

- promoting safe practice
- maintaining up-to-date knowledge and competence, and awareness of developments in practice
- enhancing skills and knowledge
- improving contributions to care and advances in practice.

For nurses there are four statutory requirements for remaining a registered practitioner:

1. Complete a minimum of 5 days (or the equivalent) of relevant study every 3 years.
2. Complete a notification of practice form every 3 years, giving details of qualifications and area of practice.
3. Use a personal professional portfolio from which a profile can be drawn for a number of purposes, including satisfying the UKCC about requirement 1.
4. After a break of 5 years or more, complete a return to practice programme, approved by a National Board, to develop knowledge and competence to an appropriate standard.

The first of these requirements became mandatory after 1 April 1995; the fourth becomes mandatory in the year 2000.

pressure sore (*syn* bedsore, decubitus ulcer) damage to integrity of skin caused by tissue distortion or skin shearing. Pressure sores are classified as either superficial or deep. *superficial pressure sores* involve destruction of the epidermis with exposure of the dermis so that microorganisms can penetrate the exposed tissue which is moist with lymph. *deep pressure* *sores* are caused by damage to the microcirculation in the deep tissues usually resulting from shearing force. The inflammatory and necrotic residue then tracks out to the skin surface destroying the dermis and epidermis. Deep sores may be infected, discharging an exudate which results in protein and fluid loss from the body. Deep sores can take many weeks or months to heal and quite often require surgical closure to prevent further debility. Pressure sores can be a source of hospital acquired infection*.

pressure sores, prevention of relief of pressure from the part by manual handling, aided lifting, moving, use of external aids, keeping the skin dry and clean, ensuring that the patient takes an adequate diet, preventing boredom. ⇒ shearing force.

pressure support ventilation (PSV) a mode of assisted ventilation, often used when weaning a patient off assisted ventilation. The machine delivers pressure support, hence additional inspired volume, when the patient takes a breath.

presystole *n* the period preceding the systole or contraction of the heart muscle—**presystolic** *adj.*

preterm *adj* ⇒ premature.

preventive nursing health visitors have traditionally been in the forefront where prevention is concerned, as have practice nurses with their role in health promotion. Focusing on a patient's potential problems highlights the preventive component of nursing.

priapism *n* prolonged penile erection in the absence of sexual stimulation.

prickly heat ⇒ miliaria.

primary complex (*syn* Ghon focus) the initial tuberculous infection in a person, usually in the lung, and manifest as a small focus of infection in the lung tissue and enlarged caseous, hilar glands. It usually heals spontaneously.

primary health care essential health care made universally accessible to individuals and their families in the community. It is perceived to be the key to the World Health Organization's goal of 'health for all by the year 2000'. *primary health care team* an interdependent group of professionals who share a common purpose and responsibility, each member clearly understanding his or her own role, and those of other team members, in offering an effective primary health care service.

primary nurse a nurse who assesses and plans a patient's care, implements it when on duty and delegates to 'an associate nurse' when off duty. The nurse is therefore responsible and accountable for the patient's nursing throughout his/her stay on the particular unit. ⇒ Primary nursing box.

primary nursing a way of organizing nursing care in which a primary* nurse has a number of patients and acts as an associate for a number of others. ⇒ Primary nursing box.

primary prevention ⇒ ill health—prevention of.

primigravida *n* a woman who is pregnant for the first time—**primigravidae** *pl.*

primipara *n* a woman who has given birth to a child for the first time—**primiparous** *adj.*

primordial *adj* primitive, original; applied to the ovarian follicles present at birth.

proband *n* the original person presenting for investigation of a genetically-inherited disease, who forms the basis for genetic study.

PRIMARY NURSING

Primary nursing is a professional model of practice, based on a belief in the therapeutic value of the nurse–patient relationship. A qualified nurse is responsible and accountable for the assessment, planning and implementation of all of the nursing care of a particular patient or group of patients for the entire duration of their stay in a particular care setting.

The nurse is supported in this role by an associate nurse who cares for the patient while the primary nurse is absent, according to the nursing plan drawn up by the primary nurse. Other nurses, including students and health care assistants, may also provide care for the patient, but this is always under the supervision and coordination of the primary nurse.

Primary nursing is not the same as named nursing—it is simply one form of named nursing, although probably the most highly developed.

See also: named nurse, team nursing.

problem-oriented records a multiprofessional system of patient records in which each patient's problem has a numbered page and entries are made using the SOAP formula–S=subjective, O=objective, A=analysis of the subjective and objective data, P=plan.

process *n* a prominence or outgrowth of any part.

procidentia *n* complete prolapse of the uterus, so that it lies within the vaginal sac but outside the contour of the body.

proctalgia *n* pain in the rectal region.

proctitis *n* inflammation of the rectum*. *granular proctitis* acute proctitis, so called because of the granular appearance of the inflamed mucous membrane.

proctocolectomy *n* surgical excision of the rectum and colon resulting in a permanent colostomy. *restorative proctocolectomy* avoids a permanent stoma: an ileal reservoir is formed and ileoanal anastomosis carried out.

proctocolitis *n* inflammation of the rectum and colon; usually a type of ulcerative colitis*.

proctoscope *n* an instrument for examining the rectum. ⇒ endoscope—**proctoscopic** *adj*, **proctoscopy** *n*.

proctosigmoiditis *n* inflammation of the rectum and sigmoid colon.

prodromal *adj* preceding, as the transitory rash before the true rash of an infectious disease.

prodrug *n* a compound with reduced intrinsic activity, but which, after absorption, is metabolized to release the active components. It avoids side-effects on the gastrointestinal tract.

professional disciplinary process nurses are expected to be self-disciplined and to act responsibly while nursing, so that they are accountable for their actions. Complaints against nurses are made to the statutory body, the United Kingdom Central Council for Nurses, Midwives and Health Visitors, where the professional conduct of a nurse is judged by peers. A nurse can have legal representation and a welfare committee is available to provide support throughout the process.

professional judgement a complex skill using cognition, intuition, a high level of professional

PROFILE

A profile can be selected from your portfolio to fit a number of different purposes. It refers to a selection of evidence extracted from the whole to meet a specific need. It is designed to be shown to others. For example, you might select a profile from your portfolio (including your CV) when applying for a new job, or for a place on a degree course, or to substantiate a claim for Accreditation of Prior Learning (APL)* or Accreditation of Prior Experiential Learning (APEL)*. Crucially, the UKCC will need to be assured that you can furnish them with a profile, should they request it, to show that you have met their requirements for professional updating, in order for periodic reregistration to take place.

See also: portfolio.

education, and experience to make a decision, often in emergency, without being conscious of using a logical process.

profile *n* ⇒ Profile box.

progesterone *n* the hormone of the corpus luteum*. Used in the treatment of functional uterine haemorrhage, and in threatened abortion. Given by intramuscular injection.

progestogen *n* any natural or synthetic progestational hormone progesterone*.

proglottis *n* a sexually mature segment of tapeworm—**proglottides** *pl.*

prognosis *n* a forecast of the probable course and termination of a disease—**prognostic** *adj.*

progress sheets a name used by some documentation systems for recording the implementation of planned nursing interventions, ongoing assessment and summative evaluation data.

Project 2000 the name given to a new system of nurse education, launched by the UKCC* in 1990. Nurses are educated to diploma level through a common foundation programme, followed by a chosen branch of nursing: care of the adult, the child, people with mental illness and people with a learning disability. Curricula are rooted in health promotion and primary health care.

projectile vomiting forceful ejection of stomach contents. Occurs shortly after feeding in babies with pyloric stenosis, when peristaltic movement is visible on the upper abdomen. Characteristic of some cerebral conditions.

projection *n* a mental mechanism occurring in normal people unconsciously, and in exaggerated form in mental illness, especially paranoia, whereby the person fails to recognize certain motives and feelings in himself but attributes them to others.

prolactin *n* a hormone secreted by the anterior pituitary, concerned with lactation and reproduction. Increased levels found in some pituitary tumours (prolactinomas) result in amenorrhoea and infertility. Treatment with bromocriptine may be effective.

prolapse *n* descent; the falling of a structure. *prolapse of an intervertebral disc (PID)* protrusion of the disc nucleus into the spinal canal. Most common in the lumbar region where it causes low back pain and/or sciatica. ⇒ backache. *prolapse of the iris* iridocele*. *prolapse of the rectum* the lower portion of the intestinal tract descends outside the external anal sphincter. *prolapse of the uterus* the uterus descends into the vagina and may be visible at the vaginal orifice. ⇒ procidentia.

proliferate *vi* increase by cell division—**proliferation** *n,* **proliferative** *adj.*

prolific *adj* fruitful, multiplying abundantly.

promontory *n* a projection; a prominent part.

pronate *vt* to place ventral surface downward, e.g. on the face; to turn (the palm of the hand) downwards ⇒ supinate *opp*—**pronation** *n.*

pronator *n* that which pronates, usually applied to a muscle. ⇒ supinator *opp.*

prone *adj* **1** lying on the anterior surface of the body with the face turned to one or other side. **2** of the hand, with the palm downwards. ⇒ supine *opp.*

prophylaxis *n* (attempted) prevention—**prophylactic** *adj.*

propranolol *n* an effective drug in the prevention or correction of cardiac arrhythmias and dysrhythmias. It reduces frequency of anginal attacks by blocking the effects of beta-receptor activation in the heart. Bronchoconstriction may occur as a side-effect in some patients. Prepared as eye drops for glaucoma.

proprietary name (*syn* brand name) the name given to, e.g., a drug by the pharmaceutical firm which produced it. The name should always be spelt with a capital letter to distinguish it from the approved name which can be used by any manufacturer. approved name *opp.*

proprioception transmission of sensory stimuli, such as those from pressure, position or stretch, arising within the body, to a proprioceptor, from which they are transmitted in the central nervous system to produce the necessary response to the stimulus.

proptosis *n* forward protrusion, especially of the eyeball.

prosector's wart ⇒ verruca.

prosody *n* a descriptive term for the phonological features of speech including rate, stress, rhythm, loudness and pitch.

prostacyclin *n* a naturally occurring substance formed by endothelial cells of blood vessel walls. It inhibits platelet aggregation and is a potent vasoconstricting agent.

prostaglandins *npl* share some of the properties of hormones, vitamins, enzymes and catalysts. All body tissues probably contain some prostaglandins. Used pharmaceutically to terminate early pregnancy, and for asthma and gastric hyperacidity.

prostate *n* a small conical gland at the base of the male bladder and surrounding the first part of the urethra—**prostatic** *adj.*

prostatectomy *n* surgical removal of the prostate* gland. *retropubic prostatectomy* the prostate is reached through a lower abdominal (suprapubic) incision, the bladder being retracted upwards to expose the prostate behind the pubis. *transurethral prostatectomy* the operation whereby chippings of prostatic tissue are cut from within the urethra using either a cold knife or electric cautery; usually restricted to small fibrous glands or to cases of prostatic carcinoma.⇒ resectoscope. *transvesical prostatectomy* the operation in which the prostate is approached through the bladder, using a lower abdominal (suprapubic) incision.

prostatic acid phosphatase an enzyme in seminal fluid secreted by the prostate gland. *prostatic acid phosphatase test* (PAP test) an increase in this enzyme in the blood is indicative of carcinoma of the prostate gland.

prostatism *n* general condition produced by hypertrophy or chronic disease of the prostate gland, characterized by the obstructive symptoms of hesitancy, a poor stream and postmicturition dribbling.

prostatitis *n* inflammation of the prostate* gland.

prostatocystitis *n* inflammation of the prostate gland and male urinary bladder.

prosthesis *n* an artificial substitute for a missing part—**prostheses** *pl*, **prosthetic** *adj*.

prosthetics *n* the branch of surgery which deals with prostheses.

prosthokeratoplasty *n* keratoplasty* in which the corneal implant is of some material other than human or animal tissue.

protamine sulphate a protein of simple structure used as an antidote to heparin*. 1 ml of 1% solution will neutralize the effects of about 1000 units of heparin.

protamine zinc insulin an insoluble form of insulin*, formed by combination with protamine (a simple protein) and a trace of zinc. It has an action lasting over 24 h, and, in association with initial doses of soluble insulin, permits a wide degree of control.

protease *n* any enzyme which digests protein: a proteolytic enzyme.

protective isolation is carried out for those patients who are rendered highly susceptible to infection by disease or treatment. ⇒ barrier nursing.

protein calorie malnutrition (PCM) (protein energy malnutrition PEM) describes a condition in which individuals have depleted body fat and protein resulting from an inadequate diet.

proteins *npl* highly complex nitrogenous compounds found in all animal and vegetable tissues. They are built up of amino* acids and are essential constituents of body tissues. Those from animal sources are of high biological value since they contain the essential amino acids. Those from vegetable sources contain not all, but some of the essential amino acids. Proteins are hydrolysed in the body to produce amino acids which are then used to build up new body proteins. ⇒ kilojoule.

proteinuria *n* albuminuria*.

proteolysis *n* the hydrolysis of the peptide bonds of proteins with the formation of smaller polypeptides—**proteolytic** *adj*.

proteolytic enzymes enzymes that promote proteolysis; they are used as a desloughing agent for leg ulcers, e.g. streptokinase and streptodornase.

proteose *n* a mixture of products from the breakdown of proteins, between protein and peptone.

Proteus *n* a bacterial genus. Gram-negative motile rods which swarm in culture. Found in damp surroundings. Sometimes a commensal of the intestinal tract. May be pathogenic, especially in wound and urinary tract infections as a secondary invader. Production of alkali turns infected urine alkaline.

prothrombin *n* a precursor of thrombin formed in the liver. The *prothrombin time* is a measure of its production and concentration in the blood. It is the time taken for plasma to clot after the addition of thrombokinase. It is inversely proportional to the amount of prothromin present, a normal person's plasma being used as a standard of comparison. Prothrombin time is lengthened in certain haemorrhagic conditions and in a patient on anticoagulant drugs. ⇒ thrombin. *prothrombin test* indirectly reveals the amount of prothrombin in blood. To a sample of oxalated blood are added all the factors needed to bring about clotting, except prothrombin. The time taken for clot to form is therefore dependent on amount of prothrombin present. Normal time is 10–12 s.

protoplasm *n* the viscid, translucent colloid* material, the essential constituent of the living cell, including the cytoplasm* and nucleoplasm—**protoplasmic** *adj.*

protozoa *npl* the smallest type of animal life; unicellular organisms. The phylum includes the genera *Plasmodium* (malarial parasites) and *Entamoeba*. The commonest protozoan infestation is *Trichomonas vaginalis*, classed with the intestinal flagellates—**protozoon** *sing*, **protozoal** *adj.*

proud flesh excessive granulation tissue.

provitamin *n* a vitamin precursor, e.g. carotene is converted into vitamin A.

proximal *adj* nearest to the head or source—**proximally** *adv.*

prune belly syndrome a rare condition found in male infants with obstructive uropathy and atrophy of the abdominal musculature. The term is descriptive. Various surgical measures are available for most types of bladder neck obstruction.

prurigo *n* a chronic, itching disease occurring most frequently in children. *prurigo aestivale* hydroa* aestivale. *Besnier's prurigo* ⇒ Besnier's.

pruritus *n* itching. *Pruritus ani* and *pruritus vulvae* are considered to be psychosomatic conditions (neurodermatitis) except in the few cases where a local cause can be found, e.g. worm infestation, vaginitis. Generalized pruritus may be a symptom of systemic disease as in diabetes, icterus, Hodgkin's disease, carcinoma, etc. It may be psychogenic—**pruritic** *adj.*

pseudoangina *n* false angina. Sometimes referred to as 'left mammary pain', it occurs in anxious individuals. Usually there is no cardiac disease present. May be part of effort* syndrome.

pseudoarthrosis *n* a false joint, e.g. due to ununited fracture; also congenital, e.g. in tibia.

pseudobulbar paralysis gross disturbance in control of tongue, bilateral hemiplegia and mental changes following on a succession of 'strokes'.

pseudocrisis *n* a rapid reduction of body temperature resembling a crisis, followed by further fever.

pseudocyesis *n* ⇒ phantom pregnancy.

pseudohermaphrodite *n* a person in whom the gonads of one sex are present, whilst the external genitalia comprise those of the opposite sex.

pseudologia fantastica a tendency to tell, and defend, fantastic lies plausibly, found in some people suffering from a psychopathic personality.

Pseudomonas *n* a bacterial genus. Gram-negative motile rods. Found in water and decomposing vegetable matter. Some are pathogenic to plants and animals and *Pseudomonas aeruginosa (pyocanea)* is able to produce disease in man. Found commonly as a secondary invader in urinary tract infections and wound infections. Produces a blue pigment (pyocyanin) which colours the exudate or pus.

pseudomucin *n* a gelatinous substance (not mucin) found in some ovarian cysts.

pseudoparalysis *n* a loss of muscular power not due to a lesion of the nervous system. *pseudoparalysis of Parrot* inability to move one or more of the extremities because of syphilitic osteochondritis: occurs in neonatal congenital syphilis.

pseudoparkinsonism *n* the signs

and symptoms of parkinsonism when they are not postencephalitic.

pseudophakia *n* presence of an artificial intraocular lens implant following cataract surgery.

pseudoplegia *n* paralysis mimicking that of organic nervous disorder but usually originating from a hysterical neurosis.

pseudopodia *npl* literally false legs; cytoplasmic projections of an amoeba or any mobile cell which help it to move. Not to be confused with cilia or microvilli which are nonretractile projections from the cell surface—**pseudopodium** *sing.*

pseudopolyposis *n* widely scattered polypi, usually the result of previous inflammation, sometimes ulcerative colitis.

psittacosis *n* disease of parrots, pigeons and budgerigars which is occasionally responsible for a form of pneumonia in man. Caused by *Chlamydia psittaci.* It behaves as a bacterium though multiplying intracellularly. Sensitive to tetracycline and macrolide antibiotics.

psoas *n* muscles of the loin. *psoas abscess* a cold abscess* in the psoas muscle, resulting from tuberculosis of the lower dorsal or lumbar vertebrae. Pressure in the abscess causes pus to track along the tough ligaments so that the abscess appears as a firm smooth swelling which does not show signs of inflammation hence the adjective 'cold'.

psoriasis *n* a genetically-determined chronic skin disease in which erythematous areas are covered with adherent scales. Although the condition may occur on any part of the body, the characteristic sites are extensor surfaces, especially over the knees and elbows. Inpatients' skin may be colonized or infected with hospital strains of *Staphylococcus aureus.* Due to the exfoliative nature of psoriasis sensitive modification of patient management is required to protect others from infection. A common cause of erythroderma—**psoriatic** *adj.*

psoriatic arthritis articular symptoms similar to those of rheumatoid arthritis occur in 3–5% of patients with psoriasis.

PSV *abbr* pressure support ventilation.

psyche *n* the Greek term for 'life force', used to describe that which constitutes the mind and all its processes, and sometimes used to describe 'self'.

psychiatric nursing ⇒ mental health nursing.

psychiatry *n* the branch of medicine devoted to the diagnosis, treatment and care of people suffering from mental illness—**psychiatric** *adj.*

psychic *adj* of the mind.

psychoanalysis *n* a method of psychotherapy in which the relationship between patient and therapist is analysed and traced back to the patient's earliest relationships. Concerned with unconscious feelings and attitudes—**psychoanalytic** *adj.*

psychochemotherapy *n* the use of drugs to improve or cure pathological changes in the emotional state—**psychochemotherapeutic** *adj.*

psychodrama *n* a method of psychotherapy whereby patients act out their personal problems by taking roles in spontaneous dramatic performances. Group discussion aims at giving the patients a greater awareness of the problems presented and possible methods of dealing with them.

psychodynamics *n* the science of the mental processes, especially of the causative factors in mental activity.

psychogenesis *n* the development of the mind.

psychogenic *adj* arising from the psyche or mind. *psychogenic symptom* originates in the mind rather than in the body.

psychogeriatric *adj* old fashioned term, pertaining to psychology as applied to geriatrics. The phrase elderly mentally ill (EMI) is now preferred.

psychological problems these can be many and varied. With nursing help, patients may be able to identify that they are experiencing excessive anxiety, depression, fear, sadness—perhaps from prolonged grieving.

psychology *n* the study of the behaviour of an organism in its environment. Medically, the study of human behaviour.

psychometry *n* the science of mental testing.

psychomotor *adj* pertaining to the motor effect of psychic or cerebral activity.

psychoneuroimmunology (PNI) *n* study of the integration of neural and immune response in relation to psychological state

psychoneurosis *n* ⇒ neurosis.

psychopath *n* one who has a psychopathic* personality—**psychopathic** *adj*.

psychopathic personality a persistent disorder or disability of mind which results in abnormally aggressive or seriously irresponsible conduct. The person lacks the ability to feel a sense of guilt for the consequences of his or her actions.

psychopathology *n* the pathology of abnormal mental processes—**psychopathological** *adj*.

psychopathy *n* any disease of the mind. The term is used by some people to denote a marked immaturity in emotional development—**psychopathic** *adj*.

psychopharmacology *n* the use of drugs which influence the affective and emotional state. The study of drugs in psychiatry.

psychophysics *n* a branch of experimental psychology dealing with the study of stimuli and sensations—**psychophysical** *adj*.

psychophysiological the physiological status determined by the current state of mind—**psychophysiology** *n*.

psychoprophylactic *adj* that which aims at preventing mental disease.

psychosexual counselling usually sought by one or both members of a partnership because one or both is not experiencing emotional and sexual satisfaction within the relationship. Psychosexual counselling of otherwise 'healthy' people is provided by specialists and is rarely available on the NHS in the UK. In a nursing context, nurses should be aware that patients whose treatment results in a negative change of body image need information to help them to adjust to changes in the emotional and sexual spheres of their living. Some of the conditions which involve such a need are: arthritis and other musculoskeletal disorders; debilitating diseases such as cancer; female cystitis resulting in a sore perineum; infections of the male and female reproductive organs; mastectomy; medical and surgical heart conditions; operations on the female reproductive organs and male genitourinary system; paraplegia; postchildbirth; poststroke; renal dialysis; stoma; and tetraplegia.

psychosis *n* the symptoms of psychosis are qualitatively different from normal experience, e.g. hallucinations and delusions. People suffering from acute psychosis do not recognize that they are ill or that their experiences are part of illness. Psychoses include schizophrenia and manic-depressive illness. ⇒ neurosis, for comparison—**psychotic** *adj*.

psychotherapy *n* a way of dealing with psychological and emotional problems by interaction between individuals or groups, usually by 'talking', but there are many different methods. Psychotherapists are not necessarily medically qualified—**psychotherapeutic** *adj. group psychotherapy* also known as 'group therapy'. With a therapist, patients are encouraged to understand and analyse their own and one another's problems.

psychotomimetics *npl syn* psychosomimetics. Drugs which produce the symptoms of a psychosis.

psychotropic *adj* that which exerts its specific effect upon the brain cells, e.g. certain drugs.

pteroylglutamic acid ⇒ folic acid.

pterygium *n* a wing-shaped degenerative condition of the conjunctiva which encroaches on the cornea—**pterygial** *adj.*

ptosis *n* a drooping, particularly that of the eyelid. ⇒ visceroptosis—**ptotic** *adj.*

ptyalin *n* salivary amylase* which is a slightly acid medium (pH 6.8) which converts starch into dextrin* and maltose*.

ptyalism *n* excessive salivation.

ptyalolith *n* a salivary calculus.

pubertas praecox premature (precocious) sexual development.

puberty *n* the age at which the reproductive organs become functionally active. It is accompanied by secondary characteristics—**pubertal** *adj.*

pubes *n* the hairy region covering the pubic bone.

pubiotomy *n* cutting the pubic bone to facilitate delivery of a live child ⇒ symphisiotomy.

pubis *n* the pubic bone or os pubis, forming the centre bone of the front of the pelvis—**pubic** *adj.*

public health the maintenance of health through attention to the social, economic, political and environmental conditions that are hazardous to it, and more positively, the encouragement of conditions which promote health.

public health nurse term used in North America and in some European countries such as Sweden and Norway to describe a community nurse, similar to a health visitor in the UK. The term is becoming more common in UK usage.

pudendal block the rendering insensitive of the pudendum by the injection of local anaesthetic. Used mainly for episiotomy and forceps delivery. ⇒ transvaginal.

pudendum *n* the external reproductive organs, especially of the female—**pudenda** *pl,* **pudendal** *adj.*

Pudenz-Hayer valve one-way valve implanted at operation for relief of hydrocephalus.

puerperal *adj* pertaining to childbirth. *puerperal psychosis* mental illnesses occurring in the puerperium*. *puerperal sepsis* infection of the genital tract occurring within 21 days of abortion or childbirth.

puerperium *n* the period immediately following childbirth to the time when involution is completed, usually 6–8 weeks—**puerperia** *pl.*

pulmonary *adj* pertaining to the lungs. Deoxygenated blood leaves the right ventricle; flows through the lungs where it becomes oxygenated and returns to the left atrium of the heart. *pulmonary embolism* an embolism* which occurs in the pulmonary arterial system: most commonly as a result of phlebothrombosis* and can be instantly fatal. Supervision of patients' deep breathing and foot exercises and the wearing of antiembolic stockings after surgery are preventive nursing interventions. *pulmonary emphysema* destruction of alveoli rendering the lung less efficient in the diffusion of gases. It can be generalized resulting from cigarette smoking; or localized, either distal to partial obstruction of a bronchiole or bronchus (obstructive emphysema), or in alveoli adjacent to a segment of collapsed lung (compensatory emphysema). *pulmonary hypertension* raised blood pressure within the pulmonary circulation, due to increased resistance to blood flow within the pulmonary vessels. It is associated with increased pressure in the right cardiac ventricle, then the atrium. It may be due to disease of the left side of the heart or in the lung. In primary pulmonary hypertension the cause is not known. It usually leads to death from congestive heart failure in 2–10 years. *pulmonary oedema* a form of 'waterlogging' of the lungs, e.g. in left ventricular failure, mitral stenosis, fluid excess in renal failure, toxic gas inhalation.

pulp *n* the soft, interior part of some organs and structures. *dental pulp* found in the pulp cavity and root canals of teeth; carries blood, nerve and lymph vessels. *digital pulp* the tissue pad of the finger tip. Infection of this is referred to as 'pulp space infection'.

pulsatile *adj* beating, throbbing.

pulsation *n* beating or throbbing, as of the heart or arteries.

pulse *n* the impulse transmitted to arteries by contraction of the left ventricle, and customarily palpated in the radial artery at the wrist. The *pulse rate* is the number of beats or impulses per minute and is about 130 in the newborn infant, 70–80 in the adult and 60–70 in old age. The *pulse rhythm* is its regularity–it can be regular or irregular; the *pulse volume* is the amplitude of expansion of the arterial wall during the passage of the wave; the *pulse force* or tension is its strength, estimated by the force needed to obliterate it by pressure of the finger. *pulse deficit* the difference in rate of the heart (counted by stethoscope) and the pulse (counted at the wrist). It occurs when some of the ventricular contractions are too weak to open the aortic valve and hence produce a beat at the heart but not at the wrist, and occurs commonly in atrial fibrillation. *pulse pressure* is the difference between the systolic and diastolic pressures. ⇒ beat.

'pulseless' disease (*syn* Takayasu's arteritis) progessive obliterative arteritis of the vessels arising from the aortic arch resulting in diminished or absent pulse in the neck and arms. Thromboendarterectomy or a bypass procedure may prevent blindness by improving the carotid blood flow at its commencement in the aortic arch.

pulsus alternans a regular pulse with alternate beats of weak and strong amplitude; a sign of left ventricular disease.

pulsus bigeminus double pulse wave produced by interpolation of extrasystoles. A coupled beat. A heart rhythm often due to excessive digitalis administration of paired beats, each pair being followed by a prolonged pause. The second weaker beat of each pair may not be strong enough to open the aortic valve, in which case it does not produce a pulse beat and the type of rhythm can then only be detected by listening at the heart.

pulsus paradoxus arterial pulsus paradoxus is alteration of the volume of the arterial pulse sometimes found in pericardial effusion. The volume becomes greater with expiration. Venous pulsus paradoxus (Kusman's sign) is an increase in the height of the venous pressure with inspiration, the reverse of normal. Sometimes found in pericardial or right ventricular disease.

pulvis *n* a powder.

punctate *adj* dotted or spotted, e.g. punctate basophilia describes the immature red cell in which there are droplets of blue-staining material in the cytoplasm—**punctum** *n,* **puncta** *pl.*

puncture *n* a stab; a wound made with a sharp pointed hollow instrument for withdrawal or injection of fluid or other substance. *cisternal puncture* insertion of a special hollow needle with stylet through the atlanto-occipital ligament between the occiput and atlas, into the cisterna magna. One method of obtaining cerebrospinal fluid. *lumbar puncture* insertion of a special hollow needle with stylet either through the space between the third and fourth lumbar vertebrae or, lower, into the subarachnoid space to obtain cerebrospinal fluid. *puncture wound* ⇒ penetrating wound.

PUO *abbr* pyrexia* of unknown origin.

pupil *n* the opening in the centre of the iris of the eye to allow the passage of light.

pupillary *adj* pertaining to the pupil.

purgative *n* a drug causing evacuation of fluid faeces. *drastic purgative* even more severe in action, when the fluid faeces may be passed involuntarily.

purin(e)s *npl* constituents of nucleoproteins from which uric acid is derived. Gout is thought to be associated with the disturbed metabolism and excretion of uric acid, and foods of high purine content are excluded in its treatment.

Purkinje's fibres conductive strands beneath the endocardium* of the ventricles*.

purpura *n* a disorder characterized by extravasation of blood from the capillaries into the skin, or into or from the mucous membranes. Manifest either by small red spots (petechiae) or large bruises (ecchymoses) or by oozing from minor wounds, the latter, in the absence of trauma, being confined to the mucous membranes. It is believed that the disorder can be due to impaired integrity of the capillary walls, or to defective quality or quantity of the blood platelets. Purpura can be caused by many different conditions, e.g. infective, toxic, allergic, etc. ⇒ Henoch-Schönlein purpura. *anaphylactoid purpura* excessive reaction between antigen and the protein globulin IgG (antibody). Antigen often unknown, but may be derived from beta-haemolytic streptococci, or drugs such as sulphonamides which may interact chemically with body proteins. *purpura haemorrhagica* (thrombocytopenic purpura) is characterized by a greatly diminished platelet count. The clotting time is normal but the bleeding time is prolonged. The patient is usually well, but intracranial haemorrhage can occur.

purulent *adj* pertaining to or resembling pus.

pus *n* a liquid, usually yellowish in colour, formed in certain infections and composed of tissue fluid containing bacteria and leucocytes. Various types of bacteria are associated with pus having distinctive features, e.g. the faecal smell of pus due to *Escherichia coli;* the green colour of pus due to *Pseudomonas aeruginosa.*

pustule *n* a small inflammatory swelling containing pus—**pustular** *adj. malignant pustule* ⇒ anthrax.

putrefaction *n* the process of rotting; destruction of organic material by bacteria—**putrefactive** *adj.*

putrescible *adj* capable of undergoing putrefaction.

PUVA *abbr* psoralen (a naturally occurring photosensitive compound) with long wavelength ultraviolet light. Used to treat psoriasis.

PVD *abbr* peripheral* vascular disease.

PVS *abbr* persistent* vegetative state.

pyaemia *n* a grave form of septicaemia in which blood-borne bacteria lodge and grow in distant organs, e.g. brain, kidneys, lungs and heart, to form multiple abscesses—**pyaemic** *adj.*

pyarthrosis *n* pus in a joint cavity.

pyelitis *n* mild form of pyelonephritis* with pyuria but minimal involvement of renal tissue. Pyelitis on the right side is a common complication of pregnancy.

pyelography *n* ⇒ urography—**pyelographic** *adj,* **pyelographically** *adv.*

pyelolithotomy *n* the operation for removal of a stone from the renal pelvis.

pyelonephritis *n* a form of renal infection which spreads outwards from the pelvis to the cortex of the kidney. Origin of infection is usually from the ureter and below, or from the bloodstream—**pyelonephritic** *adj.*

pyeloplasty a plastic operation on the kidney pelvis. ⇒ hydronephrosis.

pyelostomy *n* surgical formation of an opening into the kidney pelvis.

pyknolepsy *n* infrequently used term to describe repeated attacks of petit mal epilepsy seen in children. Attacks may number a hundred or more in a day.

pylephlebitis *n* inflammation of the veins of the portal system secondary to intraabdominal sepsis.

pylethrombosis *n* an intravascular blood clot in the portal vein or any of its branches.

pyloric stenosis mostly a congenital condition in which there is thickening of the sphincter muscle between the pylorus of the stomach and the duodenum. The characteristic feature is projectile* vomiting and failure to gain weight. Surgical treatment is required after correction of fluid and electrolyte imbalance.

pyloroduodenal *adj* pertaining to the pyloric sphincter and the duodenum.

pyloromyotomy *n* (*syn* Ramstedt's operation) incision of the pyloric sphincter muscle as in pyloroplasty.

pyloroplasty *n* a plastic operation on the pylorus designed to widen the passage.

pylorospasm *n* spasm of the pylorus; usually due to the presence of a duodenal ulcer.

pylorus *n* the opening of the stomach into the duodenum, encircled by a sphincter muscle—**pyloric** *adj.*

pyocolpos *n* pus in the vagina.

pyodermia, pyoderma *n* chronic cellulitis of the skin, manifesting itself in granulation tissue, ulceration, colliquative necrosis or vegetative lesions—**pyodermic** *adj.*

pyogenic *adj* pertaining to the formation of pus.

pyometra *n* pus retained in the uterus and unable to escape through the cervix, due to malignancy or atresia—**pyometric** *adj.*

pyonephrosis *n* distension of the renal pelvis with pus—**pyonephrotic** *adj.*

pyopericarditis *n* pericarditis* with purulent effusion.

pyopneumothorax *n* pus and gas or air within the pleural sac.

pyorrhoea *n* a flow of pus, usually referring to that caused by periodontal* disease, *pyorrhoea alveolaris.*

pyosalpinx *n* a uterine tube containing pus.

pyothorax *n* pus in the pleural cavity.

pyramidal *adj* applied to some conical eminences in the body. *pyramidal cells* nerve cells in the preRolandic area of the cerebral cortex, from which originate impulses to voluntary muscles. *pyramidal tracts* in the brain and spinal cord transmit the fibres arising from the pyramidal cells to the voluntary muscles.

pyrexia *n* ⇒ fever, hyperpyrexia, hyperthermia, hypothermia—**pyrexial** *adj.*

pyridoxine *n* vitamin* B_6; may be connected with the utilization of unsaturated fatty acids or the synthesis of fat from proteins. Deficiency may lead to dermatitis and neuritic pains. Used to treat nausea of pregnancy and radiation sickness, muscular dystrophy, pellagra, the premenstrual syndrome, etc.

pyrogen *n* a substance capable of producing fever—**pyrogenic** *adj.*

pyromania *n* an uncontrollable impulse to set fire to things. May occur on several occasions before apprehension—**pyromanic** *adj.*

pyrosis *n* (*syn* heartburn, waterbrash) eructation of acid gastric contents into the mouth, accompanied by a burning sensation felt behind the sternum.

pyrotherapy *n* production of fever by artificial means. ⇒ hyperthermia.

pyuria *n* pus in the urine—**pyuric** adj.

Q

Q fever a febrile disease caused by *Coxiella burnetti*. Human infection transmitted from sheep and cattle in which the organism does not produce symptoms. Pasteurization of milk kills *Coxiella burnetti*.

quadriceps *n* the quadriceps extensor femoris muscle of the thigh which possesses four heads and is composed of four parts.

quadriplegia *n* ⇒ tetraplegia—**quadriplegic** *adj*.

quadruple vaccine ⇒ vaccine.

qualitative *adj* pertaining to quality. *qualitative research* describes a research study based on observation and/or interviews to ascertain people's opinions, feelings or beliefs ⇒ quantitative* research.

quality assurance the attempt to measure the standard of care provided by professionals for consumers. Some of the schedules used include consumer satisfaction. ⇒ benchmarking, clinical audit, cost effectiveness, Monitor, Performance Indicators, quality circles, Qualpacs.

quality circles an initiative to improve the quality of care in a specific area. The nurses in a clinical area are guided by a nurse experienced in this process, to investigate a nursing intervention systematically and relate it to good standards of practice.

Qualpacs *n* a quality assurance programme for nurses. Trained personnel observe for 2 h, up to five randomly selected patients. A further 1 to 2 h is spent reviewing the nursing records and listening to handover reports. A numerical score is given for each of the 68 items in the schedule.

quantitative *adj* pertaining to quantity. *quantitative research* describes a research study based on gained facts and statistics ⇒ qualitative* research.

quarantine *n* a period of isolation* of infected or potentially infected people in order to prevent spread to others. It is usually the same period as the longest incubation period for the specific disease.

quartan *adj* the word applied to intermittent fever with paroxysms occurring every 72 h (fourth day).

Queckenstedt's test performed during lumbar puncture. Compression on the internal jugular vein produces a rise in CSF pressure if there is no obstruction to circulation of fluid in the spinal region.

quelling reaction swelling of the capsule of a bacterium when exposed to specific antisera. The test identifies the genera, species or subspecies of bacteria causing a disease.

quickening *n* the first perceptible fetal movements felt by the mother, usually at 16–18 weeks' gestation.

quicksilver *n* mercury.

quiescent *adj* becoming quiet. Used especially of a skin disease which is settling under treatment.

quinine *n* the chief alkaloid of cinchona, once the standard treatment for malaria. For routine use and prophylaxis, synthetic antimalarials are now preferred, but with the increasing risk of drug-resistant malaria, quinine is coming back into use in some areas. The drug also has some oxytocic action and has been employed as a uterine stimulant in labour. The main use is in management of 'night cramps' where it is given as 300–600 mg of bisulphate.

quininism *n* headache, noises in the ears and partial deafness, disturbed vision and nausea arising from an idiosyncratic reaction to, or long-continued use of quinine.

quinsy *n* ⇒ peritonsillar* abscess.

quotient *n* a number obtained by division. *intelligence quotient* ⇒ intelligence. *respiratory quotient* the ratio between inspired oxygen and expired carbon dioxide during a specified time.

R

rabid *adj* infected with rabies.

rabies *n* (*syn* hydrophobia) fatal infection in man caused by a virus; infection follows the bite of a rabid animal, e.g. dog, cat, fox, vampire bat. It is of worldwide distribution; vaccines are available—**rabid** *adj.*

racemose *adj* resembling a bunch of grapes.

rad *n* a unit of measurement of absorbed radiation. Now replaced by the gray*.

radial keratectomy surgical reshaping of the cornea to correct refractive error, sometimes performed with a surgical blade but more commonly using lasers (photorefractive* keratectomy).

radiation electromagnetic waves, including X-ray, infrared and ultraviolet rays and visible light rays. Radiation can be ionizing* or nonionizing. Ionizing radiation has the ability to damage tissue and is used therapeutically for cancer treatment.

radical *adj* pertaining to the root of a thing. *radical operation* usually extensive so that it is curative, not palliative.

radiculography *n* X-ray of the spinal nerve roots after rendering them radiopaque to locate the site and size of a prolapsed intervertebral disc—**radiculogram** *n.*

radioactive *adj* emitting radiation due to instability of the atomic nuclei. *radioactive gold* used for investigation of liver disease. *radioactive iodine* (^{181}I) a dose, which is subsequently measured, concentrates in the thyroid gland. An overactive gland concentrates 45% of the dose in 4 h, an underactive gland less than 20% in 48 h. *radioactive technetium* used for investigation of visceral lesions.

radiobiology *n* the study of the effects of radiation on living tissue—**radiobiological** *adj,* **radiobiologically** *adv.*

radiocaesium *n* a radioactive form of the element caesium used in radiation treatment of disease.

radiocarbon *n* a radioactive form of the element carbon used for research into metabolism etc.

radiograph *n* a photographic image formed by exposure to X-rays; the correct term for an 'X-ray'—**radiographic** *adj.*

radiographer *n* a person who is qualified in the techniques of diagnostic or therapeutic radiography.

radiography *n* the use of imaging techniques to create images of the body from which medical diagnosis can be made (diagnostic radiography).

radioiodine uptake test ⇒ radioactive (iodine).

radioisotope *n* (*syn* radionuclide) forms of an element which have the same atomic number but different mass numbers, exhibiting the property of spontaneous nuclear disintegration. When taken orally or by injection, can be traced by a Geigercounter. *radioisotope scan* pictorial representation of the amount and distribution of radioactive isotope present in a particular organ.

radiologist *n* a medical specialist in diagnosis by the use of X-rays and other allied imaging techniques. Some radiologists use imaging techniques to help them carry out interventional techniques.

radiology *n* the branch of medical science dealing with the diagnosis of disease, using X-rays and other allied imaging techniques—**radiological** *adj,* **radiologically** *adv.*

radiomimetic *adj* produces effects similar to those of radiotherapy.

radionuclide *n* ⇒ radioisotope.

radiosensitive *adj* affected by radiation. Applied to tumours responsive to radiation.

radiotherapist *n* a medical specialist in the treatment of disease by X-rays and other forms of radiation.

radiotherapy *n* the treatment of proliferative disease, especially cancer, by X-rays and other forms of radiation.

radium *n* a radioactive element occurring in nature, and still occasionally used in radiotherapy.

radon seeds capsules containing radon radioactive gas produced by the decay of radium atoms. Used in radiotherapy.

RA latex test for rheumatoid arthritis; discerns the presence in the blood of rheumatoid factor.

rale *n* abnormal sound heard on auscultation of lungs when fluid is present in bronchi.

Ramsay Hunt syndrome herpes zoster of the ear lobe with facial paralysis and loss of taste.

Ramstedt's operation ⇒ pyloromyotomy.

ranula *n* a cystic swelling beneath the tongue due to blockage of a duct—**ranular** *adj.*

rape *n* heterosexual or homosexual intercourse against the will of the victim. Full penetration of the vagina (or other orifice) by the penis and ejaculation of semen is not necessary to constitute rape. Most rapes include force and violence, but acquiescence because of verbal threats should not be interpreted as consent. Incidents of rape are underreported to the police because of the gruelling process of having to give evidence in court. If women are admitted to hospital, a police surgeon examines them and takes the necessary specimens in the presence of a policewoman who provides psychological support while interviewing to collect the necessary data requested by the law. There are voluntary agencies to assist raped women to regain confidence and rebuild their lives. Male rape, the rape of a man by another man, is increasingly recognized.

raphe *n* a seam, suture, ridge or crease; the median furrow on the dorsal surface of the tongue.

rapport *n* a sense of mutuality, understanding and respect for each other: it is an essential component of a nurse/patient relationship.

rarefaction *n* becoming less dense, as applied to diseased bone—**rarefied** *adj.*

rash *n* skin eruption. *nettle rash* ⇒ urticaria.

Rashkind's septostomy when the pulmonary and systemic circulations do not communicate, an artificial atrial septal communication is produced by passing an inflatable balloon-ended catheter through the foramen ovale, filling the balloon with contrast media and pulling it back into the right atrium.

RAST *abbr* radioallergosorbent test. It is an allergen-specific IgE measurement.

rat-bite fever a relapsing fever caused by *Spirillum minus* or by *Streptobacillus moniliformis.* The blood Wassermann* test is positive in the spirillary infection.

rationalization *n* a mental process whereby a person justifies his or her behaviour after the event, so that it appears more rational or socially acceptable.

Raynaud's disease idiopathic trophoneurosis. Paroxysmal spasm of the digital arteries producing pallor or cyanosis of fingers or toes, and occasionally resulting in gangrene. Disease of young women.

Raynaud's phenomenon ⇒ hand-arm vibration syndrome.

RBC *abbr* red blood cell or corpuscle. ⇒ blood.

RCN *abbr* Royal* College of Nursing.

RCN Continuing Education Points (CEPs) ⇒ RCN CEPs box.

RDS *abbr* respiratory* distress syndrome.

reaction *n* **1** response to a stimulus. **2** a chemical change, e.g. acid or alkaline reaction to litmus paper. *allergic reaction* ⇒ allergy.

RCN CONTINUING EDUCATION POINTS (CEPS)

CEPs are most helpfully thought of as a form of professional currency, and in this they complement the academic currency offered by CATS* points. They are, however, the only form of credit directly relevant to nurses and their practice. They provide evidence that their holder has:

- a commitment to continuing professional development
- improved his or her knowledge and skills in a defined area of practice
- successfully undertaken assessment related to practice
- developed skills in independent study
- attended an educational event approved by the RCN
- undertaken continuing education of high quality that meets the standards of the RCN.

Currently, there are three ways in which you can gain CEPs:

1. RCN Nursing Update—RCN's assessed updating initiative, which comprises a programme televised on BBC 2, between 05.30 and 06.00, every Tuesday throughout the year, accompanied by a distance learning supplement, available free monthly with Nursing Standard.
2. RCN CE Articles—assessed distance learning articles published regularly in Nursing Standard and other specialist journals.
3. RCN Approved Educational Events, approved for their quality, currency and relevance, which include conferences, study days and distance learning packs.

CEPs provide credible evidence of professional updating, and this evidence can be offered to anyone who needs assurance that you are keeping abreast of developments in your area of practice. 10 CEPs is the equivalent of 1 day of effort, in terms of learning.

Initiatives for which CEPs are awarded have a strong focus on enhancing practice, and the fact that they emanate from the RCN Institute is a guarantee of high quality learning opportunities.

reagent *n* an agent capable of participating in a chemical reaction, so as to detect, measure, or produce other substances. *reagent strips* a strip is impregnated with particular chemicals to detect the presence of particular substances in, e.g. urine and faeces. One strip may test for several substances.

reagin *n* IgE antibody.

reality orientation (RO) a form of therapy useful for withdrawn, confused and depressed patients: they are frequently reminded of their name, the time, place, date and so on. Reinforcement is provided by clocks, calendars and signs prominently displayed in the environment.

rebore *n* ⇒ disobliteration.

recalcitrant *adj* refractory. Describes medical conditions which are resistant to treatment.

recall *n* part of the process of memory. Memory consists of memorizing, retention and recall.

recannulation *n* reestablishment of the patency of a vessel.

receptaculum *n* receptacle, often acting as a reservoir. *receptaculum chyli* the pear-shaped commencement of the thoracic duct in front of the first lumbar vertebra. It receives digested fat from the intestine.

receptive aphasia a type of aphasia* characterized by problems in language comprehension, occurring with varying degrees of severity. Patients may also exhibit expressive language difficulties. ⇒ expressive aphasia.

receptor *n* sensory afferent nerve ending capable of receiving and transmitting stimuli.

recessive *adj* receding; having a tendency to disappear. *recessive trait* a genetically controlled character or trait which is expressed when the specific allele* which determines it is present at both paired chromosomal loci (i.e. 'in double dose'). When the specific allele is present in single dose the characteristic is not manifest as its presence is concealed by the dominant allele at the partner locus. The exception is for X-linked genes in males, in which the single recessive allele on the X-chromosome will express itself so that the character is manifest. ⇒ Mendel's law.

recipient *n* a person who receives something from a donor such as blood, bone marrow or an organ. ⇒ blood groups.

Recklinghausen's disease a name given to two conditions: (a) osteitis fibrosa cystica, the result of overactivity of the parathyroid glands (hyperparathyroidism) resulting in decalcification of bones and formation of cysts (b) multiple neurofibromatosis*, the tumours can be felt beneath the skin along the course of nerves. There may be pigmented spots (café au lait) on the skin and there may also be phaeochromocytoma.

recliner's reflux syndrome this is due to severe disturbance of the antireflux mechanism which allows stomach contents to leak at any time whatever position the patient is in, although it is most likely to happen when the patient lies down or slumps in a low chair.

recombinant DNA DNA which is produced by deliberately piecing together (recombining chemically) the genic DNA of two different organisms. It is used for the study of the structure and function of both normal and abnormal genes and so, e.g. of the molecular basis of human genetic disorders. Its practical applications are in diagnosis (including prenatal diagnosis) and in the manufacture of synthetic agents such as insulin and growth hormone.

recrudescence *n* the return of symptoms.

recruitment *n* apparent paradox seen in deaf patients, with patient not hearing quiet sounds then, with increasing loudness of the sound, the patient suddenly hears it very loudly.

rectal bladder a term used when the ureters are transplanted into the rectum, which is closed with the establishment of a proximal colostomy, in cases of severe disease of the urinary bladder.

rectal varices haemorrhoids*.

rectocele *n* prolapse* of the rectum, so that it lies outside the anus. Usually reserved for herniation of anterior rectal wall into posterior vaginal wall caused by injury to the levator muscles at childbirth. Repaired by a posterior colporrhaphy. ⇒ procidentia.

rectopexy *n* surgical fixation of a prolapsed rectum.

rectoscope *n* an instrument for examining the rectum. ⇒ endoscope—**rectoscopic** *adj.*

rectosigmoid *adj* pertaining to the rectum and sigmoid portion of colon.

rectosigmoidectomy *n* surgical removal of the rectum and sigmoid colon.

rectouterine *adj* pertaining to the rectum and uterus.

rectovaginal *adj* pertaining to the rectum and vagina.

rectovesical *adj* pertaining to the rectum and bladder.

rectum *n* the lower part of the large intestine between the sigmoid* flexure and anal canal—**rectal** *adj,* **rectally** *adv.*

recumbent *adj* lying or reclining—**recumbency** *n. recumbent position* lying on the back with the head supported on a pillow: the knees are flexed and parted to facilitate inspection of the perineum.

recurrent abortion ⇒ abortion.

Redivac drainage tube a proprietary closed suction drainage system used for the drainage of wounds in the postoperative period. The amount of exudate is visible in the drainage container. ⇒ wound drains.

referred pain pain occurring at a distance from its source, e.g. pain felt in the upper limbs from angina pectoris, that from the gallbladder felt in the scapular region.

reflection *n* consciously and systematically thinking about personal actions. The ability to review, analyse and evaluate situations, during or after events. *reflective practice* a means of monitoring professional and personal competence by consciously thinking about actions during or after events ⇒ Reflective practice box.

REFLECTIVE PRACTICE

Reflective practice is an active process whereby the professional can gain an understanding of how historical, social, cultural, cognitive and personal experiences have contributed to professional knowledge acquisition and practice. An examination of such factors yields an opportunity to identify new potentials within practice, thus challenging the constraints of habituated thoughts and practices. The process of reflection can be guided by a model and may be facilitated by the use of a strategy such as a form of supervision. Through the exploration of individual and social behaviour and experiences, there is scope to gain insights to challenge and guide professional activities.

reflex 1 *adj* literally, reflected or thrown back; involuntary, not able to be controlled by the will. *reflex action* an involuntary motor or secretory response by tissue to a sensory stimulus, e.g. sneezing, blinking, coughing. The testing of various reflexes provides valuable information in the localization and diagnosis of diseases involving the nervous system. *reflex zone therapy, reflexology* treatment of the feet for disorders in other parts of the body whether or not these disorders have resulted in signs and symptoms. 2 *n* a reflex action. *accommodation reflex* constriction of the pupils and convergence of the eyes for near vision. *conditioned reflex* a reaction acquired by repetition or practice. *corneal reflex* a reaction of blinking when the cornea is touched.

reflexology *n* a complementary* therapy which may be available through the NHS but, more often, people may attend a reflexologist privately. Rather like an acupuncture chart, the soles of the feet are mapped out to correspond with various body organs. Skilled hands touching the various parts can become aware of malfunction in body organs and can apply therapeutic massage accordingly.

reflux *n* backward flow.

refraction *n* the bending of light rays as they pass through media of different densities. In normal vision, the light rays are so bent that they meet on the retina—**refractive** *adj.*

refractory *adj* resistant to treatment; stubborn, unmanageable; rebellious.

regeneration *n* renewal of injured tissue.

regional ileitis (*syn* Crohn's disease) a nonspecific chronic recurrent granulomatous disease affecting mainly young adults and characterized by a necrotizing, ulcerating inflammatory process, there usually being an abrupt demarcation between it and healthy bowel. There can be healthy bowel ('skip' area) intervening between two diseased segments. The colon, rectum and anus may also be involved.

regression *n* in psychiatry, reversion to an earlier stage of development, becoming more childish. Occurs in dementia, especially senile dementia, or in childhood itself, e.g. following the birth of a sibling.

regurgitation *n* backward flow, e.g. of stomach contents into, or through, the mouth.

REHAB *abbr* ⇒ Rehabilitation Evaluation of Hall and Baker.

rehabilitation *n* a planned programme in which the convalescent or disabled person progresses towards, or maintains, the maximum degree of physical and psychological independence of which he or she is capable. ⇒ habilitation.

Rehabilitation Evaluation of Hall and Baker (REHAB) a broad assessment system developed by two psychologists; can be used by nurses. Information is requested about everyday living skills, work skills and any disturbed or deviant behaviour.

Reiter protein complement fixation (RPCF) test a test for syphilis; uses an extract prepared from cultivatable treponemata.

Reiter's syndrome a condition in which arthritis occurs together with conjunctivitis and urethritis (or cervicitis in women). It is commonly, but not always, a sexually transmitted infection and should be considered as a cause of knee effusion in young men when trauma has not occurred.

rejection *n* 1 the act of excluding or denying affection to another person. 2 an immune reaction against grafted tissue or organs, leading to the destruction of implanted grafts.

relapsing fever louse-borne or tick-borne infection caused by spirochaetes of the genus *Borrelia.* Prevalent in many parts of the world. Characterized by a febrile period of a week or so, with apparent recovery, followed by a further bout of fever.

relationship *n* the state of being related. In the case of people, it can be a family relationship decreed by custom, the quality of which is mainly determined by the emotional bonding between the people in the relationship. The degree of emotional involvement is shown by using such words as 'acquaintanceship', 'friendship', 'close friendship'. ⇒ personal relationship.

relaxant *n* that which reduces tension. ⇒ muscle.

relaxation techniques these are being incorporated into health education programmes. They include progressive muscle relaxation, visual guided imagery, yoga, zen, and meditation. ⇒ autogenic therapy, biofeedback, hypnosis.

relief of pressure ⇒pressure sores, prevention of.

relaxin *n* polypeptides secreted by the ovaries to soften the cervix and loosen the ligaments in preparation for birth.

REM *abbr* rapid eye movement.

REM sleep ⇒ paradoxical sleep.

remission *n* the period of abatement of a fever or other disease.

remittent *adj* increasing and decreasing at periodic intervals.

remote afterloading a method of delivering brachytherapy* radiation to treat cancer without risk to staff. ⇒ Selectron*.

renal *adj* pertaining to the kidney. *renal adenocarcinoma* cancer of the kidney. *renal asthma* hyperventilation of lungs occurring in uraemia as a result of acidosis. *renal calculus** stone in the kidney. *renal erythropoetic factor* an enzyme released in response to renal (and therefore systemic) hypoxia. Once secreted into the blood, it reacts with a plasma globulin to produce erythropoietin. *renal failure* can only be described within the context of whether it is acute or chronic. Acute renal failure (ARF) occurs when previously healthy kidneys suddenly fail because of a variety of problems affecting the kidney and its circulation. This condition is potentially reversible. Chronic renal failure (CRF) occurs when irreversible and progressive pathological destruction of the kidney leads to terminal or end stage renal disease (ESRD). This process usually takes several years but once ESRD is reached, death will follow unless the patient is treated with some type of dialysis or renal transplant. ⇒ crush syndrome, tubular necrosis, uraemia. *renal function tests* ⇒ kidney function tests. *renal glycosuria* occurs in patients with a normal blood sugar and a lowered renal threshold for sugar. *renal oedema* inefficient kidney filtration disturbing the electrolyte balance and resulting in oedema*. *renal rickets* ⇒ rickets. *renal transplant* kidney* transplant. *renal uraemia* uraemia* following kidney disease itself, in contrast to uraemia from failure of the circulation of the blood (extrarenal uraemia).

renin *n* an enzyme released into the blood from the kidney cortex in response to sodium loss. It reacts with angiotensinogen (a plasma protein fraction) to produce angiotensin I, which in turn is converted into angiotensin II by an enzyme in the lungs. Excessive production of renin results in hypertensive kidney disease.

rennin *n* milk curdling enzyme found in the gastric juice of human infants and ruminants. It converts caseinogen into casein, which in the presence of calcium ions is converted to an insoluble curd.

reovirus *n* previously called respiratory enteric orphan virus*, one of a group of RNA-containing viruses which can infect the respiratory and intestinal tracts without causing serious disease.

repetitive strain injury (RSI) (*syn* work related upper limb disorder) the definition of this condition is controversial. It usually refers to pain and discomfort in the upper limbs as a result of repetitive movements or constrained posture. It encompasses a variety of symptoms, including tenderness, tingling and numbness, swelling, etc. Some clinicians include similar signs and symptoms in lower limbs.

replogle tube a double lumen aspiration catheter, attached to low pressure suction apparatus.

repression *n* one of the mental* defence mechanisms. It is an unconscious process whereby unacceptable thoughts, impulses and painful experiences are forced into, and remain in the unconscious.

reproductive system the organs and tissues necessary for reproduction. In the male it includes the testes, vas deferens, prostate gland, seminal vesicles, urethra and penis. In the female it includes the ovaries, uterine tubes, uterus, vagina and vulva.

RES *abbr* reticuloendethelial* system (mononuclear phagocytic system).

research *n* systematic investigation of data, reports and observations to establish facts or principles. *qualitative research* involves answering the question 'what *sorts* of things are there in the world?' and may include identifying individual and/or group beliefs, values and opinions. *quantitative research* involves answering the question 'how *many* of these things are there in the world?' and usually includes counting and identifying the number of times that things occur. Qualitative and quantitative methods may be combined in a research study.

resection *n* surgical excision. *submucous resection (of nasal septum)* incision of nasal mucosa, removal of deflected nasal septum, replacement of mucosa.

resectoscope *n* an instrument passed along the urethra; it permits resection of tissue from the base of the bladder and prostate under direct vision. ⇒ prostatectomy.

resectotome *n* an instrument used for resection.

reservoirs of infection the human ones are the hands, nose, skin and bowel; they have a natural flora which under certain circumstances can become pathogenic.

residential care a term used for provision of care for frail elderly people. It can be provided in long-stay wards, in local authority old people's homes or in independent homes for elderly people.

residual *adj* remaining. *residual air* the air remaining in the lung after forced expiration. *residual urine* urine remaining in the bladder after micturition.

resins *npl* water-insoluble solid or semisolid amorphous organic polymers that can occur naturally or be manufactured synthetically. *ion exchange resins* ⇒ ion.

resistance *n* power of resisting. In psychology the name given to the force which prevents repressed thoughts from reentering the conscious mind from the unconscious. *resistance to* *infection* the capacity to withstand infection. ⇒ immunity. *peripheral resistance*⇒ peripheral.

resolution *n* the subsidence of inflammation; describes the earliest indications of a return to normal, as when, in lobar pneumonia, the consolidation begins to liquefy.

resonance *n* the musical quality elicited on percussing a cavity which contains air. *vocal resonance* is the reverberating note heard through the stethoscope when the patient is asked to say 'one, one, one' or '99'.

resorption *n* the act of absorbing again, e.g. absorption of (a) callus following bone fracture (b) roots of the deciduous teeth (c) blood from a haematoma.

respiration *n* the process whereby there is gaseous exchange between a cell and its environment—**respiratory** *adj. external respiration* involves the absorption of oxygen from the air in the alveoli into the lung capillaries, and excretion of carbon dioxide from the blood in the lung capillaries into the air in the lungs. *internal* or *tissue respiration* is the reverse process—blood vessels supplying the cells carry oxygen which passes from the blood into the tissue cells, and carbon dioxide from the cells passes into the blood in vessels draining the cells. *paradoxical respiration* occurs when the ribs on one side are fractured in two places. During inspiration air is drawn into the unaffected lung via the normal route and also from the lung on the affected side. During expiration air is forced from the lung on the unaffected side, some of which enters the lung on the affected side, resulting in inadequate oxygenation of blood. ⇒ abdominal breathing, anaerobic respiration, Cheyne-Stokes respiration, resuscitation.

respirator *n* **1** an apparatus worn over the nose and mouth and designed to purify the air breathed through it. **2** an apparatus which artifically and rhythmically inflates and deflates the lungs when the natural nervous or muscular control of respiration is impaired, as in anterior poliomyelitis. The apparatus works by creation of negative pressure around the thorax (tank respirators).

respiratory distress syndrome (RDS) *neonatal respiratory distress syndrome (NRDS)* dyspnoea in the newly born. Due to failure of secretion of protein-lipid complex (pulmonary surfactant) by type II pneumocytes in the tiny air spaces of the lung on first entry of air. Causes atelectasis. Formerly called hyaline membrane disease. Environmental temperature control, oxygen and mechanical ventilation are used in treatment. Artificial surfactants* may be sprayed into the trachea using an endotracheal tube and syringe. Clinical features include severe retraction of the chest wall with every breath, cyanosis, an increased respiratory rate and an expiratory grunt. ⇒ lecithins. *adult respiratory distress syndrome* (ARDS) acute respiratory failure due to noncardiogenic pulmonary oedema.

respiratory failure a term used to denote failure of the lungs to oxygenate the blood adequately. *acute respiratory failure* denotes respiratory insufficiency secondary to an acute insult to the lung; hypoxaemia develops, frequently terminating in bronchopneumonia. *acute or chronic respiratory failure* hypoxaemia resulting from chronic obstructive airways disease such as chronic bronchitis and emphysema.

respiratory function tests tests employed to determine the efficiency of ventilation within the lungs. These include: peak flow, tidal volume (TV), vital capacity (VC) and inspiratory capacity.

respiratory syncytial virus (RSV) causes severe respiratory infection with occasional fatalities in very young children. Infections are less severe in older children.

respiratory quotient ⇒ quotient.

respiratory system deals with gaseous exchange. Comprizes the nose, nasopharynx, larnyx, trachea, bronchi, lungs and pulmonary circulation.

resuscitation *n* restoration to life of one who is apparently dead (collapsed or shocked)—**resuscitative** *adj.*

restless leg syndrome restless legs characterized by paraesthesiae like creeping, crawling, itching and prickling.

restlessness *n* inability to keep still. Often accompanies a raised body temperature, hypovolaemia or a state of anxiety.

retardation *n* 1 the slowing of a process which has already been carried out at a quicker rate or higher level. 2 arrested growth or function from any cause.

retching *n* straining at vomiting.

retention *n* 1 retaining of facts in the mind. 2 accumulation of that which is normally excreted. *retention cyst* a cyst* caused by blocking of a duct. ⇒ ranula. *retention of urine* accumulation of urine within the bladder due to interference of nerve supply, obstruction or psychological factors.

reticular *adj* resembling a net.

reticulocyte *n* a young circulating red blood cell which still contains traces of the nucleus and endoplasmic reticulum which were present in the cell when developing in the bone marrow.

reticulocytosis *n* an increase in the number of reticulocytes in the blood indicating over-active red blood cell formation in the marrow.

reticuloendothelial system (RES) a widely scattered system of cells and organ functions, of common ancestry and fulfilling many vital functions, e.g. defence against infection, antibody, blood cell and bile pigment formation and disposal of cell breakdown products. Main sites of reticuloendothelial cells are bone marrow, spleen, liver and lymphoid tissue.

retina *n* the light-sensitive internal coat of the eyeball, consisting of eight superimposed layers, seven of which are nervous and one pigmented. It is fragile, translucent and of a pinkish colour—**retinal** *adj.*

retinitis *n* inflammation of the retina. *retinitis pigmentosa* a noninflammatory, familial, degenerative condition which progresses to blindness, for which the word retinopathy is becoming more widely used.

retinoblastoma *n* a malignant tumour of the neuroglial element of the retina, occurring in children. Some cases are due to a chromosomal abnormality which may be indicated by low blood levels of an enzyme—esterase D.

retinol *n* ⇒ vitamin A.

retinopathy *n* any noninflammatory disease of the retina. ⇒ retinitis. *retinopathy of prematurity (ROP)* retinal, vascular disease affecting premature infants.

retinoscope *n* instrument for measuring refractive errors in order to prescribe spectacles.

retinotoxic *adj* toxic to the retina.

retractile *adj* capable of being drawn back, i.e. retracted.

retractor *n* a surgical instrument for holding apart the edges of a wound to reveal underlying structures.

retrobulbar *adj* pertaining to the back of the eyeball. *retrobulbar* *neuritis* inflammation of that portion of the optic nerve behind the eyeball.

retrocaecal *adj* behind the caecum, e.g. a retrocaecal appendix.

retroflexion *n* the state of being bent backwards. ⇒ anteflexion *opp.*

retrograde *adj* going backward. *retrograde pyelography* ⇒ pyelography.

retrolental fibroplasia ⇒ fibroplasia.

retroocular *adj* behind the eye.

retroperitoneal *adj* behind the peritoneum.

retropharyngeal *adj* behind the pharynx.

retroplacental *adj* behind the placenta.

retropubic *adj* behind the pubis.

retrospection *n* morbid dwelling on the past.

retrosternal *adj* behind the breast bone.

retrotracheal *adj* behind the trachea.

retroversion *n* turning backward. ⇒ anteversion *opp. retroversion of the uterus* tilting of the whole of the uterus backward with the cervix pointing forward—**retroverted** *adj.*

revascularization *n* the regrowth of blood vessel into a tissue or organ after deprivation of its normal blood supply.

reverse barrier nursing ⇒ barrier nursing.

Reye syndrome a syndrome comprising acute encephalopathy, cerebral oedema and fatty infiltration of the liver and other organs. It often follows a viral infection and presents with vomiting, progressing to impaired consciousness and jaundice. The condition is often fatal, although full recovery may follow early diagnosis.

Rh *abbr* Rhesus factor. ⇒ blood groups.

rhabdomyolisis *n* sporadic myoglobinurea: a group of disorders characterized by muscle injury leading to degenerative changes. *nontraumatic rhabdomyolisis* ⇒ crush syndrome.

rhagades *npl* superficial elongated scars radiating from the nostrils or angles of the mouth found in congenital syphilis.

Rhesus factor (Rh) antigen on red blood cell surface ⇒ blood groups.

Rhesus incompatability, isoimmunization this problem arises when a Rhesus negative mother carries a Rhesus positive fetus. During the birth there is mixing of fetal and maternal bloods. The mother's body then develops antibodies against the rhesus positive blood. If a subsequent fetus is also Rhesus positive, maternal antibodies will attack the fetal blood supply causing severe haemolysis. May also occur after abortion*, trauma or antepartum* haemorrhage.

rheumatic *adj* pertaining to rheumatism.

rheumatic fever ⇒ rheumatism.

rheumatism *n* a nonspecific term embracing a diverse group of diseases and syndromes which have in common, disorder or diseases of connective tissue and hence usually present with pain, or stiffness, or swelling of muscles and joints. The main groups are rheumatic fever, rheumatoid arthritis, ankylosing spondylitis, nonarticular rheumatism, osteoarthritis and gout. *acute rheumatism* (*syn* rheumatic fever), a disorder, tending to recur but initially commonest in childhood, classically presenting as fleeting polyarthritis of the larger joints, pyrexia and carditis within 3 weeks following a streptococcal throat infection. Atypically, but not infrequently, the symptoms are trivial and ignored, but carditis may be severe and result in permanent cardiac damage. *nonarticular* *rheumatism* involves the soft tissues and includes fibrositis, lumbago, etc.

rheumatoid *adj* resembling rheumatism. *rheumatoid arthritis* a disease of unknown aetiology, characterized by a chronic polyarthritis mainly affecting the smaller peripheral joints, accompanied by general ill health and resulting eventually in varying degrees of crippling joint deformities and associated muscle wasting. It is not just a disease of joints because every system may be involved in some way, therefore many rheumatologists prefer the term 'rheumatoid disease'. It has an autoimmune component. *rheumatoid factors* macrogammaglobulins found in most people with severe rheumatoid arthritis. They affect not only joints but also lung and nerve tissues and small arteries. It is not yet known whether they are the cause of, or the result of, arthritis. ⇒ pneumoconiosis, Still's disease.

rheumatology *n* the science or the study of the rheumatic diseases.

rhinitis *n* inflammation of the nasal mucous membrane.

rhinology *n* the study of diseases affecting the nose—**rhinologist** *n*.

rhinophyma *n* nodular enlargement of the skin of the nose.

rhinoplasty *n* operation to correct nasal deformity.

rhinorrhoea *n* nasal discharge.

rhinoscopy *n* inspection of the nose using a nasal speculum or nasendoscope—**rhinoscopic** *adj*.

rhinosinusitis *n* inflammation of the nose and adjacent sinuses.

Rhinosporidium *n* a genus of fungi parasitic to man.

rhinovirus *n* there are about 100 different varieties which can cause the common cold.

rhizotomy *n* surgical division of a root; usually the posterior root of a spinal nerve. *chemical rhizotomy* accomplished by injection of a chemical, often phenol*.

rhodopsin *n* the visual purple contained in the retinal rods. Its colour is preserved in darkness; bleached by daylight. Its formation is dependent on vitamin* A.

rhomboid *adj* diamond shaped.

rhonchus *n* an adventitious sound heard on auscultation of the lung. Passage of air through bronchi obstructed by oedema or exudate produces a musical note.

riboflavine *n* a constituent of the vitamin* B group.

ribonuclease *n* an enzyme that catalyses the depolymerization of ribonucleic acid. Can be made synthetically.

ribonucleic acid (RNA) nucleic acids found in all living cells. On hydrolysis they yield adenine, guanine, cytosine, uracil, ribose and phosphoric acid. They play an important part in protein synthesis.

ribs *npl* the 12 pairs of bones which articulate with the 12 dorsal vertebrae posteriorly and form the walls of the thorax. The upper seven pairs are *true ribs* and are attached to the sternum anteriorly by costal cartilage. The remaining five pairs are the *false ribs* the first three pairs of these do not have an attachment to the sternum but are bound to each other by costal cartilage. The lower two pairs are the *floating ribs* which have no anterior articulation. *cervical ribs* are formed by an extension of the transverse process of the 7th cervical vertebra in the form of bone or a fibrous tissue band; this causes an upward displacement of the subclavian artery. A congenital abnormality.

rice-water stool the stool of cholera*. The 'rice grains' are small pieces of desquamated epithelium from the intestine.

rickets *n* a disorder of calcium and phosphorus metabolism associated with a deficiency of vitamin D, and beginning most often in infancy and early childhood between the ages of 6 months and 2 years. There is proliferation and deficient ossification of the growing epiphyses of bones, producing 'bossing', softening and bending of the long weight-bearing bones, muscular hypotonia, head sweating and, if the blood calcium falls sufficiently, tetany. *fetal rickets* achondroplasia*. *renal rickets* a condition of decalcification (osteoporosis) of bones associated with chronic kidney disease and clinically simulating rickets, occurs in later age groups and is characterized by excessive urinary calcium loss. *vitamin D resistant rickets* due to disease of the lower extremities producing short legs. Genetic illness. No deficiency of vitamin D. Serum levels of phosphorus low. No associated renal disease. Thought to be due to a defect in the tubular reabsorption of phosphorus and a lowered calcium absorption from the gut causing secondary hyperthyroidism and a vitamin D abnormality.

Rickettsia *n* small pleomorphic parasitic microorganisms which have their natural habitat in the cells of the gut of arthropods. Some are pathogenic to mammals and man, in whom they cause the typhus group of fevers. They are smaller in size than bacteria and larger than the viruses. Many of their physiological characteristics resemble the bacteria, but like the viruses they are obligate intracellular parasites.

rickety rosary a series of protuberances (bossing) at junction of ribs and costal cartilages in children suffering from rickets*.

Riedel's thyroiditis a chronic fibrosis of the thyroid gland; ligneous goitre.

Rift valley fever one of the mosquito*-transmitted haemorrhagic fevers.

rigor *n* a sudden chill, accompanied by severe shivering. The body temperature rises rapidly and remains high until perspiration ensues and causes a gradual fall in temperature. *rigor mortis* the stiffening of the body after death.

ringworm *n* (*syn* tinea) generic term used to describe contagious infection of the skin by a fungus, because the common manifestations are circular (circinate) scaly patches. ⇒ dermatophytes.

Rinne's test testing of air conduction and bone conduction hearing, by tuning fork.

risk factor any factor which causes a person or a group of people to be vulnerable to disease, injury or complications. Known health risk factors are smoking, high consumption of alcohol, obesity, lack of exercise, lack of dietary fibre, and drugs abuse. ⇒ bedrest–complications of, Norton scale.

RIST *abbr* (radioimmunosorbent test) measures total serum IgE.

risus sardonicus the spastic grin of tetanus*.

rite of passage a customary ritual enacted to confirm that a person has been accepted into a particular group.

river blindness a form of onchocerciasis*.

RNA *abbr* ribonucleic* acid.

RO *abbr* reality* orientation.

rodent ulcer a basal cell carcinoma on the face or scalp which, although locally invasive, does not give rise to metastases.

role *n* the characteristic social behaviour of a person in relation to others in the group, e.g. the role of the nurse vis-à-vis that of the doctor. *role conflict* a person can experience conflict when enacting the various roles, e.g. the role of being a parent may conflict at times with that of being a nurse. *role playing* can be used in an educational programme when a student nurse assumes the role of a patient/client so that other students may practise lifting* and handling or communication* skills. It can be used therapeutically, e.g. in psychiatric nursing, to help patients see themselves as others see them and to understand intrapsychic conflict.

Romberg's sign a sign of ataxia*. Inability to stand erect (without swaying) when the eyes are closed and the feet together. Also called 'Rombergism'.

rosacea *n* a skin disease which shows on flush areas of the face. In areas affected there is chronic dilation of superficial capillaries and hypertrophy of sebaceous follicles, often complicated by a papulopustular eruption.

rose bengal a staining agent used to detect diseased corneal and conjunctival epithelium.

roseola *n* the earliest manifestation of secondary syphilis. This syphilide is a faint, pink spot, widespread in distribution except for the skin over the hands and face.

rotator *n* a muscle having the action of turning a part.

rotaviruses *npl* viruses associated with gastroenteritis in children and infants. Related to, but easily distinguished from, reoviruses*.

Roth spots round white spots in the retina in some cases of bacterial endocarditis; thought to be of embolic origin.

roughage *n* an old-fashioned term which does not describe fibre adequately and should not be used. 'Nonstarch polysaccharides' better describes the complex mixture of substances which have a wide range of effects on the gastrointestinal tract. ⇒ nonstarch polysaccharides, bran.

rouleaux *n* a row of red blood cells which, when aggregated, resemble a stack of coins. Seen in disorders such as inflammatory diseases.

roundworm *n* (*Ascaris lumbricoides*) look like earth worms. Worldwide distribution. Parasitic to man. Eggs passed in stools; ingested; hatch in bowel, migrate through tissues, lungs and bronchi before returning to the bowel as mature worms. During migration worms can be coughed up which is unpleasant and frightening. Heavy infections can produce pneumonia. A tangled mass can cause intestinal obstruction or appendicitis. The best drug for treatment is piperazine. Roundworm of the cat and dog is called *Toxocara*.

Roux-en-Y operation originally the distal end of divided jejunum was anastomosed to the stomach, and the proximal jejunum containing the duodenal and pancreatic juices was anastomosed to the jejunum about 75 mm below the first anastomosis. The term is now used to include joining of the distal jejunum to a divided bile duct, oesophagus or pancreas, in major surgery of these structures.

Rovsing's sign pressure in the left iliac fossa causes pain in the right iliac fossa in appendicitis.

Royal College of Nursing (RCN) the world's largest professional union of nurses, with more than 300 000 members. It is run by nurses for nurses. The RCN is a major contributor to the development of nursing practice and standards of care, is a provider of education through the RCN Institute and is a registered charity. It is governed by the RCN Council and is incorporated by a Royal Charter.

RPCF *abbr* Reiter* protein complement fixation.

RSI *abbr* repetitive* strain injury.

RSV *abbr* respiratory* syncytial virus.

rubefacients *npl* substances which, when applied to the skin, cause redness (hyperaemia).

rubella *n* (*syn* German measles) an acute, infectious disease, with an incubation period of 14–21 days. Caused by a virus and spread by droplet infection. There is mild fever, a pink, maculopapular rash and enlarged occipital and posterior cervical glands. Complications are rare, except when contracted in the early months of pregnancy, when it may produce fetal deformities. It is occasionally followed by a painful arthritis.

Rubenstein-Taybi syndrome a constellation of abnormal findings first described in 1963. It includes mental and motor retardation, broad thumbs and toes, growth retardation, susceptibility to infection in the early years and characteristic facial features.

rubor *n* redness; usually used in the context of being one of the four classical signs of inflammation the others being calor*, dolor*, tumor*.

Ryle's tube a long fine tube with a weighted tip which is passed via the nose into the stomach: it is classified as a nasogastric tube. The rationale for its use is to empty the stomach and keep it empty, accomplished by continuous or intermittent suction. Fluid replacement will be by intravenous drip. Mouth care and psychological support are necessary for this unpleasant nursing intervention. The amount of gastric aspirate and the time of aspiration are recorded on an intake and output chart.

S

saccharides *npl* one of the three main classes of carbohydrates (i.e. sugars).

sacculation *n* appearance of several saccules.

saccule *n* a minute sac—**saccular, sacculated** *adj*.

saccus decompression drainage of excess endolymph* from the vestibular labyrinth to the subarachnoid space where it flows to join the cerebrospinal fluid. Performed for patients with MeniËre's disease.

sacral *adj* pertaining to the sacrum.

sacroanterior *adj* describes a breech presentation in midwifery. The fetal sacrum is directed to one or other acetabulum of the mother—**sacroanteriorly** *adv*.

sacrococcygeal *adj* pertaining to the sacrum* and the coccyx*.

sacroiliac *adj* pertaining to the sacrum* and the ilium*.

sacroiliitis *n* inflammation of a sacroiliac joint. Involvement of both joints characterizes such conditions as ankylosing spondylitis, Reiter's syndrome and psoriatic arthritis.

sacrolumbar *adj* pertaining to the sacrum* and the loins*.

sacroposterior *adj* describes a breech presentation in midwifery. The fetal sacrum is directed to one or other sacroiliac joint of the mother—**sacroposteriorly** *adv*.

sacrum *n* the triangular bone lying between the fifth lumbar vertebra and the coccyx. It consists of five vertebrae fused together, and it articulates on each side with the innominate bones of the pelvis, forming the sacroiliac joints—**sacral** *adj*.

SAD *abbr* seasonal* affective disorder.

saddle nose one with a flattened bridge; often a sign of congenital syphilis*.

sadism *n* the obtaining of pleasure from inflicting pain, violence or degradation on another person, or on the sexual partner. ⇒ masochism *opp*.

sagittal *adj* resembling an arrow. In the anteroposterior plane of the body. *sagittal suture* the immovable joint formed by the union of the two parietal bones.

salbutamol *n* a bronchodilator which relieves asthma, chronic bronchitis and emphysema. Does not produce cardiovascular side-effects when inhaled in the recommended dose.

Salem nasogastric tube a tube which has a double lumen to allow swallowed air to escape. It is used in whole gut irrigation.

salicylamide *n* a mild analgesic similar in action to the salicylates, but less likely to cause gastric disturbance.

salicylates *npl* widely used group of NSAIDs* with analgesic and antipyretic properties. They include acetylsalicylic acid (aspirin).

salicylic acid has fungicidal and bacteriostatic properties, and is used in a variety of skin conditions. The plaster is used to remove corns and warts.

saline *n* a solution of salt and water. Normal or physiological saline is a 0.9% solution with the same osmotic pressure as that of blood. ⇒ hypertonic, isotonic.

saliva *n* the secretion of the salivary glands (spittle). It contains water, mucus and ptyalin*—**salivary** *adj.*

salivary *adj* pertaining to saliva. *salivary calculus* a stone formed in the salivary ducts. *salivary glands* the glands which secrete saliva, i.e. the parotid, submaxillary and sublingual glands.

salivation *n* an increased secretion of saliva.

Salk vaccine a preparation of killed poliomyelitis virus used as an antigen to produce active artificial immunity to poliomyelitis. It is given by injection.

Salmonella *n* a genus of bacteria. Gram-negative rods. Parasitic in many animals and man in whom they are often pathogenic. Some species, such as *Salmonella typhi,* are host-specific, infecting only man, in whom they cause typhoid fever. Others, such as *Salmonella typhimurium,* may infect a wide range of host species, usually through contaminated foods. *Salmonella enteritidis* a motile Gram-negative rod, widely distributed in domestic and wild animals, particularly rodents, and sporadic in man as a cause of food poisoning.

salpingectomy *n* excision of a uterine tube.

salpingitis *n* acute or chronic inflammation of the uterine tubes. ⇒ hydrosalpinx, pyosalpinx.

salpingogram *n* radiological examination of patency of the uterine tubes by retrograde introduction of contrast medium into the uterus and along the tubes—**salpingographic** *adj,* **salpingographically** *adv.*

salpingo-oophorectomy *n* excision of a uterine tube and ovary.

salpingostomy *n* the operation performed to restore tubal patency.

salpinx a tube, especially the uterine tube or the eustachian tube.

salt *n* ⇒ sodium chloride.

salve *n* an ointment.

Samaritans *npl* a voluntary befriending telephone service available at all hours to suicidal or despairing people who phone in.

sandfly *n* an insect (*Phlebotomus*) responsible for short, sharp, pyrexial fever called 'sandfly fever' of the tropics. Likewise transmits leishmaniasis*.

sanguineous *adj* pertaining to or containing blood.

saphenous *adj* apparent; manifest. The name given to the two main veins in the leg, the internal and the external, and to the nerves accompanying them.

sapraemia *n* a general bodily reaction to circulating toxins and breakdown products of saprophytic (nonpathogenic) organisms, derived from one or more foci in the body.

saprophyte *n* free-living microorganisms obtaining food from dead and decaying animal or plant tissue—**saprophytic** *adj.*

sarcoid *adj* a term applied to a group of lesions in skin, lungs or other organs, which resemble tuberculous foci in structure, but the true nature of which is still uncertain.

sarcoidosis *n* a granulomatous disease of unknown aetiology in which histological appearances resemble tuberculosis. May affect any organ of the body, but most commonly presents as a condition of the skin, lymphatic glands or the bones of the hand.

sarcoma *n* malignant growth of mesodermal tissue (e.g. connective tissue, muscle, bone)—**sarcomata** *pl,* **sarcomatous** *adj.*

sarcomatosis *n* a condition in which sarcomata are widely spread throughout the body.

Sarcoptes *n* a genus of Acerina. *Sarcoptes scabiei* is the itch mite which causes scabies*.

sartorius *n* the 'tailor's muscle' of the thigh, since it flexes one leg over the other.

satisfaction *n* a positive feeling. *job satisfaction* a term which is used when people, including nurses, experience positiveness in relation to their work: lack of it can lead to low morale.⇒ burnout syndrome. *consumer satisfaction* ⇒ quality assurance.

scab *n* a dried crust forming over an open wound.

scabies *n* a parasitic skin disease caused by the itch mite. Highly contagious.

scald *n* an injury caused by moist heat.

scalenus syndrome pain in arm and fingers, often with wasting, because of compression of the lower trunk of the brachial plexus behind scalenus anterior muscle at the thoracic outlet.

scalp *n* the hair-bearing and fairly moveable skin which covers the cranium. *scalp cooling* the application of a cap made of coils through which flows cold water or malleable ice packs: research shows that it prevents doxorubicin-induced alopecia in some patients, but most find the treatment unpleasant.

scan *n* an image built up by movement along or across the object scanned, either of the detector or of the imaging agent, to achieve complete coverage, e.g. ultrasound* scan, CAT* scan, MRI.

scanning speech a form of dysarthria occurring in disseminated sclerosis. The speech is jumpy or staccato or slow.

scaphoid *n* boat-shaped, as a bone of the tarsus and carpus. *scaphoid abdomen* concavity of the anterior abdominal wall, often associated with emaciation.

scapula *n* the shoulder-blade, a large, flat triangular bone—**scapular** *adj*.

scar *n* (*syn* cicatrix) the dense, avascular white fibrous tissue, formed as the end-result of healing, especially in the skin. ⇒ disfigurement, keloid.

scarification *n* the making of a series of small, superficial incisions or punctures in the skin to allow a vaccine to enter the body.

scarlet fever *n* infectious disease with an incubation period of 2–4 days. Follows infection by a strain of Group A β–haemolytic streptococcus. Occurs mainly in children. Begins commonly with a throat infection, leading to fever and the outbreak of a punctate erythematous rash on the skin of the trunk. Characteristically the area around the mouth escapes (circumoral pallor). Usually treated with penicillin.

SCAT *abbr* sheep cell agglutination test. Rheumatoid factor in the blood is detected by the sheep cell agglutination titre.

SCBU *abbr* special* care baby unit.

Scheuermann's disease osteochondritis* of the spine affecting the ring epiphyses of the vertebral bodies. Occurs in adolescents.

Schick test a test used to determine a person's susceptibility or immunity to diphtheria. It consists of the injection of 2 or 3 minims of freshly prepared toxin beneath the skin of the left arm. A similar test is made into the right arm, but in this the serum is heated to 75°C for 10 min, in order to destroy the toxin but not the protein. A positive reaction is recognized by the appearance of a round red area on the left arm within 24–48 h, reaching its maximum intensity on the fourth day, then gradually fading with slight pigmentation and desquamation. This reaction indicates susceptibility or absence of immunity. No reaction indicates that the subject is immune to diphtheria. Occasionally a pseudoreaction occurs, caused by the protein of the toxin; in this case the redness appears on both arms, hence the value of the control.

Schilder's disease a genetically determined degenerative disease associated with mental disability.

Schilling test estimation of absorption of radioactive vitamin B_{12} for confirmation of pernicious anaemia.

Schistosoma *n* (*syn* Bilharzia) a genus of blood flukes which require fresh water snails as an intermediate host before infesting humans. *Schistosoma haematobium* is found mainly in Africa and the Middle East. *Schistosoma japonicum* is found in Japan, the Philippines and Eastern Asia. *Schistosoma mansoni* is indigenous to Africa, the Middle East, the Caribbean and South America.

schistosomiasis *n* (*syn* bilharziasis) infestation of the human body by *Schistosoma* which enter via the skin or mucous membrane. A single fluke can live in one part of the body, depositing eggs frequently for many years. Treatment is with Praziquantel. Prevention is by chlorination of drinking water, proper disposal of human waste and eradication of fresh water snails. Schistosomiasis is a serious problem in the tropics and the Orient. The eggs are irritating to the mucous membranes which thicken and bleed causing anaemia, together with pain and dysfunction of the afflicted organ: fibrosis of mucous membranes can cause obstruction.

schistosomicide *n* any agent lethal to *Schistosoma*–**schistosomicidal** *adj.*

schizophrenia *n* a psychotic disorder, one of the commonest psychiatric illnesses. Patients will display one or more of the following groups of symptoms for a prolonged period (at least 6 months): auditory hallucinations; delusions, which may be paranoid; disorder of thought with loss of normal association of ideas; loss of emotional responsiveness. Symptoms may be subgrouped into *catatonic schizophrenia,* characterized by episodes of immobility with muscular rigidity or stupor, interspersed with periods of acute excitability; *simple schizophrenia,* characterized by apathy and withdrawal–hallucinations and delusions are absent; and *paranoid schizophrenia,* where hallucinations and paranoid delusions are present.

schizophrenic *adj* pertaining to schizophrenia*.

Schlatter's disease (*syn* Osgood-Schlatter's disease) osteochondritis* of the tibial tubercle.

Schlemm's canal a lymphaticovenous canal in the inner part of the sclera, close to its junction with the cornea, which it encircles.

Scholz's disease a genetically determined degenerative disease associated with learning disability.

Schönlein's disease Henoch*-Schönlein purpura.

school nurse an RGN who has undertaken a further course on the health care of school-age children and who is responsible for monitoring growth and development, for screening out the abnormal and who has responsibility for children with *special* educational needs.

Schultz-Charlton test a blanching produced in the skin of a patient showing scarlatinal rash, around an injection of serum from a convalescent case, indicating neutralization of toxin by antitoxin.

sciatica *n* pain in the line of distribution of the sciatic nerve (buttock, back of thigh, calf and foot). ⇒ backache.

scintillography *n* (*syn* scintiscanning) visual recording of radioactivity over selected areas after administration of suitable radioisotope, e.g. to diagnose cancer.

scirrhous *adj* hard; resembling a scirrhus. Describes malignant tumours that are hard.

scirrhus *n* a carcinoma which provokes a considerable growth of hard, connective tissue; a hard carcinoma of the breast.

scissor leg deformity the legs are crossed in walking following double hip-joint disease, or as a manifestation of Little's disease (spastic cerebral diplegia).

scissors gait ⇒ gait.

sclera *n* the 'white' of the eye; the opaque bluish-white fibrous outer coat of the eyeball covering the posterior five-sixths; it merges into the cornea at the front—**sclerae** *pl,* **scleral** *adj.*

sclerema *n* a rare disease in which hardening of the skin results from the deposition of mucinous material.

scleritis *n* inflammation of the sclera*.

sclerocorneal *adj* pertaining to the sclera* and the cornea*, as the circular junction of these two structures.

scleroderma *n* a disease in which localized oedema of the skin is followed by hardening, atrophy, deformity and ulceration. Occasionally it becomes generalized, producing immobility of the face, contraction of the fingers; diffuse fibrosis of the myocardium, kidneys, digestive tract and lungs. When confined to the skin it is termed morphoea. ⇒ collagen, dermatomyositis.

sclerosis *n* a word used in pathology to describe abnormal hardening or fibrosis of a tissue. ⇒ multiple sclerosis, tuberous sclerosis.

sclerotherapy *n* injection of a sclerosing agent for the treatment of varicose veins. When, after the injection, rubber pads are bandaged over the site to increase localized compression, the term *compression sclerotherapy* is used. Sclerotherapy for oesophageal varices involves the use of an oesophagoscope, either rigid or flexible—**sclerotherapeutic** *adj,* **sclerotherapeutically** *adv.*

sclerotic *adj* pertaining to or exhibiting the symptoms of sclerosis.

scolex *n* the head of the tapeworm by which it attaches itself to the intestinal wall, and from which the segments (proglottides) develop.

scoliosis *n* lateral curvature of the spine, which can be congenital or acquired and is due to abnormality of the vertebrae, muscles and nerves. *idiopathic scoliosis* is characterized by a lateral curvature together with rotation and associated rib hump or flank recession.

scorbutic *adj* pertaining to scorbutus, the old name for scurvy*.

scotoma *n* a blind spot in the field of vision. May be normal or abnormal—**scotomata** *pl.*

scrapie *n* a virus disease of sheep and goats.

screening *n* a preventive measure to identify potential or incipient disease. It is carried out in such places as clinics for antenatal care, breast screening, cervical cytology, hypertension, well men and well women. Also a common name for fluroscopy units. ⇒ ill health—prevention of.

scrofula *n* tuberculosis of bone or lymph gland—**scrofulous** *adj.*

scrofuloderma *n* an exudative and crusted skin lesion, often with sinuses, resulting from a tuberculous lesion, underneath, as in bone or lymph glands. Rare in Europe but common in the tropics.

scrotum *n* the pouch in the male which contains the testes—**scrotal** *adj.*

scurf *n* a popular term for dandruff*.

scurvy *n* a deficiency disease caused by lack of vitamin* C (ascorbic acid). Clinical features include fatigue and haemorrhage. Latter may take the form of oozing at the gums or large ecchymoses. Tiny bleeding spots on the skin around hair follicles are characteristic. In children painful subperiosteal haemorrhage (rather than other types of bleeding) is pathognomonic.

scybala *npl* rounded, hard, faecal lumps—**scybalum** *sing.*

seasonal affective disorder (SAD) a significant depressed mood which coincides with the onset of winter and lifts with the arrival of spring. In some areas near the Arctic Circle there is a higher rate of suicide in winter than in summer. Daily treatment with light to supplement exposure to natural light has been found to relieve symptoms.

sebaceous *adj* literally, pertaining to fat; usually refers to sebum*. *sebaceous cyst* (*syn* wen) a retention cyst in a sebaceous (oil-secreting) gland in the skin. Such cysts are most commonly found on the scalp, scrotum and vulva. *sebaceous glands* the cutaneous glands which secrete an oily substance called 'sebum'. The ducts of these glands are short and straight and open into the hair follicles.

seborrhoea *n* greasy condition of the scalp, face, sternal region and elsewhere due to overactivity of sebaceous* glands. The seborrhoeic type of skin is especially liable to conditions such as alopecia, seborrhoeic dermatitis, acne, etc.

sebum *n* the normal secretion of the sebaceous* glands; it contains fatty acids, cholesterol and dead cells.

seclusion *n* a nursing intervention for mentally ill patients: they are isolated in a special room to decrease stimuli which might be causing or exacerbating their emotional distress.

secondary *adj* 2nd in order. *secondary care* care that requires admission to hospital, rather than provided in the community. ⇒ primary* care, tertiary* care. *secondary tumour* refers to spread of primary growth in neoplasm; can occur via blood, lymph, tissue extension or through a body cavity. ⇒ neoplasm, metastases.

secretin *n* a hormone produced in the duodenal mucosa, which causes a copious secretion of pancreatic juice.

secretion *n* a fluid or substance, formed or concentrated in a gland and passed into the alimentary tract, the blood or to the exterior.

secretory *adj* involved in the process of secretion: describes a gland which secretes.

secular beliefs not overtly or specifically religious. Words such as spirit, spiritual and spirituality are used in a nonreligious context, for instance, summing up a person who is undergoing a stressful period one might say 'but he's in good spirits': the term is concerned with hopefulness, optimism and positiveness. Those who use words in this way often have strong nonreligious beliefs/convictions which guide their concepts of right and wrong that affect everyday living. ⇒ spiritual beliefs.

sedation *n* the production of a state of lessened functional activity.

sedative *n* any agent which lessens functional activity by acting on the nervous system. Includes drugs such as the benzodiazepines* which have sedating effects. ⇒ hypnotic, narcotic.

segment *n* a small section; a part—**segmental** *adj,* **segmentation** *n.*

segregation *n* in genetics, the separation from one another of two alleles, each carried on one of a pair of chromosomes; this happens at meiosis* when the haploid, mature germ cells (the egg and the sperm) are made.

Seldinger catheter a special catheter and guide wire for insertion into an artery, along which it is passed, e.g. to the heart.

Selectron *n* a proprietary device used to deliver brachytherapy* by remote controlled afterloading. The radioactive sources are propelled along tubes connecting the Selectron to previously placed applicators in body cavities such as cervix, vagina, bronchus.

self-catheterization both male and female patients can be taught to pass a nonretaining catheter into the urinary bladder to evacuate urine intermittently.

self-image the total concept of what one believes oneself to be vis-à-vis one's role in society.

self-infection the unwitting transfer of microorganisms from one part of the body to another in which it produces an infection.

self-injurious behaviour ⇒ parasuicide.

self-retaining catheter a catheter* which, when inserted into the urinary bladder, can be anchored there by inflation of a tiny balloon surrounding the tip.

sella turcica pituitary* fossa.

semen *n* the secretion from the testicles and accessory male organs, e.g. prostate. In the fertile male, it contains spermatozoa*.

semicircular canals three membranous semicircular tubes contained within the bony labyrinth of the internal ear. They are concerned with appreciation of the body's position in space.

semicomatose *adj* describes a condition bordering on the unconscious.

semilunar *adj* shaped like a crescent or half moon. *semilunar cartilages* the crescentic interarticular cartilages of the knee joint (menisci).

seminal *adj* pertaining to semen.

seminiferous *adj* carrying or producing semen.

seminoma *n* a malignant tumour of the testis—**seminomata** *pl,* **seminomatous** *adj.*

semipermeable *adj* describes a membrane which is selectively permeable to some substances in solutions, but not to others ⇒ osmosis.

senescence *n* normal changes of mind and body in increasing age—**senescent** *adj.*

Sengstaken tube incorporates a balloon which after being positioned in the lower oesophagus is inflated to apply pressure to bleeding oesophageal varices.

senile *adj* suffering from senescence* complicated by morbid processes commonly called degeneration—**senility** *n* ⇒ dementia.

senna *n* leaves and pods of a purgative plant from Egypt and India. Once used extensively as 'black draught' or compound senna mixture.

sensation *n* consciousness of perceiving a state or condition of one's body or any part of it; one's senses; one's mind or its emotions.

senses *npl* the five special senses–hearing, seeing, smelling, tactile feeling and tasting.

sensible *n* **1** endowed with the sense of feeling. **2** detectable by the senses.

sensitivity training group in a supportive atmosphere members learn about what occurs during their interactions with others. They can test and refine new behavioural responses in the light of feedback about previously evoked reactions: they are encouraged to enact the positively modified behaviours in circumstances other than the group.

sensitization *n* rendering sensitive. Persons may become sensitive to a variety of substances which may be food (e.g. shellfish), bacteria, plants, chemical substances, drugs, sera, etc. Liability is much greater in some persons than others. ⇒ allergy, anaphylaxis.

sensorineural *adj* pertaining to sensory neurones. *sensorineural deafness* a discriminating term for nerve deafness*.

sensory *adj* pertaining to sensation. *sensory nerves* those which convey impulses to the brain and spinal cord.

sensory deprivation absence of usual sensory stimuli, e.g. for patients in intensive care units. Continued sensory deprivation may lead to mental changes, such as anxiety, depression and visual/auditory hallucinations.

sensory impairment/loss reduced function or total loss of any of the five special senses i.e. sight, hearing, smell, taste and touch.

sepsis *n* the state of being infected with pus-producing organisms—**septic** *adj.*

septal haematoma haematoma of nasal septum following surgery or trauma.

septic abortion ⇒ abortion.

septicaemia *n* the persistence and multiplication of living bacteria in the bloodstream—**septicaemic** *adj.*

septoplasty *n* an operation to straighten the nasal septum (conserving cartilage and bone) by remodelling and positioning it in the midline.

septum *n* a partition between two cavities, e.g. between the nasal cavities and between the left and right sides of the heart—**septa** *pl,* **septal, septate** *adj.*

sequela *n* pathological consequences of a disease.—**sequelae** *pl.*

sequestrectomy *n* excision of a sequestrum*.

sequestrum *n* a piece of dead bone which separates from the healthy bone but remains within the tissues—**sequestra** *pl.*

serology *n* the branch of science dealing with the study of sera and blood—**serological** *adj.*

seropurulent *adj* containing serum* and pus*.

serosa *n* a serous membrane*, e.g. the peritoneal covering of the abdominal viscera—**serosal** *adj.*

serositis *n* inflammation of a serous membrane*.

serotonin *n* a product of tryptophan metabolism. Liberated by blood platelets after injury and found in high concentrations in many body tissues including the CNS. It is a vasoconstrictor, inhibits gastric secretion, stimulates smooth muscle. Serves as a central neurotransmitter and is a precursor of melatonin*. Together with histamine it may be concerned in allergic reactions. Called also 5-hydroxytryptamine and 5-HT. Seven subtypes are known.

serous *adj* pertaining to serum*. *serous membrane* ⇒ membrane.

serpiginous *adj* snakelike, coiled, irregular; used to describe the margins of skin lesions, especially ulcers and ringworm.

Serratia *n* a genus of Gram-negative bacilli capable of causing infection in humans. It is an endemic hospital resident.⇒ infection.

serration *n* a saw-like notch—**serrated** *adj.*

serum *n* the clear fluid which forms when blood clots and the corpuscles and fibrin have been removed—**sera** *pl. serum glutamic oxaloacetic transaminase (SGOT)* enzyme normally present in serum and also found in heart, liver and muscle tissue. It is released into the serum as a result of tissue damage and hence its increased presence may be due to myocardial infarction or acute liver disease. *serum sickness* ⇒ anaphylaxis.

sex education an essential part of any health education programme. It includes teaching about the male and female body so that the learner can understand expressing sexuality and recognize the onset of puberty: knowledge about personal relationships including those that are heterosexual, homosexual and bisexual: knowledge about contraception, sexually transmitted diseases, pregnancy, childbirth, bonding, parenting and family living.

sexism *n* a belief that members of one sex are superior to members of the other, and thereby have advantages over them. It leads to discrimination and can act as a limiting factor in, e.g. educational and professional development.

sex-linked *adj* refers to genes which are located on the sex chromosomes or, more especially, on the X-chromosome. To avoid confusion it is now customary to refer to the latter genes (and the characteristics determined by them) as X-linked.

sexual abuse performing a sexual act with a child or with an adult against the person's wishes. The most common type of sexual abuse occurs between a father (or father figure) and daughter. ⇒ incest.

sexual counselling ⇒ counselling, psychosexual counselling.

sexual dysfunction a lack of desire or the ability to achieve coitus in one or both partners. A woman can experience dyspareunia, frigidity, perineal soreness from cystitis, vaginal infection, vaginal dryness and vaginismus. A man may experience inability to produce an erection, sustain an erection, or experience premature ejaculation.

sexual intercourse coitus*.

sexuality *n* the sum of the structural, functional and psychological attributes as they are expressed by one's gender-identity and sexual behaviour.

sexuality, expressing increasingly in a nursing context, the term is being accepted as an activity of living. It includes the many ways in which a person expresses gender to other people, by the clothes, perfume, jewellery, toilet articles used; make-up worn, behaviour, attitude to, and behaviour with, members of the opposite sex. ⇒ homosexuality, lesbianism, sexuality.

sexually transmitted disease (STD) previously called venereal disease. The currently preferred term is genitourinary* medicine (GUM).

sexual preference denotes a person's sexual attraction towards people of the same sex (homosexuality), the opposite sex (heterosexuality) or both sexes (bisexuality). It may be transitory or life-long.

sexual problems ⇒ sexual dysfunction.

sharps *n* include used needles, razor blades, giving sets, central venous lines and cannulae. They should be put immediately into a rigid sharps' container of distinctive colour which is disposed of when three-quarters full. It is sealed in such a way that used needles cannot be recovered for use by injecting drug abusers. Arrangements have to be made for safe disposal of those used by diabetic people, district nurses, at health centres and doctors' surgeries.

shaving *v* some surgeons request a hair-free operation site; shaving is still the most commonly used method of achieving this. Scanning electron micrographs have shown that every skin shave causes epidermal damage, therefore it should be done immediately prior to surgery to reduce colonization of damaged areas. It is preferable to use a disposable razor with foam rather than soap; or an electric razor with a removable head which can be disinfected.

shearing force when any part of the supported body is on a gradient, the deeper tissues near the bone 'slide' towards the lower gradient while the skin remains at its point of contact with the supporting surface because of friction which is increased in the presence of moisture. The deep blood vessels are stretched and angulated, thus the deeper tissues become ischaemic with consequent necrosis. ⇒ pressure sores.

shelf operation an operation to deepen the acetabulum in congenital dislocation of the hip joint, involving the use of a bone graft. Performed at 7–8 years, after failure of conservative treatment.

shiatsu *n* a form of massage by thumbs, fingers and palms, without the use of instruments, mechanical or otherwise, to apply pressure to the human skin to correct internal malfunctioning, promote and maintain health and treat specific diseases.

Shigella *n* a genus of bacteria containing some of the organisms causing dysentery. *Shigella flexneri* a pathogenic, Gram-negative rod, which is the most common cause of bacillary dysentery epidemics, and sometimes infantile gastroenteritis. It is found in the faeces of cases of dysentery and carriers, whence it may pollute food and water supplies.

shin bone the tibia, the medial bone of the foreleg.

shingles *n* a condition arising when the infecting agent (herpes zoster virus) attacks sensory nerves causing severe pain and the appearance of vesicles along the nerve's distribution (usually unilateral). ⇒ herpes zoster virus.

Shirodkar's operation placing of a purse-string suture around an incompetent cervix during pregnancy. It is removed when labour starts.

shock *n* circulatory disturbance produced by severe injury or illness and due in large part to reduction in blood volume (hypovolaemic, oligaemic). There is discrepancy between the circulating blood volume and the capacity of the vascular bed. Initial cause is reduction in circulating blood volume; perpetuation is due to vasoconstriction, therefore vasoconstrictor drugs are not given. Its features include a fall in blood pressure, rapid pulse, pallor, restlessness, thirst and a cold clammy skin. *cardiogenic shock* occurs as a result of an acute heart condition such as myocardial* infarction. *neurogenic shock* can occur as a result of severe fright after hearing bad news or seeing a horrifying sight.

shivering *v* an involuntary response occurring while the core body temperature is rising, either as a result of the release of pyrogens after injury, including surgery; or infection.

shortsightedness *n* ⇒ myopia.

shoulder girdle formed by the clavicle and scapula on either side.

shoulder lift ⇒ Australian lift.

'show' *n* a popular term for the bloodstained vaginal discharge at the commencement of labour.

shunt *n* a term applied to the passage of blood through other than the usual channel.

sialagogue *n* an agent which increases the flow of saliva.

sialogram *n* radiographic image of the salivary glands and ducts, after injection of a contrast medium—**sialography** *n,* **sialographic** *adj,* **sialographically** *adv.*

sialolith *n* a stone in a salivary gland or duct.

SIB *abbr* self-injurious* behaviour.

sibling *n* one of a family of children having the same parents.

sick building syndrome a recently recognized condition affecting those who work in open-plan offices. The symptoms include lethargy, headache, dry itching skin and dry throat.

sickle-cell anaemia ⇒ anaemia.

sickness certificate in the UK, when a person is ill and unable to go to work, a self-certification form is completed and forwarded to the employer. Absence from the 5th day onwards is notified by a doctor's signature on a sickness certificate, and if necessary, thereafter at a time interval as determined by the doctor on the certificate.

sick role a sociological term which signifies changes in a person's role because he or she is ill. In acute illness the person is relieved of usual activities and responsibilities, and can accept assistance from, and perhaps dependence on, others. In exchange, the person complies with the treatment and relinquishes the sick role at an appropriate time. The concept is less useful when considering a person with chronic illness.

side-effect any physiological change other than the desired one from drug administration, e.g. the antispasmodic drug propantheline causes the side-effect of dry mouth in some patients. The term also covers undesirable drug reactions. Some are predictable, being the result of a known metabolic action of the drug, e.g. yellowing of skin and eyes and bone and formation of striae with corticosteroids; loss of hair with cyclophosphamide. Unpredictable reactions can be: (a) immediate: anaphylactic shock, angioneurotic oedema (b) erythematous: all forms of erythema, including nodosum and multiforme and purpuric rashes (c) cellular eczematous rashes and contact dermatitis (d) specific e.g. light-sensitive eruptions with ledermycin and griseofulvin.

siderosis *n* excess of iron in the blood or tissues. Inhalation of iron oxide into the lungs can cause one form of pneumoconiosis*.

SIDS *abbr* sudden* infant death syndrome. ⇒ cot death.

sigmoid *adj* shaped like the letter S. ⇒ flexure.

sigmoidoscope *n* an instrument for visualizing the rectum and sigmoid flexure of the colon. ⇒ endoscope—**sigmoidoscopic** *adj,* **sigmoidoscopy** *n.*

sigmoidostomy *n* the formation of a colostomy in the sigmoid* colon.

sign *n* any objective evidence of disease.

significant other a term used to designate the person that the patient or client wants the nursing staff to consult when relevant, for instance when making arrangements for transfer or discharge; or to be notified in the case of emergency.

sign language a form of nonverbal language using the hands and upper body to make signs whereby deaf people can communicate with each other and with family members and friends. When a profoundly deaf person who uses sign language is admitted to hospital, special arrangements need to be made so that a person skilled in using sign language is present most of the time. ⇒ finger spelling.

silicone *n* an organic compound which is water-repellant. *silicone foam dressing* a soft durable substance fits exactly the contours of an open granulating wound in which it encourages healing. Silicone implants may be used in breast reconstruction following mastectomy or to increase the breast size.

silicosis *n* a form of pneumoconiosis* or 'industrial dust disease' found in metal grinders, stoneworkers, etc.

silver nitrate in the form of small sticks, is used as a caustic for warts.

silver sulphadiazine silver derivative of sulphadiazine. Topical bacteriostatic agent, used to control bacterial infection in burns patients.

Sim's position an exaggerated left lateral position with the right knee well flexed and the left arm drawn back over the edge of the bed. Used for demonstration of vaginal prolapse and stress incontinence ⇒ speculum.

SIMV *abbr* synchronized intermittent mandatory ventilation.

sinew *n* a ligament or tendon.

sinoatrial node ⇒ node.

sinus *n* **1** a hollow or cavity, especially the nasal sinuses. **2** a channel containing blood, especially venous blood, e.g. the sinuses of the brain. **3** a recess or cavity within a bone. **4** any suppurating tract or channel. *sinus arrhythmia* an increase of the pulse rate on inspiration, decrease on expiration. Appears to be normal in some children. *sinus rhythm* the normal heart rhythm beginning in the sinoatrial* node. Its electrical activity can be demonstrated on an ECG* strip. ⇒ cavernous, pilonidal.

sinusitis *n* infection in paranasal sinuses.

sinusoid *n* a dilated channel into which arterioles or veins open in some organs and which take the place of the usual capillaries.

sitz-bath *n* a hip bath.

Sjögren-Larsson syndrome genetically determined congenital ectodermosis. Associated with mental subnormality.

Sjögren syndrome deficient secretion from lacrimal, salivary and other glands, mostly in postmenopausal women. There is keratoconjunctivitis, dry tongue and hoarse voice. Thought to be due to an autoimmune process. Also called keratoconjunctivitis sicca.

skeleton *n* the bony framework of the body, supporting and protecting the soft tissues and organs and providing an attachment for muscles—**skeletal** *adj. appendicular skeleton* the bones forming the upper and lower extremities. *axial skeleton* the bones forming the head and trunk.

Skene's glands two small glands at the entrance to the female urethra; the paraurethral glands.

skills *npl* a complex of abilities required to carry out a particular task which may be of a cognitive, affective or psychomotor nature, or a mix of these.

skin *n* the tissue which forms the outer covering of the body; it consists of two main layers: (a) the epidermis, or cuticle, forming the outer coat (b) the dermis, or cutis vera, the inner or true skin, lying beneath the epidermis. *skin patch* the topical application of a drug-impregnated adhesive patch. The drug is absorbed gradually so that its blood level is maintained throughout each 24 h. *skin shedding* skin is continually shedding its outer keratinized cells as scales. As the skin has a natural bacterial flora, the scales are a potential source of infection for susceptible patients. ⇒ psoriasis.

skull *n* the bony framework of the head ⇒ cranium.

sleep *n* a naturally altered state of consciousness occurring in humans in a 24 h biological rhythm. A *sleep cycle* consists of orthodox* sleep and paradoxical* sleep: each cycle lasts approximately 60–90 min, and needs to be completed for the person to gain benefit. *sleep apnoea* ⇒ apnoea. *sleep deprivation* a cumulative condition arising when there is interference with a person's established rhythm of paradoxical* sleep. It leads to sleep deficit. It can result in slurred rambling speech, irritability, disorientation, slowed reaction time, malaise, progressing to illusions, delusions, paranoia and hyperactivity.

sleeping pills a general term which includes sedatives*, hypnotics*, narcotics*. When discontinued, return to natural sleep pattern can take 6–8 weeks.

sleeping sickness a disease endemic in Africa, characterized by increasing somnolence caused by infection of the brain by trypanosomes. ⇒ trypanosomiasis.

sleeplessness *n* some people take a long time, 30–90 minutes, to get off to sleep; others have one or more wakeful periods during the night, and yet others experience early morning wakening. Detailed assessment data will reveal a patient's or client's individual sleeping habits.

sleepwalking ⇒ somnambulism.

slipped disc *n* prolapsed intervertebral disc. ⇒ prolapse.

slipped epiphysis displacement of an epiphysis, especially the upper femoral one. ⇒ epiphysis.

slough *n* tissue which becomes necrosed and separates from the healthy tissue.

slow release drugs drug formulations which do not dissolve in the stomach but in the small intestine where the drug is slowly released and absorbed. Some drugs are now incorporated into a skin patch, which after application permits slow release.

slow virus *n* an infective agent which only produces infection after a long latent period and many cases may never develop overt symptoms but may still be a link in the chain of infectivity. ⇒ Creutzfeldt-Jakob disease.

small-for-dates ⇒ low birthweight.

smallpox *n* (*syn* variola) caused by a virus: eradicated following WHO world-wide campaign. Prophylaxis against the disease is by vaccination. ⇒ vaccinia.

smear *n* a film of material spread out on a glass slide for microscopic examination. *cervical smear* microscopic examination of cells scraped from the cervix to detect carcinoma-in situ. ⇒ carcinoma.

smegma *n* the sebaceous secretion which accumulates beneath the prepuce and clitoris. It should be removed by uncircumcized males retracting the prepuce before washing the penis. There is research evidence that the partners of circumcized men are less likely to develop cervical cancer.

Smith-Petersen nail a trifid, cannulated metal nail used to provide internal fixation for intracapsular fractures of the femoral neck.

smokers' blindness (*syn* tobacco amblyopia) absorption of cyanide in the nicotine of smoke. The sight gets worse, colour vision goes, the victim can go blind. Cyanide prevents absorption of vitamin B_{12}. Injection of hydroxycobalamin is therapeutic.

smoking, passive *v* involuntary inhalation of smoke from tobacco products by nonsmokers. Associated with an increased incidence of smoking-related diseases, such as lung cancer, coronary heart disease, hypertension, bronchitis and emphysema; may also trigger asthma. Health promotion to prevent passive smoking in children who live in a household with smokers is currently an issue.

snare *n* a surgical instrument with a wire loop at the end; used for removal of polypi*.

Snellen's test types a chart for testing visual acuity.

snoring *v* flaccid muscles in the upper respiratory tract are thought to be responsible for turbulent airflow and hence snoring. Loud snoring may be associated with upper airway closure (sleep apnoea*), resulting in repetitive awakenings and severe sleep disturbance.

snow *n* solid carbon dioxide. Used for local freezing of the tissues in minor surgery. ⇒ cryosurgery.

snuffles *n* a snorting inspiration due to congestion of nasal mucous membrane. It is a sign of early congenital (prenatal) syphilis when the nasal discharge may be purulent or bloodstained.

social class the classification of people into social groups. Currently in use in the UK is the Registrar General's model based on occupation. The information is used to analyse health and other data noting comparisons between the social classes.

social isolation a term which can be applied to one person, a family or a group of people. Those 'isolated' do not interact with other human beings in the usual pattern, for any one of a number of reasons.

socially clean a term used when articles require to be scrupulously clean, a condition achieved without using disinfectants. To prevent nosocomial infection it must characterize all articles which patients use, including baths, bath mats, showers, sieved water outlets, sinks and washbowls. ⇒ asepsis, disinfection.

sociocultural *adj* pertaining to culture in its sociological setting.

sociology *n* the scientific study of interpersonal and intergroup social relationships—**sociological** *adj*.

sociomedical *adj* pertaining to the problems of medicine as affected by sociology.

sodium bicarbonate a domestic antacid, given for heartburn etc. For prolonged therapy alkalis that cause less rebound acidity are preferred.

sodium chloride salt, present in body tissues. Used extensively in shock and dehydration as intravenous normal saline, or as dextrose saline in patients unable to take fluids by mouth. Used orally as replacement therapy in Addison's disease, in which salt loss is high. When salt is lost from the body, there is compensating production of renin*.

sodium citrate an alkaline diuretic very similar to potassium citrate. Used also as an anticoagulant for stored blood, and as an addition to milk feeds to reduce curdling.

sodium picosulphate a laxative.

soft drugs a term used in relation to drugs misuse. It is thought that early solvent* abuse and the use of cannabis* can predispose to abuse of hard* drugs.

soft sore the primary ulcer of the genitalia occurring in the venereal disease chancroid.

soft tissue rheumatism *syns* fibrositis*, muscular rheumatism. ⇒ backache.

solar plexus a large network of sympathetic (autonomic) nerve ganglia and fibres, extending from one adrenal gland to the other. It supplies the abdominal organs.

solute *n* that which is dissolved in a solvent.

solution *n* a fluid which contains a dissolved substance or substances. *saturated solution* one in which the maximum possible quantity of a particular substance is dissolved and further additions of the substance remain undissolved.

solvent *n* an agent which is capable of dissolving other substances (solutes). The component of a solution which is present in excess. *solvent abuse* previously called glue* sniffing. Inhalation of volatile substances to produce euphoria. Signs include lingering smell on clothes and hair, changed behaviour, and spots around the nose and mouth. ⇒ hard drugs, soft drugs.

solvent abuse the practice of inhaling the vapours of toluene, a constituent of glues, solvents and aerosols. The sniffers are commonly adolescents. Redness and blistering around the mouth and nose may be evidence. Intoxication results.

somatic *adj* pertaining to the body. *somatic cells* body cells, as distinct from germ cells. *somatic nerves* nerves controlling the activity of striated, skeletal muscle.

somatostatin *n* growth hormone release-inhibiting hormone (GH-RIH). It has been used to block the nocturnal surges of growth hormone which have been implicated in the pathogenesis of the dawn* phenomenon.

somatotropin *n* ⇒ growth hormone.

somnambulism *n* (*syn* sleepwalking) a state of dissociated consciousness in which sleeping and waking states are combined. Considered normal in children but as an illness in adults.

Somogyi phenomenon posthypoglycaemic hyperglycaemia; a direct result of low free-insulin levels in the blood. The evening insulin injection does not give constant levels throughout the night but peaks in the early hours, then declines. ⇒ dawn phenomenon.

Sonicaid *n* proprietary name for diagnostic ultrasound machine used to detect movement inside body.

Sonne dysentery bacillary dysentery caused by infection with *Shigella sonnei* (Sonne bacillus), the commonest form of dysentery in the United Kingdom. The organism is excreted by cases and carriers in their faeces, and contaminates hands, food and water, from which new hosts are infected.

sonograph *n* graphic record of sound waves.

sonography *n* the process by which a sonograph is recorded and interpreted; considered safer than X-rays for pregnant women.

soporific *adj, n* (describes) an agent which induces profound sleep.

sordes *npl* dried, brown crusts which form in the mouth, especially on the lips and teeth, in illness.

souffle *n* puffing or blowing sound. *funic souffle* auscultatory murmur of pregnancy. Synchronizes with the fetal heartbeat and is caused by pressure on the umbilical cord. *uterine souffle* soft, blowing murmur which can be auscultated over the uterus after the fourth month of pregnancy.

sound *n* an instrument to be introduced into a hollow organ or duct to detect a stone or to dilate a stricture.

source isolation is for patients who are sources of microorganisms which may spread from them to infect others. *strict source isolation* is for highly transmissible and dangerous diseases. *standard source isolation* is for other communicable diseases.

soya bean a highly nutritious legume*. It contains high-quality protein and little starch. Is useful in diabetic preparations. Soya protein is a constituent of soya milk used as a substitute for cow's milk by strict vegetarians (vegans) and by persons with cow's milk allergy.

spansules *n* a chemically prepared formulation for drugs designed to obtain controlled release via oral route.

spasm *n* convulsive, involuntary muscular contraction.

spasmodic colon megacolon*.

spasmodic dysmenorrhoea ⇒ dysmenorrhoea.

spasmolytic *adj, n* current term for antispasmodic drugs—**spasmolysis** *n.*

spastic *adj* in a condition of muscular rigidity or spasm, e.g. spastic diplegia (Little's disease). *spastic dystonic syndrome* abnormality of gait and foot posture usually due to brain damage at birth. Difficult to treat because imbalance in various opposing muscles has developed over a long period. *spastic gait* ⇒ gait. *spastic paralysis* results mainly from upper motor neurone lesions. There are exaggerated tendon reflexes.

spasticity *n* condition of rigidity or spasm of muscle.

spatial appreciation the ability to perceive the space relationships of things in the environment, one to the other, and to one's body. Defects can cause a person to, for instance, put a glass down before it is safely over the table, consequently it lands on the floor.

spatula *n* a flat flexible knife with blunt edges for making poultices and spreading ointment. *tongue spatula* a rigid, blade-shaped instrument for depressing the tongue.

special care baby unit (SCBU) usually reserved for preterm, sick and small-for-dates babies, mostly requiring the use of high techology which is available in these units.

specialist nursing practice a new level of nursing practice agreed by the UKCC as part of its framework for postregistration education and practice (PREP). The specialist practitioner is a nurse who demonstrates higher levels of clinical decision-making and who is involved in monitoring and developing nursing practice programmes of study leading to a specialist practice. Qualifications are at degree level ⇒ advanced nursing practice, clinical nurse specialist.

special needs a phrase usually applied to the particular (educational) needs of a child or adult with a learning disability. It can also apply to individuals who do not have a learning disability, e.g. the special educational needs of a child who is particularly gifted. ⇒ statement* of special educational needs.

species *n* a systematic category, subdivision of genus. Natural groups of organisms actually or potentially interbreeding but biologically different so that they are reproductively isolated from one another. The individuals within a species group have common characteristics and generally differ fairly clearly from those of a related species.

specific *adj* special; characteristic; peculiar to. *specific disease* one that is always caused by a specified organism. *specific dynamic action* ⇒ action. *specific* *gravity* the weight of a substance, as compared with that of an equal volume of water, the latter being represented by 1000.

specimens *npl* substances which are sent to the laboratory for analysis of contents or for culture to discover the infecting bacteria. They include blood, cerebrospinal fluid, faeces, pus, urine, sputum, swabs from nose, mouth and vagina. ⇒ biopsy.

SPECT *abbr* single photon emission computed tomography*.

spectrophotometer *n* a spectroscope combined with a photometer for quantitatively measuring the relative intensity of different parts of a light spectrum—**spectrophotometric** *adj.*

spectroscope *n* an instrument for observing spectra of light.

speculum *n* an instrument used to hold the walls of a cavity apart, so that the interior of the cavity can be examined. *Sim's speculum* used when examination is performed in the Sim's position*. *Cuscoe's speculum* used when examination is performed in the lithotomy position*—**specula** *pl.*

speech mechanism involves the processes of breathing, phonation, articulation, resonance and rhythm. It is disturbed in various combinations in dysarthria* and aphasia*.

speech pathology includes such conditions as stammering, stuttering, slurring, explosive and staccato speech. Aphasia, dysarthria and dysphasia may be part of the illness for which the affected person is in the care of the health service.

speech therapy the profession responsible for the assessment, diagnosis and treatment of speech and language disorders in children and adults. Known as speech pathologists in the USA and Australia. The professional body governing the profession in the UK is the Royal College of Speech and Language Therapists.

sperm *n* an abbreviated form of the word spermatozoon* or spermatozoa. *sperm count* a test for infertility. If there are less than 60 million sperm in an ejaculation of semen there is accompanying sterility: between 300 and 500 million is normal.

spermatic *adj* pertaining to or conveying semen. *spermatic cord* suspends the testicle in the scrotum and contains the spermatic artery and vein and the vas deferens.

spermaticidal *adj* lethal to spermatozoa*.

spermatogenesis *n* the formation and development of spermatozoa—**spermatogenetic** *adj.*

spermatorrhoea *n* involuntary discharge of semen without orgasm.

spermatozoon *n* a mature, male reproductive cell—**spermatozoa** *pl.*

spermicide, spermatocide *n* an agent that kills spermatozoa—**spermicidal** *adj.*

sphenoid *n* a wedge-shaped bone at the base of the skull containing a cavity, the sphenoidal sinus—**sphenoidal** *adj.*

spherocyte *n* round red blood cell, as opposed to biconcave—**spherocytic** *adj.*

spherocytosis *n* (*syn* acholuric jaundice) a heredofamilial genetic disorder transmitted as a dominant gene, i.e. with a one in two chance of transmission. It exists from birth but can remain in abeyance throughout life; sometimes discovered by 'accidental' examination of the blood. Can also be seen in some fibrin disorders, e.g. haemoglobinopathies ⇒ jaundice.

sphincter *n* a circular muscle, contraction of which serves to close an orifice; may be under voluntary or involuntary control.

sphincterotomy *n* surgical division of a muscular sphincter.

sphingomyelinase *n* an essential enzyme in lipid metabolism and storage.

sphygmocardiograph *n* an apparatus for simultaneous graphic recording of the radial pulse and heart-beats—**sphygmocardiographic** *adj,* **sphygmocardiographically** *adv.*

sphygmograph *n* an apparatus attached to the wrist, over the radial artery, which records the movements of the pulse beat—**sphygmographic** *adj.*

sphygmomanometer *n* an instrument used for measuring the blood pressure.

spica *n* **1** a bandage applied in a figure-of-eight pattern. **2** the application of a plaster cast to hold a joint at the required angle and position, e.g. hip, shoulder or thumb. *double hip spica* enclosure of both lower limbs and lower trunk in a plaster cast. The toes are exposed for observation of complications such as swelling, blanching, cyanosis, inability to move them, lack of sensation in them. *shoulder spica* enclosure of an upper limb and upper trunk in a plaster cast. Digits observed as for double hip spica. *single spica* enclosure of one lower limb and the lower trunk in a plaster cast. See double hip spica re observation of digits.

spicule *n* a small, spike-like fragment, especially of bone.

spider angioma a branched pattern of dilated capillaries arising from a central point, resembling a spider's web. ⇒ naevus, telangiectasis.

spigot *n* glass, wooden or plastic peg used to close a tube.

spina bifida a congenital defect in which there is incomplete closure of the neural canal, usually in the lumbosacral region. *spina bifida occulta* the defect does not affect the spinal cord or meninges. It is often marked externally by pigmentation, a haemangioma, a tuft of hair or a lipoma which may extend into the spinal canal. *spina bifida cystica* an externally protruding spinal lesion. It may vary in severity from meningocele to myelomeningocele. The condition can be detected in utero in mid-pregnancy by an increased concentration of alphafetoprotein in the amniotic fluid or maternal blood, or by ultrasonography, reducing the number of children born with 'open' defects.

spinal *adj* pertaining to the spine. *spinal anaesthetic* a local anaesthetic solution is injected into the subarachnoid space, so that it renders the area supplied by the selected spinal nerves insensitive. *spinal canal* → vertebral canal. *spinal caries* disease of the vertebral bones. *spinal column* ⇒ vertebral column. *spinal cord* the continuation of nervous tissue of the brain down the spinal canal to the level of the first or second lumbar vertebra. *spinal nerves* 31 pairs leave the spinal cord and pass out of the spinal canal to supply the periphery.

spine *n* **1** a popular term for the bony spinal or vertebral column. **2** a sharp process of bone—**spinous, spinal** *adj.*

spinhaler *n* a sophisticated nebulizer (atomizer) which delivers a preset dose of the contained drug.

Spirillum *n* a bacterial genus. Cells are rigid screws or portions of a turn. Common in water and organic matter. *Spirillum minus* is found in rodents and may infect man, in whom it causes one form of rat*-bite fever—**spirilla** *pl,* **spirillary** *adj.*

spiritual beliefs a person may choose a system of beliefs ascribed by a particular religion:

may be a modified version of these, arrived at after questioning, thinking and reasoning. Some people after going through this process develop strong nonreligious beliefs to guide their concept of right and wrong, and to find meaning in human life on earth. ⇒ secular beliefs.

spiritual distress when a person's spiritual beliefs are derived from a particular religion which transmits relevant practices in some of the everyday living activities, e.g. the way in which food is prepared; the type of food eaten; periods of fasting; attending public worship; praying; handwashing; perineal toilet and even the type of clothes, it is natural that they will be distressed when these religion-based activities are not carried out, as, e.g. in hospital. These are points to have in mind when assessing patients' religious/ spiritual concepts.

spirochaetaemia *n* spirochaetes in the bloodstream. This kind of bacteraemia occurs in the secondary stage of syphilis and in the syphilitic fetus—**spirochaetaemic** *adj.*

spirochaete *n* a bacterium having a spiral shape. *Treponema pallidum*, which causes syphilis, is an example—**spirochaetal** *adj.*

spirograph *n* an apparatus which records the movement of the lungs—**spirographic** *adj*, **spirographically** *adv.*

spirometer *n* an instrument for measuring the capacity of the lungs—**spirometric** *adj*, **spirometry** *n.*

Spitz-Holter valve a regulatory valve used as part of a drainage system designed to treat hydrocephalus* by draining cerebrospinal fluid from a lateral ventricle to the right atrium or peritoneal cavity.

splanchnic *adj* pertaining to or supplying the viscera.

splanchnicectomy *n* surgical removal of the splanchnic nerves, whereby the viscera are deprived of sympathetic impulses. Performed rarely for the relief of certain kinds of visceral pain.

splanchnology *n* the study of the structure and function of the viscera*.

spleen *n* a lymphoid, vascular organ immediately below the diaphragm, at the tail of the pancreas, behind the stomach. It can be enlarged in reactive and neoplastic conditions affecting the reticuloendothelial system.

splenectomy *n* surgical removal of the spleen.

splenic anaemia ⇒ anaemia.

splenitis *n* inflammation of the spleen*.

splenocaval *adj* pertaining to the spleen and inferior vena cava, usually referring to anastomosis of the splenic vein to the latter.

splenomegaly *n* enlargement of the spleen.

splenoportal *adj* pertaining to the spleen and portal vein.

splenoportogram *n* radiographic demonstration of the spleen and portal vein after injection of contrast medium—**splenoportographical** *adj*, **splenoportographically** *adv.*

splenorenal *adj* pertaining to the spleen and kidney, as anastomosis of the splenic vein to the renal vein; a procedure carried out in some cases of portal hypertension.

SPOD *abbr* sexual problems of the disabled. A department which offers help to disabled people: it is part of the Royal Association of Disability and Rehabilitation.

spondyl(e) *n* a vertebra*.

spondylitis *n* inflammation of one or more vertebrae—**spondylitic** *adj. ankylosing spondylitis* a condition characterized by ossification of the spinal ligaments and ankylosis of sacroiliac joints. It occurs chiefly in young men.

spondylography *n* a method of measuring and studying the degree of kyphosis by directly tracing the line of the back.

spondylolisthesis *n* forward displacement of lumbar vertebra(e)—**spondylolisthetic** *adj*.

spondylosis deformans degeneration of the whole intervertebral disc, with new bone formation at the periphery of the disc. Commonly called 'osteoarthritis of spine'.

spongioblastoma multiforme a highly malignant rapidly growing brain tumour.

sporadic *adj* scattered; occurring in isolated cases; not epidemic—**sporadically** *adv*.

spore *n* a phase in the life cycle of a limited number of bacterial genera where the vegetative cell becomes encapsulated and metabolism almost ceases. These spores are highly resistant to environmental conditions such as heat and desiccation. The spores of important species such as *Clostridium tetani* and *Clostridium botulinum* are ubiquitous so that sterilization procedures must ensure their removal or death.

sporicidal *adj* lethal to spores—**sporicide** *n*.

sporotrichosis *n* a chronic, fungal infection caused by *Sporothrix schenkii*, a species found in soil and decaying vegetation. Usually an abscess or ulcer develops, then lymphatic spread occurs. Enters the skin by traumatic injury (particularly amongst agricultural workers).

sporulation *n* the formation of spores by bacteria.

spotted fever an acute febrile disease caused by Rickettsia rickettsii and transmitted by ticks. Also known as Rocky Mountain spotted fever, as this was where it was initially recognised.

sprain *n* injury to the soft tissues surrounding a joint, resulting in discolouration, swelling and pain.

Sprengel's shoulder deformity congenital high scapula, a permanent elevation of one or both shoulders, often associated with other congenital deformities, e.g. the presence of a cervical rib or the absence of vertebrae.

sprue *n* a chronic malabsorption disorder associated with glossitis, indigestion, weakness, anaemia and steatorrhoea.

spurious diarrhoea the leakage of fluid faeces past a solid impacted mass of faeces. More likely to occur in children and the elderly.

sputum *n* (*syn* spittle) expelled from the lower respiratory tract by the force of coughing. Bacteria in the tract are enmeshed in the excessive mucus being secreted by an inflamed, diseased membrane so that sputum can be infectious and purulent. ⇒ cough, postural drainage.

squamous *adj* scaly. *squamous epithelium* the nonglandular epithelial covering of the external body surfaces. *squamous carcinoma* carcinoma arising in squamous epithelium; epithelioma.

squint *n* ⇒ strabismus.

SSPE *abbr* subacute* sclerosing panencephalitis.

staff development all registered nurses should have access to staff development or continuing professional development to maintain and enhance their knowledge, experience and skills.

staff nurse the title accorded registered general nurses working in the clinical areas.

stagnant loop syndrome stagnation of contents of any surgically created 'loop' of intestine with consequent increase in bacterial population and interference with absorption of food.

stammering *n* a disorder characterized by dysfluency of speech with sound, syllable and/or word repetitions. The term is used synonymously with stuttering. May occur developmentally or following brain injury.

St Anthony's fire a disease characterized by either (a) a burning sensation and later gangrene of the extremities or (b) convulsions. It is due to a mixture of mycotoxins*.

stapedectomy *n* operation performed for patients with otosclerosis.

stapes *n* the stirrup-shaped medial bone of the middle ear. *mobilization of stapes* forcible pressure applied to stapes to restore its mobility. Gain in hearing not permanent, but a stapedectomy can be done later—**stapedial** *adj*.

Staphylococcus *n* a genus of bacteria. Gram-positive cocci occurring in clusters. May be saprophytes* or parasites*. Common commensals of man, in whom they are responsible for much minor pyogenic infection, and a lesser amount of more serious infection. Produce several exotoxins. These include leucocidins which kill white blood cells and haemolysins which destroy red blood cells. A common cause of hospital cross infection—**staphylococcal** *adj*. *Staphylococcus epidermis* one of the most common microorganisms causing bacteraemia in patients who have had bone marrow transplant. The organism is frequently resistant to all antimicrobials except vancomycin.

staphyloma *n* a protrusion of the cornea or sclera of the eye—**staphylomata** *pl*.

starch *n* the carbohydrate present in potatoes, rice, maize, pasta, etc.

stasis *n* stagnation; cessation of motion. *intestinal stasis* sluggish bowel contractions resulting in constipation.

statement of special educational needs used in relation to educational provision for children with a learning disability. A statement of the special educational needs of a particular child may be drawn up, following formal assessment, in order to determine whether the child's needs can be met in mainstream schooling, perhaps with additional staff provision, or in special schools.

status *n* state; condition. *status asthmaticus* repeated attacks of asthma* without any period of freedom between spasms. *status epilepticus* describes epileptic seizures following each other almost continuously. *status lymphaticus* is a condition found postmortem in patients who have died without apparent cause. The thymus may be found hypertrophied with increase in lymphatic tissue elsewhere.

STD *abbr* sexually* transmitted disease.

steatorrhoea *n* excessive fat in the faeces due to malabsorption from the gut, characterized by the passage of pale, bulky, greasy, foul-smelling stools.

steatosis *n* inability of hepatocyte* to metabolize fatty acids; fatty droplets appear in the cytoplasm* of the hepatocyte. Found especially in liver disease.

stegomyia *n* a genus of mosquitoes, some of which transmit the malaria* parasite. Found in most tropical and subtropical countries.

Stein-Leventhal syndrome secondary amenorrhoea, infertility, bilateral polycystic ovaries and hirsutism occurring in the second or third decades of life. Sometimes treated by wedge resection of ovary.

Steinmann's pin wide diameter pin for heavy skeletal traction. An alternative to the use of a Kirschner wire.

stellate *adj* star-shaped. *stellate ganglion* a large collection of nerve cells (ganglion) on the sympathetic chain in the root of the neck. *stellate ganglionectomy* surgical removal of the stellate ganglion: sometimes performed for Menière's disease, when the attacks of vertigo are crippling and are unrelieved by conventional treatment.

Stellwag's sign occurs in exophthalmic goitre (thyrotoxicosis). The affected person does not blink as often as usual, and the eyelids close only imperfectly when he or she does so.

stenosis *n* narrowing of a channel or opening—**stenoses** *pl,* **stenotic** *adj. pyloric stenosis* **1** narrowing of the pylorus due to scar tissue formed during the healing of a duodenal ulcer. **2** congenital hypertrophic pyloric stenosis due to a thickened pyloric sphincter muscle. ⇒ pyloromyotomy.

stercobilin *n* the brown pigment of faeces; it is derived from the bile pigments.

stercobilinogen *n* ⇒ urobilinogen.

stercoraceous *adj* pertaining to or resembling faeces—**stercoral** *adj.*

stereotactic surgery electrodes and cannulae are passed to a predetermined point in the brain for physiological observation or destruction of tissue in diseases such as paralysis agitans, multiple sclerosis and epilepsy. Intractible pain can be relieved by this method. ⇒ pallidectomy, thalamotomy—**stereotaxy** *n.*

stereotype *n* a generalization about a behaviour, individual or a group; can be the basis for prejudice.

sterile *adj* free from microorganisms—**sterility** *n.*

sterilization *n* **1** treatment which achieves the killing or removal of all types of microorganisms, including spores, through the use of heat, radiation, chemicals or filtration. ⇒ autoclave. **2** rendering incapable of reproduction.

Steri-Strip proprietary sterile skin closure strips; wound edges are brought within 3 mm (to allow for drainage); strips of adhesive are placed across the wound with space between. Lastly a strip is placed on either side, parallel to the wound.

sternal puncture insertion of a special guarded hollow needle wth a stylet, into the body of the sternum for aspiration of a bone marrow sample.

sternoclavicular *adj* pertaining to the sternum* and the clavicle*.

sternocleidomastoid muscle a strap-like neck muscle arising from the sternum and clavicle, and inserting into the mastoid process of temporal bone ⇒ torticollis.

sternocostal *adj* pertaining to the sternum* and ribs.

sternotomy *n* surgical division of the sternum*.

sternum *n* the breast bone—**sternal** *adj.*

steroids *npl* a term embracing a naturally occurring group of chemicals allied to cholesterol and including sex hormones, adrenal cortical hormones, bile acids, etc. By custom it often now implies the natural adrenal glucocorticoids, i.e. hydrocortisone and cortisone, or synthetic analogues such as prednisolone and prednisone. Synthetic preparations are given orally or topically for a wide range of inflammatory conditions. The benefits must always be weighed against the likely side-effects of high or sustained doses.

sterol *n* a solid alcohol. Cholesterol and many hormones secreted by the adrenal cortex and the gonads are examples. Component of the plasma membrane*.

stertor *n* loud snoring; sonorous breathing—**stertorous** *adj.*

stethoscope *n* an instrument used for listening to the various body sounds, especially those of the heart and chest—**stethoscopic** *adj,* **stethoscopically** *adv.*

Stevens-Johnson syndrome severe variant of the allergic response erythema* multiforme. It is an acute hypersensitivity state and can follow a viral or bacterial infection or drugs such as long-acting sulphonamides, some anticonvulsants and some antibiotics. In some cases no cause can be found. Lung complications during the acute phase can be fatal. Mostly it is a benign condition, and there is complete recovery.

stigma *n* a defining characteristic of a person or an action usually perceived negatively by others—**stigmata**, **stigmas** *pl.*

stilboestrol *n* an orally active synthetic oestrogen, indicated in all conditions calling for oestrogen therapy. Large doses are given in prostatic carcinoma.

stilette *n* a wire or metal rod for maintaining patency of hollow instruments.

stillbirth *n* birth of a baby, after 24 weeks' gestation, that shows no sign of life. Parents, and other siblings if relevant, need opportunity to grieve for this occurrence.

stillborn *n* born dead after 24 weeks' gestation.

Still's disease systemic juvenile chronic polyarthritis, characterized by swollen joints, fever, rashes and enlargement of the spleen, liver and lymphatic nodes and glands. Occurs in infants and young children. There may also be pericarditis. Treatment is with physiotherapy, anti-inflammatory drugs and sometimes steroids.

stimulant *n* an agent, usually artificial, which excites or increases function.

stimulus *n* anything which excites functional activity in an organ or part.

Stokes-Adams syndrome a fainting (syncopal) attack, commonly transient, which occurs in patients with heart block. If severe, may take the form of a convulsion, or patient may become unconscious.

stoma *n* the mouth; any opening, e.g. opening of the bowel or ureters on to the abdominal surface. ⇒ colostomy, ileostomy, ureterostomy—**stomata** *pl,* **stomal** *adj.*

stomach *n* the most dilated part of the digestive tube, situated between the oesophagus (cardiac orifice) and the beginning of the small intestine (pyloric orifice); it lies in the epigastric, umbilical and left hypochondriac regions of the abdomen. The wall is composed of four coats: serous, muscular, submucous and mucous. *stomach pH electrode* an apparatus used to measure gastric contents in situ.

stomatitis *n* inflammation of the mouth. *angular stomatitis* fissuring in the corners of the mouth consequent upon riboflavine deficiency. Sometimes misapplied to: (a) the superficial maceration and fissuring at the labial commisures in perlËche and (b) the chronic fissuring at the site in elderly persons with sagging lower lip or malapposition of artificial dentures. *aphthous stomatitis* recurring crops of small ulcers in the mouth. Relationship to herpes simplex suspected, but not proven ⇒ aphthae. *gangrenous stomatitis* ⇒ cancrum oris.

stone *n* calculus; a hardened mass of mineral matter.

stool *n* faeces*. An evacuation of the bowels.

stove-in chest an injury which may involve multiple anterior or posterior fractures of the ribs (causing paradoxical breathing) and fractures of sternum, or a mixture of such fractures.

strabismus *n* (*syn* squint) uncoordinated action of the muscles of the eyeball, such that the visual axes of the two eyes fail to meet at the objective point. The most common are *convergent squint* when the eyes turn towards the medial line, and *divergent squint* when the eyes turn outwards.

strangulated hernia ⇒ hernia.

strangulation *n* constriction which impedes the circulation—**strangulated** *adj.*

Strassman operation a plastic operation to make a bicornuate uterus a near normal shape.

stratified *adj* arranged in layers.

stratum *n* a layer or lamina, e.g. the various layers of the epithelium of the skin, i.e. stratum granulosum, stratum lucidum.

strawberry tongue a characteristic of scarlet* fever. The tongue is thickly furred with projecting red papillae. As the fur disappears the tongue is vividly red like an overripe strawberry.

Streptobacillus *n* pleomorphic bacterium which may be Gram-positive in young cultures.

Streptococcus *n* a genus of bacteria. Gram-positive cocci, often occurring in chains of varying length. Require enriched media for growth and the colonies are small. Saprophytic and parasitic species. Pathogenic species produce powerful exotoxins including leucocidins which kill white blood cells and haemolysins which kill red blood cells. In man streptococci are responsible for numerous infections such as scarlatina, tonsillitis, erysipelas, endocarditis and wound infections in hospital, with rheumatic fever and glomerulonephritis as possible sequelae—**streptococcal** *adj.*

streptodornase *n* an enzyme used with streptokinase* in liquefying pus and blood clots.

streptokinase *n* an enzyme derived from cultures of certain haemolytic streptococci. Plasminogen activator. Used with streptodornase*. Its fibrinolytic effect has been used as thrombolytic therapy to speed removal of intravascular fibrin.

streptolysins *npl* exotoxins produced by streptococci. Antibody produced in the tissues against streptolysin may be measured and taken as an indicator of recent streptococcal infection.

Streptothrix *n* a filamentous bacterium which shows true branching. ⇒ Streptobacillus.

stress *n* the response of the body to any agent threatening physical or emotional wellbeing. Selye called such agents stressors and said that they could be physical, physiological, psychological or sociocultural. ⇒ genuine stress incontinence.

stressors *npl* any agent which causes physical or mental wear and tear of the human body. They can be categorized as structural, physiological, psychological and sociocultural.

striae *npl* streaks; stripes; narrow bands. *striae gravidarum* lines which appear, especially on the abdomen, as a result of stretching of the skin in pregnancy or severe obesity; due to rupture of the lower layers of the dermis. They are red at first and then become silvery-white—**stria** *sing,* **striated** *adj.*

stricture *n* a narrowing, especially of a tube or canal, due to scar tissue or tumour.

stridor *n* a harsh sound in breathing, caused by air passing through constricted air passages—**stridulous** *adj.*

stroke *n* ⇒ cerebrovascular accident.

stroma *n* the interstitial or foundation substance of a structure.

Strongyloides *n* a genus of intestinal worms that can infest man.

strongyloidiasis *n* infestation with *Strongyloides stercoralis*, usually acquired through the skin from contaminated soil, but can be through mucous membrane. At the site of larval penetration there may be an itchy rash. As the larvae migrate through the lungs there may be pulmonary symptoms with larvae in sputum. There may be varying abdominal symptoms. Because of autoinfective life cycle, treatment aims at complete elimination of the parasite. Thiabendazole 25 mg per kg twice daily for 2 days; given either as a suspension or tablets which should be chewed. Driving a car is inadvisable during therapy.

strontium *n* a metallic element chemically similar to calcium and present in bone. Isotopes of strontium are used in radioisotope scanning of bone to detect abnormalities.

strontium-90 a radioactive isotope with a relatively long half-life (28 years). It is incorporated into bone tissue where turnover is slow. It is the most dangerous constituent of atomic fall-out.

strychnine *n* a poisonous alkaloid made from the seeds of the nux vomica plant. Once used as a central nervous system stimulant.

Stryker bed a proprietary, turning bed, constructed so that a patient can be rotated as required to the prone or supine position. Used mainly for spinal conditions and burns.

student's elbow olecranon bursitis*.

stupor *n* a state of marked impairment, but not complete loss of consciousness. The victim shows gross lack of responsiveness, usually reacting only to noxious stimuli—**stuporous** *adj*.

Sturge-Weber syndrome (*syn* naevoid amentia) a genetically determined congenital ectodermosis, i.e. a capillary haemangioma above the eye may be accompanied by similar changes in vessels inside the skull giving rise to epilepsy and other cerebral manifestations.

St Vitus' dance ⇒ chorea.

stye *n* (*syn* hordeolum) an abscess in the follicle of an eyelash.

styloid *adj* long and pointed; resembling a pen or stylus.

styptic *n* an astringent applied to stop bleeding. A haemostatic.

subacute *adj* moderately severe. Often the stage between the acute and chronic phases of disease. *subacute bacterial endocarditis* septicaemia due to bacterial infection of a heart valve. Petechiae of the skin and embolic phenomena are characteristic. The term infective endocarditis is now preferred, since other microorganisms may be involved. *subacute combined degeneration of the spinal cord* a complication of untreated pernicious anaemia (PA) and affects the posterior and lateral columns. *subacute sclerosing panencephalitis (SSPE)* a slow* virus infection caused by the measles virus: characterized by diffuse inflammation of brain tissue.

subarachnoid haemorrhage bleeding, usually from a ruptured intracranial aneurysm into the subarachnoid space accompanied by sudden, severe headache and often by vomiting and a stiff neck. Blood is present in the CSF. Cerebral angiography reveals the site of bleeding which may be resolved by surgery.

subarachnoid space the space beneath the arachnoid membrane, between it and the pia mater. It contains cerebrospinal fluid.

subcarinal *adj* below a carina*,

usually referring to the carina tracheae.

subclavian *adj* beneath the clavicle.

subclinical *adj* insufficient to cause the classical identifiable disease.

subconjunctival *adj* below the conjunctiva—**subconjunctivally** *adj.*

subconscious *adj, n* that portion of the mind outside the range of clear consciousness, but capable of affecting conscious mental or physical reactions.

subcostal *adj* beneath the rib.

subcutaneous *adj* beneath the skin—**subcutaneously** *adv. subcutaneous oedema* is demonstrable by the 'pitting' produced by pressure of the finger.

subcuticular *adj* beneath the cuticle, as a subcuticular abscess.

subdural *adj* beneath the dura mater; between the dura and arachnoid membranes. *subdural haematoma* the bleeding comes from a small vein or veins lying between the dura and brain. It develops slowly and may present as a space-occupying lesion with vomiting, papilloedema, fluctuating level of consciousness, weakness and usually a hemiplegia on the opposite side to the clot. Finally there is a rise in blood pressure and a fall in pulse rate.

subendocardial *adj* immediately beneath the endocardium.

subhepatic *adj* beneath the liver.

subinvolution *adj* failure of the gravid uterus to return to its normal size within a normal time after childbirth. ⇒ involution.

subjective *adj* internal; personal; arising from the senses and not perceptible to others.⇒ objective *opp.*

sublimate *n* a solid deposit resulting from the condensation of a vapour.

sublimation *n* one of the mental* defence mechanisms whereby unacceptable instinctive drives are unconsciously diverted to and expressed through personally approved and socially accepted behaviour.

subliminal *adj* inadequate for perceptible response. Below the threshold of consciousness. ⇒ liminal.

sublingual *adj* beneath the tongue.

subluxation *n* incomplete dislocation of a joint. ⇒ luxation.

submandibular *adj* below the mandible.

submaxillary *adj* beneath the lower jaw.

submucosa *n* the layer of connective tissue beneath a mucous membrane—**submucous, submucosal** *adj.*

submucous *adj* beneath a mucous membrane. *submucous resection (SMR)* removal of a deflected nasal septum and an operation performed on adults to relieve severe nasal obstruction, or to gain access to a bleeding point or nasal polyps.

suboccipital *adj* beneath the occiput; in the nape of the neck.

subperiosteal *adj* beneath the periosteum of bone.

subphrenic *adj* beneath the diaphragm.

substance misuse 1 a general term which includes hard drugs, soft drugs and solvent abuse. 2 an all-inclusive term which describes abuse of alcohol, amphetamines, barbiturates, cannabis, cocaine, heroin, morphine and sleeping pills. The most recent additions are Ecstasy and temazepam.

subsultus *adj* muscular tremor. *subsultus tendinum* twitching of tendons and muscles particularly around the wrist in severe fever, such as typhoid.

succus *n* a juice, especially that secreted by the intestinal glands and called *succus entericus.*

succussion *n* splashing sound

produced by fluid in a hollow cavity on shaking the patient, e.g. liquid content of dilated stomach in pyloric stenosis. *hippocratic succussion* the splashing sound, on shaking, when fluid accompanies a pneumothorax.

sucrose *n* a disaccharide obtained from sugar cane, sugar beet and maple syrup. It is normally hydrolysed into dextrose and fructose in the body.

sucrosuria *n* the presence of sucrose in the urine.

sudamina *n* sweat rash.

Sudan blindness a form of onchocerciasis*.

sudden infant death syndrome (SIDS) (*syn* cot death) the unexpected sudden death of an infant, usually occurring overnight while sleeping in a cot. The commonest mode of death in infants between the ages of 1 month and 1 year, neither clinical nor postmortem findings being adequate to account for death. Overheating, sleeping in the prone position, and being in an environment where people smoke have all been implicated as risk factors. Parents/carers are now recommended to put babies to sleep on their backs, at the foot of the cot to prevent them wriggling under bedclothes, and in a well-ventilated room.

sudor *n* sweat—**sudoriferous** *adj.*

suggestibility *n* abnormal susceptibility to suggestion. May be heightened in hospital patients due to the dependence on others that illness brings, in children and in people with learning disabilities.

suggestion *n* the implanting in a person's mind of an idea which he accepts fully without logical reason. Suggestion is utilized when the idea of recovery is given to, and accepted by, a patient. In psychiatric practice suggestion is used as a therapeutic measure sometimes under hypnosis or narcoanalysis.

suicide *n* intentional taking of one's own life. Usually related to depression. Attitudes to suicide are culturally determined. Not now a crime in UK but stigma persists. ⇒ parasuicide.

sulcus *n* a furrow or groove, particularly those separating the gyri or convolutions of the cortex of the brain—**sulci** *pl.*

sulphaemoglobin *n* abnormal haemoglobin pigment. ⇒ sulphmethaemoglobin.

sulphaemoglobinaemia *n* a condition of circulating sulphmethaemoglobin* in the blood.

sulphmethaemoglobin *n* (*syn* sulphaemoglobin) a sulphide oxidation product of haemoglobin*, produced in vivo by certain drugs. This compound cannot transport oxygen or carbon dioxide and, not being reversible in the body, is an indirect poison.

sulphonamides *npl* a group of bacteriostatic agents, effective orally, but must be maintained in a definite concentration in the blood. They are antimetabolites: they inhibit formation of folic acid, which for many organisms is an essential metabolite.

sulphones *npl* a group of synthetic drugs (of which dapsone* is the best-known), useful for treating leprosy and sometimes tuberculosis.

sulphonylureas *npl* sulphonamide* derivatives that are oral hypoglycaemic agents. They increase insulin output from a functioning pancreas so that injections of insulin may be unnecessary. Of chief value in 'middle-age onset' diabetes.

sulphur *n* an insoluble yellow powder once used extensively as sulphur ointment for scabies. Still used in lotions and baths for acne and other skin disorders.

sunstroke *n* ⇒ heatstroke.

superego according to Freud, one of the three main aspects of the personality (the other two are id* and ego*); the part of the mind concerned with morality and self-criticism, it operates at a partly conscious, but mostly unconscious, level and corresponds roughly to what is called 'conscience'.

superior *adj* in anatomy, the upper of two parts—**superiorly** *adj*.

supernumerary *n* in excess of the normal number; additional.

superovulation *n* process used in various assisted conception techniques. Ovarian activity is controlled, follicular growth encouraged and ovulation stimulated at a specified time using a complex programme of hormone injections. It may be preceded by a period of down-regulation*. Progress is monitored by ultrasound scan.

supinate *vt* turn or lay face or palm upward ⇒ pronate *opp*.

supinator *n* that which supinates, usually applied to a muscle ⇒ pronator *opp*.

supine *adj* **1** lying on the back with face upwards. **2** of the hand, with the palm upwards. ⇒ prone *opp*.

support *n* can be of a physical nature as when the hands are placed over an abdominal wound during coughing. It can be of a psychological nature as when a nurse listens actively to a patient, or holds the hand of someone who is dying. It can be of a social nature as when a district nurse arranges for a voluntary visitor to spend time with a lonely housebound patient.

support worker ⇒ health* care assistant.

suppository *n* medicament in a base that melts at body temperature. Inserted into the rectum.

suppression *n* in psychology, one of the mental* defence mechanisms. Voluntarily forcing painful thoughts out of the mind; it can precipitate a neurosis.

suppuration *n* the formation of pus—**suppurative** *adj*, **suppurate** *vi*.

supraclavicular *adj* above the collar bone (clavicle).

supracondylar *adj* above a condyle.

supraorbital *adj* above the orbits. *supraorbital ridge* the ridge covered by the eyebrows.

suprapubic *adj* above the pubis.

suprarenal *adj* above the kidney. ⇒ adrenal.

suprasternal *adj* above the breast bone (sternum).

surfactant *n* a mixture of phospholipids, chiefly lecithin* and sphingomyelin secreted into the pulmonary alveoli: it reduces the surface tension of pulmonary fluids, contributing to the elastic properties of pulmonary tissues. Can be instilled via a tracheal catheter for respiratory distress syndrome. ⇒ pneumocytes, zinc.

surgeon *n* a person qualified to carry out surgical operations. By custom the title is Mr, Mrs or Ms, as opposed to those practising medicine* who are called Dr.

surgery *n* that branch of medicine which treats diseases, deformities and injuries, wholly or in part, by manual or operative procedures.

surgical emphysema air in the subcutaneous tissue planes following the trauma of surgery or injury.

surrogate motherhood currently a highly controversial concept. A surrogate is a substitute, so the term means that a substitute woman conceives and produces a baby for another woman. Many emotional, ethical and legal problems surround the concept.

susceptibility *n* the opposite of resistance. Includes a state of reduced capacity to deal with infection.

suspensory bandage applied so that it supports and suspends the scrotum*.

suture *n* **1** the junction of cranial bones. **2** in surgery, a suture is a stitch used to close a wound, either deep, of the layers, or superficial.

swab *n* **1** a small piece of cotton wool or gauze. **2** a small piece of sterile cotton wool, or similar material, on the end of a shaft of wire or wood, enclosed in a protecting tube. It is used to collect material for bacteriological examination.

swallowing *v* a complex biological activity initiated voluntarily by placing food on the tongue. When it is sufficiently chewed, the tip of the tongue is placed against the hard palate, then by learned behaviour the larynx is elevated and backward movement of the tongue forces food through the isthmus of the fauces into the pharynx. Constriction of the pharyngeal walls, closure of the glottis by backward movement of the epiglottis, propels food into the oesophagus, along which it travels by peristaltic action to the stomach. Food is prevented from entering the nasal cavities by upward movement of the soft palate. *dysphagia* difficulty in swallowing.

sweat *n* the secretion from the sudoriferous glands.

sweat test a petri dish prepared with agar, silver nitrate and potassium chromate. With palm of hand pressed to this, excessive chlorides in sweat give distinctive white print, as in cystic fibrosis.

sycosis barbae (*syn* barber's itch) a pustular folliculitis* of the beard area in men. Now rare due to antibiotics and improved hygiene.

sycosis nuchae a folliculitis* at the nape of the neck which leads to keloid thickening (acne keloid).

symbiosis *n* a relationship between two or more organisms in which the participants are of mutual aid and benefit to one another. ⇒ antibiosis *opp.*—**symbiotic** *adj.*

symblepharon *n* adhesion of the lid to the eyeball.

Syme's amputation amputation just above the ankle joint. Provides an endbearing stump.

sympathectomy *n* surgical excision or chemical blockade of part of the sympathetic nervous system.

sympathetic nervous system one of the two portions of the autonomic nervous system. It is composed of a chain of ganglia on either side of the vertebral column in the thoracolumbar region and sends fibres to all plain muscle tissue. Said to be responsible for the 'fight or flight' response via its transmitter noradrenaline.

sympatholytic *n* a drug which opposes the effects of the sympathetic nervous system.

sympathomimetic *adj* capable of producing changes similar to those produced by stimulation of the sympathetic nerves.

symphisiotomy *n* cutting of the connective tissue of the symphisis pubis to facilitate delivery of a baby when caesarian section is impractical or dangerous.

symphysis *n* a fibrocartilaginous union of bones—**symphyseal** *adj.*

symptom *n* a subjective phenomenon or manifestation of disease—**symptomatic** *adj.* *symptom complex* a group of symptoms which, occurring together, typify a particular disease or syndrome.

symptomatology *n* **1** the branch of medicine concerned with symptoms. **2** the combined symptoms typical of a particular disease.

Synacthen test intramuscular infusion of Synacthen normally produces pituitary stimulation for increased secretion of steroid hormones by the adrenal cortex, measured by estimation of plasma cortisol. Lack of response denotes inactivity of adrenal cortex as in Addison's disease.

synapse, synapsis *n* the point of communication between two adjacent neurones.

synchronized intermittent mandatory ventilation (SIMV) a mode of assisted ventilation. May be used when weaning a patient off ventilation. The machine allows spontaneous respiration but also provides mandatory rate and volume which are synchronized with the patient's breaths. The ventilator rate is gradually reduced as the patient breathes alone more and more.

syncope *n* (*syn* faint) literally, sudden loss of strength. Caused by reduced cerebral circulation often following a fright, when vasodilation is responsible. May be symptomatic of cardiac arrhythmia, e.g. heart block.

syndactyly, syndactylism, syndactylia *n* webbed fingers or toes—**syndactylous** *adj.*

syndrome *n* a group of symptoms and/or signs which, occurring together, produce a pattern or symptom complex, typical of a particular disease.

synechia *n* abnormal union of parts, especially adhesion of the iris to the cornea in front, or the lens capsule behind—**synechiae** *pl.*

synergism, synergy *n* the harmonious working together of two agents, such as drugs, microorganisms, muscles, etc—**synergic** *adj.*

synergist *n* an agent cooperating with another. One partner in a synergic action.

synergistic action ⇒ action.

synkinesis *n* the ability to carry out precision movements.

synovectomy *n* excision of synovial membrane. Frequently used for rheumatoid arthritis.

synovial fluid the fluid secreted by the membrane lining a joint cavity.

synovial membrane ⇒ membrane.

synovioma *n* a tumour of synovial membrane benign or malignant.

synovitis *n* inflammation of a synovial membrane.

synthesis *n* the process of building complex substances from simpler substances by chemical reactions—**synthetic** *adj.*

syphilide *n* a syphilitic skin lesion.

syphilis *n* caused by *Treponema pallidum*. Infection is acquired or it may be congenital when it is prenatal. *acquired syphilis* manifests in: (a) the primary stage, appears 4–5 weeks (or later) after infection when a primary chancre associated with swelling of local lymph glands appears (b) the secondary stage in which the skin eruption (syphilide) appears (c) the third stage occurs 20 years after initial infection. Gummata appear, or neurosyphilis* and cardiovascular syphilis supervene. The commonest types of nervous system involvement are general paralysis of the insane and tabes dorsalis (locomotor ataxia). Cardiovascular involvement produces aortic aneurysm and impairment or destruction of the aortic valve—**syphilitic** *adj. congenital syphilis* is acquired by the fetus from the infected mother.

syringe *n* a device for injecting, instilling or withdrawing fluids.

syringomyelia *n* an uncommon, progressive disease of the nervous system of unknown cause, beginning mainly in early adult life. Cavitation and surrounding fibrous tissue reaction, in the upper spinal cord and brain stem, interfere with sensation of pain and temperature, and sometimes with the motor pathways. The characteristic symptom is painless injury, particularly of the exposed hands. Touch sensation is intact. ⇒ Charcot's joint.

syringomyelocele *n* the most severe form of meningeal hernia (spina* bifida). The central canal is dilated and the thinned out posterior part of the spinal cord is in the hernia.

systemic *adj* relating to the body as a whole ⇒ circulation.

systole *n* the contraction phase of the cardiac cycle, as opposed to diastole*—**systolic** *adj.*

systolic murmur a cardiac murmur occurring between the first and second heart sounds due to valvular disease, e.g. mitral systolic murmur.

T

TAB *abbr* a vaccine containing killed *Salmonella typhi, S. paratyphi A* and *S. paratyphi B;* and used to produce active artificial immunity in man, against typhoid* and paratyphoid* fever.

tabes *n* wasting away—**tabetic** *adj. tabes dorsalis* is a variety of neurosyphilis in which the posterior (sensory) roots of the spinal cord are infected with *Treponema pallidum.* ⇒ Charcot's joint, locomotor ataxia. *tabes mesenterica* is tuberculosis of the mesenteric and retroperitoneal lymph nodes.

taboparesis *n* a condition of general paralysis of the insane in which the spinal cord shows the same lesions as in tabes* dorsalis.

tachycardia *n* excessively rapid action of the heart. *paroxysmal tachycardia* a temporary but sudden marked increase in frequency of heartbeats, because the conducting stimulus is originating in an abnormal focus.

tachyphasia *n* extreme rapidity of flow of speech occurring in some mental disorders.

tachypnoea *n* abnormal frequency of respiration—**tachypnoeic** *adj.*

tactile *adj* pertaining to the sense of touch.

Taenia *n* a genus of flat, parasitic worms; cestodes or tapeworms. *Taenia echinococcus* the adult worm lives in the dog's intestine (the definitive host) and man (the intermediate host) is infested by swallowing eggs from the dog's excrement. These become embryos in the human small intestine, pass via the bloodstream to organs, particularly the liver, and develop into hydatid cysts. *Taenia saginata* larvae present in infested, undercooked beef; the commonest species in Britain. In man's (the definitive host) intestinal lumen they develop into the adult tapeworm, which by its four suckers attaches itself to the gut wall. *Taenia solium* resembles *Taenia saginata* but has hooklets as well as suckers. Commonest species in Eastern Europe. The larvae are ingested in infested, undercooked pork; man can also be the intermediate host for this worm by ingesting eggs which, developing into larvae in his stomach, pass via the bowel wall to reach organs, and there develop into cysts. In the brain these may give rise to epilepsy.

taenia *n* a flat band. *taenia coli* three flat bands running the length of the large intestine and consisting of the longitudinal muscle fibres, leading to a pouched appearance.

taeniacide *n* an agent that destroys tapeworms—**taeniacidal** *adj.*

taeniafuge *n* an agent that expels tapeworms.

Takayasu's arteritis 'pulseless'* disease

talc a naturally occurring soft white powder, consisting of magnesium silicate. Used extensively as a dusting powder, prior to the donning of surgical gloves.

talipes *n* any of a number of deformities of the foot and ankle.

talus *n* the second largest bone of the ankle, situated between the tibia* proximally and the calcaneus distally, thus directly bearing the weight of the body.

tamponade *n* the surgical use of tampons to control haemorrhage or absorb secretions. ⇒ cardiac tamponade.

tampon shock syndrome ⇒ toxic shock syndrome.

tapeworm *n* ⇒ Taenia.

tapotement *n* (*syn* tapping) percussion in massage. It includes *beating* with the clenched hand; *clapping* with the palm of the hand; *hacking* with the little finger side of the hand, and *punctuation* with the tips of the fingers.

tapping *n* **1** ⇒ aspiration. **2** ⇒ tapotement.

tarsalgia *n* pain in the foot.

tarsometatarsal *adj* pertaining to the tarsal and metatarsal region.

tarsoplasty *n* any plastic operation to the eyelid.

tarsorrhaphy *n* suturing of the lids together in order to protect the cornea when it is anaesthetised, or to allow healing.

tarsus *n* **1** the seven small bones of the foot. **2** the thin elongated plates of dense connective tissue found in each eyelid, contributing to its form and support—**tarsal** *adj.*

tartar *n* the deposit, calculus, which forms on the teeth.

taste *n* one of the five senses*. Taste receptors or buds are distributed on the tongue which result in four perceptions: sweet, bitter, sour and salty. Taste can be distorted, particularly after cancer treatment, and relatives need to understand that their effort at providing a nutritious meal can be rejected after the first tasting, purely as a manifestation of a change in taste.

Tay-Sachs' disease the primary defect appears to be a deficiency of the enzyme β-D-*N*-acetylhexosamidase which leads to a massive accumulation of a specific lipid substance called GM_2, or Tay-Sachs ganglioside, hence the alternative name, gangliosidosis.

Tay's choroiditis ⇒ choroiditis.

T-bandage used to hold a dressing on the perineum in position.

TBI *abbr* ⇒ total body irradiation.

T cell a lymphocyte which is derived from the thymus and is responsible for cell-mediated immunity.

T-cytotoxic cells T cells that are activated by T-helper* cells and which circulate in the blood and lymphatic systems, searching for the body cells displaying antigens to which they have been sensitized (also called CD8 cells). Main target are virus infected cells but also attack cells infected by intracellular bacteria.

T-helper cell a T cell that activates B cells to release antibodies and killer T cells to destroy cells having a specific antigenic makeup (also called T4 or CD4 cells).

tears *npl* the secretion formed by the lacrimal gland. They contain the enzyme lysozyme* which acts as an antiseptic.

team nursing ⇒ Team nursing box.

teeth *npl* the structures used for mastication. The deciduous, milk or primary set, 20 in number, is shed by the age of 7 years, and is normally replaced by the permanent or secondary teeth. The permanent set, 32 in number, is usually complete in the late teens. When charting the teeth in the patient's records the primary dentition is designated by the letters A-E so that the upper left incisor and last molar are described as A and E, thus:

upper right	*upper left*
EDCBA	ABCDE
EDCBA	ABCDE
lower right	*lower left*

The permanent or secondary teeth are designated by number so that the upper left central incisor and the last molar or wisdom tooth are described as 1 and 8, thus:

upper right	*upper left*
87654321	12345678
87654321	12345678
lower right	*lower left*

⇒ mouth care.—**tooth** *sing.* *bicuspid teeth* ⇒ bicuspid. *canine* or *eye teeth* have a sharp fang-like edge for tearing food. ⇒ canine. *Hutchinson's teeth* have a notched edge and are characteristic of congenital syphilis. *incisor teeth* have a knife-like edge for biting food. *premolar* and *molar teeth* have a squarish termination for chewing and grinding food. *teething* discomfort, often associated with the signs of inflammation, during the eruption of teeth in infants. *wisdom teeth* are the last molar teeth, one at either side of each jaw.

tegument *n* the skin or covering of the animal body.

telangiectasis *n* dilatation of the capillaries on a body surface.

teletherapy *n* treatment using a source of radiation that is remote from the patient, e.g. X-rays, cobalt—**teletherapeutic** *adj*, **teletherapeutically** *adv*.

temazepam *n* short-acting benzodiazepine*.

temperament *n* the habitual mental attitude of the individual.

temperature *n* ⇒ body temperature, clinical thermometer, clinical thermometry.

temple *n* that part of the head lying between the outer angle of the eye and the top of the earflap.

temporal *adj* relating to the temple. *temporal bones* one on each side of the head below the parietal bone, containing the middle ear.

temporomandibular *adj* pertaining to the temporal region or bone, and the lower jaw.

temporomandibular joint syndrome (TMJ) pain in the region of the temporomandibular joint frequently caused by malocclusion of the teeth, resulting in malposition of the condylar heads in the joint and abnormal muscle activity, and by bruxism.

TEN *abbr* toxic* epidermal necrolysis.

Tenckhoff catheter a silicone-coated tube with spaced perforations in the last 7 cm of the tube, suitable for continuous ambulatory peritoneal dialysis*.

TEAM NURSING

Team nursing is a method of care delivery designed to provide maximum continuity of patient-centred care. A small team of nurses, working together but led by one registered nurse, is responsible and accountable for the assessment, planning and implementation of the care of a particular group of patients for the length of time they require care in a particular setting.

It differs from patient allocation or primary nursing in that it is based on the belief that a small group of nurses working together can give better care than if working individually, using the skills of all the team members to the benefit of each patient, but retaining continuity of care.

Effective verbal and written communication between the team members is vital.

See also: primary nursing, named nurse.

tendon *n* a firm, white, fibrous inelastic cord which attaches muscle to bone—**tendinous** *adj.*

tendonitis *n* inflammation of a tendon.

tenesmus *n* painful, ineffectual straining to empty the bowel or bladder.

tenoplasty a reconstructive operation on a tendon—**tenoplastic** *adj.*

tenorrhaphy *n* the suturing of a tendon.

tenosynovitis *n* inflammation of the thin synovial lining of a tendon sheath, as distinct from its outer fibrous sheath. It may be caused by mechanical irritation or by bacterial infection.

tenotomy *n* division of a tendon.

teratogen *n* anything capable of disrupting fetal growth and producing malformation. Classified as drugs, poisons, radiations, physical agents such as ECT, infections, e.g. rubella, and rhesus and thyroid antibodies. ⇒ dysmorphogenic—**teratogenic, teratogenetic** *adj,* **teratogenicity, teratogenesis** *n.*

teratology *n* the scientific study of teratogens and their mode of action—**teratological** *adj,* **teratologically** *adv.*

teratoma *n* a tumour of embryonic origin and composed of various structures, including both epithelial and connective tissues; most commonly found in the ovaries and testes, the majority being malignant—**teratomata** *pl,* **teratomatous** *adj.*

tertiary *adj* third in order. *tertiary care* hospital care in a specialized, regional centre, e.g. specializing in cardiac surgery or cancer treatment. ⇒ primary* care, secondary* care.

tertiary prevention ⇒ ill health, prevention of.

testicle *n* ⇒ testis—**testicular** *adj.*

testicles, self-examination of currently advocated to check for the appearance of lumps or irregularities which may be signs of testicular tumour. Cancer of the testicles is a major contributor to young, male mortality but, if detected at an early stage, has a high chance of effective treatment and cure. After a bath or shower to relax the scrotal skin, roll each testicle with the hand from the same side of the body gently between the thumb and fingers to feel any deviation from normal.

testis *n* one of the two glandular bodies contained in the scrotum of the male; they form spermatozoa and also the male sex hormones. *undescended testis* the organ remains within the bony pelvis or inguinal canal. ⇒ cryptorchism, testicles—self-examination of—**testes** *pl.*

testosterone *n* the hormone derived from the testes and responsible for the development of the secondary male characteristics. Used to treat male underdevelopment, e.g. premature closure of epiphyses in prepubescent males.

test-tube baby one produced by in* vitro fertilization.

tetanus *n* (*syn* lockjaw) disease caused by *Clostridium tetani,* an anaerobe commonly found in ruminants and manure. Affected patients develop a fear of water and muscle spasms. Tetanus toxoid injections produce active immunity. ATS injection produces passive immunity—**tetanic** *adj.*

tetany *n* condition of muscular hyperexcitability in which mild stimuli produce cramps and spasms. Found in parathyroid deficiency and alkalosis. Associated in infants with gastrointestinal upset and rickets.

tetracoccus *n* coccal bacteria arranged in cubical packets of four.

tetracycline *n* a broad spectrum antibiotic related to both chlortetracycline and oxytetracycline and used for similar purposes. As a rule it causes fewer gastrointestinal disturbances. There is less absorption of oral tetracyline when the stomach is full, or contains aluminium, calcium and magnesium. Causes fluorescence in body cells. This disappears rapidly from normal cells when the drug is discontinued and is retained by cancerous cells for 24–30 h after dosage ceases.

tetradactylous *adj* having four digits on each limb.

tetradecapeptide *n* a peptide* containing 14 amino acids.

tetralogy *n* a series of four. *tetralogy of Fallot* ⇒ Fallot's tetralogy.

tetraplegia *n* (*syn* quadriplegia) paralysis of all four limbs—**tetraplegic** *adj.*

thalamotomy *n* usually operative (stereotactic) destruction of a portion of thalamus. Can be done for intractable pain.

thalamus *n* a paired collection of grey matter at the base of the cerebrum. Sensory impulses from the whole body pass through on their way to the cerebral cortex—**thalami** *pl,* **thalamic** *adj.*

thalassaemias *npl* a group of defects resulting from reduced synthesis of globin chains producing haemolytic anaemia. It is inherited in an autosomal recessive pattern. There are three classifications: (a) *minor,* denotes the carrier and he/she is asymptomatic (b) *intermediate,* a very mild form which may require an occasional blood transfusion (c) *major,* a severe form in which the affected bone marrow produces fetal type haemoglobin. The breakdown of haemoglobin and recurrent blood transfusions lead to iron overload which is treated with chelating agents such as desferrioxamine.

thanatology *n* the scientific study of death, including its aetiology and diagnosis.

theca *n* an enveloping sheath, especially of a tendon—**thecal** *adj. theca vertebralis* the membranes enclosing the spinal cord.

thenar *adj* pertaining to the palm of the hand and the sole of the foot. *thenar eminence* the palmar eminence below the thumb.

theophylline *n* a diuretic related to caffeine* but more powerful. It is used mainly as its derivative aminophylline in the treatment of congestive heart failure, dyspnoea and asthma.

therapeutics *n* the branch of medical science dealing with the treatment of disease—**therapeutic** *adj,* **therapeutically** *adv.*

therapeutic touch the use of touch* as a therapeutic intervention in its own right, rather than as a necessary function of nursing activity. It may involve therapeutic massage or simply bodily contact, such as a pat, handshake or embrace, indicating empathy and support.

therapy *n* treatment of a physical or psychological condition. ⇒ occupational therapy, physiotherapy.

thermal *adj* pertaining to heat.

thermogenesis *n* the production of heat—**thermogenetic** *adj.*

thermography *n* the detection of minute differences in temperature over regions of the body using an infrared device (thermograph) sensitive to radiant heat. It is a technique which can be used to study blood flow disorders, the viability of skin grafts and the early detection of breast cancer through screening programmes.

thermolabile *adj* capable of being easily altered or discomposed by heat.

thermolysis *n* heat-induced chemical dissociation. Dissipation of body heat—**thermolytic** *adj.*

thermometer *n* ⇒ clinical thermometer—**thermometric** *adj.*

thermophile *n* a microorganism accustomed to growing at a high temperature—**thermophilic** *adj.*

thermostable *adj* unaffected by heat. Remaining unaltered at a high temperature, which is usually specified—**thermostability** *n.*

thermotherapy *n* heat treatment. ⇒ hyperthermia.

thiamine *n* vitamin B_1. Coenzyme concerned in carbohydrate metabolism. Deficiency results in beri-beri, affecting metabolism and nerve and muscle tissues.

thiazides *npl* saluretic diuretic group of drugs ⇒ diuretics.

Thiersch skin graft a very thin skin graft.

thirst *n* awareness of a dry mouth; part of the symptomatology of dehydration*. ⇒ mouth care.

Thomas' splint a metal splint shaped like a hairpin, with a padded ring at the opened end which is placed in the armpit or groin. Used for emergency treatment or transporting a patient with a fractured arm or leg.

thoracentesis *n* aspiration of the pleural cavity.

thoracic *adj* pertaining to the thorax. *thoracic duct* a channel conveying lymph (chyle) from the receptaculum* chyli in the abdomen to the left subclavian vein. *thoracic inlet syndrome* ⇒ cervical rib.

thoracoplasty *n* an operation on the thorax in which the ribs are resected to allow the chest wall to collapse and the lung to rest; used in the treatment of tuberculosis. Since the advent of antituberculous drugs it is rarely necessary.

thoracoscope *n* an instrument which can be inserted into the pleural cavity through a small incision in the chest wall, to permit inspection of the pleural surfaces and division of adhesions by electric diathermy. *thorascopic sympathectomy* destruction of the sympathetic ganglia with low power unipolar diathermy through laparoscopic incisions. Performed for hyperhydrosis of the hands, axillae and feet, and for advanced Raynaud's phenomenon—**thoracoscopic** *adj,* **thoracoscopy** *n.*

thoracotomy *n* surgical exposure of the thoracic cavity.

thorax *n* the chest cavity—**thoracic** *adj.*

threadworm *n Enterobius vermicularis.* Tiny threadlike worms that infest man's intestine. Females migrate to anus to lay eggs, thus spread of, and reinfestation is easy. The whole family should be treated simultaneously using piperazine over a week, together with hygiene measures to prevent reinfestation. A further course after a 10 day interval is advisable to deal with worms that have since hatched, as the eggs are not affected by the drug.

threonine *n* an essential amino* acid.

thrill *n* vibration as perceived by the sense of touch.

thrombectomy *n* surgical removal of a thrombus from within a blood vessel.

thrombin *n* not normally present in circulating blood; generated from prothrombin (factor II). The extrinsic and intrinsic pathways lead to production of thrombin. The extrinsic pathway is tested by the prothrombin time (PT). The intrinsic pathway involves principally factors IX and VIII among others. The partial thromboplastin time (PTT) or a modification called the partial thromboplastin time with kaolin (PTTK) detects abnormalities in this pathway. ⇒ blood, Christmas disease, haemophilia.

thromboangiitis *n* clot formation within an inflamed vessel. *thromboangiitis obliterans* ⇒ Buerger's disease.

thromboarteritis *n* inflammation of an artery with clot formation.

thrombocyte *n* (*syn* platelet) small, disc-shaped cellular fragment present in the blood. Plays a vital part in the clotting of blood. ⇒ blood clotting.

thrombocythaemia *n* a condition in which there is an increase in circulating blood platelets which can stimulate clotting within blood vessels. ⇒ thrombocytosis.

thrombocytopenia *n* a reduction in the number of platelets in the blood which can result in spontaneous bruising and prolonged bleeding after injury—**thrombocytopenic** *adj.*

thrombocytopenic purpura a syndrome characterized by a low blood platelet count, intermittent mucosal bleeding and purpura. It can be symptomatic, i.e. secondary to known disease or to certain drugs; or idiopathic, a rare condition of unknown cause (purpura haemorrhagica) occurring principally in children and young adults. In both forms the bleeding time is prolonged.

thrombocytosis *n* an increase in the number of platelets in the blood. It can arise in the course of chronic infections and cancers.

thromboembolism *n* embolism or clot which detaches from a blood clot and is carried to another part of the body in the bloodstream to block a blood vessel—**thromboembolic** *adj.*

thromboendarterectomy *n* removal of a thrombus and atheromatous plaques from an artery.

thromboendarteritis *n* inflammation of the inner lining of an artery with clot formation.

thrombogenic *adj* capable of clotting blood—**thrombogenesis, thrombogenicity** *n.*

thrombokinase *n* ⇒ thromboplastin.

thrombolytic *adj* pertaining to disintegration of a blood clot—**thrombolysis** *n. thrombolytic therapy* the attempted removal of preformed intravascular fibrin occlusions using fibrinolytic agents.

thrombophlebitis *n* inflammation of a vein associated with the formation of a thrombus—**thrombophlebitic** *adj. thrombophlebitis migrans* recurrent episodes of thrombophlebitis in various sites.

thromboplastin *n* (*syn* thrombokinase) chemical released from damaged tissue which initiates extrinsic pathway or coagulation system. An enzyme which converts prothrombin into thrombin. *intrinsic thromboplastin* produced by the interaction of several factors during the clotting of blood. Much more active than tissue thromboplastin. *tissue thromboplastin* thromboplastic enzymes are present in many tissues, and tissue extracts are used in clotting experiments and in the estimation of prothrombin time.

thrombosis *n* the intravascular formation of a blood clot—**thromboses** *pl,* **thrombotic** *adj.*

thrombus *n* an intravascular blood clot—**thrombi** *pl.*

thrush *n* ⇒ candidiasis.

Thudichum's speculae a range of nasal speculae for examination of the anterior part of the nose.

thymectomy *n* surgical excision of the thymus*.

thymocytes *n* cells found in the dense lymphoid tissue in the lobular cortex of the thymus gland—**thymocytic** *adj.*

thymoleptic *n* a term for drugs primarily exerting their effect on the brain, thus influencing 'feeling' and behaviour.

thymoma *n* a tumour arising in the thymus—**thymomata** *pl.*

thymosin *n* hormone secreted by

the epithelial cells of the thymus gland. Provides the stimulus for lymphocyte production within the thymus; confers on lymphocytes elsewhere in the body the capacity to respond to antigenic stimulation.

thymus *n* a lymphoid gland lying behind the breast bone and extending upward as far as the thyroid gland. It is well developed in infancy and attains its greatest size towards puberty; the lymphatic tissue is then replaced by fatty tissue. It has an immunological role. Autoimmunity is thought to result from pathological activity of this gland—**thymic** *adj.*

thyrocalcitonin *n* ⇒ calcitonin.

thyroglossal *adj* pertaining to the thyroid gland and the tongue. *thyroglossal cyst* a retention* cyst caused by blockage of the thyroglossal duct: it appears on one or other side of the neck. *thyroglossal duct* the fetal passage from the thyroid gland to the back of the tongue where its vestigial end remains as the foramen caecum. In this area thyroglossal cyst or fistula can occur.

thyroid *n* the ductless gland found on both sides of the trachea. It secretes thyroxine, which controls the rate of metabolism. The commercial material is prepared from the thyroid gland of the ox, sheep or pig, dried and reduced to powder and adjusted in strength to contain 0.1% of iodine as thyroxine. Used to treat hypothyroidism, i.e. myxoedema and cretinism. *thyroid antibody test* the presence and severity of autoimmune thyroid disease is diagnosed by the levels of thyroid antibody in the blood. *thyroid-stimulating hormone (TSH) test* radioimmunoassay of the level of thyroid-stimulating hormone in the serum. Useful in diagnosing mild hypothyroidism. The thyroid also secretes calcitonin involved in calcium metabolism.

thyroidectomy *n* surgical removal of the thyroid* gland.

thyroiditis *n* inflammation of the thyroid gland. Autoimmune thyroiditis or Hashimoto's disease is a firm goitre ultimately resulting in hypothyroidism. ⇒ Riedel's thyroiditis.

thyrotoxic crisis the sudden worsening of symptoms in a patient with thyrotoxicosis; may occur immediately after thyroidectomy if the patient is not properly prepared.

thyrotoxicosis *n* one of the autoimmune thyroid diseases. A condition due to excessive production of the thyroid gland hormone (thyroxine*), usually due to a thyroid stimulating immunoglobulin, and resulting classically in anxiety, tachycardia, sweating, increased appetite with weight loss, fine tremor of the outstretched hands, and prominence of the eyes (Graves' disease). It is much commoner in women than in men. In older patients cardiac irregularities may be a prominent feature. Thyrotoxicosis may also be due to increased thyroxine production by a single thyroid nodule or a multinodular goitre—**thyrotoxic** *adj.*

thyrotrophic *adj* describes a substance which stimulates the thyroid gland, e.g. thyrotrophin (thyroid stimulating hormone, TSH) secreted by the anterior pituitary gland.

thyroxine *n* the principal hormone of the thyroid gland. It raises the basal metabolic rate. Thyroxine is used in the treatment of hypothyroidism.

TIA *abbr* transient* ischaemic attacks.

tibia *n* the shin-bone; the larger of the two bones in the lower part of the leg; it articulates with the femur*, fibula* and talus*—**tibial** *adj.*

tibiofibular *adj* pertaining to the tibia and the fibula.

tic *n* purposeless, involuntary, spasmodic muscular movements and twitchings, due partly to habit, but often associated with a psychological factor.

tic douloureux (trigeminal neuralgia) spasms of excruciating pain in the distribution of the trigeminal nerve.

tick *n* a blood-sucking parasite, larger than a mite. Some of them are involved in the transmission of relapsing fever, typhus, etc.

tidal volume the volume of air which passes in and out of the lungs in normal quiet breathing.

Tietze syndrome costochondritis* which is self-limiting and of unknown aetiology. There is no specific treatment. Differential diagnosis is myocardial infarction.

tincture *n* the solution of a drug in alcohol.

tinea *n* a group of skin infections caused by a variety of fungi. ⇒ ringworm. Each is named after the area of the body affected, i.e. *tinea barbae* sycosis* barbae. *tinea capitis* ringworm of the head. *tinea corporis* (*syn* circinata) ringworm of the body. *tinea cruris* (*syn* dhobie itch) ringworm of the crutch area. *tinea incognita* unrecognized ringworm to which topical corticosteroids have been inappropriately applied, obscuring the usual signs of ringworm. *tinea pedis* ringworm of the foot.

tine test a multiple puncture test using disposable equipment. The plastic holder has four small tines coated with undiluted tuberculin. The reaction is read in 48–72 h using a grading system I to N.

tinnitus *n* a buzzing, thumping or ringing sound in the ears.

tintometer *n* an apparatus for measuring the degree of redness in the skin, an early sign of hyperaemia* which may progress to inflammation.

tissue *n* a collection of cells or fibres of similar function, forming a structure. *tissue repair* ⇒ healing, wound dressings. *tissue respiration* ⇒ respiration.

titration *n* volumetric analysis by aid of standard solutions to determine the concentation of a substance in solution.

titre *n* a standard of concentration per volume, as determined by titration. Unit of measure used to assess antibody concentration in serum.

TMJ *abbr* temporomandibular* joint syndrome.

TNM system a method of staging the extent of the malignant process. The initial letters indicate three significant factors, Tumour, Nodes (lymph) and Metastases (distant).

tobacco amblyopia ⇒ smokers' blindness.

tocography *n* process of recording uterine contractions using a tocograph or a parturiometer.

tocopherol *n* synthetic vitamin E, similar to that found in wheatgerm oil. It has been used in habitual abortion, and empirically in many other conditions with varying success.

token economy a part of some behaviour* modification programmes; the person is rewarded by tokens for desired behaviour: these are then exchanged for commodities or services of the person's choice.

tolerance *n* ability to resist the application or administration of a substance, usually a drug. One may have to increase the dose of the drug as tolerance develops, e.g. nitrites. *exercise tolerance* exercise accomplished without pain or marked breathlessness. American Heart Association's classification of functional capacity: Class I no symptoms on ordinary effort; Class II slight disability on ordinary effort (in Britain it is usual to subdivide this class into Class IIa able to carry on with normal housework under difficulty and Class IIb cannot manage shopping or bedmaking except very slowly); Class III marked disability on ordinary effort which prevents any attempt at housework; Class IV symptoms at rest or heart failure.

tomography *n* a technique of using X-rays to create an image of a specific, thin layer through the body (rather than the whole body)—**tomographic** *adj,* **tomograph** *n,* **tomographically** *adv.*

tone *n* the normal, healthy state of tension.

tongue *n* the mobile muscular organ contained in the mouth and attached to the hyoid bone; it is concerned with speech, mastication, swallowing and taste. ⇒ strawberry tongue.

tonic *adj* used to describe a state of continuous, as opposed to intermittent, muscular contraction (clonic). *tonic, tonic-clonic seizures* ⇒ epilepsy.

tonography *n* continuous measurement of blood, or intraocular, pressure. *carotid compression tonography* normally occlusion of one common carotid artery causes an ipsilateral fall of intraocular pressure. Used as a screening test for carotid insufficiency.

tonometer *n* an instrument for measuring intraocular pressure.

tonsillectomy *n* removal of the tonsils. *tonsillectomy position* the three quarters prone position to prevent inhalation (aspiration) pneumonia and asphyxiation.

tonsillitis *n* inflammation of the tonsils.

tonsilloliths *npl* concretions arising in the body of the tonsil.

tonsillopharyngeal *adj* pertaining to the tonsils* and pharynx*.

tonsils *npl* small patches of lymphoid tissue, one on each side, covered by mucous membrane, embedded in the fauces between the palatine arch; composed of about 10–18 lymph follicles—**tonsillar** *adj.*

tophus *n* a small, hard concretion forming on the ear lobe, on the joints of the phalanges, etc. in gout—**tophi** *pl.*

topical *adj* describes the local application of such things as anaesthetics, drugs, powders and ointments to skin and mucous membrane.

topography *n* a description of the regions of the body—**topographical** *adj,* **topographically** *adv.*

torsion *n* twisting.

torticollis *n* (*syn* wryneck) a painless contraction of one sternocleidomastoid* muscle. The head is slightly flexed and drawn towards the contracted side, with the face rotated over the other shoulder.

total body irradiation (TBI) a treatment used in the early treatment of some cancers. Usually carried out prior to bone marrow transplantation.

total parenteral nutrition (TPN) solutions containing all essential nutrients administered by a central venous line: only liquids and low density solutions are administered. ⇒ parenteral feeding.

total patient care 1 a therapeutic programme for a patient to which members of several professional groups contribute. **2** a term used to signify inclusion of the physical, psychological and social dimensions of the person who requires nursing.

touch *n* one of the five special senses*. There is increasing awareness of the value of therapeutic touch in nursing. ⇒ therapeutic touch.

tourniquet *n* an apparatus for the

compression of the blood vessels of a limb. Designed for compression of a main artery to control bleeding. It is also often used to obstruct the venous return from a limb and so facilitate the withdrawal of blood from a vein. Tourniquets vary from a simple rubber band to a pneumatic cuff.

toxaemia *n* a generalized poisoning of the body by the products of bacteria or damaged tissue—**toxaemic** *adj.*

toxic *adj* poisonous, caused by a poison. *toxic epidermal necrolysis (TEN)* a syndrome in which the appearance is of scalded skin. It can occur in response to drug reaction, staphylococcal infection, systemic illness, and it can be idiopathic. *toxic shock syndrome* (*syn* tampon shock syndrome) a recently recognized cluster of signs and symptoms which occur in some women who use tampons. There is high temperature, vomiting and diarrhoea. *Staphylococcus aureus* is present in the vagina of about 5% of women; it produces a toxin and the victim develops blood poisoning. Tampons are thought to encourage production of toxin by acting as a plug. The condition is sometimes fatal.

toxicity *n* the quality or degree of being poisonous.

toxicology *n* the science dealing with poisons, their mechanisms of action and antidotes to them—**toxicological** *adj,* **toxicologically** *adv.*

toxicomania *n* WHO definition: Periodic or chronic state of intoxication produced by repeated consumption of a drug harmful to the individual or society. Characteristics are: (a) uncontrollable desire or necessity to continue consuming the drug and to try to get it by all means (b) tendency to increase the dose (c) psychological and physical dependency as a result.

toxin *n* a product of bacteria that damages or kills cells.

Toxocara *n* genus of roundworm of the cat and dog. Man can be infested (toxocariasis) by eating with hands soiled from these pets. Can exist for several months in soil contaminated by infected faeces from dogs or cats. The worms cannot become adult in man (incorrect host) so the larval worms wander through the body, attacking mainly the liver and the eye. Treatment is unsatisfactory, but the condition usually clears after several months.

toxoid *adj* a toxin altered in such a way that it has lost its poisonous properties but retained its antigenic properties. *toxoid antitoxin* a mixture of toxoid and homologous antitoxin in floccule form, used as a vaccine, e.g. in immunization against diphtheria or tetanus.

Toxoplasma *n* a protozoon whose natural host in the UK is the domestic cat. Cats' faeces are allegedly the source of most human infections in this country and, like another possible source, undercooked meat, should be avoided by pregnant women.

toxoplasmosis *n Toxoplasma* parasites which, commonly occurring in mammals and birds, may infect man. Intrauterine fetal and infant infections are often severe, producing encephalitis, convulsions, hydrocephalus and eye diseases, resulting in death or, in those who recover, mental retardation and impaired sight. Infection in older children and adults may result in pneumonia, nephritis or skin rashes. Skull X-ray reveals flecks of cerebral calcification. Skin and antibody tests confirm the diagnosis.

TPI test *Treponema pallidum* immobilization test: a modern, highly specific test for syphilis in which syphilitic serum immobilizes and kills spirochaetes grown in pure culture.

TPN *abbr* total* parenteral nutrition.

TPR *abbr* temperature, pulse and respiration.

trabeculae *npl* the fibrous bands or septa projecting into the interior of an organ, e.g. the spleen; they are extensions from the capsule surrounding the organ—**trabecula** *sing*, **trabecular** *adj.*

trabeculotomy *n* operation for glaucoma. It aims to create a channel through the trabecular meshwork from the canal of Schlemm to the angle of the anterior chamber.

trace elements metals and other elements which are regularly present in very small amounts in the tissues and known to be essential for normal metabolism (e.g. copper, cobalt, manganese, fluorine, etc.).

tracer *n* a substance or instrument used to gain information about metabolic processes. Radioactive tracers can be used to investigate thyroid disease or possible brain tumours.

trachea *n* (*syn* windpipe) the fibrocartilaginous tube lined with mucous membrane passing from the larynx* to the bronchi*. It is about 115 mm long and about 25 mm wide—**tracheal** *adj.*

tracheitis *n* inflammation of the trachea; most commonly the result of a viral infection such as the common cold ⇒ acute bronchitis.

trachelorrhaphy *n* operative repair of a uterine cervical laceration.

tracheobronchial *adj* pertaining to the trachea* and the bronchi*.

tracheobronchitis *n* inflammation of the trachea and bronchi ⇒ acute bronchitis.

tracheooesophageal *adj* pertaining to the trachea* and the oesophagus*. *tracheooesophageal fistula* usually occurs in conjunction with oesophageal atresia. The fistula usually connects the distal oesophagus to the trachea.

tracheostomy *n* fenestration in the anterior wall of the trachea by removal of cartilage from the third and fourth rings, for establishment of a safe airway with the aid of a tracheostomy tube. May be temporary or permanent—**tracheostome** *n.*

tracheotomy vertical slit in the anterior wall of the trachea at the level of the third and fourth cartilaginous rings.

trachoma *n* contagious inflammation affecting conjunctiva, cornea and eyelids. It is due to *Chlamydia trachomatis* which, though resembling a virus, behaves like a bacterium, though it multiplies intracellularly: it is sensitive to sulphonamides and antibiotics. If untreated, trachoma leads to blindness—**trachomatous** *adj.*

traction *n* a drawing or pulling on the patient's body. A steady pulling exerted on some part of the body by means of weights and pulleys. ⇒ Balkan beam, Braun's frame, Bryant's traction, halopelvic traction, Milwaukee brace.

tractotomy *n* incision of a nerve tract for relief of intractable pain.

trade union an association of workers in a trade, or a group of allied trades, or a profession, for promotion and protection of their common interests. ⇒ Royal College of Nursing.

tragus *n* the projection in front of the external auditory meatus—**tragi** *pl.*

trait *n* an inherited or developed mental or physical individual characteristic.

trance *n* a term used for hypnotic sleep and for certain self-induced stuporous states.

tranquillizers *npl* drugs used to relieve anxiety or combat psychotic symptoms without significant sedation. These drugs do not affect a basic disease, but reduce symptoms so that the patient feels more comfortable and is more accessible to help from psychotherapy. Greatly exaggerate the effects of alcohol. Minor tranquillizers–benzodiazepines. Major tranquillizers–antipsychotics or neuroleptics.

transabdominal *adj* through the abdomen, as the transabdominal approach for nephrectomy–**transabdominally** *adv*.

transactional analysis a form of psychotherapy predicated on the theory that interrelationships between people can be analysed in terms of transactions with each other as representing 'child', 'adult' and 'parent'. The goal is to give the adult ego decision-making power over the child and parent egos.

transaminase tests *aspartate aminotransferase (AST),* released by the brain, kidney, lungs and red blood cells. Formerly serum glutamic oxalacetic transaminase test. *alanine aminotransferase (ALT),* indicates when liver cell damage has occurred. Formerly glutamic pyruvic transaminase test.

transamniotic *adj* through the amniotic membrane and fluid, as a transamniotic transfusion of the fetus for haemolytic disease.

transcultural nursing in multicultural societies a nurse's knowledge of such factors as the customs and perceptions of health, ill health, diet, birth, circumcision, contraception, marriage, religion and death, can alert him or her to actual or potential health needs or problems.

transcutaneous *adj* through the skin, e.g. absorption of applied drugs or the monitoring of the oxygen and carbon dioxide content of blood in skin vessels. *transcutaneous electrical nerve stimulation (TENS)* a noninvasive method of pain relief; four electrodes are placed on either side of the spine to control a mild electric current from a battery-operated apparatus which can be controlled by the patient.

transection *n* the cutting across or mechanical severance of a structure.

transfrontal *adj* through the frontal bone; an approach used for hypophysectomy.

transfusion *n* the introduction of fluid into the tissue or into a blood vessel. *blood transfusion* the intravenous replacement of lost or destroyed blood by compatible citrated human blood. Also used for severe anaemia with deficient blood production. Fresh blood from a donor or stored blood from a blood bank may be used. It can be given 'whole', or with some plasma removed ('packed-cell' transfusion). If incompatible blood is given severe reaction follows. ⇒ autologous blood transfusion, blood groups. *intrauterine transfusion* of the fetus endangered by Rhesus incompatibility. Rh-negative blood is transfused directly into the abdominal cavity of the fetus, on one or more occasions. This enables the induction of labour to be postponed until a time more favourable to fetal welfare.

transient ischaemic attacks (TIA) ⇒ drop attacks, vertebrobasilar insufficiency.

translocation *n* transfer of a segment of a chromosome to a different site on the same chromosome (shift) or to a different one. Can be a direct or indirect cause of congenital abnormality.

translucent *adj* intermediate between opaque and transparent.

translumbar *adj* through the lumbar region. Route used for injecting aorta prior to aortography.

transmethylation *n* a process in the metabolism of amino acids in which a methyl group is transferred from one compound to another.

transmural *adj* through the wall, e.g. of a cyst, organ or vessel.

transperitoneal *adj* across or through the peritoneal cavity. ⇒ dialysis.

transplacental *adj* through the placenta—**transplacentally** *adv.*

transposition *n* **1** displacement of any internal organ to the other side of the body. **2** the operation which attaches a piece of tissue to one part of the body from another, delaying complete separation until it has become established in its new location. *transposition of the great vessels* a congenital abnormality of the heart in which the aorta and the pulmonary artery are transposed, with the aorta arising from the right ventricle and the pulmonary artery from the left ventricle.

transonic *adj* allowing the passage of ultrasound.

transplant *n* customarily refers to the surgical operation of grafting an organ, which has been removed from a person who has been declared braindead, or from a living relative. If the recipient's malfunctioning organ is removed and the transplant is placed in its bed it is referred to as an *orthotopic transplant* (e.g. liver and heart). If the transplanted organ is not placed in its normal anatomical site the term *heterotopic transplant* is used. The word also refers to transplantation of healthy bone marrow to treat inborn errors such as: immune deficiency; the deficiency anaemias such as thalassaemia and aplastic anaemia; and mucopolysaccharidoses, a group of diseases in which the enzyme that breaks down body mucus is absent—**transplant** *vt,* **transplantation** *n.* ⇒ graft.

transrectal *adj* through the rectum, as a transrectal injection into a tumour—**transrectally** *adv.*

transsphenoidal *adj* through the sphenoid bone; an approach used for hypophysectomy.

transthoracic *adj* across or through the chest, as in transthoracic needle biopsy of a lung mass, transthoracic echocardiography.

transudate *n* a fluid that has passed out of the cells either into a body cavity (e.g. ascitic fluid in the peritoneal cavity) or to the exterior (e.g. serum from the surface of a burn).

transurethral *adj* by way of the urethra.

transvaginal *adj* through the vagina, as an incision to drain the uterorectal pouch, transvaginal injection into a tumour, pudendal block or culdoscopy—**transvaginally** *adv.*

transventricular *adj* through a ventricle. Term used mainly in cardiac surgery—**transventricularly** *adv.*

transvesical *adj* through the bladder, by custom referring to the urinary bladder—**transvesically** *adv.*

trauma *n* **1** bodily injury. **2** emotional shock—**traumatic** *adj.*

traumatologist *n* a surgeon who specializes in traumatology.

traumatology *n* the branch of surgery dealing with injury caused by accident—**traumatological** *adj,* **traumatologically** *adv.*

Trematoda *n* a class of parasitic worms which include many pathogens of man such as the *Schistosoma* of schistosomiasis.

tremor *n* involuntary trembling. *intention tremor* an involuntary tremor which only occurs on attempting voluntary movement; a characteristic of multiple sclerosis.

trench foot (*syn* immersion foot) occurs in frostbite* or other conditions of exposure where there is deprivation of local blood supply and secondary bacterial infection.

Trendelenburg's operation ligation of the long saphenous vein in the groin at its junction with the femoral vein. Used in cases of varicose veins.

Trendelenburg's position lying on an operating or examination table, with the head lowermost and the legs raised.

Trendelenburg's sign a test of the stability of the hip, and particularly of the ability of the hip abductors (gluteus medius and minimus) to steady the pelvis upon the femur. Normally, when one leg is raised from the ground the pelvis tilts upwards on that side, through the hip abductors of the standing limb. If the abductors are inefficient (e.g. in poliomyelitis, severe coxa vara and congenital dislocation of the hip), they are unable to sustain the pelvis against the body weight and it tilts downwards instead of rising.

trephine *n* an instrument with sawlike edges for removing a circular piece of tissue, such as the cornea or skull.

Treponema *n* a genus of slender spiral-shaped bacteria which are actively motile. Best visualized with dark-ground illumination. Cultivated in the laboratory with great difficulty. *Treponema pallidum* is the causative organism of syphilis; *Treponema pertenue* the spirochaete that causes yaws; *Treponema carateum* the spirochaete that causes pinta.

treponematosis *n* the term applied to the treponemal diseases.

treponemicide *n* lethal to *Treponema*–**treponemicidal** *adj*.

Trexler isolator a flexible film, negative pressure, bed isolator for dangerous infections such as viral haemorrhagic disease or immunocompromized patients.

triage *n* a system of priority classification of patients in any emergency situation. *triage nurse* the nurse given this specific responsibility in an accident and emergency department.

triangular bandage useful for arm slings, for securing splints, in first aid work and for inclusive dressings of a part, as a whole hand or foot.

TRIC *abbr* trachoma inclusion conjunctivitis. The organism responsible for TRIC is *Chlamydia trachomatis,* which also causes urethritis and genital tract disease. ⇒ conjunctivitis.

triceps *n* the three-headed muscle on the back of the upper arm.

trichiasis *n* abnormal ingrowing eyelashes causing irritation from friction on the eyeball.

trichinosis *n* a disease caused by eating undercooked pig meat infected with *Trichinella spiralis* (the trichina worm). The female worms living in the small bowel produce larvae which invade the body and, in particular, form cysts in skeletal muscles; the usual symptoms are diarrhoea, nausea, colic, fever, facial oedema, muscular pains and stiffness.

trichomonacide *n* lethal to the protozoa belonging to the genus *Trichomonas.*

Trichomonas *n* a protozoan parasite of man. *Trichomonas vaginalis* produces infection of the urethra and vagina often associated with profuse discharge (leucorrhoea). The organism is best recognized by microscopic examination of the discharge. ⇒ protozoa.

trichomoniasis *n* a sexually transmitted infection caused by *Trichomonas vaginalis.* Inflammation of the vagina and often profuse discharge in women. Inflames urethra in males.

trichophytosis *n* infection with a species of the fungus *Trichophyton,* e.g. ringworm* of the hair or skin.

trichuriasis *n* infestation with *Trichuris trichiura.*

Trichuris *n* a genus of nematodes. *Trichuris trichiura* the whipworm.

tricuspid *adj* having three cusps. *tricuspid valve* that between the right atrium and ventricle of the heart.

trigeminal *adj* triple; separating into three sections, e.g. the trigeminal nerve, the fifth cranial nerve, which has three branches, supplying the skin of the face, the tongue and teeth. *trigeminal neuralgia* ⇒ tic douloureux.

trigger finger a condition in which the finger can be actively bent but cannot be straightened without help; usually due to a thickening on the tendon which prevents free gliding.

trigone *n* a triangular area, especially applied to the bladder base, bounded by the ureteral openings at the back and the urethral opening at the front—**trigonal** *adj.*

triiodothyronine *n* a thyroid hormone that plays a part in maintaining the body's metabolic process.

trimester *n* a period of 3 months. Used particularly to distinguish the three trimesters of pregnancy.

triple antigen contains diphtheria, whooping cough and tetanus antigens. Given as part of the routine immunization programme for infants. ⇒ immunization.

triple duty nurse in the UK where there are many outlying rural areas, one nurse is employed. She is qualified as a community nurse, a midwife and a health visitor.

triple test a Dreiling tube is passed through the mouth into the duodenum and pancreatic function tests are carried out. In these, the enzymes secretin and pancreozymin are given to stimulate the pancreas and the juice is aspirated as it flows into the duodenum. It is possible to recognize a tumour in the pancreas from analysis of the volume and chemistry of this juice. Some of the juice is then examined by the pathologist using Papanicolaou's method to show cancer cells and thirdly, the radiologist performs a hypotonic duodenogram which, unlike the conventional barium meal, frequently demonstrates tumours of the pancreas or ampulla. The test takes 2 h to complete.

triple vaccine ⇒ vaccines.

triploid *adj* possessing three chromosomal sets. ⇒ genome, haploid.

trismus *n* spasm in the muscles of mastication.

trisomy *n* the presence in triplicate of a chromosome that should normally be present only in duplicate. This increases the chromosome number by one (single trisomy), e.g. to 47 in man. *trisomy 18* ⇒ Edward syndrome. *trisomy 21* ⇒ Down syndrome.

trocar *n* a pointed rod which fits inside a cannula*.

trochanters *npl* two processes, the larger one (*trochanters major)* on the outer, the other (*trochanters minor)* on the inner side of the femur between the shaft and neck; they serve for the attachment of muscles—**trochanteric** *adj.*

trochlea *n* any part which is like a pulley in structure or function—**trochlear** *adj.*

trophic *adj* pertaining to nutrition.

trophoblastic tissue cells covering the embedding ovum and concerned with the nutrition of the embryo.

Trousseau's sign ⇒ carpopedal spasm.

trypanosomiasis *n* disease produced by infestation with *Trypanosoma.* In man this may be with *Trypanosoma rhodesiense* in East Africa or *Trypanosoma gambiense* in West Africa, both transmitted by the tsetse fly, and with *Trypanosoma cruzii,* transmitted by bugs, in South America. In West Africa infection of the brain commonly produces the symptomatology of 'sleeping sickness'.

tryptophan *n* one of the essential amino* acids necessary for growth. It is a precursor of serotonin*. Adequate levels of tryptophan may compensate for deficiencies of niacin and thus mitigate pellagra.

tsetse fly a fly of the genus *Glossina,* the vector of *Trypanosoma* in Africa. The *Trypanosoma* live part of their life cycle in the flies and are transferred to new hosts, including man, in the salivary juices when the fly bites for a blood meal.

T-tube T-shaped tube which is used to drain the common bile duct after surgery or after myringotomy to ventilate the middle ear and allow drainage of secretions in glue ear. ⇒ wound drains.

tubal *adj* pertaining to a tube. *tubal abortion* ⇒ abortion. *tubal ligation* tying of both uterine tubes as a means of sterilization. *tubal pregnancy* ⇒ ectopic pregnancy.

tubegauz *n* a soft tubular woven bandage available in a variety of sizes–may be used as a protective covering on limbs or digits.

tubercle *n* **1** a small rounded prominence, usually on bone. **2** the specific lesion produced by *Mycobacterium tuberculosis.*

tuberculide, tuberculid *n* a small lump. Metastatic manifestation of tuberculosis*, producing a skin lesion, e.g. papulonecrotic tuberculide, rosacea-like tuberculide.

tuberculin *n* a sterile extract of either the crude (old tuberculin) or refined (PPD) complex protein constituents of the tubercle bacillus. Its commonest use is in determining whether a person has or has not previously been infected with the tubercle bacillus, by injecting a small amount into the skin and reading the reaction, if any, in 48–72 h; negative reactors have escaped previous infection. ⇒ Mantoux reaction.

tuberculoid *adj* resembling tuberculosis*. Describes one of the two types of leprosy.

tuberculoma *n* a caseous tubercle, usually large, its size suggesting a tumour.

tuberculosis *n* a specific infective disease caused by *Mycobacterium tuberculosis* (Koch's tubercle bacillus)–**tubercular, tuberculous** *adj. avian tuberculosis* endemic in birds and rarely seen in man. *bovine tuberculosis* endemic in cattle and transmitted to man via infected cow's milk ⇒ bovine. *human tuberculosis* endemic in man and the usual cause of pulmonary and other forms of tuberculosis. *miliary tuberculosis* a generalized acute form in which, as a result of bloodstream dissemination, minute, multiple tuberculous foci are scattered throughout many organs of the body.

tuberculostatic *adj* inhibiting the growth of *Mycobacterium tuberculosis.*

tuberosity *n* a bony prominence.

tuberous sclerosis (*syn* epiloia) an inherited sclerosis of brain tissue resulting in mental disability. It may be associated with epilepsy.

Tubigrip *n* a supporting elastic tubular bandage. Available in a variety of sizes. Generally applied to limbs to reduce swelling or give support.

tuboovarian *adj* pertaining to or involving both tube and ovary, e.g. tuboovarian abscess.

tubular necrosis acute necrosis of the renal tubules which may follow crush syndrome, severe burns, hypotension, intrauterine haemorrhage and dehydration. The urine flow is greatly reduced and acute renal* failure develops.

tubule *n* a small tube. *collecting tubule* straight tube in the kidney medulla conveying urine to the kidney pelvis. *convoluted tubule* coiled tube in the kidney cortex. *seminiferous tubule* coiled tube in the testis. *uriniferous tubule* nephron*.

tularaemia *n* (*syn* deer-fly fever, rabbit fever, tick fever) an endemic disease of rodents, caused by *Pasteurella tularensis;* transmitted by biting insects and acquired by man either in handling infected animal carcasses or by the bite of an infected insect. Suppuration at the inoculation site is followed by inflammation of the draining lymph glands and by severe constitutional upset—**tularaemic** *adj.*

tulle gras a nonadhesive dressing for wounds. Gauze impregnated with soft paraffin and sterilized.

tumescence *n* a state of swelling; turgidity.

tumor *n* **1** swelling; usually used in the context of being one of the four classical signs of inflammation calor*, dolor*, rubor*. **2** *Am* tumour.

tumour *n* a swelling. A mass of abnormal tissue which resembles the normal tissues in structure, but which fulfils no useful function and which grows at the expense of the body. Benign, simple or innocent tumours are encapsulated, do not infiltrate adjacent tissue or cause metastases and are unlikely to recur if removed. A malignant tumour is not encapsulated and will infiltrate adjacent tissue and cause metastases. ⇒ cancer. *tumour marker* a substance linked to a specific tumour, which is detectable in the blood and by which the progress of the disease and treatment can be monitored.—**tumorous** *adj.*

tunica *n* a lining membrane; a coat. *tunica adventitia* the outer coat of an artery. *tunica intima* the lining of an artery. *tunica media* the middle muscular coat of an artery.

tunnel reimplantation operation a surgical procedure used to reimplant the ureter.

turbinate *adj* shaped like a top or inverted cone. *turbinate bone* three on either side forming the lateral nasal walls.

turbinectomy *n* removal of turbinate* bones.

turgid *adj* swollen; firmly distended, as with blood by congestion—**turgescence** *n,* **turgidity** *n.*

Turner syndrome a condition of multiple congenital abnormalities in females, with infantile genital development, webbed neck, cubitus valgus and, often, aortic coarctation. The ovaries are almost completely devoid of germ cells and there is failure of pubertal development. Most females with Turner syndrome have a single sex chromosome, the X, and thus only 45 chromosomes in their body cells.

tussis *n* a cough.

tympanic membrane ⇒ eardrum.

tympanites, tympanism *n* (*syn* meteorism) abdominal distension due to accumulation of gas in the intestine.

tympanoplasty *n* any reconstructive operation on the middle ear designed to improve hearing. Normally carried out in ears damaged by chronic suppurative otitis media with associated conductive deafness—**tympanoplastic** *adj.*

tympanotomy *n* elevation of eardrum to inspect the middle ear.

type A behaviours behaviours characterized by high competitiveness resulting in compulsive working schedules: believed by some to be associated with an increased risk of coronary heart disease.

type B behaviours behaviours which display minimal aggression and hostility; not highly competitive and believed to have a lower risk of heart disease.

typhoid fever an infectious fever usually spread by contamination of food, milk or water supplies with *Salmonella typhi,* either directly by sewage, indirectly by flies or by faulty personal hygiene. Symptomless carriers harbouring the germ in the gallbladder and excreting it in their stools are the main source of outbreaks of disease in the UK. The average incubation period is 10–14 days. A progressive febrile illness marks the onset of the disease, which develops as the germ invades lymphoid tissue, including that of the small intestine (Peyer's patches) to profuse diarrhoeal (pea soup) stools which may become frankly haemorrhagic; ultimate recovery usually begins at the end of the third week. A rose-coloured rash may appear on the upper abdomen and back at the end of the first week. ⇒ TAB.

typhus *n* an acute infectious disease characterized by high fever, a skin eruption and severe headache. It is a disease of war, famine or catastrophe, being spread by lice, ticks or fleas. It is only sporadic in Britain. Infecting organism is *Rickettsia prowazekii,* sensitive to sulphonamides and antibiotics.

tyramine *n* an amine present in several foodstuffs, especially cheese. It has a similar effect in the body to adrenaline*, consequently patients taking drugs in the monoamine* oxidase inhibitor (MAOI) group should not eat cheese, otherwise a dangerously high blood pressure may result.

tyrosine *n* an amino acid essential for growth. Combines with iodine to form thyroxine.

tyrosinosis *n* a congenital condition in which there is abnormal metabolism of phenylalinine into tyrosine.

U

UHBI *abbr* upper hemibody irradiation*.

UKCC *abbr* United* Kingdom Central Council for Nursing, Midwifery and Health Visiting.

ulcer *n* destruction of either mucous membrane or skin from whatever cause, producing a crater or indentation. An inflammatory reaction occurs and if it penetrates a blood vessel, bleeding ensues. If the ulcer is in the lining of a hollow organ it can perforate through the wall.

ulcerative *adj* pertaining to or of the nature of an ulcer. ⇒ colitis.

ulcerogenic *adj* capable of producing an ulcer.

Ullrich syndrome ⇒ Noonan syndrome.

ulna *n* the inner bone of the forearm.

ultrasonic *adj* relating to mechanical vibrations of very high frequency (above 30 000 Hz). In *diagnostic ultrasound* information is derived from echoes which occur when a controlled beam of this energy crosses the boundary between adjacent tissues of differing physical properties.

ultrasonography *n* production of a visible image from the use of ultrasound. A controlled beam is directed into the body. The echoes of reflected ultrasound are used to build up an electronic image of the various structures of the body. Routinely offered during pregnancy to detect fetal abnormalities. *real-time ultrasonography* an ultrasound imaging technique involving rapid pulsing to enable continuous viewing of movement to be obtained, rather than stationary images—**ultrasonograph** *n*, **ultrasonographically** *adv*.

ultrasound *n* sound waves with a frequency of over 20 000 Hz and inaudible to the human ear.

umbilical cord the navel string attaching the fetus to the placenta.

umbilical hernia ⇒ hernia.

umbilicated *adj* having a central depression, e.g. a smallpox vesicle.

umbilicus *n* (*syn* navel) the abdominal scar left by the separation of the umbilical cord after birth—**umbilical** *adj*.

unconsciousness *n* state of being unconscious; insensible.

'underarm pill' ⇒ levonorgestrel

underwater seal a tube is anchored in the pleural cavity and connected to a long glass tube which, after passing through a cork, is immersed in water in a bottle. Another short glass tube through the cork introduces air on to the water surface, thus air can escape from the pleural cavity and bubble through the water, but air cannot enter the pleural cavity, as long as the bottle is lower than the cavity. This is now achieved with disposable suction bottles but the principle is the same.

undine *n* a small, thin glass flask used for irrigating the eyes.

undulant fever brucellosis*.

unemployment *n* unable to gain paid employment. There are two groups to be considered—those who have previously been employed, and school-leavers who have been unable to get a job. It has enormous social consequences. More than one member of a family may be unemployed; there may be inadequate income; unstructured daytime living; lack of purpose and self-esteem; and hopelessness may result as succeeding applications are rejected. These factors together with many others may contribute to an increase in illness, parasuicides, premature deaths and suicides.

unguentum *n* ointment.

unicellular *adj* consisting of only one cell.

unilateral *adj* relating to or on one side only—**unilaterally** *adv.*

uniocular *adj* pertaining to, or affecting one eye.

uniovular *adj* (*syn* monovular) pertaining to one ovum, as uniovular twins (identical). ⇒ binovular *opp.*

United Kingdom Central Council (UKCC) for Nursing, Midwifery and Health Visiting the statutory body which, together with four national boards representing England, Northern Ireland, Scotland and Wales, resulted from the Nurses, Midwives and Health Visitors Act 1979. It has responsibility for education, training regulations and the professional conduct of nurses, midwives and health visitors. The UKCC is also responsible for maintaining a single register—Parts 1 to 9 are concerned with different statutory nursing qualifications; Part 10 is for registered midwives; Part 11 is for registered health visitors, and Parts 12 to 15 for the different branches of diploma level courses. ⇒ UKCC Code of Conduct, p. xiv.

unipolar depression ⇒ depression.

upper respiratory tract infections (URTI) the upper respiratory tract is the commonest site of infection in all age groups. The infections include rhinitis—usually viral—sinusitis, tonsillitis, adenoiditis, pharyngitis, otitis media and croup (acute laryngotracheobronchitis). Such infections seldom require hospital treatment, with the exception of epiglottitis which can be rapidly fatal.

urachus *n* the stemlike structure connecting the bladder with the umbilicus in the fetus; in postnatal life it is represented by a fibrous cord situated between the apex of the bladder and the umbilicus, known as the median umbilical ligament—**urachal** *adj.*

uraemia *n* a clinical syndrome due to renal failure resulting from either disease of the kidneys, or from disorder or disease elsewhere in the body which induces kidney dysfunction and which results in gross biochemical disturbance in the body, including retention of urea and other nitrogenous substances in the blood (azotaemia). Depending on the cause it may or may not be reversible. The fully developed syndrome is characterized by nausea, vomiting, headache, hiccough, weakness, dimness of vision, convulsions and coma. ⇒ renal—**uraemic** *adj.*

uraemic snow ⇒ uridrosis.

urate *n* any salt of uric acid; such compounds are present in the blood, urine and tophi*; deposits of sodium urate.

urea *n* the chief nitrogenous end-product of protein metabolism; it is excreted in urine of which it is the main nitrogenous constituent. Can be given as an osmotic diuretic by intravenous infusion to reduce intracranial and intraocular pressure and topically to moisturize, soften and smooth dry, rough skin.

ureter *n* the tube passing from

each kidney to the bladder for the conveyance of urine; its average length is from 25–30 cm—**ureteric, ureteral** *adj.*

ureterectomy *n* excision of a ureter.

ureteritis *n* inflammation of a ureter.

ureterocolic *adj* pertaining to the ureter* and colon*, usually indicating anastomosis of the two structures.

ureterocolostomy *n* (*syn* uterocolic anastomosis) surgical transplantation of the ureters from the bladder to the colon so that urine is passed by the bowel.

ureteroileal *adj* pertaining to the ureters* and ileum* as the anastomosis necessary in ureteroileostomy (ileal conduit).

ureteroileostomy *n* ⇒ ileoureterostomy.

ureterolith *n* a calculus* in the ureter.

ureterolithotomy *n* surgical removal of a stone from a ureter.

ureterosigmoidostomy *n* ureterocolostomy*.

ureterostomy *n* the formation of a permanent fistula through which the ureter discharges urine. ⇒ cutaneous, ileoureterostomy, rectal bladder.

ureterovaginal *adj* pertaining to the ureter* and vagina*.

ureterovesical *adj* pertaining to the ureter* and urinary bladder*.

urethra *n* the passage from the bladder through which urine is excreted—**urethral** *adj.*

urethritis *n* inflammation of the urethra. *nonspecific urethritis* ⇒ nongonococcal urethritis.

urethrocele *n* prolapse of the urethra, usually into the anterior vaginal wall.

urethrography *n* radiological examination of the urethra. Can be an inclusion with cystography either retrograde (ascending) or during micturition—**urethrographic** *adj,* **urethrograph** *n,* **urethrographically** *adv.*

urethrometry *n* measurement of the urethral lumen using a urethrometer—**urethrometric** *adj,* **urethrometrically** *adv.*

urethroplasty *n* any plastic operation on the urethra—**urethroplastic** *adj.*

urethroscope *n* an instrument designed to allow visualization of the interior of the urethra—**urethroscopic** *adj,* **urethroscopically** *adv.*

urethrostenosis *n* urethral stricture*.

urethrotomy *n* incision into the urethra; usually part of an operation for stricture.

urgency *n* a strong desire to pass urine, which, if not responded to immediately, may lead to urge incontinence*.

uric acid an acid formed in the breakdown of nucleoproteins in the tissues, the end-product of purine metabolism, and excreted in the urine. It is relatively insoluble and excessive amounts are liable to give rise to stones. Present in excess in the blood in gout, and also in a deficiency occurring in male infants, which may manifest as early as 4 months, and which can lead to self-destructive behaviour, cerebral palsy and mental retardation.

uridrosis *n* (*syn* uraemic snow) excess of urea in the sweat; it may be deposited on the skin as fine white crystals.

urinalysis *n* examination and analysis of the urine.

urinary *adj* pertaining to urine. *urinary bladder* a muscular distensible bag situated in the pelvis. It receives urine from the kidneys via two ureters and stores it until the volume causes reflex evacuation through the urethra. *urinary system* comprises two kidneys, two ureters, one urinary bladder and one urethra. The kidneys filter the urine from the blood; the ureters convey the urine to the bladder, which stores it until there is sufficient volume to elicit the desire to pass urine and it is then conveyed to the exterior by the urethra. *urinary tract infection (URI)* the most common hospital-acquired infection. It occurs most frequently in the presence of an indwelling catheter. The most common infecting agent is *Escherichia coli*, suggesting that autogenous infection via the periurethral route is the commonest pathway.

urination *n* → micturition.

urine *n* the amber-coloured fluid which is excreted from the kidneys at the rate of about 1500 ml every 24 h in the adult; it is slightly acid and has a specific gravity of 1005–1030.

urinometer *n* an instrument for estimating the specific gravity of urine.

urobilin *n* a brownish pigment formed by the oxidation of urobilinogen and excreted in the faeces. Sometimes found in urine left standing in contact with air.

urobilinogen *n* (*syn* stercobilinogen) a pigment formed from bilirubin* in the intestine by the action of bacteria. It may be reabsorbed into the circulation and converted back to bilirubin in the liver and re-excreted in the bile or urine. Elevated levels in urine may indicate liver abnormalities.

urobilinuria *n* the presence of increased amounts of urobilin in the urine. Evidence of increased production of bilirubin in the liver, e.g. after haemolysis.

urochrome *n* the yellow pigment which gives urine its normal colour.

urodynamics *n* the use of sophisticated equipment to measure bladder function. Particularly useful in diagnosing the cause of urinary incontinence.

urogenital *adj* (*syn* urinogenital) pertaining to the urinary and the genital organs.

urography *n* (*syn* pyelography) radiographic visualization of the renal pelvis and ureter by injection of a contrast medium. The medium may be injected into the blood stream whence it is excreted by the kidney (intravenous urography) or it may be injected directly into the renal pelvis (antegrade via percutaneous injection) or ureter by way of a fine catheter introduced through a cystoscope (retrograde or ascending urography)—**urographic** *adj*, **urographically** *adv*. *intravenous urography (IVU)* demonstration of the urinary tract following an intravenous injection of a contrast medium.

urologist *n* a person who specializes in disorders of the female urinary tract and the male genitourinary tract.

urology *n* that branch of science which deals with disorders of the female urinary tract and the male genitourinary tract—**urological** *adj*, **urologically** *adv*.

uropathy *n* disease in any part of the urinary system.

urostomy *n* a word sometimes used to encompass conditions described by complex but specific words such as cutaneous ureterostomy, ileoureterostomy, rectal bladder, ureterocolostomy.

URTI *abbr* upper* respiratory tract infection.

urticaria *n* (*syn* nettlerash, hives) an allergic skin eruption characterized by multiple, circumscribed, smooth, raised, pinkish, itchy weals, developing very suddenly, usually lasting a few days and leaving no visible trace. Common provocative agents in susceptible subjects are ingested foods such as shellfish, injected sera and contact with, or injection of, antibiotics such as penicillin and streptomycin. ⇒

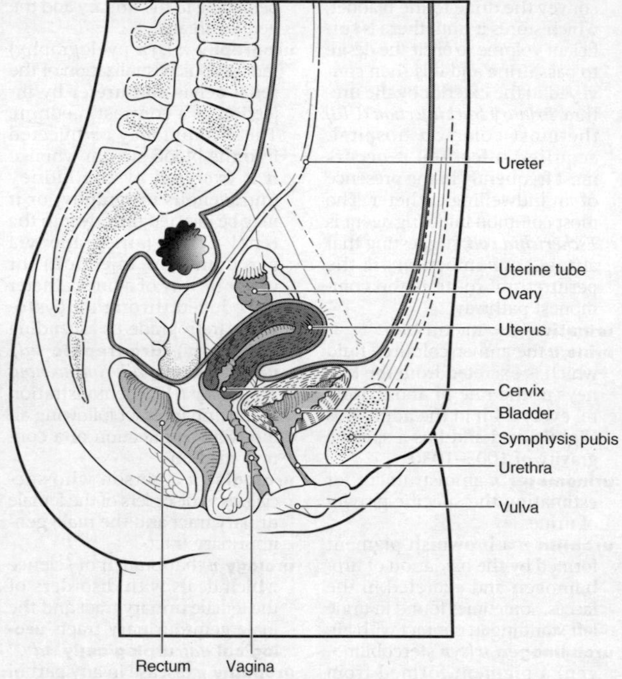

■ **Fig. 10** The normal position of the uterus, i.e. anteverted (leaning forward) and anteflexed (bent forward over the bladder).

angiooedema. *factitial urticaria*⇒ dermographia.

uterine tubes (*syn* fallopian tubes, oviducts) two tubes opening out of the upper part of the uterus. Each measures 10 cm and the distal end is fimbriated and lies near the ovary. Their function is to convey the ova into the uterus.

uteroplacental *adj* pertaining to the uterus* and placenta*.

uterorectal *adj* pertaining to the uterus* and the rectum*.

uterosacral *adj* pertaining to the uterus* and sacrum*.

uterosalpingography *n* (*syn* hysterosalpingography) radiological examination of the uterus and uterine tubes involving retrograde introduction of a contrast medium during fluoroscopy. Used to investigate patency of uterine tubes.

uterovaginal *adj* pertaining to the uterus* and the vagina*.

uterovesical *adj* pertaining to the uterus* and the urinary bladder*.

uterus *n* the womb; a hollow muscular organ in the pelvic cavity (see Fig. 10) into which a fertilized ovum implants and is retained during development, and from which the fetus is expelled through the vagina.

When the ovum is not fertilized, the endometrial lining of the uterus is shed, resulting in menstrual flow. ⇒ bicornuate–**uteri** *pl,* **uterine** *adj.*

UTI *abbr* urinary* tract infection.

uvea *n* the pigmented part of the eye, including the iris, ciliary body and choroid–**uveal** *adj.*

uveitis *n* inflammation of the uvea*.

uvula *n* the central, tag-like structure hanging down from the free edge of the soft palate.

uvulectomy *n* excision of the uvula.

uvulitis *n* inflammation of the uvula.

V

vaccination *n* originally described the process of inoculating persons with discharge from cowpox to protect them from smallpox. Now applied to the inoculation of any antigenic material for the purpose of producing active artificial immunity.

vaccines *npl* suspensions or products of infectious agents, used chiefly for producing active immunity. *triple vaccine* protects against diphtheria, tetanus and whooping-cough. In addition to these, *quadruple vaccine* protects against poliomyelitis ⇒ immunization. ⇒ Salk, TAB, BCG.

vaccinia *n* virus used to confer immunity against smallpox. Its origins are obscure but it is probably a cowpox-smallpox hybrid–**vaccinial** *adj.*

vacuum extractor **1** an instrument used to assist delivery of the fetus. **2** an instrument used as a method of abortion.

VADAS *abbr* voice* activated domestic appliance system.

vagal *adj* pertaining to the vagus* nerve.

vagina *n* literally, a sheath; the musculomembranous passage extending from the cervix uteri to the vulva–**vaginal** *adj.*

vaginismus *n* painful muscular spasm of the vaginal walls resulting in dyspareunia or painful coitis.

vaginitis *n* inflammation of the vagina. It can be caused by anaerobes, *Chlamydia trachomatis, Escherichia coli, Gardenerella vaginalis,* herpes simplex virus, *Neisseria gonorrhoeae, Trichomonas vaginalis* and yeasts, particularly *Candida albicans.* There should be adequate history taking at the initial assessment, followed by physical examination and bacteriological tests so that a correct diagnosis of the cause can lead to appropriate treatment. *senile vaginitis* can cause adhesions which may obliterate the vaginal canal. ⇒ Trichomonas.

vagolytic *adj* that which neutralizes the effect of a stimulated vagus nerve.

vagotomy *n* surgical division of the vagus nerves; done in conjunction with gastroenterostomy in the treatment of peptic ulcer or pyloroplasty.

vagus nerve the parasympathetic pneumogastric nerve; the 10th cranial nerve, composed of both motor and sensory fibres, with a wide distribution in the neck, thorax and abdomen, sending important branches to the heart, lungs, stomach, etc.–**vagi** *pl,* **vagal** *adj.*

valgus, valga, valgum *adj* exhibiting angulation away from the midline of the body, e.g. hallux* valgus.

valine *n* one of the essential amino* acids, α-aminoisovalerianic acid.

Valsalva manoeuvre the maximum intrathoracic pressure achieved by forced expiration against a closed glottis; occurs in such activities as lifting heavy objects or straining at stool: the glottis narrows simultaneously with contraction of the abdominal muscles.

values *npl* principles of living

which are distilled from life's experience; they guide behaviour and in a nursing context are manifested in the integrity of a nurse's work. ⇒ beliefs, secular beliefs.

valve *n* a fold of membrane in a passage or tube permitting the flow of contents in one direction only—**valvular** *adj.*

valvoplasty *n* a plastic operation on a valve, usually reserved for the heart; to be distinguished from valve replacement or valvotomy—**valvoplastic** *adj.*

valvotomy, valvulotomy *n* incision of a stenotic valve, by custom referring to the heart, to restore normal function.

valvulitis *n* inflammation of a valve, particularly in the heart.

valvulotomy *n* ⇒ valvotomy.

Van den Bergh's test estimation of serum bilirubin*. Direct positive reaction (conjugated) occurs in obstructive and hepatic jaundice. Indirect positive reaction (unconjugated) occurs in haemolytic jaundice.

vanyl mandelic acid (VMA) *n* a metabolite of adrenaline* (epinephrine) which is excreted in the urine. Levels of VMA detected in a 24-hour collection of urine can be used to assess the function of the adrenal medulla.

Vaquez's disease polycythaemia* vera.

varicella *n* ⇒ chickenpox—**varicelliform** *adj.*

varicella zoster hyperimmune globulin (VZIG) a blood product which when injected produces immunity to varicella and zoster.

varices *npl* dilated, tortuous (or varicose) veins. ⇒ varicose veins—**varix** *sing.*

varicocele *n* varicosity of the veins of the spermatic cord.

varicose ulcer (*syn* gravitational ulcer) an indolent type of ulcer* which occurs in the lower third of a leg afflicted with varicose* veins.

varicose veins dilated veins, the valves of which become incompetent so that blood flow may be reversed. Most commonly found in the lower limbs where they can result in a gravitational ulcer; in the rectum, when the term 'rectal varices' (haemorrhoids) is used; and in the lower oesophagus, when they are called oesophageal varices.

variola *n* ⇒ smallpox.

varioloid *n* attack of smallpox modified by previous vaccination.

varix *n* ⇒ varices.

varus, vara, varum *adj* displaying displacement or angulation towards the midline of the body, e.g. coxa vara.

vas *n* a vessel or duct—**vasa** *pl.* *vas deferens* the excretory duct of the testis. *vasa vasorum* the minute nutrient vessels of the artery and vein walls.

vascular *adj* supplied with vessels, especially referring to blood vessels.

vascularization *n* the acquisition of a blood supply; the process of becoming vascular. Occurs during the healing process.

vasculitis *n* (*syn* angiitis) inflammation of a blood vessel.

vasculotoxic *adj* any substance which brings about harmful changes in blood vessels.

vasectomy *n* surgical excision of part of the vas deferens, usually for sterilization.

vasoconstrictor *n* any agent which causes a narrowing of the lumen of blood vessels.

vasodilator *n* any agent which causes a widening of the lumen of blood vessels.

vasoepididymostomy *n* anastomosis of the vas deferens to the epididymis.

vasomotor nerves nerves which cause changes in the calibre of the blood vessels, usually constriction.

vasopressin *n* formed in the hypothalamus. Passes down the nerves in the pituitary stalk to be stored in the posterior lobe of the pituitary gland. It is the antidiuretic hormone (ADH). A synthetic preparation, desmopressin, is available which can be given intranasally or by injection in diabetes insipidus*.

vasopressor *n* a drug which increases blood pressure usually, but not always, by vasoconstriction of arterioles.

vasospasm *n* constricting spasm of vessel walls—**vasospastic** *adj.*

vasovagal attack faintness, pallor, sweating, feeling of fullness in epigastrium. When part of the postgastrectomy syndrome it occurs a few minutes after a meal.

VBI *abbr* vertebrobasilar* insufficiency.

VDRL test *abbr* for Venereal Disease Research Laboratory test, a serological flocculation test for syphilis.

vector *n* a carrier of disease.

vegetations *npl* growths or accretions composed of fibrin and platelets occurring on the edge of the cardiac valves in endocarditis.

vegetative *adj* pertaining to the nonsporing stage of a bacterium.

vehicle *n* an inert substance in which a drug is administered, e.g. water in mixtures.

vein *n* a vessel conveying blood from the capillaries back to the heart. It has the same three coats as an artery, the inner one being fitted with valves—**venous** *adj.*

Velpeau's bandage an arm to chest bandage for a fractured clavicle.

vena *n* a vein*. *vena cava* one of two large veins (inferior and superior) which return venous blood to the right atrium of the heart—**venae** *pl.*

venepuncture (venipuncture) *n* puncture of a vein for introduction of a drug or fluid or withdrawal of blood. When performed on children, a topical anaesthetic cream (EMLA) may be applied in advance. Research has revealed that the traditional method of flexing the arm after venepuncture is more likely to cause bruising than maintaining pressure over a swab with the arm extended.⇒ intravenous.

venereal *adj* pertaining to or caused by sexual intercourse. *venereal disease* ⇒ sexually transmitted disease. The term 'venereal disease' was replaced by 'sexually transmitted disease' and currently 'genitourinary* medicine' is preferred. ⇒ contact tracing.

venereology *n* the study and treatment of sexually-transmitted disease.

venesection *n* (*syn* phlebotomy) a clinical procedure, formerly by opening the cubital vein with a scalpel (now usually by venepuncture), whereby blood volume is reduced in congestive heart failure.

venoclysis *n* the introduction of nutrient or medicinal fluids into a vein.

venography *n* (*syn* phlebography) radiological examination of the venous system involving injection of a contrast medium—**venographic** *adj,* **venograph** *n,* **venographically** *adv.*

venom *n* a poisonous fluid produced by some scorpions, snakes and spiders.

venotomy *n* incision of a vein. ⇒ venesection.

venous *adj* pertaining to the veins.

ventilator *n* apparatus for providing assisted ventilation. Built-in controls can vary the mode of ventilation, between one or even a combination of the following: intermittent* positive pressure ventilation (IPPV), synchronized* intermittent mandatory ventilation (SIMV), mandatory minute volume (MMV), pressure* support ventilation (PSV) or continuous* positive airways pressure (CPAP).

Ventimask *n* a proprietary oxygen therapy mask incorporating a Venturi* device to provide controlled oxygen enrichment of inspired gas.

Ventouse extraction use of the vacuum* extractor in obstetrics.

ventral *adj* pertaining to the abdomen or the anterior surface of the body—**ventrally** *adv.*

ventricle *n* a small belly-like cavity—**ventricular** *adj. ventricle of the brain* four cavities filled with cerebrospinal fluid within the brain. *ventricle of the heart* the two lower muscular chambers of the heart.

ventricular puncture a highly skilled method of puncturing a cerebral ventricle for a sample of cerebrospinal fluid.

ventricular septal defect (VSD) a communication between the right and left ventricles of the heart.

ventriculocysternostomy *n* artificial communication between cerebral ventricles and subarachnoid space. One of the drainage operations for hydrocephalus.

ventriculoscope *n* an instrument via which the cerebral ventricles can be examined—**ventriculoscopic** *adj,* **ventriculoscopically** *adv.*

ventriculostomy *n* an artificial opening into a ventricle. Usually refers to a drainage operation for hydrocephalus.

ventrosuspension *n* fixation of a displaced uterus to the anterior abdominal wall.

Venturi *n* a device used in e.g. oxygen therapy masks to allow preset and constant oxygen enrichment of air for inspiration.

venule *n* a small vein.

Veress needle a sharp needle with a blunt-ended trochar which has a lateral hole; it is used for a pneumoperitoneum. When the trochar projects from the needle the gut is pushed safely away from the needle point.

vermicide *n* an agent which kills intestinal worms—**vermicidal** *adj.*

vermiform *adj* wormlike. *vermiform appendix* the vestigial, hollow, wormlike structure attached to the caecum*.

vermifuge *n* an agent which expels intestinal worms.

vernix caseosa the fatty substance which covers the skin of the fetus in utero and keeps it from becoming sodden by the liquor amnii*. This becomes absorbed in the postmature fetus leading to drying and cracking of the newborn's skin.

verruca *n* wart. ⇒ condyloma—**verrucae,** *pl,* **verrucous, verrucose** *adj. verruca necrogenica* (postmortem wart, prosector's wart) develops as result of accidental innoculation with tuberculosis while carrying out a postmortem. *verruca plana* the common multiple, flat, tiny warts often seen on children's hands, knees and face. *verruca plantaris* a flat wart on the sole of the foot. Highly contagious. *verruca seborrhoeica (syn* basal cell papilloma) the brown, greasy wart seen in seborrhoeic subjects, commonly on the chest or back, which increase with ageing. *verruca vulgaris* the common wart of the hands or feet, of brownish colour and rough pitted surface, caused by human papillomavirus type 2.

version *n* turning applied to the manoeuvre to alter the position of the fetus in utero to facilitate labour. *cephalic version* turning the child so that the head presents. *external cephalic version (ECV)* the turning of the fetus with both hands on the abdomen. The technique is safer with the use of ultrasound and tachographic monitoring. *internal version* is turning the child by one hand in the uterus, and the other on the patient's abdomen. *podalic version* turning the child to a breech presentation. This version may be external or internal.

vertebra *n* one of the irregular bones making up the spinal column—**vertebrae** *pl,* **vertebral** *adj.*

vertebral column (*syn* spinal column) made up of 33 vertebrae, articulating with the skull above and the pelvic girdle below. The vertebrae are so shaped that they enclose a cavity (spinal* canal, neural canal) which houses the spinal* cord.

vertebrobasilar insufficiency (VBI) a syndrome caused by lack of blood to the hindbrain. May be progressive, episodic or both. Clinical manifestations include giddiness and vertigo, nausea, ataxia, drop* attacks and signs of cerebellar disorder such as nystagmus.

vertex *n* the top of the head.

vertigo *n* giddiness, dizziness; a subjective sense of imbalance, often rotary—**vertiginous** *adj.*

vesical *adj* pertaining to the urinary bladder.

vesicant *n* a blistering substance.

vesicle *n* **1** a small bladder, cell or hollow structure. **2** a skin blister—**vesicular** *adj,* **vesiculation** *n.*

vesicostomy *n* ⇒ cystostomy.

vesicoureteric *adj* pertaining to the urinary bladder* and ureter*. Vesicoureteric reflux can cause pyelonephritis.

vesicovaginal *adj* pertaining to the urinary bladder and vagina*.

vesiculitis *n* inflammation of a vesicle, particularly the seminal vesicles.

vesiculopapular *adj* pertaining to or exhibiting both vesicles and papules.

vessel *n* a tube, duct or canal, holding or conveying fluid, especially blood and lymph.

vestibule *n* **1** the middle part of the internal ear, lying between the semicircular canals and the cochlea. **2** the triangular area between the labia minora—**vestibular** *adj.*

vestigial *adj* rudimentary; indicating a remnant of something formerly present.

viable *adj* capable of living a separate existence. Used in relation to a fetus. In English law this is after 24 weeks' gestation—**viability** *n.*

Vibrio *n* a genus of curved, motile microorganisms. *Vibrio cholerae,* or the *comma vibrio,* causes cholera.

vicarious *adj* substituting the function of one organ for another. *vicarious menstruation* bleeding from the nose or other part of the body when menstruation is abnormally suppressed.

Vigilon *n* a proprietary wound dressing which is a thin sheet of breathable copolymer gel. It freely transports gases and fluids and can absorb approximately its own weight in exudate. It is also claimed that it absorbs some shearing force and has a cooling effect which helps to reduce pain.

villus *n* a microscopic fingerlike projection; found in the small intestine—**villi** *pl.*

Vincent's angina infection and ulceration of the mouth or throat by a spirochaete and a bacillus. To be differentiated from Ludwig's* angina.

viraemia *n* the presence of virus in the blood—**viraemic** *adj. maternal viraemia* can cause fetal damage.

viral haemorrhagic fevers fevers which occur mainly in the tropics; they are often transmitted by mosquitoes or ticks;

sufferers may have a petechial skin rash. Examples are chikungunya, ebola, dengue, Lassa fever, Marburg disease, Rift valley fever and yellow fever.

viral hepatitis ⇒ hepatitis.

viricidal *adj* lethal to a virus—**viricide** *n*.

virilism *n* the appearance of secondary male characteristics in the female.

virology *n* the study of viruses and the diseases caused by them—**virological** *adj*.

virulence *n* infectiousness; the disease-producing power of a microorganism; the power of a microorganism to overcome host resistance—**virulent** *adj*.

virus *n* very small microorganisms, parasitic within living cells. They differ from bacteria in having only one kind of nucleic acid, either DNA or RNA; in lacking the apparatus necessary for energy production and protein synthesis; and by not reproducing by binary fission but by independent synthesis of their component parts which are then assembled. They cause many kinds of acute and chronic diseases in man, and can cause tumours in animals. Some of the more important groups are: (a) *poxviruses,* e.g. smallpox, molluscum contagiosum (b) *herpesviruses,* e.g. herpes simplex virus, cytomegalovirus, varicella-zoster virus, Epstein-Barr virus (c) *adenoviruses,* (d) *papovaviruses,* e.g. polyoma virus, which can cause tumours in laboratory animals (e) *reoviruses,* e.g. rotaviruses (f) *togaviruses,* e.g. yellow fever virus (g) *picornaviruses* (h) *myxoviruses* (i) *paramyxoviruses* (j) *rhabdoviruses,* e.g. rabies virus (k) *coronaviruses,* e.g. some common cold viruses (l) *arenaviruses,* e.g. Lassa fever virus. Groups a-d are DNA viruses, groups e-l are RNA viruses. Those viruses which are spread by arthropods—insects and ticks—are known as arboviruses, these include reoviruses, togaviruses and rhabdoviruses.

viscera *npl* the internal organs—**viscus** *sing,* **visceral** *adj*.

visceroptosis *n* downward displacement or falling of the abdominal organs.

viscid *adj* sticky, glutinous, mainly used to describe sputum.

visiting *v* refers to the time at which visitors can visit patients in hospital. It varies throughout the country from stipulated periods to a more liberal policy. Visiting can help to prevent boredom*, institutionalization and to encourage rehabilitation. In sick children's units, open visiting is usually allowed and parents enabled to be resident with their child. Visitors of terminally-ill patients, children and people in long-stay wards are encouraged to participate in the nursing of their relatives to relieve their feelings of helplessness.

visual *adj* pertaining to vision. *visual acuity* ⇒ acuity. *visual field* the area within which objects can be seen. *visual* purple the purple pigment in the retina of the eye, which is called rhodopsin.

vital capacity the maximum amount of air expelled from the lungs after a deep inspiration. ⇒ forced vital capacity.

vitallium *n* an alloy which can be left in the tissues in the form of nails, plates, tubes, etc.

vitalograph *n* apparatus for measuring the forced* vital capacity.

vitalograph emergency respirator an aspirator suitable for resuscitation. It is portable and has a pump handle so that it does not require a power source and can be operated with one hand.

vitamins *npl* essential organic compounds essential for growth and health, present in certain foodstuffs. Most vitamins function as coenzymes, e.g. in metabolism.

vitamin A (*syn* retinol) a fat-soluble vitamin found in liver and egg-yolk. In its provitamin form, β carotene, it is present in carrots, cabbage, lettuce, tomatoes and other fruits and vegetables: in the body it is converted into retinol. It is essential for healthy skin and mucous membranes: it aids night vision. Deficiency can result in stunted growth and night blindness.

vitamin B refers to any one of a group of water-soluble vitamins of the vitamin B complex, all chemically related and often occurring in the same foods ⇒ biotin, cyanocobalamin, folic acid, nicotinic acid, pantothenic acid, pyridoxine, riboflavine, thiamine.

vitamin B_1 thiamine*.

vitamin B_6 pyridoxine*.

vitamin B_{12} cyanocobalamin*.

vitamin C ascorbic* acid.

vitamin D a fat-soluble vitamin cholecalciferol (vitamin D_3); production in the body is dependent on ultraviolet light acting on a provitamin form. Good sources are oily fish and dairy produce. Deficiency in childhood results in rickets. *vitamin D resistant rickets* ⇒ rickets.

vitamin E a group of chemically related compounds known as tocopherols*. A fat-soluble vitamin which functions as an antioxidant, it protects polyunsaturated fatty acids and hence helps maintain cell membranes. Deficiency seen in infants who are premature or small for gestational age may manifest as haemolytic blood disease.

vitamin K essential in the formation of blood clotting factors. Synthesized by coliform bacteria of large intestine.

vitiligo *n* a skin disease of probable autoimmune origin characterized by areas of complete loss of pigment.

vitrectomy *n* surgical removal of the vitreous humor from the vitreous chamber of the eye.

vitreous *adj* resembling jelly. *vitreous chamber* the cavity inside the eyeball and behind the lens. *vitreous humor* the jelly-like substance contained in the vitreous chamber.

VMA ⇒ vanyl mandelic acid.

vocal cords membranous folds stretched anteroposteriorly across the larynx. Sound is produced by their vibration as air from the lungs passes between them.

voice activated domestic appliance system (VADAS) computerised system for switching on or off domestic appliances such as lights, kettle, telephone, each 'instruction' to the computer being controlled by the user's voice. Enables severely impaired individual, e.g. someone with a high spinal fracture, to live as independently as possible, without relying on interventions by helpers.

voiding *n* emptying, usually of the urinary bladder. *prompted voiding* used for institutionalized patients by inviting them to empty their bladder. *timed voiding* a fixed voiding schedule, determined by the baseline frequency/volume chart. Often used for elderly people who may be debilitated or for those with neurogenic* bladder.

volatile *adj* evaporating rapidly.

volition *n* the will to act.

Volkmann's ischaemic contracture a flexion deformity of the wrist and fingers from fixed contracture of the flexor muscles in the forearm. The cause is ischaemia of the muscles by injury or obstruction to the brachial artery, near the elbow.

voluntary *adj* under the control of the will; free and unrestricted; as opposed to reflex or involuntary.

voluntary organisations a group of people who join in an unpaid capacity to serve a particular cause such as providing a library service to inpatients, running a hospital shop, taking a trolley shop to the wards, organizing a coffee shop in the outpatients' department. Other voluntary organisations are concerned with providing help to patients suffering from a particular condition, and their families.

volvulus *n* a twisting of a section of bowel, so as to occlude the lumen: a cause of intestinal obstruction.

vomit *n* ejection of the stomach contents through the mouth; sickness. ⇒ projectile.

vomiting of pregnancy ⇒ hyperemesis gravidarum.

vomitus *n* vomited matter.

von Recklinghausen's disease Recklinghausen's* disease.

von Willebrand's disease an inherited bleeding disease due to deficiencies relating to the factor VIII proteins in plasma. The inheritance is autosomal dominant, affecting both sexes, and is essentially a disorder of the primary haemostatic mechanism with deranged platelet-endothelial cell interaction. In severe cases von Willebrand's disease results in a clotting defect resembling haemophilia*.

VSD *abbr* ventricular* septal defect.

vulva *n* the external genitalia of the female—**vulval** *adj.*

vulvectomy *n* excision of the vulva.

vulvitis *n* inflammation of the vulva.

vulvovaginal *adj* pertaining to the vulva* and the vagina*.

vulvovaginitis *n* inflammation of the vulva and vagina.

vulvovaginoplasty *n* operation devised for congenital absence of the vagina, or acquired disabling stenosis—**vulvovaginoplastic** *adj.*

VZIG *abbr* varicella* zoster hyperimmune immunoglobulin.

W

Waldeyer's ring a lymphatic circle surrounding the pharynx.

ward rounds traditionally refers to doctors' rounds when, e.g. a consultant, registrar and houseman visit each patient to monitor response to treatment. The ward sister or charge nurse may accompany these rounds. Where primary nursing is being practised, the primary nurse accompanies the round.

warfarin *n* the oral anticoagulant of choice. Coumarin derivative.

wart *n* ⇒ verruca.

Wasserman test carried out in the diagnosis of syphilis. It is a complement-fixation test and is not entirely specific. ⇒ TPI test.

waterbrash *n* ⇒ pyrosis.

Waterhouse-Friderichsen syndrome shock with widespread skin haemorrhages occurring in meningitis, especially meningococcal. There is bleeding in the adrenal glands.

Waterston's operation anastomosis of the right pulmonary artery to the ascending aorta. Used as a palliative measure in the treatment of Fallot's* tetralogy in the young child.

WBC *abbr* white blood cell or corpuscle. ⇒ blood.

weal *n* a superficial swelling on the skin surface, characteristic of urticaria, nettle-stings, etc.

weaning *v* usually taken to mean the period when an infant's sucking skills gradually give way to manipulating thickened food placed on the tongue and swallowing it. He gradually learns to control the spoon and trace the spatial pathway from plate to mouth. An increasing proportion of the infant's nutritional requirements are met in this way, rather than from milk alone. Weaning is not recommended before the age of 4 months. As solid foods are introduced the skill of chewing before swallowing is acquired. The word 'weaning' is also used in the sense of helping to withdraw a person from something on which he is dependent, e.g. a respirator.

Weber's test a tuning fork test for the diagnosis of deafness.

Wegener's granulomatosis Weil-Felix test an agglutination reaction used in the diagnosis of the typhus group of fevers. Patient's serum is titrated against a heterologous antigen.

Weil's disease spirochaetosis icterohaemorrhagica, a type of jaundice with fever caused by a leptospire voided in the urine of rats. A disease of miners, sewer workers, etc. who work in dirty water but increasingly found in people who practise water sports.

well baby clinic mothers are encouraged to bring their new babies during the early years for monitoring by health visitors. Health promotion and immunization* are available. ⇒ prevention of: accidents*, ill health*, infection*.

well man clinic a clinic, usually at the GP's surgery, where men are encouraged to have an annual health check which might include measurement of blood pressure, weight, assessment of diet and alcohol use and health promotion. ⇒ risk factors, testicles, self-examination of, smegma.

well woman clinic a clinic, usually at the GP's surgery, where women are encouraged to have an annual health check which might include measurement of blood pressure, weight, cervical smear, breast awareness education. ⇒ Pap test, perineal toilet, risk factors, breast, self-examination of, smegma.

wen *n* ⇒ sebaceous.

Wertheim's hysterectomy an extensive operation for removal of carcinoma of the cervix, where the uterus, cervix, upper vagina, tubes, ovaries and regional lymph glands are removed.

Western blot a method of testing for HIV* infection. The test is usually not carried out until two positive results have been gained from the less specific ELISA* test.

Wharton's jelly a jelly-like substance contained in the umbilical cord.

wheezing *v* a type of dyspnoea* audible as a whistling sound, often only detectable by stethoscope, and usually present on inspiration and expiration.

whipworm *n Trichuris trichiura,* a roundworm which infests the intestine of man in the humid tropics. Eggs are excreted in the stools. The worms do not normally produce symptoms, but heavy infestations of over 1000 worms cause blood diarrhoea, anaemia and prolapse of the rectum.

white asphyxia ⇒ asphyxia.

white leg thrombophlebitis* occurring in women after childbirth.

whitlow *n* ⇒ paronychia.

whole body vibration an occupational disease which affects drivers of certain vehicles, e.g. tractors, helicopters and some ships. There is discomfort from interference with the natural resonance of organs and may lead to osteoarthritis of the spine.

whooping cough ⇒ pertussis.

Widal test an agglutination reaction for typhoid fever. The patient's serum is put in contact with *Salmonella typhi.* The result is positive if agglutination occurs, proving the presence of antibodies in the serum.

Wilms' tumour the commonest abdominal tumour of childhood (also known as a nephroblastoma), and one which usually affects the kidneys. Usually diagnosed during the preschool period. Prognosis is uncertain and depends on the stage of the tumour and child's age at onset of diagnosis and treatment. The treatment involves removal of the kidney and surrounding infiltrated tissue, chemotherapy, and radiotherapy.

Wilson's disease hepaticolenticular degeneration with choreic movements. Due to disturbance of copper metabolism. No urinary catecholamine excretion. Associated with mental subnormality. Can be treated with BAL and penicillamine. Asymptomatic relatives can be given prophylactic penicillamine.

windpipe *n* ⇒ trachea.

withdrawal *n* **1** a particular group of symptoms experienced by people when giving up a substance such as alcohol, hard or soft drugs, sleeping pills, smoking or solvents to which they have been addicted. **2** a negative coping behaviour when a person becomes increasingly socially isolated. **3** an unreliable method of contraception. ⇒ coitus.

womb *n* the uterus.

Wood's light special ultraviolet light used for the detection of ringworm.

woolsorters' disease ⇒ anthrax.

work related upper limb disorder repetitive* strain injury.

World Health Organization (WHO) an agency of the United Nations affiliated to other organizations concerned with worldwide health and welfare. For administrative purposes the world is divided into 6 regions, each having a regional office. The headquarters is in Geneva, Switzerland.

worms *npl* ⇒ ascarides, Taenia, *Trichuris*.

wound *n* most commonly used when referring to injury to the skin or underlying tissues or organs by a blow, cut, missile or stab. It also includes injury to the skin caused by chemicals, cold, friction, heat, pressure and rays; and manifestation in the skin of internal conditions, e.g. pressure sores and ulcers.

wound drains most commonly used in surgical wounds. They may be inserted as a therapeutic measure, e.g. to drain an abscess, or prophylactically, e.g to prevent blood clotting and forming a haematoma, or in case of the escape of bile. Drainage may be active where the drain is attached to suction apparatus producing a 'closed wound suction'. ⇒ healing, T-tube.

wound dressings proprietary materials of different substances applied to surgical or medical wounds. Modern dressings aim to be permeable to water vapour and gases but not to bacteria or liquids; this retains serous exudate which is actively bactericidal. They do not adhere to the wound surface and on removal do not damage new tissue. ⇒ Lyofoam C, OpSite.

wound healing ⇒ healing, moist wound healing.

wrist *n* the carpus.

wrist drop paralysis of the muscles which raise the wrist because of damage to the radial nerve.

wryneck *n* ⇒ torticollis.

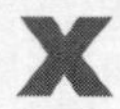

xanthelasma *n* a variety of xanthoma. *xanthelasma palpebrarum* small yellowish plaques appear on the eyelids.

xanthine *n* dioxypurine found in liver, muscle, pancreas and urine. An intermediate found in the formation of urate from guanine, excreted in the urine.

xanthoma *n* a collection of cholesterol under the skin producing a yellow discoloration—**xanthomata** *pl.*

xenon *n* a rare gas that is chemically inert, but which can induce general anaesthesia.

Xenopsylla *n* a genus of fleas. *Xenopsylla cheopis* is the rat flea that transmits bubonic plague.

xeroderma *n* (xerodermia) dryness of the skin ⇒ ichthyosis. *xeroderma pigmentosum* (Kaposi's disease) a familial dermatosis probably caused by photosensitization. Pathological freckle formation (ephelides) may give rise to keratosis and potentially fatal neoplastic growth.

xerophthalmia *n* dryness and ulceration of the cornea which may lead to blindness. Associated with lack of vitamin* A.

xerosis *n* dryness. *xerosis conjunctivae* ⇒ Bitot's spots.

xerostomia *n* dry mouth.

X-rays short rays of electromagnetic spectrum. The word is popularly used for radiographs*.

xylose test more convenient than fat balance and equally as accurate. Xylose is given orally and its urinary excretion is measured. Normally 25% of loading dose is excreted. Less than this indicates malabsorption syndrome.

XXY syndrome Klinefelter* syndrome.

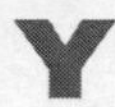

yaws *n* a tropical disease which resembles syphilis so closely that they may be one and the same disease but modified by differences of climate, social habit and hygiene. Pinta (S. America) and bejel (Transjordan) may be similar variants. All these diseases are caused by an identical spirochaete and produce a positive Wassermann test in the blood. Syphilis, alone, is a venereal disease. The general term for the group is 'treponematosis'.

yeast *n* saccharomyces. A unicellular fungus which will cause fermentation and which reproduces by budding only. Commonly used to make bread and in the brewing industry. Brewer's yeast is said to be rich in vitamin B complex.

yellow fever an acute febrile illness of tropical areas, caused by a group B arbovirus and spread by a mosquito (*Aedes aegypti*). Characteristic features are jaundice, black vomit and anuria. An attenuated virus variant known as 17D is prepared as vaccine for immunization.

yolk *n* the stored nutrient of the ovum.

yttrium 90 (^{90}Y) a radioactive isotope of yttrium. Used in the treatment of malignant effusions.

Z

ZIFT *abbr* zygote* intrafallopian transfer.

Zimmer aids there are now several designs of Zimmer frames to help patients to regain or retain independence for walking.

zinc *n* a trace element which is essential for cell multiplication and successful wound healing. Zinc absorption is reduced by alcohol and the contraceptive pill.

zinc oxide a widely used mild astringent, present in calamine lotion and cream, Lassar's paste, Unna's paste and many other dermatological applications.

Zollinger-Ellison syndrome *n* the presence of ulcerogenic tumour of the pancreatic islets of Langerhans, hypersecretion of gastric acid, fulminating ulceration of oesophagus, stomach, duodenum and jejunum. Frequently accompanied by diarrhoea. Diagnosed by peroral biopsy.

zona *n* a zone; a girdle; herpes zoster. *zona pellucida* the vitelline membrane surrounding the ovum.

zonula ciliaris suspensory ligament attaching the periphery of the lens of the eye to ciliary body.

zonule *n* small zone, belt or girdle. Zonula.

zonulolysis *n* breaking down the zonula ciliaris–sometimes necessary before intracapsular extraction of the lens–**zonulolytic** *adj.*

zoonosis *n* disease in man transmitted from animal. Abbattoir and farm workers are at risk–**zoonoses** *pl.*

zygoma *n* the cheekbone–**zygomatic** *adj.*

zygote *n* the fertilized ovum. *zygote intra-fallopian transfer* process used in assisted conception. Mature ova are retrieved. After mixing with sperm, fertilization is awaited and the resultant zygote placed within the uterine tube.

Appendices

Contents

Appendix 1

SI units and the metric system

Basic units

The SI has seven basic units.

Name of SI unit	Symbol for SI unit	Quantity
metre	m	length
kilogram	kg	mass
second	s	time
mole	mol	amount of substance
ampere	A	electric current
kelvin	°K	thermodynamic temperature
candela	cd	luminous intensity

Derived units

Derived units are obtained by appropriate combinations of basic units:

– unit area results when unit length is multiplied by unit length
– unit density results when unit weight (mass) is divided by unit volume

Name of SI unit	Symbol for SI unit	Quantity
joule	J	work, energy, quantity of heat
pascal	Pa	pressure
newton	N	force

Appendix 1

Decimal multiples and submultiples

Multiples and submultiples of units

	Multiplication factor	*Prefix*	*Symbol*
1 000 000 000 000	10^{12}	tera	T
1 000 000 000	10^{9}	giga	G
1 000 000	10^{6}	mega	M
1 000	10^{3}	kilo	k
100	10^{2}	hecto	h
10	10^{1}	deca	da
0.1	10^{-1}	deci	d
0.01	10^{-3}	centi	c
0.001	10^{-3}	milli	m
0.000 001	10^{-6}	micro	μ
0.000 000 001	10^{-9}	nano	n
0.000 000 000 001	10^{-12}	pico	p
0.000 000 000 000 001	10^{-15}	femto	f
0.000 000 000 000 000 001	10^{-18}	atto	a

Rules for using units

a. The symbol for a unit is unaltered in the plural and should not be followed by a full stop except at the end of a sentence:

   5 cm *not* 5 cm. or 5 cms.

b. The decimal sign between digits is indicated by a full stop in typing. No commas are used to divide large numbers into groups of three, but a half-space (whole space in typing) is left after every third digit. If the numerical value of the number is less than 1 unit, a zero should precede the decimal sign:

   0.1234 456 *not* .123,456

c. The SI symbol for 'day' (i.e. 24 hours) is 'd', but urine and faecal excretions of substances should preferably be expressed as 'per 24 hours':

   g/24 h

d. 'Squared' and 'cubed' are expressed as numerical powers and not by abbreviation:

   square centimetre is cm2 *not* sq. cm.

Commonly used measurements

a. Temperature is expressed as degrees Celsius (°C) and the standard thermometer is graded 32–42°C.

   1° Celcius = 1° Centigrade

b. The calorie is replaced by the joule:

   1 calorie = 4.2 J.
   1 Calorie (dietetic use) = 4.2 kilojoules = 4.2 kJ.

The previous 1000 Calorie reducing diet is expressed (approximately) as a 4000 kJ diet.

1 g of fat provides	38 kJ
1 g of protein provides	17 kJ
1 g of carbohydrate provides	16 kJ

c. Equivalent concentration mEq/l is commonly used for reporting results of monovalent electrolyte measurements (sodium, potassium, chloride and bicarbonate). It is not part of the SI system and should be replaced by molar concentration – in these examples mmol/l.

   For these four measurements, the numerical value will not change.

d. The SI unit of pressure is the pascal (Pa). Blood gas measurements should be given in the SI unit kPa instead of mmHg.

   1 mmHg = 133.32 Pa.
   1 kPa = 7.5006 mmHg

   Column measurement will be *retained* in clinical practice *as at present.*

   blood pressure (in mmHg)
   cerebrospinal fluid (in mmH_2O)
   central venous pressure (in cmH_2O)

Appendix 2

Measurements

Metric

Linear measure

		1 millimetre	=	0.039 in
10 mm	=	1 centimetre	=	0.394 in
10 cm	=	1 decimetre	=	3.94 in
10 dm	=	1 metre	=	39.37 in
1000 m	=	1 kilometre	=	0.6214 mile

Square measure

		1 sq centimetre	=	0.155 sq in
10 000 cm^2	=	1 sq metre	=	1.196 sq in
100 m^2	=	1 are	=	119.6 sq yd
100 ares	=	1 hectare	=	2.471 acres
100 ha	=	1 sq kilometre	=	0.386 sq miles

Cubic measure

		1 cu centimetre	=	0.061 in^3
1000 cu cm	=	1 cu decimetre	=	0.035 ft^3
1000 cu dm	=	1 cu metre	=	1.308 yd^3

Capacity measure

		1 millilitre	=	0.002 pt
10 ml	=	1 centilitre	=	0.018 pint
10 cl	=	1 decilitre	=	0.176 pt
10 dl	=	1 litre	=	1.76 pt
1000 l	=	1 kilolitre	=	220.0 gall

Weight

		1 milligram	=	0.015 grain
10 mg	=	1 centigram	=	0.154 grain
10 cg	=	1 decigram	=	1.543 grain
10 dg	=	1 gram	=	15.43 grain
			=	0.035 oz
1000 g	=	1 kilogram	=	2.205 lb
1000 kg	=	1 tonne (metric ton)	=	0.984 (long) ton

Temperature

°Fahrenheit = (9/5 × x°C) +32
°Centigrade = 5/9 × (x°F − 32)
where x is the temperature needing converting

Imperial

Linear measure

1 inch	=	25.4	mm
1 foot	=	0.305	mm
1 yard	=	0.914	m
1 mile	=	1.61	km

Square measure

1 square inch	=	6.452	cm^2
1 square foot	=	9.29	dm^2
1 square yard	=	0.836	m^2
1 acre	=	4047	m^2
1 square mile	=	259	ha

Cubic measure

1 cubic inch	=	16.4	cm^3
1 cubic foot	=	0.0283	m^3
1 cubic yard	=	0.765	m^3

Capacity measure

1 fluid ounce	=	28.4	cm^3
1 pint	=	0.568	l
1 quart	=	1.136	l
1 gallon	=	4.546	l

Weight

1 grain	=	64.8	mg
1 dram	=	1.772	g
1 ounce	=	28.35	g
1 pound	=	0.4536	kg
1 stone	=	6.35	kg
1 quarter	=	12.7	kg
1 hundred weight	=	50.8	kg
1 ton	=	1.016	tonnes
1 short ton	=	0.907	tonnes

Appendix 3

Conversion charts

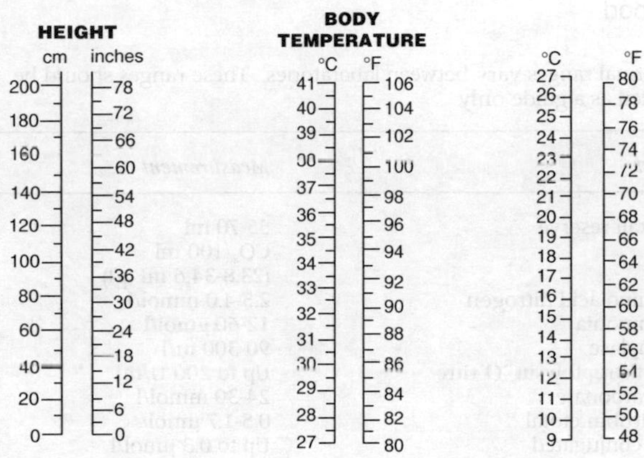

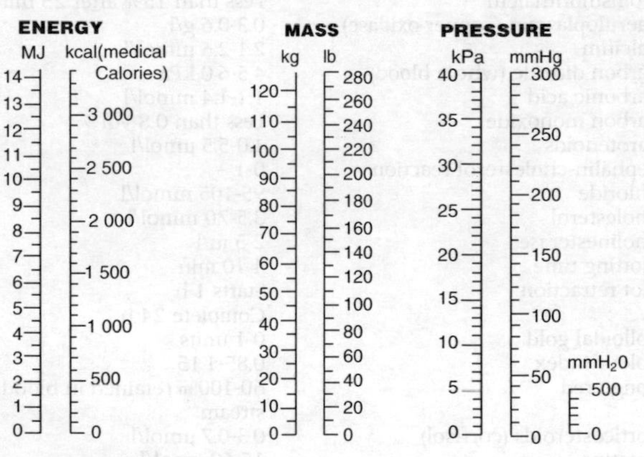

Appendix 4

Normal characteristics

Blood

Normal ranges vary between laboratories. These ranges should be taken as a guide only

Test	*Measurement*
Alkali reserve	55-70 ml CO_2/100 ml (23.8-34.6 mEq/l)
Amino acid nitrogen	2.5-4.0 mmol/l
Ammonia	12-60 μmol/l
Amylase	90-300 iu/l
Antistreptolysin `O`titre	Up to 200 U/ml
Bicarbonate	24-30 mmol/l
Bilirubinætotal	0.5-1.7 μmol/
conjugated	Up to 0.3 μmol/l
Bleeding time	1-6 min
Blood volume	Approx 1/12 or 8% body weight
Bromsulphthalein	Less than 15% after 25 min
Caeruloplasmin (copper oxidase)	0.3-0.6 g/l
Calcium	2.1-2.6 mmol/l
Carbon dioxide (whole blood)	4.5-6.0 kPa
Carbonic acid	1.1-1.4 mmol/l
Carbon monoxide	Less than 0.8 vol %
Carotenoids	1.0-5.5 μmol/l
Cephalin-cholesterol reaction	0-1 +
Chloride	95-105 mmol/l
Cholesterol	3.5-7.0 mmol/l
Cholinesterase	2-5 iu/l
Clotting time	4-10 min
Clot retraction	Starts 1 h Complete 24 h
Colloidal gold	0-1 units
Colour index	0.85-1.15
Congo red	60-100% retained in blood stream
Corticosteroids (cortisol)	0.3-0.7 μmol/l
Creatine	15-60 μmol/l
Creatine kinase	4-60 iu/l
Creatinine	60-120 μmol/l
Copper	13-24 μmol/l

Test	*Measurement*
Erythrocyte sedimentation rate (ESR)	
Men	3-5 mm/1 h: 7-15 mm/2 h (Westergren)
Women	7-12 mm/1 h: 12-17/2 h (Westergren)
Fatty acids (free)	0.3-0.6 mmol/l
Folic acid	greater than 3 ng/ml
Gamma-glutamyl-transpeptidase	5-30 iu/l
Glucose (whole blood, fasting)	
venous	3.0-5.0 mmol/l
capillary (arterial)	3.3-5.3 mmol/l
Glucose tolerance	max. 180 mg/100 ml returns fasting $1\frac{1}{2}$h
Haemoglobin	12–18 g/dl
Haptoglobins	20–110 μmol/l
Hydrogen ion activity exponent (pH)	7.36-7.42
Hydrogen ion concentration	35-44 nmol/l
Icetric index	4-6U
Iron	
Men	13-32 μmol/l
Women	Approx. 3.25 μmol/l less
Iron-binding capacity (total)	45-70 μmol/l
Kahn	negative
Ketones	0.06-0.2 mmol/l
Lactate	0.75-2.0 mmol/l
Lactate dehydrogenase	
total	60-250 iu/l
'heart specific'	50-150 iu/l
Lead (whole blood)	0.5-1.7 μmol/l
LE cells	None
Leucine aminopeptidase	1-3 μmol/h/ml
Lipase	18-280 iu/l
Lipids (total)	4.5-10g/l
β-Lipoproteins	3.5-6.5 g/l
Magnesium	0.7-1.0 mmol
Methaemoglobin	None
5′-Nucleotidase	2.15 iu/l
Osmolality	275-295 mosmol/kg
Oxygen (whole blood)	11-15 kPa
Oxygen capacity	14.4-24.7 ml
Oxygen combining power	
Men	17.8-22.2 ml
Women	16.1-18.9 ml
Paul-Bunnell	Agglutination up to 1:20
CO^2	4.5-6.0 kPa
pH	7.36-7.42
Phosphotase	
Acid-total	3.5-20 iu/l
Acid-prostatic	0-3.5 iu/l
Alkaline-total	20-90 iu/l

Test	*Measurement*
Phosphate (inorganic)	0.8-1.4 mmol/l
Phospholipids	
(as fatty acids)	5.0-9.0 mmol/l
(as phosphorus)	1.9-3.2 mmol/l
Platelets	200-500 × 10^9/l
PO_2 (whole blood)	11-15 kPa
Potassium	3.8-5.0 mmol/l
Protein	
— total	62-80 g/l
— albumin	35-50 g/l
— globulin (total)	18-32 g/l
— gammaglobulin	7-15 g/l
Fibrinogen	2-4 g/l
— A-G ratio	1.5:1-2.5:1
Protein-bound iodine	0.3-0.6 µmol/l
Prothrombin time	11-18 s
Pyruvate (fasting)	0.05-0.08 mmol/l
Red cell count	4.0-6.0 × 10^{12}/l
Red cell fragility	Haemolysis slight 0.44% NaCl Haemolysis complete 0.3% NaCl
Sodium	136-148 mmol/l
Sulphaemoglobin	None
Thymol	
flocculation	0-±
turbidity	0-4 units
Thyroxine	0.04-0.85 µmol/l
Transaminase	
alanine (at 25°C)	4-12 iu/l
aspartate (at 25°C)	5-15 iu/l
Transferrin	0.12-0.2 g/l
Triglyceride	0.3-1.8 mmol/l
Urea	3.0-6.5 mmol/l
Uric acid	0.1-0.45 µmol/l
Vitamin A	1.0-3.0 mmol/l
Vitamin B_{12}	150-800 pg/ml
Vitamin C	0.7-1.4 mg/100ml
Wasserman reaction (WR)	Negative
White cell count	4.0-10.0 × 10^9/l
Zinc sulphate reaction	2.8 units

Cerebrospinal fluid

Pressure (adult)	50 to 200 mm water
Cells	0 to 5 lymphocytes/mm^3
Glucose	3.3-4.4 mmol/l
Protein	100-400 mg/l

Faeces

Normal fat content

Daily output on normal diet	less than 7g
Fat (as stearic acid)	11-18 mmol/24 h

Urine

Total quantity per 24 hours	1000 to 1500ml
Specific gravity	1.012 to 1.030
Reaction	pH 4 to 8

Average amounts of inorganic and organic solids in urine each 24 hours

Calcium	2.5 –7.5 mmol
Creatinine	9–17 mmol
5H1AA	15–75 μmol
HMMA*	10–35 μmol
Hydroxyproline	0.08–0.25 mmol
Magnesium	3.3–5.0 mmol
Oestriol	varies widely during pregnancy—μmol
Phosphate	15–50 mmol
Urea	250–500 mmol
17-ketosteroids:	
Men	8 to 15 mg/24 hours
Women	5 to 12 mg/24 hours

*4-Hydroxy-3-methoxy mandelic acid.

Appendix 5

Weights and heights

Weight for age, birth to 5 years, sexes combined.
Means for boys are 0.05 to 0.15 kg heavier and for girls 0.05 to 0.15 kg lighter.

	Weight (kg)		
Age (months)	*Standard*	*80% Standard*	*60% Standard*
0	3.4	2.7	2.0
1	4.3	3.4	2.5
2	5.0	4.0	2.9
3	5.7	4.5	3.4
4	6.3	5.0	3.8
5	6.9	5.5	4.2
6	7.4	5.9	4.5
7	8.0	6.3	4.9
8	8.4	6.7	5.1
9	8.9	7.1	5.3
10	9.3	7.4	5.5
11	9.6	7.7	5.8
12	9.9	7.9	6.0
13	10.2	8.1	6.2
14	10.4	8.3	6.3
15	10.6	8.5	6.4
16	10.8	8.7	6.6
17	11.0	8.9	6.7
18	11.3	9.0	6.8
19	11.5	9.2	7.0
20	11.7	9.4	7.1
21	11.9	9.6	7.2
22	12.05	9.7	7.3
23	12.2	9.8	7.4
24	12.4	9.9	7.5
25	12.6	10.1	7.6
26	12.7	10.3	7.7
27	12.9	10.5	7.8

Age (months)	Weight (kg) Standard	80% Standard	60% Standard
28	13.1	10.6	7.9
29	13.3	10.7	8.0
30	13.5	10.8	8.1
31	13.7	11.0	8.2
32	13.8	11.1	8.3
33	14.0	11.2	8.4
34	14.2	11.3	8.5
35	14.4	11.5	8.6
36	14.5	11.6	8.7
37	14.7	11.8	8.8
38	14.85	11.9	8.9
39	15.0	12.05	9.0
40	15.2	12.2	9.1
41	15.35	12.3	9.2
42	15.5	12.4	9.3
43	15.7	12.6	9.4
44	15.85	12.7	9.5
45	16.0	12.9	9.6
46	16.2	12.95	9.7
47	16.35	13.1	9.8
48	16.5	13.2	9.9
49	16.65	13.35	10.0
50	16.8	13.5	10.1
51	16.95	13.65	10.2
52	17.1	13.8	10.3
53	17.25	13.9	10.4
54	17.4	14.0	10.5
55	17.6	14.2	10.6
56	17.7	14.3	10.7
57	17.9	14.4	10.75
58	18.05	14.5	10.8
59	18.25	14.6	10.9
60	18.4	14.7	11.0

Appendix 5

Desirable weights for men and women aged 25 years and over according to height and frame, based on measurements made in indoor clothing without shoes.

Height (metres) **Men**	*Weight (kg)* *Small frame*	*Medium frame*	*Large frame*
1.550	51–54	54–59	57–64
1.575	52–56	55–60	59–65
1.600	53–57	56–62	60–67
1.625	55–58	58–63	61–69
1.650	56–60	59–65	63–71
1.675	58–62	61–67	64–73
1.700	60–64	63–69	67–75
1.725	62–66	64–71	68–77
1.750	64–68	66–73	70–79
1.775	65–70	68–75	72–81
1.800	67–72	70–77	74–84
1.825	69–74	72–79	76–86
1.850	71–76	74–82	78–88
1.875	73–78	76–84	81–90
1.900	74–79	78–86	83–93

Height (metres)	Weight (kg) Small frame	Medium frame	Large frame
Women			
1.425	42–44	44–49	47–54
1.450	43–46	45–50	48–55
1.475	44–48	46–51	49–57
1.500	45–49	47–53	51–58
1.525	46–50	49–54	52–59
1.550	48–51	50–55	53–61
1.575	49–53	51–57	55–63
1.600	50–54	53–59	57–64
1.625	52–56	54–61	59–66
1.650	54–58	56–63	60–68
1.675	55–59	58–65	62–70
1.700	57–61	60–67	64–72
1.725	59–63	62–69	66–74
1.750	61–65	63–70	68–76
1.775	63–67	65–72	69–79

Appendix 6

Vitamins

Vitamin and Reference Nutrient Intake (RNI)	*Sources*	*Function*
Fat-soluble		
A (retinol) 700 µg/day male 600 µg/day female (retinol equivalents)	Liver, kidney, oily fish, egg yolk contain retinol. Carrots, green vegetables, apricots mangoes, tomatoes, milk, butter and cheese contain carotenes.	Normal devt of bones and teeth. Antiinfective. Essential for healthy skin and mucous membranes. Aids night vision.
D (calciferol) 10 µg/day for the housebound	Oily fish, egg yolk, butter, fortified margarine. Ultra-violet rays of sunlight.	Antirachitic. Assists absorption and metabolism of calcium and phosphorus.
E (tocopherol)	Wheat germ, egg yolk, milk, cereals, liver, green vegetables.	An antioxidant. May protect against cancer and heart disease.
K	Green leafy vegetables	Antihaemorrhagic. Essential for the production of prothrombin.
Water-soluble		
Thiamin (vitamin B_1) 1.0 mg/day male 0.8 mg/day female	Milk, offal, eggs, pork, fortified breakfast cereals, vegetables, Fruit, wholegrain cereals.	Important for metabolism of carbohydrate, fat and alcohol. Requirement increases with increase in carbohydrate intake.
Riboflavin (vitamin B_2) 1.3 mg/day male 1.1 mg/day female	Milk and milk products, offal, fortified breakfast cereals.	Steady and continuous release of energy from carbohydrates.

Properties	*Deficiencies*
Synthesized in the body from carotenes present in the diet. Can be stored in liver. High doses are teratogenic.	Poor growth. Rough dry skin and mucous membranes encouraging infection. Lessened ability to see in poor light. Xerophthalmia and eventual blindness.
Produced in the body by action of sunlight on ergosterol in skin.	Rickets in children: osteomalacia in adults. Develops in those who are not exposed to sun, such as the housebound.
	Rare. Can develop in premature infants and malabsorption syndrome.
Only absorbed in presence of bile. Synthesized by intestinal bacteria.	Delayed clotting time. Liver damage.
Destroyed by excessive heat.	Beri-beri. Neuritis. Poor growth in children. Wernicke–Korsakov syndrome when deficiency occurs with alcoholism.
Destroyed by sunlight.	Fissures at corner of mouth and tongue inflammation. Vascularization of cornea.

Vitamin and Reference Nutrient Intake (RNI)	*Sources*	*Function*
Niacin (nicotinic acid equivalent) 17 mg/day male 13 mg/day female	Meat, fish, pulses, wholegrains, fortified breakfast cereals. Can be synthesized from the amino acid tryptophan.	Energy metabolism. Part of coenzymes NAD and NADP involved in oxidation and reduction reactions.
B_6 (pyridoxine) 1.4 mg/day male 1.2 mg/day female	Meat, fish, wholegrains, eggs.	Protein metabolism. Requirement related to protein intake.
B_{12} (cobalamin) 1.5 mg/day	Animal products, meat, eggs, fish dairy products. Not found in plants.	Essential for red blood cell formation. Needed for nerve myelination.
Folate 200 µg/day	Green vegetables, fortified breakfast cereals, yeast, extract, liver.	Assists production of red blood cells and protein synthesis.
C (ascorbic acid) 40 mg/day	Fresh fruit: oranges lemons grapefruit blackcurrants; green leaf vegetables, potatoes. turnips, rose hip syrup.	Formation of bones, connective tissue, teeth and red blood cells.

Properties	*Deficiencies*
	Pellagra: dermatitis diarrhoea dementia
Used therapeutically for a range of conditions.	Rare. Metabolic abnormalities and convulsions.
Requires intrinsic factor secreted by gastric cells for absorption.	Megaloblastic anaemia. Irreversible neurological damage. Supplements necessary for strict vegetarians and vegans.
Supplement recommended proir to conception and during first 3 months of pregnancy to incidence of Neural Tube Defect.	Megaloblastic anaemia and growth retardation.
Destroyed by cooking in the presence of air and by plant enzymes released when cutting and grating raw food. Lost by long storage.	Sore mouth and gums. Capillary bleeding, scurvy. Delayed wound healing.

Minerals and trace elements

Reference Nutrient Intake (RNI) (adults) (9–50 year)	*Sources*	*Function*
Calcium 700 mg/day +550 mg during lactation	Milk and dairy products. Green leafy vegetables, white bread.	Necessary for bone formation and teeth. Blood clotting. Normal muscle and nerve function.
Iodine 140 µg/day	Sea food; iodized salt, milk.	Synthesis of thyroid hormones, thyroxine and triiodothyronine essential for body metabolism and circulation.
Iron 8.7 mg/day male 14.8 mg/day female	Liver, kidney, red meat, egg yolk, wholegrains, dark green vegetables, raisins, treacle, cocoa, molasses.	Component of haemoglobin, myoglobin and many enzymes.
Magnesium 300 mg/day male 270 mg/day female	Cereals and green vegetables.	Influences many enzymes; essential for carbohydrate and protein metabolism. Important role in calcium homeostasis.
Potassium 3500 mg/day	Fruit, vegetables, meat, wholegrains.	Principal intracelluler electrolyte; influences muscle contraction and nerve excitability.
Sodium 1600 mg/day	Table salt, milk, meat, vegetables, pre-prepared foods, cheese.	Principal extracellular fluid, important for regulating water balance.
Zinc 9.5 mg/day male 7.0 mg/day female	Red meats, eggs , wholegrains.	Present in all tissues. Wound healing. Immune system. Sexual and physical development.

Properties	*Deficiencies*
Absorption helped by vitamin D and parathyroid hormone.	Bone diseases: osteomalacia, rickets. Tetany.
Stored by thyroid gland. Radioisotope used in scanning.	Goitre. Cretinism.
Absorption aided by vitamin C. Inhibited by phytates and tanin in diet. Greater demand during pregnancy.	Anaemia. Fatigue. Lethargy and poor growth in children.
	Unlikely, mainly in cases of chronic malabsorption and chronic renal failure. Will be accompanied by hypocalcaemia.
Kidney controls secretion and absorption.	Due to poor dietary intake rare. Can occur following prolonged use of diuretics and purgatives causing muscular weakness, depression, confusion, arrhythmias and cardiac arrest.
Lost through fever, sweat and diarrhoea. High intake may be linked to hypertension.	Weakness, abdominal cramps, faintness.
	Fatigue. Retarded growth and sexual maturity.

Appendix 7

Drugs and the law

The main Acts governing the use of medicines are the Medicines Act 1968 and the Misuse of Drugs Act 1971.

The Misuse of Drugs Act 1971

This Act imposes controls on those drugs liable to produce dependence or cause harm if misused. The substance cited in Schedule 2 of the Act are known as 'Controlled Drugs' or 'CDs' and include:

amphetamine
cocaine
codeine injection
dexamphetamine
dextromoramide
diamorphine (heroin)
dihydrocodeine injection
dipipanone (diconal)
fentanyl
methadone
methylphenidate
morphine
pethidine
phenazocine

Note also the controls which apply to Schedule 3 drugs such as buprenorphine and, very recently, temazepam.

Registered medical practitioners and registered dentists may prescribe preparations containing controlled drugs. However, the Misuse of Drugs (Notification of and Supply to Addicts) Regulations 1973 state that medical practitioners may not prescribe, administer or supply controlled drugs to addicted persons as a means of treating their addiction, unless specifically licensed to do so. This is to ensure that addicts will be referred for treatment to a hospital or clinic.

A prescription involving controlled drugs must fulfil the following conditions:

1. Patient's name and address specified in ink.
2. Signed and dated by prescriber.
3. Dose and dosage form, e.g. tab, cap etc. to be specified.
4. Total quantity to be supplied written in words and figures.

N.B. All above in the doctor's handwriting (computer-generated prescriptions are not permitted).

Accurate records must be kept by general practitioners, dentists and hospital staff of all purchases, amounts of drugs issued and dosages given. In hospital the following controls are imposed:

1. Special double locked cupboard for controlled drugs alone.
2. Key kept and carried by ward sister or deputy.
3. Supplies can be obtained by prescription signed by a medical officer, and the drugs can only be given under such written instructions. Ward stocks of controlled drugs in frequent use can also be ordered in special Controlled Drugs Order Books. Each order must be signed by the sister-in-charge.
4. Written record of each dose is made stating date, patient's name, time administered and dosage. This record is signed by nurse giving drug and another nurse who has checked the source of the drug as well as the dosage against the prescription.

All containers used for controlled drugs must bear special labels to distinguish them clearly. The hospital pharmacist checks the contents of the CD cupboard at regular intervals against the record books. Any discrepancies require full investigation.

The Medicines Act 1968

Under this Act, medicines are divided into three groups:

Prescription Only Medicines (POM) (apart from Controlled Drugs)
Pharmacy Only Medicines (P)
General Sales List Medicines (GSL)

The POM list includes most of the potent drugs in common use, from antibiotics to hypnotics. The list is too extensive to permit reference to individual drugs as it includes most medicines which should not be used without medical supervision.

Pharmacy Only Medicines are drugs supplied under control and supervision of a registered pharmacist. Representative drugs include ibruprofen, antihistamines and glyceryl trinitrate.

The General Sales List includes commonly used drugs such as aspirin and paracetamol, available through any retail outlet.

These distinctions of POM, P and GSL medicines do not apply to hospitals where it is accepted practice that medicines are supplied only on prescription.

Appendix 8

Drug and measurement calculations

Acknowledgements

The measurement section was compiled from Henney CR et al 1995 *Drugs in nursing practice,* 5th edn. (Churchill Livingstone, Edinburgh) and the formulae from Havard M 1994 *A nursing guide to drugs,* 4th edn. (Churchill Livingstone, Edinburgh) with permission.

The introduction of metrication into medical practice has altered the way in which drug dosages and concentrations, patient data (including height, weight and body surface area), drug levels in the body and other measurements are expressed.

Weight

The unit of weight is the kilogram (kg), made up of 1000 grams (g); each gram is composed of 1000 milligrams (mg). Each milligram is composed of 1000 micrograms (μ or mcg).

Whenever drugs are prescribed in microgram dosages it is good practice to write the units in full, i.e. Digoxin 250 micrograms, as the use of the contracted terms μg or mcg may in practice be mistaken for mg and as this dose is one thousand times greater disastrous consequences may follow.

Drug dosages are often described in terms of unit dose per kg of body weight, i.e. mg/kg, μg/kg etc. This method of dosage is frequently used in paediatric medicine and allows dosages to be tailored to the individual patient's size.

Volume

The unit of volume is the litre which is denoted by the symbol 'l'. One litre comprises 1000 millilitres (ml). The symbols 'l' or 'ml' account for almost all measurements expressed in unit volume for the prescription and administration of drugs.

Concentration

When expressing concentration of dosages of a medicine in liquid form, several methods are available:

Unit weight per unit volume

This describes the unit of weight of a drug contained in unit volume, e.g. 1 mg in 1 ml; 2 mg in 1 l; 40 mg in 2 ml etc. Examples of drugs in common use expressed in these terms: diazepam injection 10 mg in 1ml; chloral hydrate mixture 1 g in 10 ml; Penicillin V suspension 250 mg in 5 ml.

Percentage (weight in volume)

This describes the weight of a drug expressed in grams (g) which is contained in 100 ml or 1 dl of solution. Common examples are lignocaine hydrochloride injection 2%: this contains 2g in each 100 ml of solution or 0.2 g (200 mg) in each 10 ml of solution or 0.02 g (20 mg) in each 1 ml of solution,etc. Calcium gluconate injection 10%: this contains 10 g in each 100 ml of solution or 1 g in each 10 ml or 0.1 g (100) mg in each 1 ml, etc.

Percentage (weight in weight)
This describes the weight of a drug expressed in grams (g) which is contained in 100 g of a solid or semi-solid medicament, e.g. ointments and creams. Examples are: Fucidin ointment 2% which contains 2 g of fucidic acid in each 100 g of ointment; Betnovate cream 25% in aqueous cream which contains 25 g of Betnovate cream mixed with 75 g of aqueous cream (overall weight 100 g).

Volume containing '1 part'
A few liquids and to a lesser extent gases, particularly those containing drugs in very low concentrations, are often described as containing 1 part per 'x'units of volume. For liquids 'parts' are equivalent to grams and volume to millimetres, e.g. adrenaline injection 1 in 1000 which contains 1 g in 1000 ml or expressed as a percentage (w/v): 0.1%.

Molar concentration
Only very occasionally are drugs in liquid form expressed in molar concentration. The mole is the molecular weight of a drug expressed in grams and a one molar (1 M) solution contains this weight dissolved in each litre. More often the term millimole (mmol) is used to describe a medicinal product. (1000 mmol = 1 mole), e.g. potassium chloride solution 15 mmol in 10 ml indicates a solution containing the molecular weight of potassium chloride in milligrams × 15 dissolved in 10 ml of solution. Molar concentrations are most commonly seen in the results of biochemical investigations.

Body height and surface area
Occasionally drug doses are expressed in terms of microgram, milligram or gram per unit of body surface area. This is frequently the case where precise dosages tailored to individual patient`s needs are required. Typical examples may be seen in cytotoxic chemotherapy or in drugs used in paediatric problems. Body surface area is expressed as square metres or m^2 and drug dosages as units/m^2 or units per square metre. Examples are: Cytarabine injection 100mg/m^2; Dacarbazine injection 250 mg/m^2.

Formulae for calculation of drug doses and drip rates

Oral drugs (solids, liquids)

$$\text{Amount required} = \frac{\text{Strength required}}{\text{Stock strength}} \times \text{Volume of stock strength}$$

Parental drugs

a. *Solutions (IM, IV injections)*

$$\text{Volume required} = \frac{\text{Strength required}}{\text{Stock strength}} \times \text{Volume of stock strength}$$

b. *Powders*

It is essential to follow the manufacturer's directions for dilution, then use the appropriate formula

c. *IV infusions*

$$\text{Rate (drops/min)} = \frac{\text{Volume of solution (mL)} \times \text{Number of drops/mL}}{\text{Time (minutes)}}$$

Macrodrip (20 drops/mL)

$$\text{Rate (drops/min)} = \frac{\text{Volume of solution (mL)} \times 20}{\text{Number of hours} \times 60}$$

Macrodrip (20 drops/mL)

$$\text{Rate (drops/min)} = \frac{\text{Volume of solution (mL)} \times 15}{\text{Number of hours} \times 60}$$

d. *Infusion pumps*

$$\text{Rate (mL/hr)} = \frac{\text{Volume (mL)}}{\text{Time (hr)}}$$

e. *IV infusions with drugs*

$$\text{Rate (mL/hr)} = \frac{\text{Amount of drug required (mg/hr)}}{\text{Total amount of drug (mg)}} \times \text{Volume of solution (mL)}$$

Note: After selecting the appropriate formula, ensure that all strengths are in the same units, otherwise convert.

1% solution contains 1 g of solute dissolved in 100 mL of solution.

1:1000 means 1g in 100 ml of solution, therefore 1g in 1000 ml is equivalent to 1 mg in 1 ml

Other useful formulae

Children's dose (Clarke's Body Weight Rule)

$$\text{Child's dose} = \frac{\text{Adult dose} \times \text{Weight of child (kg)}}{\text{Average Adult Weight (70 kg)}}$$

Children's dose (Clarke's Body Surface Area Rule)

$$\text{Child's dose} = \frac{\text{Adult dose} \times \text{Surface Area of Child}}{\text{Surface Area of Adult (1.7 m}^2\text{)}}$$

Appendix 9

Useful addresses

Organizations

British Red Cross
9 Grosvenor Crescent
London, SW1X 7EJ
Tel. 0171-235-5454

Chartered Society of Physiotherapy
14 Bedford Row
London, WC1R 4ED
Tel. 0171-242-1941

College of Occupational Therapists
6/8 Marshalsea Road
London, SU1 1HL
Tel. 0171-357-6480

Commission for Racial Equality
Elliot House
10-12 Allington Street
London, SW1E 5EH
Tel. 0171-828-7022

Commonwealth Nurses Federation
c/o **International Department**
Royal College of Nursing
20 Cavendish Square
London, W1M 0AB
Tel. 0171-409-3333

Department of Health
(Public Enquiry Office)
Room 444
Richmond House
79 Whitehall
London, SW1A 2NS
Tel. 0171-210-4850

Department of Health
(Northern Ireland)
Dundonald House
Upper Newtownards Road
Belfast, BT4 3SB
Tel. 01232-520-500

The English National Board for Nursing, Midwifery & Health Visiting
Victory House
170 Tottenham Court Road
London, W1T 0HA
Tel. 0171-388-3131

Equal Opportunities Commission
Overseas House
Quay Street
Manchester, M3 3HN
Tel. 0161-833-9244

Health Education Authority
Hamilton House
Mabledon Place
London, WC1H 9TX
Tel. 0171-383-3833

Health & Safety Executive
2 Southwark Bridge
London, SE1 9HS
Tel. 0171-717-6000

Health Service Ombudsman
Church House
Great Smith Street
London, SW1P 3BW
Tel. 0171-276-3000

Health Visitors' Association
50 Southwark Street
London, SE1 1UN
Tel. 0171-378-7255

Institute of Complementary Medicine
PO Box 194
London, SE15 1QZ
Tel. 0171-237-5165

International Confederation of Midwives
10 Barley Mow Passage
Chiswick, W4 4PH
Tel. 0181-995-1332

International Council of Nurses (ICN)
Geneva
Switzerland
Tel. 0041-22-731-1960

Skillshare Africa
3 Belvoir Street
Leicester, LE1 6SL
Tel. 01162-541-862

The King's Fund
11–13 Cavendish Square
London, W1M 0AN
Tel. 0171-307-2400

National Association of Theatre Nurses
22 Mount Parade
Harrogate, HG1 1BX
Tel. 01423-508-079

The National Board for Nursing, Midwifery & Health Visiting for Northern Ireland
RAC House
79 Chichester Street
Belfast, BT1 4JE
Tel. 01232-238-152

The National Board for Nursing, Midwifery & Health Visiting for Scotland
22 Queen Street
Edinburgh, EH2 1JX
Tel. 0131-226-7371

Nurses Welfare Service
Victoria Chambers
16/18 Strutton Ground
London, SW1P 2HP
Tel. 0171-222-1563/4

Nursing and Midwfery Staffs Negotiating Council
Staff Side Secretary
20 Cavendish Square
London, W1M 0AB
Tel. 0171-491-4447

Royal College of Midwives
15 Mansfield Street
London, W1M 0BE
Tel. 0171 580 6523/5

Royal College of Nursing of the United Kingdom
20 Cavendish Square
London, W1M 0AB
Tel. 0171-409-3333
(**RCN Institute** also at this address)

Royal College of Nursing
(Scottish Board)
42 South Oswald Road
Edinburgh, EH9 2HH
Tel. 0131-662-1010

Royal College of Nursing
(Northern Ireland)
17 Windsor Avenue
Belfast, BT9 6EE
Tel. 01232-668-236

Royal College of Nursing
(Welsh Board)
Ty Maeth
King George V Drive East
Cardiff, CF4 4XZ
Tel. 01222-751-373/7

Royal Commonwealth Society
New Zealand House
Haymarket
London, SW1Y 4TQ
Tel: 0171-930-6733

Royal National Pension Fund for Nurses
Burdett House
15 Buckingham Street
London, WC2N 6ED
Tel. 0171-839-6785

Royal Society of Health
38a St Georges Drive
London, SW1Y 4BH
Tel. 0171-630-0121

Society & College of Radiographers
2 Carriage Row
183 Eversholt Street
London, NW1 1BU
Tel. 0171-391-4500

Scottish Home and Health Dept.
St. Andrew's House
Regent Road
Edinburgh, EH1 3DE
Tel. 0131-556-8400

Society of Chiropodists & Podiatrists
53 Welbeck Street
London, W1M 7HE
Tel. 0171-486-3381

UK Central Council for Nursing, Midwifery & Health Visiting
23 Portland Place
London, W1N 3AF
Tel. 0171-637-7181

UNISON (Head Office)
1 Mabledon Place
London, WC1H 9HA
Tel. 0171-388-2366

VSO
317 Putney Bridge Road
London, SW15 2PN
Tel. 0181-780-2266

Welsh National Board for Nursing, Midwifery & Health Visiting
13th Floor
Pearl Assurance House
Greyfriars Road
Cardiff, CF1 3AG
Tel. 01222-395-535

Associations

Action for Sick Children (formerly Nat. Assoc. for the Welfare of Children in Hospital)
Argyle House
29–31 Euston Road
London, NW1 2SP
Tel. 0171-833-2041

Alcoholics Anonymous
PO Box 1
Stonebow House
Stonebow
York, YO1 2NJ
Tel. 01904-644-026

Association of British Paediatric Nurses (ABPN)
PO Box 14
Ashton-Under-Lyne
Lancs. OL5 9WW
Tel. 01224-821-289

Association of Carers
20-25 Glasshouse Yard
London, EC1A 4JS
Tel. 0171-490-8818

Aschma Society (merged with Asthma Research Council to become National Ashma Campaign)
Providence House
Providence Place
London, N1 0NT
Tel. 0171-226-2260

Breast Care & Mastectomy Association
15-19 Britton Street
London, SW3 3TZ
Tel. 0171-867-8275 (admin)
Tel. 0171-867-1103 (helpline)

British Association for Cancer United Patients BACUP
3 Bath Place
Rivington Street
London, EC2 3JR
Tel. 0171-696-9003

British Colostomy Association
15 Station Road
Reading, RG1 1LG
Tel. 01734-391-537

British Deaf Association
38 Victoria Place
Carlisle
Cumbria, CA1 1HU
Tel. 01228-488-44

British Diabetic Association
10 Queen Anne Street
London, W1M 0BD
Tel. 0181-323-1531

British Epilepsy Association
Anstey House
40 Hanover Square
Leeds, LS3 1BE
Tel. 0113-243-9393

Capability (formerly Spastics Society)
12 Park Crescent
London, W1N 4EQ
Tel. 0171-636-5020
Tel. 0800-626-216 (helpline)

Coeliac Society
PO Box 220
High Wycombe
Bucks. HP11 2HY
Tel. 0494-437-278

Cruse
Cruse House
126 Sheen Road
Richmond
Surrey, TW9 1UR
Tel. 0181-940-4818

Disabled Living Foundation
380-384 Harrow Road
London, W9 2HU
Tel. 0171-289-6111

Haemophilia Society
123 Westiminster Bridge Road
London, SE1 7HR
Tel. 0171-928-2020

Ileostomy Association (now Ileostomy & Internal Pouch Support Group)
Amblehurst House
PO Box 23
Mansfield, NG18 4TT
Tel. 01623-280-99

Leukaemia Society
14 Kingfisher Court
Venny Bridge
Pinhoe
Exeter, EX4 8JN
Tel. 0392-464-848

McMillan Cancer Relief
Anchor House
15-19 Britten Street
London, SW3 3TZ
Tel. 0171-351-7811

Malcolm Sargent Cancer Fund for Children
14 Abingdon Road
London, W8 6AF
Tel. 0171-937-4548 (admin)
Tel. 0171-937-4405 (appeals)

MIND - National Association for Mental Health
15-19 Broadway
London, E15 4BQ
Tel. 0181-519-2122

Multiple Sclerosis Society
25 Eppie Road
Fulham
London, SW4 QP
Tel. 0171-736-6267

National Childbirth Trust (NCT)
Alexandra House
Oldham Terrace
London, W3 6NH
Tel. 0181-992-867

National Society for the Prevention of Cruelty to Children (NSPCC)
67 Curtain Road
London, EC2A 3NH
Tel. 0171-825-2500

Royal National Institute for the Blind (RNIB)
224 Great Portland Place
London, W1N 6AA
Tel. 0171-388-1266

Royal National Institute for the Deaf (RNID)
19-23 Featherstone Street
London, EC1Y 8SL
Tel. 0171-296-8000

St John Ambulance Association & Brigade
1 Grosvenor Crescent
London, SW1X 7EF
Tel. 0171-235-5231

Sickle Cell Society
54 Station Road
London, NW10 4UA
Tel. 0181-961-7795

Stillbirth & Neonatal Death Society (SANDS)
28 Portland Place
London, W1N 4DE
Tel. 0171-436-7940

Terrence Higgins Trust
52-54 Greys Inn Road
London, WC1X 8JU
Tel. 0171-242-1010
Tel. 1200 2200 (helpline)
Tel. 0171-831-0330

World Health Organization
Avenue Appia
1211 Geneva 27
Switzerland
Tel. 0041-22-791-2111

Appendix 10

Abbreviations in Nursing – Degrees, Diplomas, Organizations

AA	Alcoholics Anonymous
ABPN	Association of British Paediatric Nurses
ACA	The Association for Continence Advice
ADFAM	Aid for Addicts and Family
AEMT	Association of Emergency Medical Technicians
AIMSW	Associate of the Institute of Medical Social Workers
ANSA	Association for Nurses in Substance Abuse
ARC	Arthritis and Rheumatism Council
ASH	Action on Smoking and Health
ASTMS	Association of Scientific Technical and Managerial Staffs
AVERT	Aids Education and Research Trust
BA	Bachelor of Arts
BACUP	British Association of Cancer United Patients
BAON	British Association of Orthopaedic Nurses
BCMA	Breast Care and Mastectomy Association
BCS	British Computer Society
BDA	British Diabetic Association
BEd	Bachelor of Education
BHMA	British Holistic Medical Association
BITA	British Intravenous Therapy Association
BMA	British Medical Association
BMJ	British Medical Journal
BN	Bachelor of Nursing
BPOG	British Psychosocial Oncology Group
BRSC	British Red Cross Society
BSc	Bachelor of Science
BSc (Soc Sc-Nurs)	Bachelor of Science (Nursing)
CATS	Credit Accumulation Transfer Scheme
CCD	Central Council for the Disabled
CCETSW	Central Council for the Education and Training of Social Work
CDSU	Communicable Diseases Surveillance Unit
CEPS	Continuing Education Points
CGLI	City and Guilds of London Institute
CLAPA	Cleft Lip and Palate Association
CLIC	Cancer and Leukaemia in Childhood Trust
CMT	Clinical Midwife Teacher
CNF	Commonwealth Nurses Federation
CNN	Certificated Nursery Nurse
COMA	The Committee on Medical Aspects of Food Policy

COSHH	Control of Substances Hazardous to Health
CPH	Certificate of Public Health
CRC	Cancer Reseach Campaign
CRMF	The Cancer Relief Macmillan Fund
CSS	Council for Science and Society
DCD	Diploma of Child Development
DCH	Diploma in Child Health
DDM	Diploma in Dermatological Medicine
DEBRA	The Dystrophic Epidermolysis Bullosa Research Association
DEN	District Enrolled Nurse
DEO	Disability Employment Officer
DipHE	Diploma in Higher Education
DHSS	Department of Health and Social Security
DipEd	Diploma in Education
DipN	Diploma in Nursing
DipNEd	Diploma in Nursing Education
DMS	Doctor of Medicine and Surgery
DN	Diploma in Nursing; District Nurse
DNA	District Nursing Association
DNE	Diploma in Nursing Education
DNT	District Nurse Teacher
DoH	Department of Health
DPH	Diploma in Public Health
DPhil	Doctor of Philosophy
EMS	Emergency Medical Service
EN	Enrolled Nurse (Scotland)
EN(G)	Enrolled Nurse (General)
EN(M)	Enrolled Nurse (Mental)
EN(MH)	Enrolled Nurse (Mental Handicap)
ENB	English National Board for Nursing, Midwifery and Health Visiting
ERASMUS	European Community Action Scheme for the Mobility of University Students
ERIC	Enuresis Resource and Information Centre
EXTEND	Exercise Training for the Elderly and/or Disabled
FETC	Further Education Teaching Certificate
FHSA	Family Health Services Authority
FNIF	Florence Nightingale International Foundation
FPA	Family Planning Association
FPC	Family Practitioner Committee
FPCert	Family Planning Certificate
FRcn	Fellow of the Royal College of Nursing
GMC	General Medical Council
GP	General Practitioner
HDSU	Hospital Sterilisation and Disinfection Unit
HEA	Health Education Authority
HFEA	Human Fertilisation and Embryology Authority

HSA	Hospital Savings Association
HV	Health Visitor
HVCert	Health Visitor's Certificate
HVT	Health Visitor Teacher
ICN	International Council of Nurses; Infection Control Nurse
ICNA	Infection Control Nurse's Association
IHF	International Hospitals Federation
INR	Index of Nursing Research
INRIG	Irish Nursing Research Interest Group
ISDD	Institute for the Study of Drug Dependence
ISRT	International Spinal Research Trust
JP	Justice of the Peace
LEA	Local Education Authority
MA	Master of Arts
MBA	Master of Business Administration
MBCS	Member of the British Computer Society
MBIM	Member of the British Institute of Management
MEd	Master of Education
MIND	National Association for Mental Health
MOEH	Medical Officer for Environmental Health
MOH	Medical Officer of Health
MPhil	Master of Philosophy
MRC	Medical Research Council
MSc	Master of Science
MSW	Medical Social Worker
MT	Midwifery Teacher
MTD	Midwife Teachers' Diploma
NA	Narcotics Anonymous
NACC	National Association for Colitis and Crohn's Disease
NACNE	National Advisory Committee on Nutrition Education
NAMCW	National Association for Maternal and Child Welfare
NAMH	National Association for Mental Health
NATN	National Association of Theatre Nurses
NAWCH	National Association for the Welfare of Children in Hospital
NCVQ	National Council for Vocational Qualifications
NDN	National District Nurse Certificate
NHC	National Hospice Council
NHI	National Health Insurance
NHS	National Health Service
NIESR	National Institute for Economic and Social Research
NINB	Northern Irish National Board for Nursing, Midwifery and Health Visiting
NNHT	Nuffield Nursing Homes Trust

NT	Nurse Teacher
NUMINE	Network of Users of Microcomputers in Nurse Education
NUS	National Union of Students
NVQ	National Vocational Qualification
ODA	Operating Department Assistant
OECD	Organisation for Economic Co-operation and Development
OHE	Office of Health Economics
OHNC	Occupational Health Nursing Certificate
ONC	Orthopaedic Nurses' Certificate
OND	Ophthalmic Nursing Diploma
OPCS	Office of Population Censuses and Surveys
OSCAR	Organisation for Sickle Cell Anaemia Research
OT	Occupational Therapist
OU	Open University
PhD	Doctor of Philosophy
PHLS	Public Health Laboratory Services
PMRAFNS	Princess Mary's Royal Air Force Nursing Service
PNA	Psychiatric Nurses Association
PT	Physiotherapist
QARANC	Queen Alexandra's Royal Army Nursing Corps
QARNNS	Queen Alexandra's Royal Naval Nursing Service
QIDN	Queen's Institute of District Nursing
QNI	Queen's Nursing Institute
RADAR	Royal Association for Disability and Rehabilitation
RCM	Royal College of Midwives
Rcn	Royal College of Nursing and National Council of Nurses of the United Kingdom
RCNT	Registered Clinical Nurse Teacher
RELATE	National Marriage Guidance Council
RFN	Registered Fever Nurse
RG	Remedial Gymnast
RGN	Registered General Nurse
RHA	Regional Health Authority
RHV	Registered Health Visitor
RM	Registered Midwife
RMN	Registered Mental Nurse
RN	Registered Nurse
RNIB	Royal National Institute for the Blind
RNMH	Registered Nurse for the Mentally Handicapped
RNPFN	Royal National Pension Fund for Nurses
RNT	Registered Nurse Tutor
RSCN	Registered Sick Children's Nurse
SCM	State Certified Midwife
SCODA	Standing Conference on Drug Abuse
SCOTEC	Scottish Technical Education Council
SEN	State Enrolled Nurse

SHHD	Scottish Home and Health Department
SHIP	Self-Help in Pain Groups
SHO	Senior House Officer
SMO	Senior Medical Officer
SNB	Scottish National Board for Nursing, Midwifery and Health Visiting
SPAPCC	Scottish Partnership Agency for Palliative and Cancer Care
SPOD	The Association to Aid the Sexual and Personal Relationships of People with a Disability
SRN	State Registered Nurse
SSRC	Social Science Research Council
ST	Speech Therapist
SVQ	Scottish Vocational Qualification
UKCC	United Kingdom Central Council for Nursing, Midwifery and Health Visiting
VOCAL	Voluntary Organizations Communication and Language
VSO	Voluntary Service Overseas
WHO	World Health Organization
WNB	Welsh National Board for Nursing, Midwifery and Health Visiting
WRVS	Women's Royal Voluntary Service

Nursing/Medical Abbreviations

AAA	Abdominal Aortic Aneurysm
AAFB	Acid Alcohol Fast Bacilli
ABG	Arterial Blood Gases
ACE	Angiotensin Converting Enzyme
ACTH	Adreno Corticotrophic Hormone
ADA	Adenosine Deaminase
ADD	Attention Deficit Disorder
ADH	Antidiuretic Hormone
ADL/ALs	Aids to Daily Living or Activities of Living
AF	Atrial Fibrillation
AFP	Alphafeto Protein
AGA	Appropriate for Gestational Age
AIDS	Acquired Immuno Deficiency Syndrome
ALL	Acute Lymphoblastic Leukaemia
ALT	Alanine Transaminase
AMI	Acute Myocardial Infarction
AML	Acute Myeloid Leukaemia
APSAC	Anistreplase
ARC	Aids Related Complex
ARDS	Adult Respiratory Distress Syndrome
ARF	Acute Renal Failure
ASD	Atrial Septal Defect
ASO	Antistreptolysin O
ASOM	Acute Suppurative Otitis Media

AST	Aspartate Transaminase
ATN	Acute Tubular Necrosis
ATP	Adenosine Triphosphate
ATS	Anti Tetanus Serum
AV	Atrioventricular (1) Node (2) Bundle
AVM	Arteriovenous Malformation
AVP	Vasopressin
AZT	Azidothymidine
BBB	(1) Bundle Branch Block (2) Blood Brain Barrier
BCC	Basal Cell Carcinoma
BCG	Bacille–Calmette–Guérin
BMR	Basal Metabolic Rate
BMT	Bone Marrow Transplant
BNF	British National Formulary
BP	(1) Blood Pressure (2) British Pharmacopoeia
BSE	(1) Breast Self-Examination (2) Bovine Spongiform Encephalopathy
CABG	Coronary Artery Bypass Grafting
CAD	Coronary Artery Disease
CAH	(1) Congential Adrenal Hyperplasia (2) Chronic Active Hepatitis
CAL	Computer Assisted Learning
CAPD	Continuous Ambulatory Peritoneal Dialysis
CAT	(1) Computerized Axial Tomography (2) Computer Assisted Tomography
CBF	Cerebral Blood Flow
CCF	Congestive Cardiac Failure
CCIE	Counter Current Immuno Electrophoresis
CCU	Coronary Care Unit
CD	Crohn's Disease
CD	Curriculum Development
CEA	Carcino Embryonic Antigen
CF	Cystic Fibrosis
CFTR	Cystic Fibrosis Transmembrane Regulator
CHI	Creatinine Height Index
CIN	Cervical Intraepithelial Neoplasia
CJD	Creutzfeldt–Jakob Disease
CLL	Chronic Lymphatic Leukaemia
CMF	Cyclophosphamide, Methotrexate, 5-Fluouracil
CML	Chronic Myeloid Leukaemia
CMV	Cytomegalovirus
CNS	Central Nervous System
COAD	Chronic Obstuctive Airways Disease
COPD	Chronic Obsructive Pulmonary Disease
CPAR	Continuous Positive Airways Pressure
CPK	Creatinine Phosphokinase
CPR	Cardiopulmonary Resuscitation
CRH	Corticotrophin-Releasing Hormone
CSF	Cerebrospinal Fluid
CSOM	Chronic Suppurative Otitis Media
CT	(1) Computerised Tomography (2) Cerebral Tumour (3) Coronary Thrombosis

CVA	Cerebrovascular Accident
CVP	Central Venous Pressure
CVS	Cardiovascular System
CXR	Chest X-Ray
DC	Direct Current
DCCT	Diabetes Control and Complications Trial
DDA	Dangerous Drugs Act
DDAVP	Desmopressin (Synthetic Vasopressin)
ddI	Dideoxyosine
DIC	Disseminated Intravascular Coagulation
DIDMOAD	Diabetes Insipidus, Diabetes Mellitus, Optic Atrophy, And Deafness
DIMS	Disorders of Initiating and Maintaining Sleep
DKA	Diabetics Ketoacidosis
DM	Diabetes Mellitus
dmft	Decayed Missing and Filled Teeth (Deciduous)
DMFT	Decayed Missing and Filled Teeth (Permanent)
DNA	Deoxyribonucleic Acid
DOES	Disorders of Excessive Somnolence
DU	Duodenal Ulcer
DVT	Deep Vein Thrombosis
EBM	Expressed Breast Milk
EBV	Epstein–Barr Virus
ECF	Extra Cellular Fluid
ECG	Electrocardiogram
ECT	Electroconvulsive Therapy
EDV	End-Diastolic Volume
EEG	Electroencephalography
ELISA	Enzyme-Linked Immunosorbent Assay
EMD	Electromechanical Dissociation
EMG	Electromyography
ENT	Ear, Nose and Throat
EOG	Electrooculogram
ERCP	Endoscopic Retrograde Cholangio Pancreatography
ERV	Expiratory Reserve Volume
ESR	Erythrocyte Sedimentation Rate
ESWL	Extracorporeal Shock Wave Lithotripsy
ET	(1) Endotracheal (2) Embryo Transfer
EUA	Examination under Anaesthetic
FBC	Full Blood Count
FBS	Fasting Blood Sugar
FET	Forced Expiratory Technique
FEV	Forced Expiratory Volume
FFA	Free Fatty Acids
FFP	Fresh Frozen Plasma
FRC	Functional Residual Capacity
FSH	Follicle Stimulating Hormone
FSHRH	Follicle Stimulating Hormone Releasing Hormone
FVC	Forced Vital Capacity

GABA	Gamma Aminobutyric Acid
GCSF	Granulocyte Colony Stimulating Factor
GFR	Glomerular Filtration Rate
GGTP	Gamma Glutamyl Transpeptidase
GH	Growth Hormone
GHIH	Growth Hormone Inhibiting Hormone
GHRH	Growth Hormone Releasing Hormone
GHRIH	Growth Hormone Release-Inhibiting Hormone
GI	Gastrointestinal
GIFT	Gamete Intrafallopian Transfer
GIS	Gastrointestinal System
GN	Glomerulo Nephritis
GnRH	Gonadotrophin Releasing Hormone
GTN	Glyceryl Trinitrate
GUS	Genitourinary System
GVHD	Graft Versus Host Disease
HAV	Hepatitis A Virus
Hb	Haemoglobin
HBGM	Home Blood Glucose Monitoring
HBsAg	Hepatitis B Surface Antigen
HBV	Hepatitis B Virus
HC	Head Circumference
HCV	Hepatitis C Virus
HCG(hCG)	Human Chorionic Gonadotrophin
HD	Huntington's Disease
HDLs	High Density Lipoproteins
HDV	Hepatitis Delta Virus
HGP	Human Genome Project
HHNK	Hyperglycaemic Hyperosmolar Nonketotic
HIV	Human Immunodeficiency Virus
HLA	Human Leucocyte Antigen
HMG(hMG)	Human Menopausal Gonadotrophin
HOCM	Hypertrophic Obstructive Cardiomyopathy
HR	Heart Rate
HRM	Human Resource Management
HRT	Hormone Replacement Therapy
HSA	Human Serum Albumin
HSV	Herpes Simplex Virus
IABP	Intraaortic Balloon Pump
IBD	Inflammatory Bowel Disease
IBS	Irritable Bowel Syndrome
ICF	Intracellular Fluid
ICP	Intracranial Pressure
ICSH	Interstitial Cell Stimulating Hormone
ICU	Intensive Care Unit
ID	(1) Intradermal (2) Identity
IDDM	Insulin Dependent Diabetes Mellitus
IGT	Impaired Glucose Tolerance
IHD	Ischaemic Heart Disease
IM	(1) Intramuscular (2) Infectious Mononucleosis
IMV	Intermittent Mandatory Ventilation

IOL	Intraocular Lens
IOP	Intraocular Pressure
IPA	Immunosupressive Acid Protein
IPPV	Intermittent Positive Pressure Ventilation
IQ	Intelligence Quotient
IRV	Inspiratory Reserve Volume
IT	Information Technology
ITCP	Idiopathic Thrombocytopenia Purpura
ITU	Intensive Therapy Unit
IU	International Units
IUCD	Intrauterine Contraceptive Device
IUGR	Intrauterine Growth Retardation
IV	Intravenous
IVF	In Vitro Fertilisation
IVI	Intravenous Infusion
IVP	Intravenous Pyelogram
IVT	Intravenous Therapy
IVU	Intravenous Urogram
JVP	Jugular Vein Pressure
KCO	Transfer Factor for Carbon Monoxide
KCTT	Kaolin Cephalin Clotting Time
KS	Kaposi's Sarcoma
KUB	Kidneys Ureters and Bladder
LAD	Left Axis Deviation
LAS	Lymphadenopathy Syndrome
LDH	Lactic Dehydrogenase
LDLs	Low Density Lipoproteins
LFT	Liver Function Test
LGA	Large for Gestational Age
LH	Luteinising Hormone
LHRH	Luteinising Hormone Releasing Hormone
LLETZ	Large Loop Excision of the Transformation Zone
LOC	Level of Consciousness
LP	Lumbar Puncture
LSD	Lysergic Acid Diethylamide
LVEDP	Left Ventriclular End-Diastolic Pressure
LVF	Left Ventricular Failure
MAC	(1) Mid-Arm Circumference (2) Mycobacterium Avium Complex
MAMC	Mid-Arm Muscle Circumference
MAOI	Mono-Amine Oxidase Inhibitor
MAST	Military Antishock Trousers
MCHC	Mean Corpuscular Haemoglobin Concentration
MCV	Mean Corpuscular Volume
ME	Myalgic Encephalopathy
MEN	Mulitple Endocrine Neoplasia
MHC	Major Histocompatability Complex
Mhg	Megacycles Per Second
MI	Myocardial Infarction

mmHg	Millimetres of Mercury
MMM	Mitozantrone, Methotrexate, Mitomycin C
mmol	Millimole
MODY	Maturity Onset Diabetes of the Young
MPQ	McGill Pain Questionnaire
MRI	Magnetic Resonance Imaging
mRNA	Messenger Ribonucleic Acid
MRSA	Multiple Resistant Staphylococcus Aureus
MS	(1) Musculoskeletal System (2) Multiple Sclerosis
MSAFP	Maternal Serum Alphafetoprotein
MSU	Midstream Specimen of Urine
NANB	Non A, Non B Viruses
NAP	Neutrophil Alkaline Phosphatase
NAS	No Added Salt
NBM	Nil (nothing) by Mouth
NCVs	Nerve Conduction Velocities
NEC	Necrotizing Enterocolitis
NG	Nasogastric
NIDDM	Non Insulin Dependent Diabetes Mellitus
NK	Natural Killer (cells)
NREM	Non Rapid Eye Movement (sleep)
NRS	Numerical Rating Scale
NSAIDs	Non Steroidal Antiinflammatory Drugs
NST	Non Shivering Thermogenesis
OCP	Oral Contraceptive Pill
OPT	Orthopantomogram
OTC	Over the Counter (remedies)
PABA	Para-Aminobenzoic Acid
PAP	Primary Atypical Pneumonia
Pap	Papanicolaou Smear Test
PAS	p-Aminosalicylic Acid
PAWP	Pulmonary Artery Wedge Pressure
PBC	Primary Biliary Cirrhosis
PCA	Patient Controlled Analgesia
PCNL	Percutaneous Nephrolithotomy
PCP	Pneumocytis Carinii Pneumonia
PCT	Prothrombin Clotting Time
PCV	Packed Cell Volume
PCWP	Pulmonary Capillary Wedge Pressure
PDA	Patent Ductus Arteriosus
PE	Pulmonary Embolus
PEEP	Positive End Expiratory Pressure
PEFR	Peak Expiratory Flow Rate
PEM	Protein-Energy Malnutrition
PET	Positron Emission Tomography
PGL	Persistent Generalized Lymphadenopathy
PICKUP	Professional, Industrial and Commercial Updating
PID	(1) Pelvic Inflammatory Disease (2) Prolapsed Intervertebral Disc

PIH	Prolactin Inhibiting Hormone
PKU	Phenylketonuria
PML	Progressive Multifocal Leukoencephalopathy
PMS	Premenstrual Syndrome
PMT	Premenstrual Tension
POAG	Primary Open Angle Glaucoma
POP	Plaster of Paris
PPAM	Pneumatic Post-Amputation Mobility
PPD	Purified Protein Derivative
PPS	Plasma Protein Solution
PR	Per Rectum
PRH	Prolactin-Releasing Hormone
PRL	Prolactin
PS	Problem Solving
PSCT	Pain and Symptom Control Team
PSD	Personal and Social Development
PT	Prothrombin Time
PTC	Percutaneous Transhepatic Cholangiography
PTCA	Percutaneous Transluminal Coronary Angioplasty
PTH	Parathormone
PTRs	Pupil/Teacher Ratios
PTT	Partial Thromboplastin Time
PUA	Pyrexia of Unknown Origin
PUVA	Psoralen + Ultra Violet Light A (photochemotherapy)
PV	Per Vagina
rDNA	Recombinant Deoxyribonucleic Acid
RAD	Right Axis Deviation
RAS	Reticular Activating System
RAST	Radio-Allergosorbent Test
RBC	Red Blood Cell
RCC	Red Cell Concentrate
RDA	Recommended Dietary Allowance
REM	Rapid Eye Movement (sleep)
RF	Rheumatic Fever
Rh	Rhesus
RHD	Rheumatic Heart Disease
RIF	Right Iliac Fossa
RNA	Ribonucleic Acid
ROM	Range of Movement (exercises)
RPE	Retinal Pigment Epithelial (cells, layer)
RS	Respiratory System
RSI	Repetitive Strain Injury
RSV	Respiratory Syncytial Virus
RTA	(1) Road Traffic Accident (2) Renal Tubular Acidosis
RV	(1) Residual Volume (2) Right Ventricle
RVF	Right Ventricular Failure
SA	(1) Sinus Arrhythmia (2) Sinoatrial (node)
SACD	Subacute Combined Degeneration
SAD	Seasonal Affective Disorder
SAH	Subarachnoid Haemorrhage

SBE	Subacute Bacterial Endocarditis
SCC	Squamous Cell Carcinoma
SCD	Sequential Pneumatic Compression Device
SDH	Subdural Haematoma
SGA	Small for Gestational Age
SGOT	Serum Glutamic Oxaloacetic Transaminase now Serum Aspartate Transferase
SI Units	Systeme International d' Unites
SIADH	Syndrome of Inappropriate Antidiuretic Hormone
SIDS	Sudden Infant Death Syndrome
SLE	Systemic Lupus Erythematosis
SLS	Social and Life Skills
SPF	Sun Protection Factor
SVT	Supraventricular Tachycardia
SWS	Slow Wave Sleep
TA-4	Tumour Associated Antigen
TB	Tuberculosis (Tubercle Bacillus)
TBW	Total Body Water
TCP	Thrombocytopenia
TED	Thromboembolic Deterrent (stockings)
TENS	Transcutaneous Electrical Nerve Stimulation
TIA	Transitory Ischaemic Attack
TIBC	Total Iron Binding Capacity
TIPS	Transjugular Intrahepatic Portosystemic Shunting
TLC	Total Lung Capacity
TNF	Tumour Necrosis Factor
tPA	Recombinant Tissue-Type Plasminogen Activator
TPN	Total Parenteral Nutrition
TPR	Temperature, Pulse, Respiration
TRH	Thyrotropin-Releasing Hormone
TSF	Triceps Skinfold Thickness
TSH	Thyrotropic-Stimulating Hormone
TT	(1) Tetanus Toxoid (2) Thrombin Clotting Time
TURP	Transurethral Resection of the Prostate Gland
TURT	Transurethral Resection of Tumour
TV	Tidal Volume
UC	Ulcerative Colitis
UGH	Uveitis + Glaucoma + Hyphaema Syndrome
URT	Upper Respiratory Tract
URTI	Upper Respiratory Tract Infection
USS	Ultra Sound Scan
UTI	Urinary Tract Infection
UVA	Ultra Violet Light A
UVB	Ultra Violet Light B
VAC	Vincristine, Adriamycin, Cyclophosphamide
VAS	Visual Analogue Scale
VDU	Visual Display Unit
VF	Ventricular Fibrillation

VMA	Vanillyl-Mandelic Acid
VRS	Verbal Rating Scale
VSD	Ventricular Septal Defect
VT	Ventricular Tachycardia
WBC	White Blood Cells/Count
ZN	Ziehl-Nielsen Stain

Appendix 11

RCN National Membership Groups

Accident and Emergency Nursing Association
Association for the Care of the Elderly (ACE)
Association of Nursing Education
Association of Nursing Students
Behavioural and Cognitive Psychotherapy Nursing Forum
Blood Transfusion Nursing Forum
Breast Care Society
Cancer Nursing Society
Child and Adolescent Mental Health Nursing Forum
Community Health Teachers Forum
Community Mental Health Nursing Forum
Community Nursing Association
Community Nursing in Learning Disabilities Forum
Community Practice Teachers Forum
Complementary Therapies in Nursing Group
Continence Care Forum
Continuing Education Teachers Forum
Critical Care Nursing Forum
Diabetes Nursing Forum
Dialysis and Transplant Nursing Forum
District Nurses Forum
Enrolled Nurse Advisory Committee
Ethics Forum
Family Planning Nursing Forum
Fertility Nurses Group
Forum for Independent Nurse Managers (INFORM)
Forum for Nurses Working in a Controlled Environment
Forum For Occupational Nurses in the NHS
Gynaecology Nursing Forum
Haemophilia Nursing Association
Health Visitors Forum
Higher Education Forum
HIV Nursing Forum
Information in Nursing Groups
Leukaemia and Bone Marrow Transplant Nursing Forum
Liaison And Discharge Planning Nurses Association
Mental Health Nursing Society
Midwifery Society
Nurse Practitioner Group
Nurses in Commissioning
Nurses in Executive Roles
Nurses in Registration and Inspection
Nurses Managing Community Services
Nurses Managing Specialist Palliative Care Services
Nursing and Care Agency Managers

Nursing in Operational Management
Occupational Health Managers
Older People Nursing and Mental Health Forum (FOCUS)
Ophthalmic Nursing Group
Orthopaedic Nursing Society
Outpatient Nurses Group
Paediatric Community Nurses Forum
Paediatric Intensive Care Nurses Forum
Paediatric Nurse Managers Forum
Pain Forum
Palliative Nursing Group
Perioperative Nursing Society
Practice Nurses Association
Psychodynamic Nursing Group
Radiology and Cardiology Nursing Forum
Rehabilitation Nurses Forum
Research Society
Respiratory Nurses Forum
Rheumatology Nursing Forum
School Nurses Forum
Society of Nursing for People with a Learning Disability
Society of Occupational Health Nursing
Society of Paediatric Nursing
Stoma Care Nursing Forum
Substance Misuse Nursing Forum
Transplant Nurses Forum
Tuberculosis Visitors Forum
Tutors in Learning Disabilities
VQ Forum

Appendix 12

Organizations that offer Scholarships and Grants

(Note: Check *exact* closing date for applications with the organization)

The Barbers Company Scholarship, National Institute of Nursing Research Award
The Administrator
National Institute of Nursing
Radcliffe Infirmary
Woodstock Road
Oxford, OX2 6HE
To enable nurses making a career in clinical nursing to undertake further education, research or a clinical project. Fees or subsistence are offered for nurses undertaking a masters or research in an academic setting in the UK or overseas. Closing date: *March*.

British Geriatrics Society
1 St. Andrews Place
London, NW1 4LB
Offer grants to attend courses, conferences and study days for nurses working with older people.

The Edwina Mountbatten Trust
1 Grosvenor Crescent
London, SW1X 7EF
Grants are made for specific projects aimed at promoting and improving the art and practice of nursing, midwifery and health visiting. No courses will be funded.

Enrolled Nurses Fund
Advisor to Enrolled Nurses
Royal College of Nursing
20 Cavendish Square
London, W1M 0AB
Not relevant for conversion course funding.

Florence Nightingale Memorial Committee
9 Grosvenor Crescent
London, SW1 7EH
Awards for postregistration study for improving standards of care for patients and clients. Any nursing, midwifery or health visiting subjects will be considered. No funding for courses except research

methods leading to a diploma. Usually advertised in nursing press in August. Closing date: *end September.*

Fulbright Commission
Fulbright House
62 Doughty Street
London, WC1N 2LS
Fulbright Scholarship Grants–to enable British lecturers and postdoctoral research scholars to spend a minimum of 3 months in USA. Candidates must demonstrate academic excellence. Subjects where there is an opportunity for collaborative innovation or international significance or a focus on Anglo-American relations are of particular interest. Closing date: *5 April.*
Fulbright Postgraduate Student Awards–must have at least a 2: 1 honours or above in first degree. Must demonstrate evidence of academic excellence and leadership qualities. Grants for a minimum of 9 months postgraduate study in USA. Subject field open. Closing: date: *October.*

The Harkness Fellowships
28 Bedford Square
London, WC1B 3EG
To encourage opinion formers and professional leaders to benefit from new ideas, practices and contacts in the USA with a view to enhancing UK development. Open to individuals active in any part of public, business or voluntary sectors. Candidates must demonstrate exceptional personal and intellectual qualities and professional achievement. Different catergories each year. Closing date: *October.*

National Asthma Campaign
Jane Saunders
Providence House
Providence Place
London, N1 0NT
Grants for applied, basic or clinical research relevant to asthma and/or related allergy. Usually awarded for 1 to 3 year period to those working in hopital and general practice, clinical care, epidemiology, environmental research and product evaluation. Closing date: *December.*

National Board for Nursing, Midwifery and Health Visiting for Scotland Edinburgh
Dr T Murphy-Black
Research and Developments Offices
NBS
22 Queen Street
Edinburgh, EH2 1NT
Grants for nurses, midwives and health visitors working in *Scotland* who wish to undertake innovative small-scale research projects resulting in a report of relevance to the NBS; pilot studies leading to full-scale research project; study tours undertaken for the purpose of gathering data to facilitate the development of a pilot programme. Closing date: *end January.*

The NHS Executive offers support for education and training in research, through regional offices of the NHS Executive, Research & Development Directorate. Please apply directly to the R & D Directorate in your area.

The Nightingale Fund Council
The Hon Secretary
The Nightingale Fund Council
108 Brancaster Lane
Purley
Surrey, CR8 1HH
Postregistration education of nurses, midwives and others who are working in a clinical, educational or possibly research field. Any recognized study that will enhance clinical or tutorial skills may be considered.

Peter Holgate Scholarship
c/o Adviser in Occupational Health Nursing
Royal College of Nursing
20 Cavendish Square
London. W1M 0AB
Awards offered in *summer* with *closing dates in October.*
a) A scholarship for full-time occupational health nursing students of the RCN Institute–forms are sent automatically with enrolment papers.
b) Student or conference grants for occupational health nursing students.
c) Grants to help occupational health nursing students to purchase course books.

Smith & Nephew Foundation Nursing Awards
Secreatry to the Trustees
Smith & Nephew Foundation
2 Temple Place
Victoria Embankment
London, WC2R 3BP
Awards are for courses, research, projects and study tours and are usually advertised in nursing journals in *January.*

Wingate Scholarships
The Administrator
Wingate Scholarships
38 Curzon Street
London, W1Y 8EY
Awards are for individuals of great potential or proven excellence who need financial support to undertake pioneering or original work of intellectual, scientific, artistic, social or environmental value and who are not eligible for funding from the usual sources. The awards are to help with the costs of a specific project, for up to 3 years. The work proposed may or may not be in the context of a higher degree but the awards are not for taught courses of any kind or for completing courses already begun. Closing date: *February.*

Winston Churchill Memorial Trust Travel Grants
15 Queens Gate Terrace
London, SW7 5PR
Open to British Citizens from all walks of life to gain a better understanding of the lives and work of people in other countries and to acquire knowledge and experience which will make them more effective in their work and in the community when they return. Different catergories each year, usually finalized in *June.*

Appendix 13

Compiling a curriculum vitae (CV)

A curriculum vitae (literally 'course of one's life') is a formal statement of educational and professional achievements. It is usually drawn up for the benefit of prospective employers when you are applying for jobs–you hope that the information given on your CV will persuade an employer to meet you because you seem to be a suitable candidate for the post.

If your CV is stored on a word processor disk it is easy to keep up it to date, or to revise it for a new application so that relevant items are highlighted. It should always include:

- your name, and the address where you can be reached
- a daytime telephone number
- your National Insurance number, if appropriate
- your career profile, stating briefly who you are and what you have done
- your career history, detailing your present position (and how long you have been in the post) and your past employment
- your education, that is, primary and secondary schools, college and/or university, with dates for each, and your professional qualifications
- any training you have undertaken, internal and external
- personal details, such as age and date of birth
- interests, selecting those which describe you best.

It is usual to use reverse chronological order in a CV so that you give your most recent educational qualification and position first. You should also supply the names and addresses of referees, preferably people from your present, or very recent, positions.

People evaluate CVs very quickly, often in less than a minute, so aim to make the right impression as quickly as possible by the way your CV looks and the way the information is organized. For example:

- Make your presentation more professional by using plain white or cream A4 paper and a conventional typeface.
- Direct the reader to the key parts of the CV by using bold for main headings and bullet points for each accomplishment (rather than wrapping information in long sections of prose).
- Make the information easier to absorb by keeping your sentences short and by using active verbs.

You can obtain an expertly written CV from a professional CV writer but you will make a better impression if you use your own words. It is a good idea, however, to get someone else to read it through for errors.

Remember, you are showing what skills and qualities you could bring to a job so, although professional and educational achievements should take precedence over, for example, descriptions of your hobbies and sports, the latter will help an employer gain a more complete picture of you as a person. Try not only to give consideration to the facts of your career (GSCEs, professional qualifications, e.t.c.) but also to a self-appraisal of your strong points and weaknesses, as you see them. Also, employers usually respect honesty so don't be afraid to offer some sort of self-criticism, if you feel it is appropriate.

Appendix 14

RCN's Association of Nursing Students (ANS)

The RCN is a large and complex organization which recognizes and values the significant contribution made by nursing students in pursuing its aims and objectives. The RCN actively facilitates and supports student involvement in all levels of RCN activity.

RCN Council have two seats specifically for nursing students: the nationally elected student member of Council and the Chair of the RCN's Association of Nursing Students. The Association of Nursing Students (ANS) exists to ensure the voice of nursing students is heard at all levels of nursing. Every student member of the RCN has automatic membership of the ANS, which has a nationally elected committee with representation from Scotland, Wales, Northern Ireland and England.

The elected members of the ANS Executive Committee serve a 2-year term of office, 1 year of which can be on a full time basis. This means that RCN nursing students are represented by nursing students who have time to facilitate actively on a local, regional and national basis.

The ANS holds a 2-day annual conference in September which is free to RCN student members. It also runs an annual student award with the prize of £1000 and administers a Scholarship Fund to which RCN students can apply for financial help with study days and elective placements.

Roz Osbourne,
Adviser to ANS

